Advances in Experimental Medicine and Biology

Volume 1187

Advances in Experimental Medicine and Biology provides a platform for scientific contributions in the main disciplines of the biomedicine and the life sciences. This series publishes thematic volumes on contemporary research in the areas of microbiology, immunology, neurosciences, biochemistry, biomedical engineering, genetics, physiology, and cancer research. Covering emerging topics and techniques in basic and clinical science, it brings together clinicians and researchers from various fields.

Advances in Experimental Medicine and Biology has been publishing exceptional works in the field for over 40 years, and is indexed in SCOPUS, Medline (PubMed), Journal Citation Reports/Science Edition, Science Citation Index Expanded (SciSearch, Web of Science), EMBASE, BIOSIS, Reaxys, EMBiology, the Chemical Abstracts Service (CAS), and Pathway Studio.

2019 Impact Factor: 2.450 5 Year Impact Factor: 2.324

More information about this series at http://www.springer.com/series/5584

Dong-Young Noh • Wonshik Han • Masakazu Toi
Editors

Translational Research in Breast Cancer

Springer

Editors
Dong-Young Noh
Department of Surgery, College of Medicine
Seoul National University
Seoul, South Korea

Wonshik Han
College of Medicine
Seoul National University College of Medicine
Seoul, Korea (Republic of)

Masakazu Toi
Graduate School of Medicine
Kyoto University Graduate School of Medicine
Kyoto, Japan

ISSN 0065-2598 ISSN 2214-8019 (electronic)
Advances in Experimental Medicine and Biology
ISBN 978-981-32-9619-0 ISBN 978-981-32-9620-6 (eBook)
https://doi.org/10.1007/978-981-32-9620-6

This Springer imprint is published by the registered company Springer Nature Singapore Pte Ltd.
The registered company address is: 152 Beach Road, #21-01/04 Gateway East, Singapore 189721, Singapore

Acknowledgement

Those listed below contributed to this publication by organizing the contents and authors of textbooks, collecting and arranging manuscripts as assistant editors.

Department of Surgery, Seoul National University College of Medicine, Seoul, Republic of Korea

Hyeong-Gon Moon
Han-Byoel Lee
Hong-Kyu Kim

Contents

Part I
Introduction

Chapter 1
Translational Research in Surgical Oncology: Introduction and My Own Experience as a Surgeon-Scientist

Dong-Young Noh

Abstract Translational research is possible when scientists have broad knowledge of not only basic research, but also clinical science, which is acquired via experience in patient care. These requirements cannot always be met by one individual, and, hence, collaboration between suitably qualified individuals is the key for the progress of translational research. However, it is vital that translational research is conducted by an investigator who has knowledge about all fields. I could be a good conductor in that sense, because as an oncology surgeon, I have considerable experience in working with patients; in addition, I have a background in biochemistry and have started my basic research laboratory. Thus, I can use these qualifications to my advantage to build a tissue bank as the first step, and initiate small-scale experiments such as estimating the DNA or protein levels in specific tissues or blood samples. Once I successfully launch good research products and publish in peer-reviewed journals, I intend to build a large research group focusing on large-scale studies on single nucleotide polymorphisms and proteomics. These translational approaches can overcome several unsolved clinical problems. Many of my research products, for example, patents and new techniques such as Mastocheck@, are designed for improving the clinical outcomes in patients.

Keywords Breast cancer · Surgical oncology · Translational research · Bioinformatics · Genomics · Proteomics

D.-Y. Noh (✉)
Department of Surgery, College of Medicine, Seoul National University, Seoul, South Korea

Gangnam CHA Medical Center, Seoul, South Korea
e-mail: dynoh@snu.ac.kr; dynoh@chamc.co.kr

D.-Y. Noh et al. (eds.), *Translational Research in Breast Cancer*, Advances in Experimental Medicine and Biology 1187,
https://doi.org/10.1007/978-981-32-9620-6_1

1.1 Introduction

Modern medical service has improved considerably due to advancements in medical science, which has enabled curation of scientific evidence and has allowed physician's access to information regarding diseases. In particular, translational research has a vital role in bridging basic science and patient concerns. One advantage of being an oncology surgeon specialized in breast cancer is the easy access to normal or diseased human tissues, along with basic knowledge of human anatomy. I started building my own human tissue bank in 1990, which now includes both cancer tissue and adjacent normal tissues. All the tissues are frozen in liquid nitrogen and stored in −70 °C or −20 °C freezers. Tissue banking is important as a resource for conducting research using diseased organs and normal tissues. The process of establishing a tissue bank starts from obtaining permission from Institutional Review Board (IRB) and patients or from normal healthy individuals. The term "translational research" had not been coined at the time when I initiated my tissue bank; however, a bed to bench, bench to bed concept existed. Nonetheless, this tissue bank formed an important resource for successful translational research.

Combining clinical practice and laboratory work was not easy for a clinician; however, once I overcame the hurdles, it turned out to be the most appropriate way of conducting translational research. In the beginning, I was able to start with a technician and rent a small part of a bench in a biochemistry laboratory owned by my colleague. My research efforts and small achievements led to the growth and development of my own laboratory. My postgraduate medical students and graduates (PhD) from basic research laboratories were the key personnel who developed ideas and conducted research in the field of translational medicine.

My postgraduate study on biochemistry as the major subject formed the basis of my translational research. My thesis was on "Purification of membranous 5' nucleotides." and "Enzyme immunoassay of a-fetoprotein using monoclonal antibodies." These studies performed by clinicians were not common in the 1980s, but are now available in the MD-PhD courses. After PhD, I spent two years in a biochemistry laboratory in Building 3 at the National Institute of Health (NIH), Bethesda, Maryland, USA, as a Fogarty international postdoctoral fellow. I consider myself lucky to be trained in both basic science and clinical practice in oncology.

During my term as a postdoctoral fellow at NIH, I concentrated only on laboratory work, without having to deal with patients or clinical work. Thus, I was able to dedicate my time completely to basic science and worked toward developing my project. I also gained the ability to design and troubleshoot my own research.

> Translational research was originally defined as follows: To improve human health, scientific discoveries must be translated into practical applications. Such discoveries typically begin at "the bench" with basic research then progress to the clinical level, or the patient's "bedside."
>
> Source: National Cancer Institute, National Institutes of Health.

Translation research has a broader meaning and has been extended to computer and cyberspace research at the bench to the bedside. Finally, translation is moving from a disconnected unidirectional approach to an engaged bidirectional partner approach between research laboratories to bedside, and from the bedside to the community. Translational science encompasses many research areas involving human, animal, organ, tissue, and cell line models. It also requires establishment of networks between community and industry. All these components should collaborate to build good communication and feedback. This concept was also built by myself, when I started the tissue bank and my laboratory as a surgeon scientist, which was before the term "translational research" was introduced worldwide. I also organized a group of patient survivors in 2000, and at the same time, I started a pink ribbon campaign on the streets of Korea. All these activities were well organized and has led to many scientific articles and social products. The first clinical aspect to consider was creation of a patient database. The data should be of good quality with standardized terms and each valuable should be as numerical as possible. Later we built a web-based database for all breast cancer patients who were operated and also followed the condition of the patients over time.

With time, the Laboratory of Breast Cancer Biology (LBCB) has transformed into a perfect translational research platform. On the clinical side, tissue and blood banking are performed at the operating room, clinical database is created using data from clinics, and all pathological data collection and tissue banking were performed at pathology laboratories; data from bioinformatics, sequencing, proteomics, and other engineering experiments are obtained from collaborators, and functional studies, animal experiments, and tissue and blood processing are performed at the Medical College of LBCB's Cancer Research Institute.

I started by establishing a cancer cell culture system as I was interested in cancer stem cell biology. Thus, I successfully established a sphere culture system and was able to generate my own cancer cell lines named SBCC1, 2, and 3, which are of epithelial origin, and NDY of mesenchymal origin. These are all mammospheres with different characteristics, expressing the epithelial marker EpCAM, with the exception of NDY, which has sarcomatous characteristics such as rapidly growing sarcospheres. All these cells grow as serial cultures and can also be transplanted in NOD/SCID mice [1, 2].

Since 2001, we are participating in the Genomic Research Center for lung and breast cancers, sponsored by the Ministry of Health and Welfare, Korea. We are continuing our genomic studies, including single nucleotide polymorphism (SNP) analysis and cDNA microarrays at the Genomic Research Center. Later in 2007, we organized a group named Translational Research Organization for Cancer (TROICA) for collaborative translational research. TROICA has enabled targeted studies such as biomarker discovery, mining of prognostic predictors, and targeted drug discovery. In addition, we were able to expand our basic research area not only to proteomics, but also to genomics and aptamer development by collaborating with the best scientists in each area in the country [3–5].

Networking between groups and individuals with the same purpose and aims is interesting and scientifically satisfying. I aim to form a competent research group in which the members enjoy their research and can share their experiences and ideas regarding research in particular and life in general. These are the features of translational research. In addition, I wish to transfer this legacy of combining basic and clinical research to my junior faculties and postgraduate students.

1.1.1 Genomics

I have generated numerous publications from translational research in the field of genomics related to SNPs, which are variations of single DNA building blocks called nucleotides in genes. For example, conversion of nucleotide C to A is a SNP. They occur once in every 300 nucleotides on average and are considered the most common type of genetic variation. Most SNPs are benign, although some may contribute to serious conditions such as breast cancer.

SNPs can be categorized into different subgroups similar to a pedigree (Fig. 1.1). Those that fall in the coding regions are of two types: synonymous SNP and non-synonymous SNP. Synonymous SNPs result in different codons, which encode the same amino acid. Hence, synonymous SNPs are ineffective, as the building blocks for proteins remain unchanged. However, missense or nonsense mutations are formed when the codon and the amino acid it encodes change.

Studies for identifying the most common non-synonymous genetic variants that are susceptible to breast cancer are limited [6]. A study showed that a novel SNP, rs1053338(K264R) in *ATXN7* at locus 3p21, is associated with susceptibility to breast cancer. AKAP9-rs6964587 was also found to be a marker of a breast cancer risk at 7q21 [7]. Both SNPs are susceptible to estrogen receptor (ER)-positive and ER-negative disease [7]. Another locus, 2q35 rs 13387042, shows strong evidence of association between rs13387042 and breast cancer in Caucasian women. This SNP is also associated with both ER-positive and ER-negative breast cancer in European women [8]. Another SNP from the same locus 2q35 was scrutinized. By genotyping 276 SNPs using the 1000 Genomes Project data, the best functional candidate, rs4442975, was found to be associated with ER+ among Europeans.

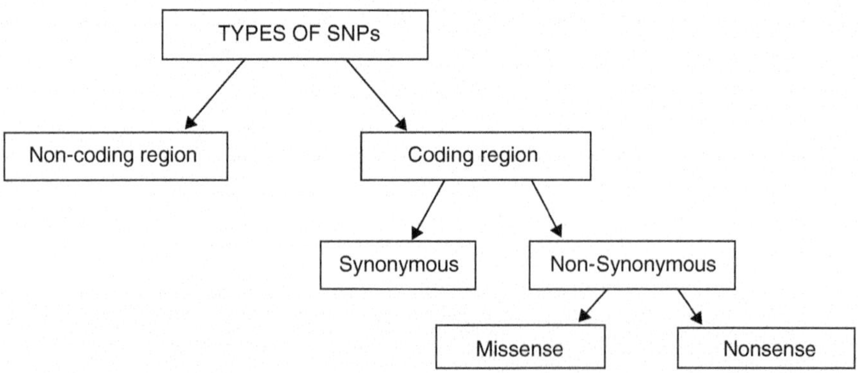

Fig. 1.1 Breast cancer exhibits consistent genetic variation

Evidence shows that the g-allele increases breast cancer susceptibility via down-regulation of *IGFBP5*, which is known to play a significant role in breast cancer biology [9]. Genome-wide association studies (GWAS) has revealed that SNP rs889312 in the 5q11.2 locus is associated with breast cancer risk in European women. Functional analysis indicated that the cancer risk alleles of four candidates (rs74345699, rs62355900, rs16886397, and rs17432750) increased MAP 3K1 transcriptional activity. Cancer risk alleles act to increase MAP 3K1 expression in vivo and might promote breast cancer cell survival [10]. Out of the 227,876 SNPs that were estimated to correlate with 77% of the known common SNPs in Europeans, five novel independent loci signaled strong and consistent evidence of association with breast cancer. Four of these contain causative genes (*FGFR2, TNRC9, MAP 3K1*, and *LSP1*). A second stage of the same research indicated that more SNPs can act as susceptibility alleles [11].

Studies have been performed to locate the single nucleotide variation that can be a critical factor for either inhibiting or accelerating tumor cell growth in breast cancer. Certain types of SNPs can be found to be significantly associated with the overall survival of patients due to their differential sensitivities toward certain drugs. Further studies on these lines will ensure better outcomes for patients with breast cancer. Initially, we hypothesized that if SNP can affect breast cancer development, it can also play a role during disease progression and may change clinicopathological features. We have observed that certain variants of *CYP1A1* and *CYP1B1* were related with onset at younger age, and that a certain haplotype of *BRCA1* showed less ER negativity and another was associated more with lymph node-negative phenotype [12].

Certain SNPs, for example those in *HER-2*, can affect tumor aggressiveness or response to therapy, and, as a result, clinical outcome. In this study, the haplotypes were not related with the risk of breast cancer; however, the most common haplotype 1 was associated with 1.5-times more frequent expression of HER-2 and showed poorer prognosis than other haplotypes [13]. We have published 23 papers regarding these SNP association studies in peer-reviewed journals.

The studies in LBCB regarding identification of SNPs for early detection of breast cancer can be summarized as follows:

- Haplotype analysis of *HER-2* polymorphism.
- Correlation between polymorphisms in DNA repair genes and susceptibility to breast cancer occurrence using SNP chip.
- Breast cancer susceptibility of innate immunity- and non-Hodgkin's lymphoma–related genes.
- *CASP8* polymorphism and breast cancer risk: A common coding variant in CASP8 is associated with breast cancer risk.

1.2 Comparative Genomic Hybridization (CGH) Array for Prognosticators

- Detecting prognostic factors in ER-positive breast cancer treated with tamoxifen using the CGH array.
- Discovery of candidate clones associated with breast cancer systemic recurrence using the CGH array.

1.2.1 Expression chip

- Investigation of differentially expressed genes and proteins during anoikis using the breast cancer cell line MCF-7.

1.2.2 Immunohistochemistry (IHC)

- Utility of Ki-67 for predicting distant metastasis in node-negative breast cancer.

Among the other examples showing how research on SNPs can translate the discoveries to the clinic, we investigated the correlation between significant SNPs in DNA repair genes in breast cancer samples and breast cancer occurrence. We evaluated the genetic polymorphisms (384 SNPs) in 38 DNA repair genes in a hospital-based case-control study 480:480). The results were translated and patented as breast cancer risk diagnosis SNP chip [14, 15]. Table 1.1 shows the results of analysis of clone with gain or loss observed in more than 50% of the 77 samples in the study [16]. For the clones selected in the analysis, a literature search, such as NCBI and PubMed, confirmed their association with cancer and finally selected eight candidate genes (Table 1.2) [16]. For the development of prognosticators after treatment of breast cancer, we attempted to identify candidate clones associated with breast cancer systemic recurrence using the CGH array and 31 pairs of breast cancer patients matched for clinicopathological characteristics of recurrence cases and recurrence-free cases after standard treatment [16] (Fig. 1.2).

Another interesting algorithm for predicting distant recurrence involved the use of clinicopathological multimarkers and a decision tree. We developed a decision tree for predicting prognosis from the 328 points of lymph node-negative breast cancer patients and 38 recurrences using clinicopathological characteristics such as age, tumor size, grade, and ER, PR, p53, c-erbB-2, and Ki-67 levels after adjuvant treatments. The results were remarkably applicable (Fig. 1.3) [17].

Table 1.1 Common regions showing gain or loss in more tnan 50% of all 77 samples

Region	Clone No.	Cytoband	Start (kb)	End (kb)	Number (%)	Cancer related genes
Gain-1	c5784	1p36.33	552,910	563,807	75 (97.4)	
Gain-2	c5242	8q24.3	145,647,141	145,761,879	46 (59.7)	CYHR1, KIFC2, FOXH1, PPP1R16A, GPT, MFSD3, RECQL4, LRRC14, LRRC24, MGC70857, KIAA1688
Gain-3	c4824	8q24.13	126,947,484	127,030,285	42(54.5)	
Gain-4	c1394	8q23.3	116,937,688	117,027,644	41 (53.2)	
Gain-5	c1437	8q24.12	119,396,534	119,465,174	41 (53.2)	SAMD12
Gain-6	c1433	8q24.21	131,335,147	131,416,013	41 (53.2)	DDEF1, DDEF1IT1
Gain-7	c2733	20q13.33	61,387,393	61,535,237	39 (50.6)	ARFGAP1, COL20A1, CHRNA4, KCNQ2
Loss-1	c5256	8p23.1	7,323,700	7,428,919	57 (74.0)	DEFB106B, DEFB105B, DEFB107B, LOC645489, FAM90A6P, FAM90A7. LOC729339, FAM90A22, FAM90A23
Loss-2	c4589	8p23.1	7,334,384	7,420,885	56 (72.7)	DEFB105B, DEFB107B, LOC645489, FAM90A6P, FAM90A7, LOC729339, FAM90A22
Loss-3	c5126	8p23.1	7,647,665	7,716,751	55 (71.4)	FAM90A19, LOC729394, FAM90A9. FAM90A10, DEFB107A
Loss-4	c5189	10q11.22	46,320,705	46,408,357	43 (55.8)	RHEBP1, SYT15
Loss-5	c710	14q32.33	105,821,330	105,907,464	39 (50.6)	IGHVIII-25-1, IGHV2–26, IGHVIII-26-1. IGHVII-26-2, IGHV7–27, IGHV4–28, IGHVII-28-1, IGHV3–29

kb kilobase

Table 1.2 Candidate gene list from candidate clones in gain and loss group

Gain/ loss	Gene	Clone No.	Cytoband	Description
Gain	NTRK1	c2168	1q21-q22	Neurotrophic tyrosine kinase, receptor, type 1
	ARHGEF11	c2168	1q21	Rho guanine nucleotide exchange factor (GEF) 11
	AHRR	c5262	5p15.3	Aryl-hydrocarbon receptor repressor
	SLC9A3	c5262	5p15.3	Solute carrier family 9 (sodium/hydrogen exchanger), member 3
	NBN	c301	8q21	Nibrin
	PPP1R1B	c2096	17q12	Protein phosphatase 1. Regulatory (inhibitor) subunit 1B (dopamine and cAMP regulated phos-phoprotein, DARPP-32)
	COL18A1	c2806	21q22.3	Collagen, type XVIII, alpha 1
Loss	IGHVIII-25-1	c710	14q32.33	Immunoglobulin heavy variable (III)-25-1

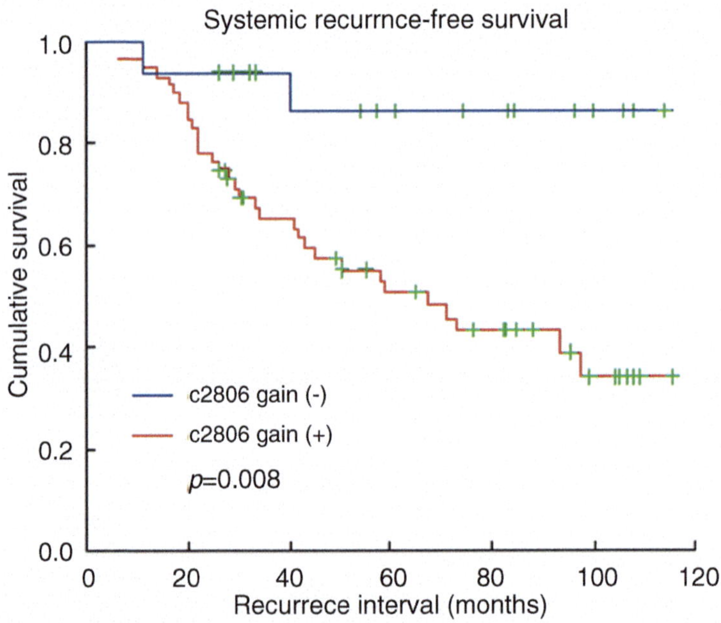

Fig. 1.2 Survival curve of systemic recurrence-free survival analysis for the clone which contains COL18A1 gene (c2806) by Kaplan-Meier test. The survival of the group with gain of c2806 clone was better than that without gain of c2806 clone and the difference of survival between two groups was statistically significant ($p = 0.008$) by log rank test [16]

Another simple and powerful prognosticator involved the use of candidate expansion using public database, dividing cases into high- and low-risk groups, which were defined as,

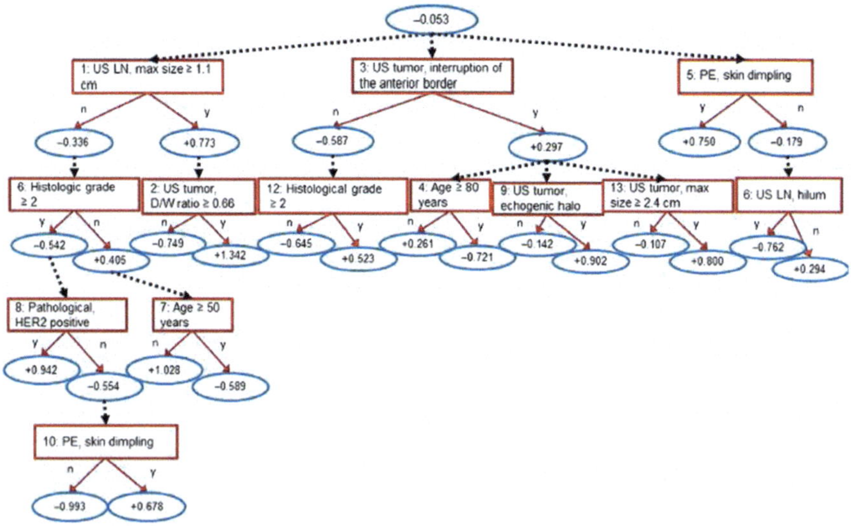

Fig. 1.3 ADTree model. The final prediction model consisted of five ADTree-based prediction models. The final prediction was calculated by calculating the mean score of the five ADTree models

High-risk group

- Ki-67 $\geq$ 10, Bcl-2 (−).
- Ki-67 $\geq$ 10, Bcl-2 (+), age < 35 years.
- Ki-67 < 10, ER (−).

Low-risk group

- Ki-67 $\geq$ 10, Bcl-2 (+), age > 35 years.
- Ki-67 < 10, ER (+).

The prognosticator model was comparable or superior to the multimarker model NPI and St. Gallen classification. Once this model is validated and applied practically to the patients, it can be a useful tool similar to oncotype or mammaprint [18].

We also attempted to identify drug responders among patients with breast cancer. After neo-adjuvant chemotherapy, we divided the responders and non-responders, identified candidate clones from two groups, and validated them using fluorescent in situ hybridization (FISH) on FFPE. FISH probes were developed for predicting chemosensitivity [19, 20].

We also prospectively compared the performance of DCE MR imaging using pharmacokinetic parameters and parametric response map (PRM) analysis for early prediction of pathological response to chemotherapy [21].

Association between PRM and Pathologic Response According to Subtype

Variable	pCR Group (n = 6)	npCR Group (n = 42)	P Value	Good Response Group (n = 38)	Minor Response Group (n = 10)	P Value
Triple negative						
PRM_{SI+}	3.8 ± 6.5*	49.6 ± 29.2†	.004	29.7 ± 28.4†	63.4 ± 18.1*	.051
PRM_{SI-}	83.5 ± 8.1*	47.3 ± 29.9†	.005	67.5 ± 28.9†	33.1 ± 19.2*	.051
PRM_{SID}	2.7 ± 1.7*	3.1 ± 1.5†	.705	2.8 ± 1.6†	3.5 ± 1.5*	.429
Hormone receptor positive						
PRM_{SI+}	8.0‡	37.9 ± 26.6§	NA	35.6 ± 25.4‖	46.6 ± 40.8#	.511
PRM_{SI-}	89.9‡	59.4 ± 27.2§	NA	61.6 ± 26.1‖	51.6 ± 41.8#	.561
PRM_{SID}	2.2‡	2.7 ± 1.5§	NA	2.8 ± 1.4‖	1.8 ± 1.5#	.264
HER2 positive						
PRM_{SI+}	20.8‡	37.9 ± 28.2**	NA	28.4 ± 33.0*	44.9 ± 15.9#	.468
PRM_{SI-}	76.3‡	58.8 ± 28.5**	NA	69.2 ± 32.8*	50.7 ± 15.9#	.417
PRM_{SID}	2.9‡	3.3 ± 1.4**	NA	2.4 ± 1.1*	4.4 ± 0.1#	.032

Note.—NA = not applicable.
* Data are means ± standard deviations, with $n = 4$.
† Data are means ± standard deviations, with $n = 10$.
‡ Data are PRM values of the case, with $n = 1$.
§ Data are means ± standard deviations, with $n = 26$.
‖ Data are means ± standard deviations, with $n = 24$.
Data are means ± standard deviations, with $n = 3$.
** Data are means ± standard deviations, with $n = 6$

1.3 Proteomics

Breast tumors are heterogeneous, with epithelial cells neighboring stromal cells [22]. To eliminate the majority of the stromal component, we collected specific epithelial cells from fresh frozen breast tissue via manual microdissection. The collected samples can be used for DNA and protein analyses without interference from stromal contamination. Another way to avoid the effect of abundant proteins is to analyze proteins after fractionation. After several steps of fractionation, the membrane and cytosolic fractions can be used separately to detect small amounts of significant proteins.

For better analysis we also collaborated with a Stanford group to develop better platforms for high-content functional proteomics [23]. I was also engaged in ICBC with Lee Hartwell of Fred Hutchinson Cancer Research Center.

The results of difference gel electrophoresis (DIGE) with membrane fractions of ER (−) and ER (+) breast cancer cell lines showed that the expression of the group ones increased 1.5-fold, while those of the others decreased. We have obtained several candidate proteins of interest, the expression of which increase and decrease by 1.5-fold in DIGE. We also analyzed the secretions released from cancer cells speculating that they may be detected in blood. Hence, we analyzed and compared the media collected from Hs578Bst (normal cell line) with that from Hs578T (cancer cell line) culture using 2D polyacrylamide gel electrophoresis (PAGE). Comparative analysis led to the identification of a specific protein, called the endorepellin LG3 fragment. The expression of this protein decreased in cancer cell media. As a next step, we verified this using plasma from normal individuals and patients with breast cancer; results showed that the levels of this protein decreased in patients with cancer.

These results were further verified using the sera of 186 patients with early breast cancer and no lymph node metastasis and those of 213 healthy controls. Again, we observed significant decrease in LG3 fragment expression in the sera of patients with cancer. We finally translated the early detector to breast cancer screening in selected cases where dense breast in young women decreased the screening sensitivity of mammography. We analyzed whether this marker can distinguish females with dense breast. In an analysis involving 109 healthy women and 142 patients with breast density grade 3 or 4, those aged below 50 years were tested for the LG3 fragment (Fig. 1.4). Results showed that dense breasts were positive for LG3 and negative with 98% specificity; although the sensitivity was 21% and accuracy was 55%, the area under the curve (AUC) was 0.6, indicating that this could be a clinically meaningful approach [24].

We also hypothesized that patients' urine might contain cancer-specific proteins that are metabolized and cleared via urine. Hence, we concentrated patients' urine and separated them on a 2D gel. The separated urinary proteins were transferred to a nitrocellulose membrane, which was incubated with the pooled serum from 10 patients with breast cancer or 10 healthy volunteers as the primary antibody. Finally, reactivity was visualized using horseradish peroxidase-conjugated antihuman immunoglobulin as the secondary antibody.

We identified several proteins using comparative analysis, which were verified and validated using western blotting and detected using normal and cancer patients' sera. Finally, we identified several autoantibodies such as alpha2-HS glycoprotein [26]. We expanded the cases to verify the individual reactivity of autoantibodies in the sera of 73 healthy controls and 81 breast cancer patients using western blotting. The results were excellent as the sensitivity was 79%, specificity was 90%, and accuracy was 84%. We attempted to develop an enzyme-linked immunosorbent assay (ELISA) kit, which is still underway, because the selection of antibody to autoantibody is challenging [25, 26].

I have successfully identified many biomarkers via genomic and proteomic approaches at LBCB. These materials have been patented and some have been further practically applied in clinical trials.

***Mastocheck*@story**

The highlight of the proteomic studies in LBCB was the development of a novel plasma protein signature using multiple reaction monitoring-based mass spectrometry for breast cancer diagnosis. Based on our previous studies, we selected 124 proteins for MRM. The proteomics signature was then validated; in total, 56 proteins were optimized for MRM. In the verification cohort, 11 proteins exhibited significantly differential expression in plasma. Three proteins (carbonic anhydrase 1 [CAH1], neural cell adhesion molecule L1-like protein [NCHL1], and apolipoprotein C-1 [APOC1]) with highest statistical significance, which yielded consistent results for patients of stage I and II breast cancer, were selected, and a 3-protein signature was developed using binary logistic regression analysis [27]. The 3-protein signature clearly showed similar performance in independent validation with relatively high sensitivity, specificity, and accuracy (71.6%, 85.3%, and 77.1%,

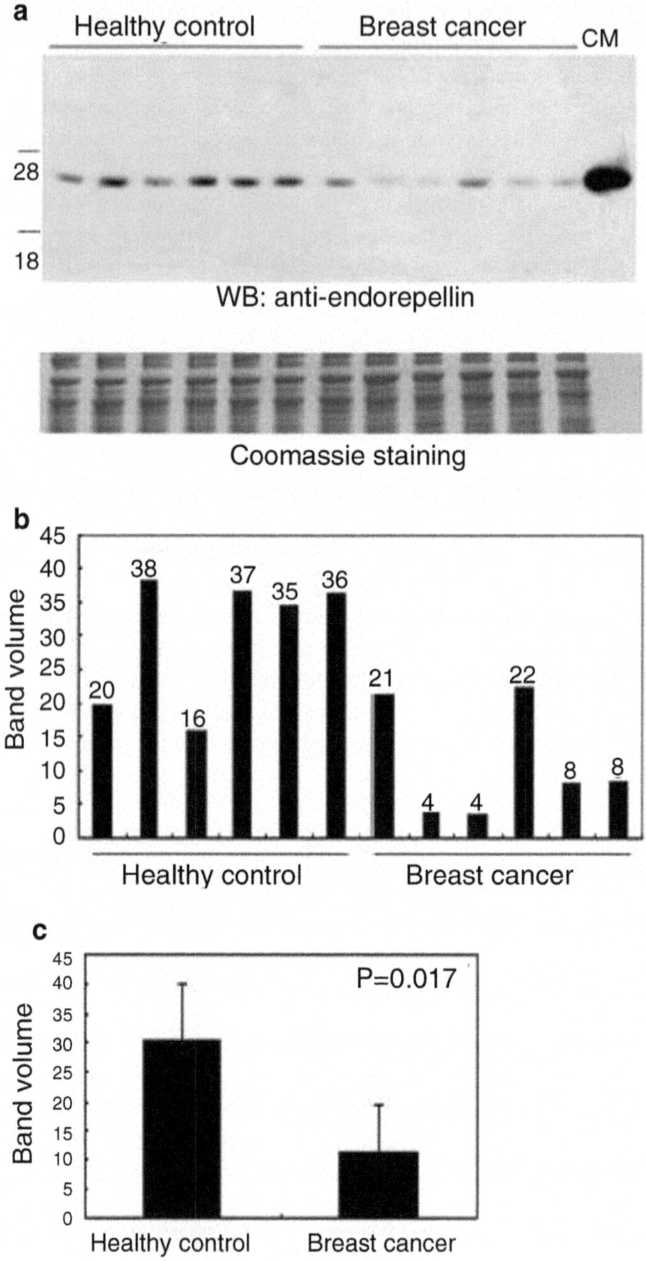

Fig. 1.4 Western blot analysis of the endorepellin LG3 fragment in plasma. Before Western blotting, all plasmas were depleted of the six abundant proteins using a MARS column as described in Sect. 1.2. (**a**) Individual plasma analyzed by Western blotting. Conditioned media (CM) of Hs578Bst was used as a positive control. The loading amount of plasma was monitored by duplicate Coomassie staining of the gels. (**b, c**) Densitometric analyses of Western blot (*t*-test; $p = 0.017$)

respectively) [28]. We decided to name the new diagnostic test for this 3-protein signature *Mastocheck@*. To evaluate the correlation with other cancers, experiments were conducted using blood samples from patients with thyroid cancer, lung cancer, colon cancer, pancreatic cancer, and ovarian cancer. As a result, it was found that *Mastocheck@* is specific to breast cancer diagnosis [28]. Based on these results, *Mastocheck@* was approved for using in early breast cancer diagnosis by the Korean Food and Drug Administration (FDA) in January 2019. In addition, it has been recognized for its usefulness as a breast cancer diagnostic marker and has obtained patents in Japan, China, and the United States as well as in Korea. Reproducibility was confirmed not only in plasma but also in experiments using serum and repeated experiments, which gives more confidence in diagnostic capabilities. Following FDA approval, *Mastocheck@* acquired the New Excellent Technology (NET) certification in September 2019 for the first time in 10 years in the field of medical science in Korea.

In order to evaluate the usefulness of *Mastocheck@* as an adjunct test, an analysis comparing to the current standard test, mammography, was performed. As a result, it was found that the use of *Mastocheck@* alone was superior to the use of the mammography alone, and when the mammography and *Mastocheck@* were used together, the sensitivity was improved by 30% and the accuracy was improved by 15% or more [29]. In the case of mammography, the diagnostic accuracy is very low for dense breasts, but it was confirmed that this limitation can be overcome by simultaneously performing *Mastocheck@* Therefore, in women with dense breasts, it is expected that the benefit of early diagnosis can be definitely obtained through *Mastocheck@*. In Fig. 1.5, ROC curves were used to compare diagnostic values of the five test combinations. As a result, mammography+*Mastocheck@* (AUC 0.846) was better than mammography alone (AUC 0.641), and it was statistically significant ($p < 0.001$) [29]. A study is underway to determine if it is useful as a test for follow-up observation after treatment of cancer, and this is to confirm how *Mastocheck@* value changes according to changes in the cancer state in the body before or after surgery. *Mastocheck@* has reached normal levels in about 70% of postoperatively and is expected to be useful as a follow-up test. We are also experimenting with many conditions of cancer and healthy individuals to increase the level of the accumulated evidence.

1.4 Data

Finally, I will introduce electronic medical record (EMR). EMR and BioEMR involve development of clinical information and trial system using standard-based data modeling of integrated biomedical EMR sources. Our strategy involves identification of not only a single powerful biomarker, but also curation and comparison of data from patients clinical records and from analyses involving SNPs, chromosomes, arrays, proteins, and imaging, to generate a constitutional marker composed

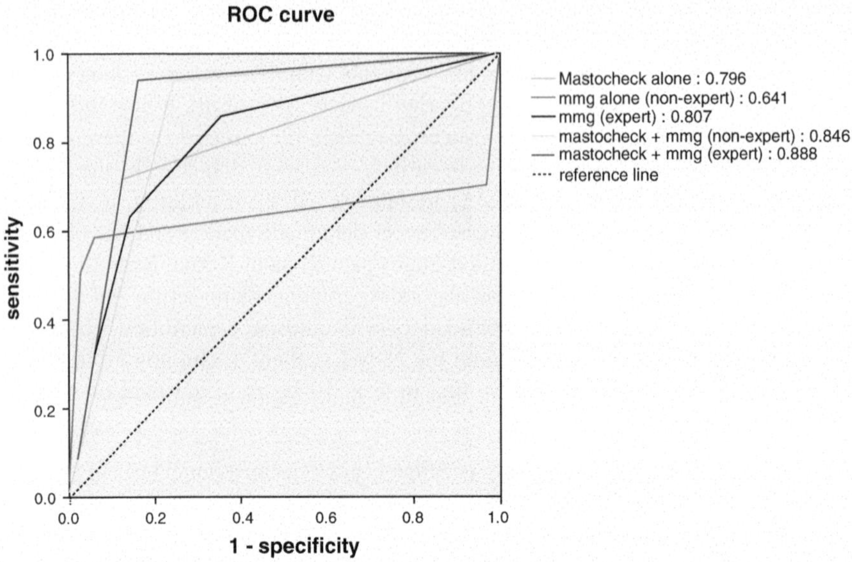

Fig. 1.5 Comparison of diagnostic accuracy when *Mastocheck@* alone, mammography (mmg) alone, and both tests combined [29]

of various components of separate origin (Fig. 1.6). If the BioEMR is completed in the future, patient records and laboratory and biological data will be assembled to generate useful information using bioinformatics tools to select drug and treatment modalities, and also disease signatures that can be followed up or used for predicting disease prognosis. This information will also be useful for clinical research and trials.

LBCB has also transitioned to a platform for next-generation sequencing for studies on gene panel and mRNA sequencing, which are underway. Clinically, we have also developed new patient-derived xenograft (PDX) mice from breast cancer patients; this model will also have an important role in translational research in the next generation [31].

The key point of translational research is collaboration. Personally, I started my small laboratory with one technician and assistance from the Department of Biochemistry in 1990. Thereafter, I was in charge of 10-year grants on national cancer genomic program with Professor Kim and was also involved in the functional proteomics group led by Prof Ryu. Subsequently, I have collaborated with numerous scientists from institutes such as SNU, KIST, POSTEC, and UNIST. Translational research can be practiced in collaboration with biotech companies such as Bio-Medieng, Macrogen, and Celemics.

I also believe in the philosophy of "deserve then desire." I had gathered insights and experience in basic research during my postgraduate and post-doctoral days. I have allowed my junior colleague and first postgraduate student, Dr. Han, to learn bioinformatics from S. Jeffrey in Stanford University when the microarray was first

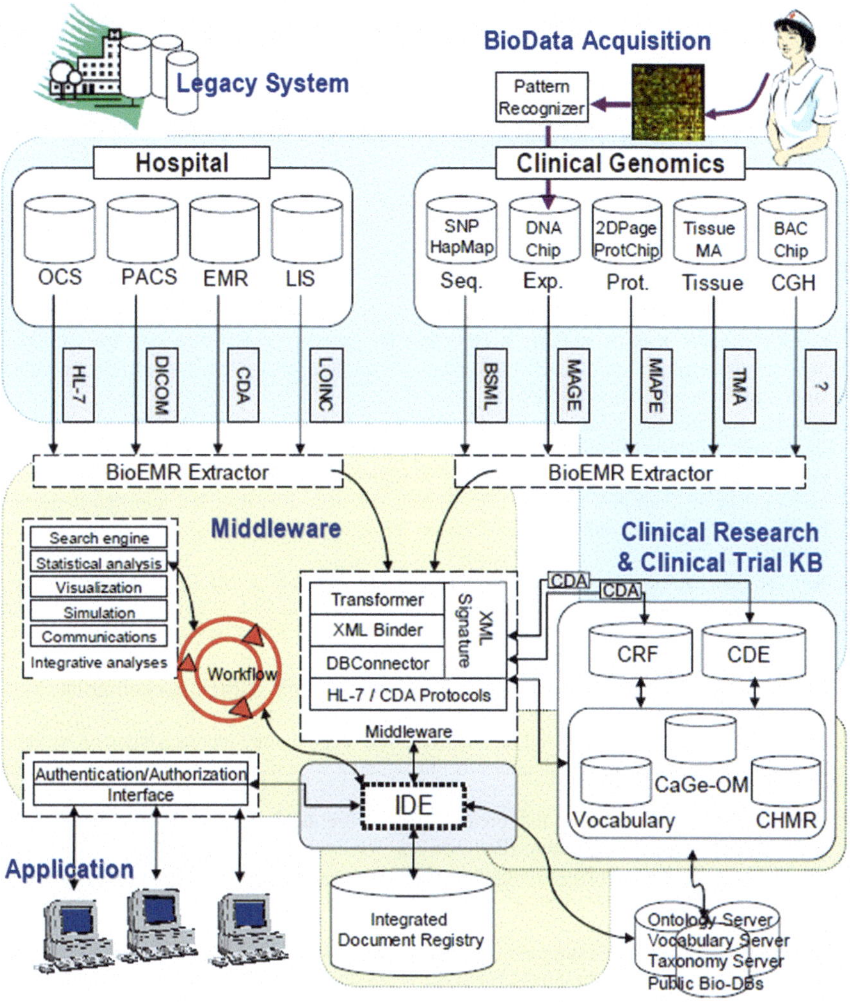

Fig. 1.6 BioEMR. Architecture of the pilot information system of integrated clinical, histopathological and genomic information [30]

introduced in the early 1990s. He is one of the best surgeon-scientists to handle genomics research and precision medicine. I have also sent Dr. Moon to Jackson Laboratories to better understand the basic science regarding generation of PDX mice. My youngest staff, Dr. Lee, who has organized the research at LBCB, might have his own research topic in the field of precision medicine in future. They are excellent researchers and good models of surgeon-scientists. They deserve it and are all contributing to the legacy of LBCB.

Acknowledgments I acknowledge Ms. Minjung Kim (Bioinformatics Laboratory, SNU) for summarizing my publications on SNP. I also thank Dr. Yumi Kim (SNUH) for the illustrations and updates on *Mastocheck@*. I thank Mr. Sangwoo Kim (Imperial College, London) for correcting the English. I also thank Dr. Hong Kyu Kim (SNUH) for collecting and editing entire chapters.

Conflict of Interest Noh DY has a stock-option for Bertis Inc.

References

1. Lee KM, Han W, Kim JB, Shin IC, Ko EY, Park IA, Lee DS, Oh KH, Noh DY. The CD49d+/high subpopulation from isolated human breast sarcoma spheres possesses tumor-initiating ability. Int J Oncol. 2012;40(3):665–72.
2. Kim HJ, Kim JB, Lee KM, Shin IC, Han WS, Ko EY, Bae JY, Noh DY. Isolation of CD24 (high) and CD24(low/−) cells from MCF-7: CD24 expression is positively related with proliferation, adhesion and invasion in MCF-7. Cancer Lett. 2007;258(1):98–108.
3. Lee YJ, Kim IS, Park SA, Kim Y, Lee JE, Noh DY, Kim KT, Ryu SH, Suh PG. Periostin-binding DNA aptamer inhibits breast cancer growth and metastasis. Mol Ther. 2013;21 (5):1004–13.
4. Kim HC, Lee JY, Sung H, Choi JY, Park SK, Lee KM, Kim YJ, Go MJ, Li L, Cho YS, Park M, Kim DJ, Oh JH, Kim JW, Jeon JP, Jeon SY, Min H, Kim HM, Park J, Yoo KY, Noh DY, Ahn SH, Lee MH, Kim SW, Lee JW, Park BW, Park WY, Kim EH, Kim MK, Han W, Lee SA, Matsuo K, Shen CY, Wu PE, Hsiung CN, Lee JY, Kim HL, Han BG, Kang D. A genome-wide association study identifies a breast cancer risk variant in ERBB4 at 2q34: results from the Seoul breast cancer study. Breast Cancer Res. 2012;14(2):R56.
5. Mun J, Kim YH, Yu J, Bae J, Noh DY, Yu MH, Lee C. A proteomic approach based on multiple parallel separation for the unambiguous identification of an antibody cognate antigen. Electrophoresis. 2010;20:3428–35.
6. Ghoussaini M, et al. Evidence that breast cancer risk at the 2q35 locus is mediated through IGFBP5 regulation. Nat Commun. 2018;9:16193.
7. Milne RL, et al. Common non-synonymous SNPs associated with breast cancer susceptibility: findings from the breast cancer association consortium. Hum Mol Genet. 2014;23 (22):6096–111.
8. Milne RL, et al. Risk of estrogen receptor-positive and -negative breast cancer and single-nucleotide polymorphism 2q35-rs13387042. J Natl Cancer Inst. 2009;101(14):1012–8.
9. Glubb DM, et al. Fine-scale mapping of the 5q11.2 breast cancer locus reveals at least three independent risk variants regulating MAP 3K1. Am J Hum Genet. 2015;96(1):5–20.
10. Han MR, Long J, Choi JY, Low SK, Kweon SS, Zheng Y, Cai Q, Shi J, Guo X, Matsuo K, Iwasaki M, Shen CY, Kim MK, Wen W, Li B, Takahashi A, Shin MH, Xiang YB, Ito H, Kasuga Y, Noh DY, Matsuda K, Park MH, Gao YT, Iwata H, Tsugane S, Park SK, Kubo M, Shu XO, Kang D, Zheng W. Genome-wide association study in east Asians identifies two novel breast cancer susceptibility loci. Hum Mol Genet. 2016;25(15):3361–71.
11. Kim HJ, Im SA, Keam B, Ham HS, Lee KH, Kim TY, Kim YJ, Oh DY, Kim JH, Han W, Jang IJ, Kim TY, Park IA, Noh DY. ABCB1 polymorphism as prognostic factor in breast cancer patients treated with docetaxel and doxorubicin noeadjuvant chemotherapy. Cancer Sci. 2015;106(1):86–93.
12. Shin A, Kang D, Choi JY, Lee KM, Park SK, Noh DY, Ahn SH, Yoo KY. Cytochrome P450 1A1 (CYP1A1) polymorphisms and breast cancer risk in Korean women. Exp Mol Med. 2007;39(3):361–6.
13. Han W, Kang D, Lee JE, Park IA, Choi JY, Lee KM, Bae JY, Kim S, Shin ES, Lee JE, Shin HJ, Kim SW, Kim Sw, Noh DY. A haplotype analysis HER-2 gene polymorphisms: association

with breast cancer risk, HER-2 protein expression in the tumor, and disease recurrence in Korea. Clin Cancer Res 2005;11(13), 4775.
14. Lee KM, Choi JY, Kang C, Kang CP, Park SK, Cho H, Cho DY, Yoo KY, Noh DY, Ahn SH, Park CG, Wei Q, Kang D. Genetic polymorphisms of selected DNARepair genes, estrogen and progesterone receptor status, and breast cancer risk cancer. Epidemiol Biomark Prev. 2005;14 (4):821–5.
15. Han W, Kim KY, Yang SJ, Noh DY, Kang D, Kwack K. SNP-SNP interactions between DNA repair genes were associated with breast cancer risk in. Cancer. 2012;118(3):594–602.
16. Hwang KT, Han W, Cho J, Lee JW, Ko E, Kim EK, Jung SY, Jeong EM, Bae JY, Kang JJ, Yang SJ, Kim SW, Noh DY. Genomic copy number alterations as predictive markers of systemic recurrencein breast cancer. Int J Cancer. 2008;123(8):1807–15.
17. Takada M, Sugimoto M, Naito Y, Moon HG, Han W, Noh DY, Kondo M, Kuroi K, Sasano H, Inamoto T, Tomita M, Toi M. Prediction of axillary lymph node metastasis in primary breast cancer patients using a decision tree-based model. BMC Med Inform Decis Mak. 2012;12(54)
18. Jung SY, Han W, Lee JW, Ko E, Kim E, Yu JH, Moon HG, Park IA, Oh DY, Im SA, Kim TY, Hwang KT, Kim SW, Noh DY. Ki-67 expression gives additional prognostic information on St. Gallen 2007 and adjuvant! online risk categories in early breast cancer. Ann Surg Oncol. 2009;16(5):1112–21.
19. Moon HG, Im SA, Han W, Oh DY, Han SW, Keam B, Park IA, Chang JM, Moon WK, Cho N, Noh DY. Estrogen receptor status confers a distinct pattern of response to neoadjuvant chemotherapy: implications for optimal durations of therapy: distinct patterns of response according to ER expression. Breast Cancer Res Treat. 2012;134(3):1133–40.
20. Hyung SW, Lee MY, Yu JH, Shin B, Jung HJ, Park JM, Han W, Lee KM, Moon HG, Zhang H, Aebersold R, Hwang D, Lee SW, Yu MH, Noh DY. A serum protein profile predictive of the resistance to neoadjuvant chemotherapy in advanced breast cancers. Mol Cell Proteomics. 2011;10(10):M111.011023.
21. Cho N, Im SA, Park IA, Lee KM, Li M, Han W, Noh DY, Moon WK. Breast cancer: early prediction of response to neoadjuvant chemotherapy using parametric response maps for MR imaging. Radiology. 2014;272(2):385.
22. Wiseman BS, Werb Z. Stromal effects on mammary gland development and breast cancer. Science. 2002;296(5570):1046–9.
23. Jessani N, Niessen S, Wei BQ, Nicolau M, Humphrey M, Ji Y, Han W, Noh DY, Yates JR 3rd, Jeffrey SS, Cravatt BF. A streamlined platform for high-content functional proteomics of primary human specimens. Nat Methods. 2005;2(9):691–7.
24. Chang JW, Kang UB, Kim DH, Yi JK, Lee JW, Noh DY, Lee C, Yu MH. Identification of circulating endorepellin LG3 fragment: potential use as a serological biomarker for breast cancer. Proteomics Clin Appl. 2008;2(1):23–32.
25. Yi JK, Chang JW, Han W, Lee JW, Ko E, Kim DH, Bae JY, Yu J, Lee C, Yu MH, Noh DY. Autoantibody to tumor antigen, alpha 2-HS glycoprotein: a novel biomarker of breast cancer screening and diagnosis. Cancer Epidemiol Biomark Prev. 2009;
26. Harris L, Fritsche H, Mennel R, Norton L, Ravdin P, Taube S, Somerfield MR, Hayes DF, Bast RC Jr. American Society of Clinical Oncology. 2007 update of recommendations for the use of tumor markers in breast cancer. J Clin Oncol. 2007;25(33):5287–312.
27. Lee HB, Kang UB, Moon HG, Lee J, Lee KM, Yi M, Park YS, Lee JW, Choi SH, Cho SH, Lee C, Han W, Noh DY. Development and validation of a novel plasma protein signature for breast cancer diagnosis by using multiple reaction monitoring-based mass spectrometry. Anticancer Res. 2015;25:6271–80.
28. Kim Y, Kang UB, Kim S, Lee HB, Moon HG, Han W, Noh DY. A validation study of a multiple reaction monitoring-based proteomic assay to diagnose breast cancer. J Breast Cancer. 2019;22(4):579–86.
29. Kim Y, Moon HG, Lee HB, Moon WK, Cho N, Chang JM, Han W, Noh DY. Efficacy of Mastocheck for screening of early breast cancer: comparison with screening mammography. J Breast Dis. 2019;7(2):59–64.

30. Park YR, Bae YJ, Kim JH. BioEMR: an integrative framework for cancer research with multiple genomic technologies. Summit Trans Bioinf. 2008;2008:81–4.
31. Moon HG, Oh K, Lee J, Lee M, Kim JY, Yoo TK, Seo MW, Park AK, Ryu HS, Jung EJ, Kim N, Jeong S, Han W, Lee DS, Noh DY. Prognostic and functional importance of the engraftment-associated genes in the patient-derived xenograft models of triple-negative breast cancers. Breast Cancer Res Treat. 2015;154(1):13–22.

Part II
Breast Cancer Biology and Cell Signaling Pathways

Chapter 2
Phosphplipase Signaling in Breast Cancer

Yu Jin Lee, Kyeong Jin Shin, Hyun-Jun Jang, Dong-Young Noh, Sung Ho Ryu, and Pann-Ghill Suh

Abstract Breast cancer progression results from subversion of multiple intra- or intercellular signaling pathways in normal mammary tissues and their microenvironment, which have an impact on cell differentiation, proliferation, migration, and angiogenesis. Phospholipases (PLC, PLD and PLA) are essential mediators of intra- and intercellular signaling. They hydrolyze phospholipids, which are major components of cell membrane that can generate many bioactive lipid mediators, such as diacylglycerol, phosphatidic acid, lysophosphatidic acid, and arachidonic acid. Enzymatic processing of phospholipids by phospholipases converts these molecules into lipid mediators that regulate multiple cellular processes, which in turn can promote breast cancer progression. Thus, dysregulation of phospholipases contributes to a number of human diseases, including cancer. This review describes how phospholipases regulate multiple cancer-associated cellular processes, and the interplay among different phospholipases in breast cancer. A thorough understanding of the breast cancer–associated signaling networks of phospholipases is necessary to determine whether these enzymes are potential targets for innovative therapeutic strategies.

Y. J. Lee · K. J. Shin · H.-J. Jang
School of Life Sciences, Ulsan National Institute of Science and Technology, Ulsan, Republic of Korea

D.-Y. Noh
Department of Surgery, College of Medicine, Seoul National University, Seoul, South Korea

Gangnam CHA Medical Center, Seoul, South Korea
e-mail: dynoh@snu.ac.kr; dynoh@chamc.co.kr

S. H. Ryu
Department of Life Sciences, Pohang University of Science and Technology, Pohang, Republic of Korea

P.-G. Suh (✉)
School of Life Sciences, Ulsan National Institute of Science and Technology, Ulsan, Republic of Korea

Korea Brain Research Institute, Daegu, Republic of Korea
e-mail: pgsuh@unist.ac.kr

D.-Y. Noh et al. (eds.), *Translational Research in Breast Cancer*, Advances in Experimental Medicine and Biology 1187,
https://doi.org/10.1007/978-981-32-9620-6_2

Keywords Phospholipid · Phospholipases · Breast cancer · Cell signaling · Proliferation · Metastasis

2.1 Introduction

Breast carcinoma is the most common malignancy worldwide after lung cancer, the fifth most common cause of cancer death, and the leading cause of cancer death in women [1]. The global burden of breast cancer exceeds that of all other cancers, and the incidence rates of breast cancer are increasing. Recently, mortality rates have exhibited a small decline, which more likely is a result of increased public awareness and early diagnosis, the implementing more affordable and effective screening programs, and advances in therapeutic techniques [2]. Nevertheless, the heterogeneity of breast cancers makes them both a fascinating and a challenging solid tumor to diagnose and treat. For example, patients with estrogen receptor (ER)-positive tumor can be treated with adjuvant endocrine therapy to suppress the growth-promoting actions of estrogen receptor alpha (ERα) [3]. Current ER-targeted pharmacological interventions include Tamoxifen and fulvestrant. Patients whose tumors express human epidermal growth factor receptor 2 (HER2) can benefit from treatment with specific antagonists of this receptor, such as Lapatinib and Trastuzumab (Herceptin) [4]. The majority of patients treated with adjuvant systemic therapy respond poorly to treatment, or go on to develop acquired resistance to hormonal therapies or HER2-targeted therapies, rendering the therapy ineffective. For the subset of patients with tumors that are ER-negative, progesterone receptor (PR)-negative, and HER2-negative (triple-negative, or basal-like cancers), there is no standard adjuvant intervention and they can be treated only with conventional chemotherapy [5]. Therefore, there is a critical need for new systemic therapies. Over the last decade, in-depth research has focused on the molecular biology of this disease, and study populations have been selected for clinical trials based on their molecular markers. Technological breakthroughs and high throughput approaches in particular have allowed researchers to probe deeply into the nature of breast cancer, revealing that this disease requires an interconnect-environment, and that the innate characteristics of the patient influence disease pathophysiology, outcome, and treatment response. Thus, focusing on personalized medicine to target disease manifestation on an individual basis will facilitate the development of more effective interventions, particularly for later stage malignancies with worse prognoses, and also in cases where resistance to existing therapies develops over time.

Phospholipases (PLC, PLD, and PLA) comprise a highly diverse group of enzymes that share the common property of hydrolyzing phospholipids, which are major components of cell membranes [6, 7]. Phospholipids, including phosphatidylcholine (PC), phosphatidylethanolamine, phosphatidylserine, phosphatidylglycerol, and phosphatidylinositol, can be broken down into various intracellular signaling moieties, such as diacylglycerol (DAG), phosphatidic acid (PA), lysophosphatidic acid (LPA), and arachidonic acid (AA) [8]. Through inter- and intracellular signaling, bioactive lipid mediators or second messengers regulate a variety of cellular physiological and pathophysiological functions, including proliferation, survival, migration, vesicle trafficking, tumorigenesis, metastasis, and inflammation [9, 10].

Each phospholipase regulates its own specific signaling pathways, but shares common signaling molecules with other members of its subfamily, acting as upstream regulators or downstream effectors. Recent findings indicate that phospholipases crosstalk with one another, which influences cell fate via the integration and fine-tuning of intracellular signals [8, 9]. To understand these complex signaling systems in the microenvironments of tumors, as well as in individual tumor cells, systematic analyses of phospholipase functions are required. In this chapter, we summarize current understanding of the various roles of phospholipases in breast tumor progression, with a focus on the signaling networks of phospholipases. We also discuss potential strategies for treating cancer by disrupting these networks, with a focus on their potential utility for aiding clinical management and prognostication, and for informing therapeutic options.

2.2 Review of Past Studies

2.2.1 Characteristics and Cellular Signaling of Phospholipases

Phospholipases are common enzymes present in a broad range of organisms, including bacteria, yeast, plants, animals, and viruses. Phospholipases can be categorized into three major classes—PLA (consisting of A1 and A2), PLC, and PLD—which are differentiated by the type of reaction that they catalyze [11, 12] (Fig. 2.1).

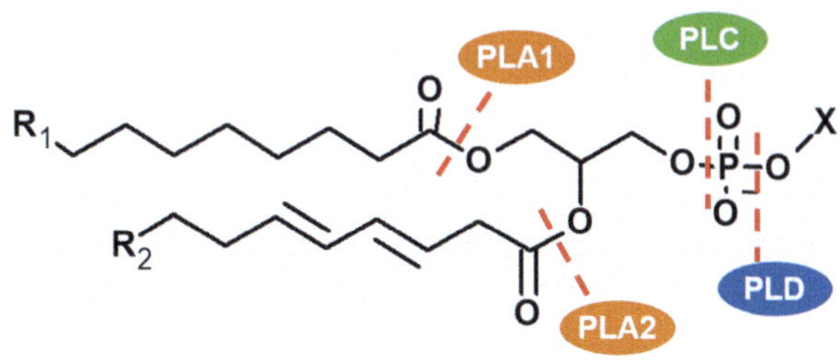

Fig. 2.1 Phospholipid structure and the site of actin of phospholipases. Phospholipids are composed of a glycerol-3-phosphate esterified at the sn-1 and sn-2 positions to nonpolar fatty acids (R1 and R2, respectively) and at the phosphoryl group to a polar head group, X. Phospholipase A1 and phospholipase A2 cleave the acyl ester bonds at sn-1 and sn-2, respectively. Phospholipase C cleaves the glycerophosphate bond, whereas phospholipase D removes the head group, X. *PLA* phospholipase A, *PLC* phospholipase C, *PLD* phospholipase D

2.2.1.1 PLC

Phosphoinositide-hydrolyzing PLC cleaves the glycerophosphate bond that links the polar head group to the glycerol backbone to produce inositol-1,4,5-triphosphate (IP3) and DAG in the cellular setting of ligand-mediated signal transduction (Fig. 2.1). DAG activates protein kinase C (PKC), whereas the binding of IP3 to its receptor triggers the release of calcium ions from intracellular stores into the cytosol [13]. Since the first report of PLC, 13 mammal PLC isozymes have been identified, and they can be divided into six subgroups: PLC-β [1–4], -γ [1 and 2], -δ [1, 3, 4, and], -ε, -ζ, and –η [1 and 2] [14] (Fig. 2.2). Interestingly, PLC isozymes have highly conserved X and Y domains which are responsible for PIP2 hydrolysis. Each PLC contains distinct regulatory domains, including the C2 domain, the EF-hand motif, and the pleckstrin homology (PH) domain [15]. Notably, each PLC subtype exhibits a unique combination of X-Y and regulatory domain, so that each PLC isozyme is regulated differently and has a different function and tissue distribution; thus, PLC-mediated signaling pathways regulate diverse biological functions [16].

The X and Y domains are usually located between the EF-hand motif and the C2 domain, and are composed of α-helices alternating with β-strands, with a structure that is similar to an incomplete triose phosphate isomerase α/β-barrel [17]. Conversely, the PH domain, although a membrane phospholipid-binding region like the C2 domain, has specific functions according to the type of isozyme. For example, he PH domain of PLC-δ1 binds PIP2 and contributes to the access of PLC-δ1 to the membrane surface [18]. In contrast, the PH domain specifically binds the heterotrimeric Gβγ subunit in PLC-β2 and PLC-β3 isozymes [19], and mediates interactions with phosphatidylinositol-3,4,5-trphosphate (PIP3) in PLC-γ1, where it is required to induce phosphoinositide 3-kinase (PI3K)-dependent translocation and activation [20]. As for the latter, it is worth noting that PLC-γ1 and PLC-γ2 isozymes contain an additional PH domain, which is split by two tandem Src homology domains, SH2 and SH3, for direct interaction with the calcium-related transient receptor potential cation channel, thereby providing a direct coupling mechanism between PLC-γ and agonist-induced calcium entry [21]. Finally, the C2 and EF-hand motifs are important for calcium regulation: the EF-hand motifs are helix-turn-helix structural domains that bind calcium ions to enhance PLC enzymatic activity [22, 23]. Interestingly, among the PLC isoenzymes, PLC-β subtypes also distinguish themselves by the presence of an elongated C-terminus, consisting of about 450 residues, which contains many of the determinants for the interaction with Gq alpha subunit as well as for other functions, such as membrane binding and nuclear localization [24–26].

The activation and regulation of PLC isozymes differ by subtype. For example, PLC-β subtypes are activated by G protein-coupled receptors (GPCRs) through several mechanisms. In contrast, PLC-γ subtypes are commonly activated by receptor tyrosine kinases (RTKs) via SH2 domain-phosphotyrosine interactions, and are subjected to phosphorylation by RTKs after the stimulation of growth factors like

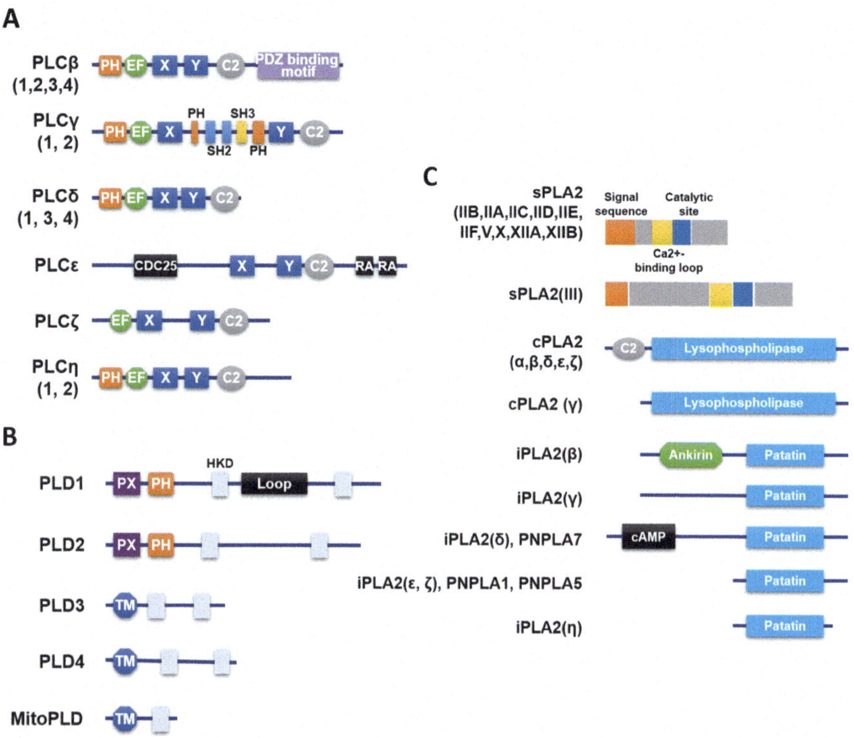

Fig. 2.2 Schematic structure of phospholipases. (**a**) Thirteen mammalian PLC isozymes are subdivided into six groups. All PLC isotypes have X and Y domains, which contain catalytic activity. Several isoforms have pleckstrin homology (PH) and a calcium-binding (C2) domain, which can regulate PLC activity. EF-hand domain is responsible for forming a flexible tether to the PH domain. PLCε has a RAS guanine nucleotide exchange factor (GEF) domain for RAP1A122 and the RA2 domain mediates interaction with GTP-bound *Ras* and RAP1A. PLCγ has SRC homology 2 (SH2) and Sh3 domains, which interact with many proteins. (**b**) In mammals, PLD1 and PLD2 hydrolyze phosphatidyl-choline (PC). PC-PLD has several conserved regions, including phox homology (PX) and PH domains, and two conserved catalytic domains (HKD). Non-PC-hydrolyzing PLD3, PLPD4, and mitochondrial PLD (mitoPLD) have recently been described. (**c**) The three major types of PLA2 include secretory PLA2 (sPLA2), cytosolic PLA2 (cPLA2), and calcium-independent PLA2 (iPLA2). Eleven sPLA2, six cPLA2, and nine iPLA2 have been found in mammals. sPLA2 has a signal sequence to target the extracellular region, a Ca2+-binding loop, and a catalytic site. cPLA1α, cPLA1β, cPLA1δ, cPLA1ε, and cPLA1ξ have a C2 domain, and a lysophospholipase-like domain. iPLA2β has Ankyrin repeats, which may mediate its oligomerization. Both iPLA2δ and PNPLA7 also have a cyclic AMP-binding domain and a patatin domain that is implicated in enzymatic activity. PLA1 has not been well characterized and has few links to cancer. *DAG* diacylglycerol, *IP3* inositol 1,4,5-triphosphate, *PA* phosphatidic acid

epidermal growth factor (EGF) and fibroblast growth factor (FGF) [15, 27]. Interestingly, PLC-ε can be activated by both GPCR and RTK systems, via distinct activation mechanisms [28]. Indeed, several GPCR ligands, such as lipoprotein A, thrombin, and endothelin, can activate PLC- ε, but PLC- ε also associates with Rap and translocates to the perinuclear area, where it interacts with activated RTKs [29]. It has been suggested that overall PLC activity may be amplified and sustained by both intracellular calcium mobilization and extracellular calcium entry. PLC-δ1and PLC-η1 are activated via GPCR-mediate calcium mobilization. In particular, the PLC-δ1 isozyme is one of the most sensitive of the PLC isozymes, suggesting that its activity is directly regulated by calcium. PLC-η1 specifically acts as a calcium sensor during the formation and maintenance of the neuronal network in the postnatal brain. Moreover, several studies have suggested positive feedback amplification of PLC signaling. Indeed, the overall PLC activity may be amplified and sustained by both intracellular calcium mobilization and extracellular calcium entry, through either a negative or a positive feedback amplification of PLC signaling [30, 31]. By these mechanisms, it has been suggested that PLC-β, PLC-γ, and PLC-ε may be primarily activated by extracellular stimuli. In contrast, activation of PLC-δ1and PLC-η1 may be secondarily enhanced by intracellular calcium mobilization serving to amplify PLC activity [32]. As for PLC-ζ, its activation and nuclear translocation mechanisms remain to be revealed.

2.2.1.2 PLD

Phosphatidylcholine-specific phospholipase D (PLD) hydrolyzes PC, the most abundant membrane phospholipid, to yield choline and the secondary messenger signaling lipid PA (Fig. 2.1). In mammals, two isoforms found in association with membrane surfaces in the cytoplasm, PLD1 and PLD2 [33, 34]. PLD3 and PLD4 are endoplasmic reticulum (ER) integral transmembrane proteins with a short N-terminal cytoplasmic tail, and the bulk of the protein, including the hypothetical catalytic domains, is present in the ER lumen [35, 36]. In contrast, PLD6 (MitoPLD) is anchored by an N-terminal transmembrane tail into the outer surface of mitochondria [37]. PLD5, on which there are no published studies, is most similar to PLD3 and PLD4, but is unlikely to have enzymatic activity because the canonical PLD enzymatic catalytic motif is not well conserved in its sequence. Enzymatic activities have also not been identified for PLD3 or PLD4, and it is possible that they have non-enzymatic functions instead. PLD6 has been reported to both hydrolyze cardiolipin, a mitochondrial-specific lipid, to PA, and to function as a endonuclease (phosphodiesterase) to generate a specialized form of micro-RNA known as piwi-interacting RNA (piRNA) [38]. For different reasons, therapeutic applications are not immediately apparent for PLD3–6; therefore, this review focuses on PLD1 and PLD2.

PLDs are ubiquitously expressed in almost all of tissues and cells of mice, and their activity is stimulated in response to various extracellular agonists, such as hormones, neurotransmitters, extracellular matrixes (ECM), and growth factors [39–41]. Clarification of the domain structure of PLDs has contributed to the elucidation of the activation mechanisms and physiological functions of PLD isozymes. Both PLD1 and PLD2 has several conserved regions, including phox homology (PX) and PH domains that are important for binding various lipids and proteins, and two conserved catalytic domains (HKD), which are essential for enzymatic activity [42, 43]. However, it has been reported that the PH domains of PLD1 and PLD2 are not required for PLD activation. One interesting domain is the "loop domain," which is found in PLD1, but not PLD2. The loop domain seems to be involved in auto-inhibition of enzymatic activity of PLD1, because deletion of this region increases basal activity, and insertion of the loop domain into recombinant PLD2 significantly reduces its basal activity [44–46].

PLD1 and -2 are widely expressed in different tissues and cell types, and are activated by a variety of GPCRs and RTKs [47]. PA generated by PLDs functions locally as a signaling messenger to regulate diverse cellular functions, including endocytosis, exocytosis, membrane trafficking, cell proliferation, and actin cytoskeleton reorganization [48]. PA can also act as a lipid anchor, recruiting PA-binding proteins to localized sites of signal transduction, examples of which include the guanine nucleotide exchange factors (GEFs) DOCK2 and SOS, which activate Rac1 and Ras, respectively [49–51]. In some instances, PA additionally activates the proteins recruited, s uch as phosphorylating phosphatidylinositol 4-phosphate (PI4P), to generate phosphatidylinositol 4,5-bisphosphate (PI(4,5)P2) and mammalian target of rapamycin (mTOR), which regulate many processes including cell hypertrophy, differentiation, and survival [52]. Finally, PA also functions as an intermediate for the production of bioactive DAG or LPA [53, 54]. Therefore, aberrant expression or activation is closely linked to human diseases including cancer, diabetes, neurodegenerative disorders, and myocardial disease.

2.2.1.3 PLA

PLA hydrolyzes the carboxylic esters at the sn-1 (PLA1) or sn-2(PLA2) positions on glycerol backbones of phospholipids to produce free fatty acids and 2-acyl lysophospholipid or 1-acyl lysophospholipid, respectively (Fig. 2.1). PLA1 can be divided into two groups according to cellular localization: intracellular and extracellular PLA1. Three members of the mammalian intracellular phospholipase A1 subfamily have been identified: PA-preferring phospholipase A1, p125, and KIAA0725p [55, 56]. These enzymes commonly contain a lipase consensus sequence. There are 10 mammalian extracellular phospholipase A1 enzymes: phosphatidylserine-selective phospholipase A1 (PS-PLA1), membrane-associated PA-selective phospholipase A1α (mPA-PLA1 α), mPA-PLA1β, pancreatic lipase, lipoprotein lipase, hepatic lipase, endothelial lipase, and pancreatic lipase–related proteins-1–3 (Fig. 2.2). These PLA1s share multiple conserved motifs, including a lipase consensus sequence, a catalytic Ser-Asp-His triad, cysteine residues, and a lipid-binding surface loop [55]. In contrast to other phospholipases, the physiological roles of PLA1 remain largely unknown, especially in mammalian.

The PLA2 family of enzymes catalyze the hydrolysis of the sn-2 bond of membrane phospholipids to release AA and lysophospholipid secondary messengers under the influence of various stimuli, including circulating hormones and growth factors. The first PLA2 was identified in snake venom, while other enzymes were discovered in other organisms. The growing superfamily of PLA2s is categorized into 14 groups based on amino acid sequences and these 14 groups are subdivided into 4 classes in mammals (Fig. 2.2). PLA2s are classified into several major types: secretory PLA2 (sPLA2), cytosolic PLA2 (cPLA2), calcium-independent PLA2 (iPLA2), platelet-activating factor acylhydrolases (PAF-AHs), lysosomal PLA2s, and adipose-specific PLA2s. They differ from each other in terms of substrate specificity, calcium requirement, and lipid modification [56, 57]. The ubiquitously expressed cPLAα 2 has high selectivity for membrane phospholipids that contain AA, which can be metabolized to growth-promoting eicosanoids. This has resulted in a number of studies that link cPLA2α activity to tumorigenesis. cPLA2α has a cytoplasmic distribution when inactive, but translocates to intracellular membranes once activated by concurrent Ca^{2+} binding and phosphorylation at serine residue 505 [58]. cPLA2α -released AA is a potent cytotoxic compound, inducing cell death through stimulation of mitochondrion-mediated apoptosis and sphingomyelin phosphodiesterase (SMase)-ceramide pathways, unless the AA is subjected to further metabolism [59]. The iPLA2 family is important for membrane homeostasis and energy metabolism, and the sPLA2 family modulates extracellular phospholipid environments.

2.2.2 Phospholipases Signaling in Cancer

Phospholipases can be activated by multiple extracellular signals, including hormones (e.g., insulin and growth hormones), growth factors (e.g., EGF and vascular endothelial growth factor [VEGF]), and lipids (e.g., LPA and sphingosine 1-phosphate [S1P]; Fig. 2.3) [14, 60–62]. These extracellular cues stimulate phospholipases through the direct activation of RTKs or GPCRs [15, 63]. Phospholipases act as key mediators of many cellular functions by generating bioactive lipids that transmit signals to a variety of downstream molecules and interactions with their binding partners. As illustrated in Fig. 2.3, phospholipases and their lipid mediators underlie complicated, multilayered signaling networks. Furthermore, lipid mediators are major participants in a variety of cellular processes related to tumorigenesis and/or metastasis, such as matrix metalloproteinase (MMP) secretion, actin cytoskeleton reorganization, migration, proliferation, growth, inflammation, and angiogenesis [14, 55, 56, 64]. The importance of phospholipases and their products (that is, lipid mediators) in key cellular functions has been characterized by cell-based analyses, and by studies using transgenic and knockout mice. Studies using transgenic and knockout mice have demonstrated that phospholipases are crucially involved in various phenotypes. Specifically, many studies on phospholipase transgenic and knockout mice have demonstrated tumor-related phenotypes, such as tumorigenesis, metastasis, and angiogenesis, in a variety of organs, including the intestine, colon, lung, and ovary (Table 2.1). The following sections discuss what have been learned from studies of cell lines and mouse models regarding the

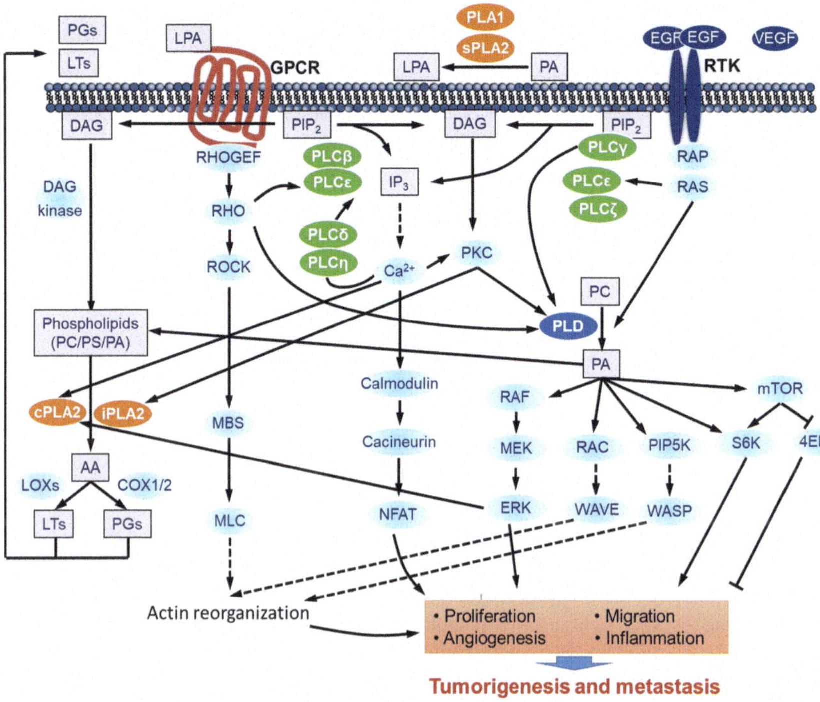

Fig. 2.3 Overview of phospholipase signaling pathways and networks in cancer. Phospholipases (PLA, PLC, PLD)-related signal pathways are closely connected with each other and essential in various tumor processes (e.g., growth, differentiation, and migration). Among PLC isozymes, PLCβ and ε are activated by G protein or small GTPase in GPCR signaling. Activity of PLCδ and η is controlled by calcium signaling induced by GPCR. PLCγ is directly phosphorylated by RTK activated by growth hormones such as EGF and VEGF. Activated PLC can cleave PIP_2 into DAG and IP_3 which are important second messengers in cellular functions. PLC-mediated signaling, IP_3-induced calcium release, and PKC activation can stimulate other phospholipases activity, PLA, and PLD. Cytosolic PLA2(cPLA2) and intracellular calcium-independent PLA2 (iPLA2) can generate AA by hydrolyzing various phospholipids (PC, PS, PA). AA is further modified into eicosanoids, including PGs and LTs by COX and LOX, respectively. PGs and LTs are released from the cell and act as autocrine and paracrine factors. In extracellular environment, membrane-associated PA-selective PLA1(mPA-PLA1) and secretory PLA2 (sPLA2) hydrolyze PA into LPA, which induces GPCR signaling in an autocrine/paracrine manner. PLD, activated by PKC, converts PC into PA, which can stimulate multiple downstream signal molecules. *PL* phospholipase, *GPCR* G-protein-coupled receptor, *RTK* receptor tyrosine kinases, *EGF* epidermal growth factor, *PIP_2* phosphatidylinositol-4,5-bisphosphate, *DAG* diacylglycerol, *IP_3* inositol-1,4,5-trisphosphate, *PKC* protein kinase C, *AA* arachidonic acid, *PC* phosphatidylcholine, *PS* phosphatidylserine, *PA* phosphatidic acid, *PGs* prostaglandins, *LTs* leukotrienes, *COX* cyclooxygenase, *LOX* lipoxygenase, *LPA* lysophosphatidic acid, *4EBP1* 4E binding protein 1, *CASP* caspase, *GEF* guanine nucleotide exchange factor, *MBS* myosin binding subunit, *MLC* myosin light chain, *NFAT* nuclear factor of activated T cells, *PIP5K* phosphatidylinositol 4-phosphate 5-kinase, *ROCK* RHO kinase, *S6K* S6 kinase, *VEGF* vascular endothelial growth factor, *WASP* Wiskott–Aldrich syndrome protein, *WAVE* WASP family protein member

Table 2.1 Cancer-related phonotypes of phospholipase transgenic and knockout mice

Gene	Types of mutation	Tissue affected	Phenotype	Refs
sPla2	Spontaneous/ Transgenic	Intestine	Increased tumor susceptibility in $Apc^{min/+}$ mice Reduced tumorigenesis in $Apc^{min/+}$ mice	[128, 131]
	Spontaneous	Colon	Inverse correlation of Pla2g2a expression level with susceptibility to carcinogen-induced colon tumor	[129]
cPla2	Knockout	Intestine	Decreased tumor number in small intestine of $Apc^{min/+}$mice	[118]
	Knockout	Lung	Decreased number of carcinogen-induced lung tumor	[127, 145]
	Knockout	Colon	Increased colonic injury and number of colon tumor by carcinogen Impaired colonic eicosanoid production	[117, 123]
	Knockout	Angiogenesis	Tumor regression and attenuated vascularity	[130]
iPla2b	Knockout	Lung metastasis	Decreased lung metastasis	[132]
	Knockout	Ovary	Reduced tumorigenesis and ascites formation from injected ovarian cancer cells	[135]
Plcb3	Knockout	Hematopoietic cells	Developed myeloproliferative disease, lymphoma, and other tumors	[86]
Plcg	Transgenic (dominant negative)	Lung metastasis	Decreased number of lung metastases in PyVmT and TRAMP models	[74]
Plcg2	Knockout	B cells	Lymphoma development in $Plc\gamma2^{-/-}$; Eμ-Myc transgenic mice	[65]
Plcd1	Knockout	Skin	Developed spontaneous skin tumor	[84]
Plce1	Knockout	Skin	Delayed onset and markedly reduced incidence of carcinogen-induced skin squamous tumors	[85]
	Knockout	Colon	Alleviates the colitis and suppresses tumorigenesis	[66]
Plcz1	Transgenic	Ovary	Developed benign ovarian teratomas	[67]
Pld1	Transgenic/ Knockout	Intestine	Accelerates tumorigenesis in $Apc^{min/+}$ mice Loss of PLD1 suppresses the intestinal tumorigenesis in $Apc^{Min/+}$ and AOM/DSS mice models	[110, 109]
	Knockout	Tumor microenvironment	Suppressed tumor growth, metastasis, and angiogenesis	[94]
Pld2	Knockout	Angiogenesis	Reduced tumor growth and tumor blood vessel formation	[111]
	Knockout	Lung metastasis	Inhibited invadopodia formation in breast cancer cells	[106]

APC adenomatous polyposis coli, *Pl* phospholipase, *PyVmT* polyomavirus middle T antigen, *TRAMP* transgenic adenocarcinoma of the mouse prostate functions of various phospholipases in breast cancer–associated processes and signaling pathways.

2.3 Current Evidence and Concepts

2.3.1 PLC and Breast Cancer

A role for PLC has recently been identified in the regulation of a number of cellular behaviors, and in the promotion of tumorigenesis by regulating cell motility, transformation, and cell growth, partly by acting as signaling intermediates for cytokines such as EGF and interleukins in cancer cells [65–67]. Aberrant expression and activation of PLC isozymes are observed in a variety of human cancers, and are related to tumor progression.

Previous studies have highlighted alteration in PLC expression levels in breast tumor cells. It has been reported that PLC-β2 is abnormally elevated in breast cancer and correlates with poor clinical outcomes, suggesting its role as a marker for breast cancer severity [68]. In addition, PLC-β2 provokes the transition from G0/G1 to S/G2/M cell cycle phase, which is important in cancer progression and inositol lipid–related modifications of the cytoskeleton architecture occurring during tumor cell division, motility, and invasion [69]. PLC-β isozymes can be activated by GPCRs, indicating that most chemokines secreted in the tumor microenvironment can activate PLC-β to increase cell migration and invasion; indeed, gain- and loss-of-function studies in tumor cells have demonstrated the functional importance of PLC-β in tumor cell migration and invasion. Recently, PLC-β1 was shown to be highly expressed in breast cancer tissues in comparison with normal mammary gland tissues. Also, there are significant differences in PLC-β1 expression between metastasis and recurrence tumor tissue, which may indicate its role in promoting migration in breast cancer [70, 71]. However, further experimental verification is necessary.

Among the PLC isozymes, PLC-γ is important because it plays a specific and key role in cell proliferation, and in migration and invasion, therefore contributing to tumorigenesis and/or metastasis [72–74]. Compared with normal mammary gland tissue, moderately or poorly differentiated breast tumors (grade 2 or 3) express higher levels of PLC-γ1. Expression is at marginally low levels in low-grade tumors compared with normal tissues. A significant association was found between PLC-γ1 expression and the risk of metastatic relapse in T1/T2, N0-stage breast cancer patients treated with chemotherapy [75]. As expected from its expression pattern, PLC-γ1 is involved in the migration and metastatic potential of breast cancer [76]. Growth factor receptors (e.g., EGFR and HER2) and their downstream molecules are associated with increased cancer proliferation and motility. The epithelial growth factor receptor (EGFR)/ErbB family is among the most notable cancer molecular targets in many epithelial tumors. ErbB2 (also known as HER2/neu) in particular is overexpressed in approximately 25% of breast cancers, and trastuzumab (Herceptin), a well-established breast cancer drug, targets ErbB2. Major downstream signaling pathways of ErbB are the mitogen-activated protein kinase (MAPK) pathway, PI3K pathway, and PLC-γ1 pathway, which lead to gene expression changes.

EGF-induced migration of breast cancer cells mainly depends on the transient activation of PLC-γ1 via ErbB2 activation. Correlatively, downregulation of PLC-γ1expression blocked Rac1 and CDC42 GTPases via IP3-induced calcium release activation, resulting in the suppression of human breast cancer cell–derived lung metastasis in a mouse model [77, 78]. In addition, PLC-γ1 has been shown to mediate the cell motility effects of growth factors including PDGF, EGF, insulin-like growth factor (IGF), and hepatocyte growth factor (HGF). A dominant-negative PLC-γ1 fragment reduced the metastatic potential of breast cancer in a transgenic mouse model. Metastasis assays also demonstrated that nude mice with PLC-γ1 knockdown exhibited inhibition of breast cancer–derived lung metastasis [79]. This result suggests that PLC-γ1 is a potential therapeutic target in the clinical treatment of tumor metastasis.

Moreover, PLC-γ1 is a target of the micro RNA (miR)-200bc/429 cluster that suppresses EGF-driven cell invasion, viability, and cell cycle progression in breast cancer [80]. The miR-200 family consists of five members. They are expressed as two separate polycistronic pri-miRNA transcripts, with miR200b-200a-429 at chromosomal location 1p36 and miR-200c-141 at chromosomal location 12p13. This shared seed sequence suggests that the clusters may share some common target genes. The miR-200 family is downregulated to undetectable levels in breast cancer cell lines with invasive and generally mesenchymal phenotypes compared with well-differentiated breast cancer cell lines. Consistent with its expression in breast cancer cell lines, the levels of the miR-200 family are approximately 10- to 22-fold lower in mesenchymal sarcomatoid regions of human primary breast cancers compared with epithelial epithelioid regions [81], and loss of the miR-200 family contributes to breast cancer progression [82]. In breast cancer, position 4915–4921 on the 3-′-untranslated region (UTR) of PLCG1 is a direct target of miR-200bc/429, and the downregulation of PLC-γ1 by miR-200bc/429 inhibits EGF-driven cell invasion. These reports suggest the mechanism by which PLC-γ1 is overexpressed in breast cancer (Table 2.2).

Furthermore, PLC-δ4 is upregulated in breast tumor cells, and its overexpression enhances cell proliferation in breast cancer cells with lower oncogenicity [83]. Patients with tumor metastasis expressed higher levels of PLC-δ4 than those with local recurrence. Significantly, breast cancer patients with higher expression levels of PLC-δ4 experience a shorter disease-free survival period, which may indicate a correlation between PLC-δ4 and recurrence in breast cancer patients.

Unlike PLC-γ and PLC-ε, the PLC-β and PLC-δ isoforms are known tumor suppressors [84, 85]. Loss of PLC-β3 in mice can result in myeloproliferative diseases, lymphoma, and other types of cancer through the regulation of signal transducer and activator of transcription 5 (STAT5) phosphorylation. Consistent with this, PLC-β3 downregulation has been observed in human chronic lymphocytic leukemia samples [86]. Furthermore, monoallelic deletion of *PLCB1* (which encodes PLC-β1) increases the risk of developing acute myeloid leukemia in patients

Table 2.2 Aberrant expression and mutation of phospholipases in breast cancer

Gene	Expression	Correlation	Refs
sPLA2	Increased	Poor prognosis	[112, 116]
cPLA2A	Increased	Poor prognosis Her2 subtype	[113, 114, 115]
PLCB1	Increased	Invasiveness	[71]
PLCB2	Increased	Poor prognosis with breast cancer malignancy	[68, 69]
PLCG1	Increased	ND	[72, 73, 75]
PLCD1	Decreased	With ER status and tumor grade	[89]
	Increased	ND	[88]
PLCD3	Increased	ND	[88]
PLCD4	Increased	ND	[83]
PLCE	Increased	ND	[71]
PLD1	Increased	ND	[91]
PLD2	Increased	ND	[93]

ND not determined, *PL* phospholipase

with myelodysplastic syndrome. The loss of PLC-δ1 expression is highly associated with its role as a tumor suppressor in esophageal squamous cell carcinoma (ESCC). In addition, decreased PLC-δ1 expression is correlated with poor clinical outcomes in patients with acute or chronic myeloid leukemia [87, 88]. Also, PLC-δ1 is downregulated via hypermethylation in breast cancer. PLC-δ1 suppressed cell migration by regulating cytoskeletal reorganization proteins [89]. Although some mechanistic details remain unclear, the position of PLCs in the vicinity of cell surface receptors that relay signals from the extracellular microenvironment may enable them to amplify downstream signals through the generation of second messengers, activating effectors such as PKC and other phospholipases to continue the propagation of mitogenic signals.

2.3.2 *PLD and Breast Cancer*

PLD-mediated signaling pathways are highly complicated; therefore, its physiological functions are diverse. Recently, increased expression of PLD enzymes, their subcellular mislocalization, and altered PLD catalytic activity have been implicated as contributing factors in several types of human cancer, such as colon, gastric, kidney, and thyroid cancers. PLD is increasingly recognized as a critical regulator of cancer progression and tumorigenesis. In malignant breast cancer, PLD activity is increased, as is the expression of PLD1 and -2 [90, 91]. PLD1 tends to be overexpressed in tumors that show high expression of cytokeratins 5/17, which are frequently associated with poor prognosis [92]. In addition, elevated PLD2 expression suppresses apoptosis and also promote tumor growth rate and chemoresistance in breast cancer [93]. PLD1 has a critical function not only in the cancer cell itself but also in the tumor microenvironment. Studies in PLD1-deficient mice showed that

PLD1 promotes tumor growth and metastasis through enhanced angiogenesis and decreased tumor cell-platelet interactions [94]. Recent genomic analyses of human cancers have revealed several unique PLD2 mutations in breast, stomach, and brain cancers, although most of the reported mutations remain to be functionally characterized [95, 96]. These studies provide initial evidence that increased PLD activity is linked to oncogenic signals and tumorigenesis.

Several mitogenic signals (such as EGF, EDGF, and FGF) and oncogenic activation (such as *v-ras*, *v-raf*, and *v-src*) stimulate PLD-mediated oncogenic signaling pathways [39–41, 97–99]. The oncogenic signaling network is mediated by the interaction between PLDs and Ras, and facilitates the activation of MAPK [100]. Furthermore, recent work has revealed that PLD2-generated PA recruits SOS1 to the plasma membrane and activates RAS, promotes cell proliferation and anti-apoptosis of cancer cells [50]. Another critical downstream target of PLD in cancer cells is the mTOR, a serine/threonine kinase known to be a key regulator in cell growth and survival signaling pathways. Because PA binds to and activates mTOR, overexpression of PLD1 or PLD2 stimulates mTOR activity, which was monitored by the phosphorylation of the mTOR enzymatic substrate S6 kinase in breast adenocarcinoma or rat fibroblasts, through PA production. PLD activation also induces c-Myc expression, which is regulated by mTOR activity, in breast adenocarcinoma, indicating the involvement of PLD-mTOR signaling pathway in cancer cell growth and survival signals [101, 102]. The mTOR inhibitor rapamycin has been used as an anti-cancer drug. However, rapamycin-based therapeutic strategies are unsuccessful in some cancer patients. Interestingly, it has been demonstrated that PA competes with rapamycin in mTOR regulation, and activation of PLD inhibits the effect of rapamycin in human breast cancer cell line. Therefore, inhibition of PLD may provide the strategy for suppressing the survival signal of rapamycin-resistant cancer cells. In normal proliferating cells, DNA-damaging agents cause apoptosis through a mechanism that involves increased expression of p53. In rat fibroblasts and MDA-MB-231 breast cancer cells, overexpression of PLD1 decreased p53 levels and apoptosis after treatment with DNA-damaging agents, suggesting that PLD activity promotes p53 degradation [103].

Many studies have detected a positive correlation between PLD activity and invasive potential. Overexpression of PLD in breast, glioblastoma, or lymphoma cells stimulates invasion, whereas expression of dominant-negative PLD prevents invasion [104]. Similarly, small-molecule PLD inhibitors (FIPI: 5-fluoro-2-indolyl des-chlorohalopemide;NOPT:N-[2-(4-oxo-1-phenyl-1,3,8-triazaspiro[4,5]dec-8-yl) ethyl]-2-naphthalenecarboxamide) and PLD siRNA also decrease tumor size and breast cancer cell metastasis formation in vivo [94]. PLD2 stimulates cell protrusion in *v-src*-transformed cells and is required for EGF-induced membrane ruffling. Elevated PA levels can reorganize actin by its regulation of RAC complexes and phosphoatidylinositol 4-phosphate 5-kinase (PIP5K). In addition to lipid-mediated activation of downstream effectors, the PX domain of PLD2 shows RHO GEF activity, which induces actin reorganization. Thus, PLD2 induces stress fiber formation by mediating nucleotide exchange for RHOA [105]. A recent study showed that PLD2 knockout inhibited lung metastases in the mammary tumor virus

(MMTV)-*Neu* transgenic mouse breast cancer model [106]. PLD2-generated PA binds to and regulates the motor protein KIF5B, which controls membrane type1 metalloproteinases (MT1-MMP, also known as MMP14) surface localization and invasion. Furthermore, increased PLD activity enhanced the ability of MDA-MB-231 breast cancer cells to migrate and invade matrigel, and PLD2 overexpression increased the invasion and metastasis of EL4 mouse lymphoma cells. In contrast, inactive PLD2 inhibited metastasis in a syngeneic mouse model [107, 108]. Taken together, these results demonstrate that PLD1 and PLD2 promote tumor progression through distinct mechanisms.

PLD2-dependent cancer metastasis is intrinsic to cancer cells, whereas PLD1 is critical for both cancer and stromal cells [94, 109, 110]. Phenotypic analysis of *PLD1* knockout mice, which are otherwise viable and normal, revealed that PLD1 expression in tumor microenvironment plays important roles in tumor growth metastasis. The tumor microenvironment consists of various types of cells, such as vascular and lymphatic endothelial cells, mesenchymal cells, and immune cells. The soluble factors, signaling cues, ECM, and mechanical cues provided by tumor microenvironmental cells can promote tumor progression by supporting tumor growth and invasion, and by protecting the tumor from host immune system attack. Angiogenesis, which is required to supply oxygen and nutrients, is one of the major aspects of tumor microenvironment contributing to tumor progression; inhibition of angiogenesis in tumors prevents tumor growth. Ghim et al. found that the ablation of PLD2 from endothelial cells led to the suppression of hypoxia-induced HIF-1α expression and VEGF secretion, and also reduced proximal tumor neovascularization [111]. Additionally, when mouse melanoma or lung cancer cells were implanted into wild-type or PLD1 knockout mice exhibited a much lower density of microvascular cells. When VEGF-coated matrigel plugs were inserted into the same mice, endothelial cells failed to migrate to the plugs in the PLD1 knockout mice, suggesting inherent defects in the migration of PLD1 knockout-derived endothelial cells. Consistent with this observation, PLD1 knockout mice showed impaired integrin signaling, manifested in a failure to properly adhere to ECM integrin ligands, such as fibronectin, vitronectin, and collagen. Therefore, PLDs in the tumor microenvironmental cells are required for both primary tumor growth and metastasis.

2.3.3 PLA and Breast Cancer

Phospholipase A2 has a role in many biological processes, including inflammation, cell growth, and cancer development. Yamashita et al. were the first to report that PLA2 levels were highly elevated in patients with various malignant tumors, and especially in breast cancer [112]. Their study indicated a possible role of PLA2 in breast cancer progression. In particular, the role of EGFR/HER2 transactivation in estrogen-induced cPLA2α activation in breast carcinoma cell lines suggests that cPLA2α activity and expression may be coupled with HER2 over-expression in tumor cells [113, 114]. Previous investigations found a correlation between the expression of intermediates in the eicosanoid signaling pathway, particularly COX-2, and the abundance of HER2 in breast carcinomas. cPLA2α expression was correlated with worse prognostic indicators, which also characterize more invasive tumors of the HER2-positive and basal-like subtypes. Elevated cPLA2α expression was associated with decreased survival in patients with luminal breast cancers, and also correlated with a reduced efficacy of endocrine therapy. This study found that cPLA2α expression was an independent predictive marker of a poor response to endocrine therapy over the first 5 years of post-treatment follow-up [113, 115]. In addition, PLA is synchronously overexpressed, and participates, in tumorigenesis by producing sufficient substrates for the metabolic cascade of COX2/PEG2 and other pathways, and is significantly correlated with a poor prognosis. Recently, higher plasma PLA2 and sPLA2 activity was detected in patients with breast cancer, particularly at late disease stages, than in healthy controls [112, 116]. Thus, plasma PLA2 activity may be a potential prognostic biomarker for patients with breast cancer. However, the functions and underlying molecular mechanisms of PLAs in breast cancer remain to be elucidated.

PLA2 has been shown to have both growth-inhibiting and growth-promoting effects [117, 118]. Its metabolite, AA, also has opposing functions in different tumor microenvironments. AA can be converted into various biologically active eicosanoid mediators including prostaglandins (PGs), hydroxyeicosatetraenoic acids (HETEs), and epoxyeicosatrienoic acids (EETs) by cytochrome P450 monooxygenase, COX isoforms, and lipoxygenases (LOXs) [119, 120]. The metabolism of AA by 15-LOX produces 15-S-hydroxyeicosatetraenoic acid (15-(S)-HETE) and prevents the proliferation of cell in culture [120, 121]. In contrast, PGE2 contributes to cell proliferation; consequently, the AA-based eicosanoid signaling pathway has been implicated in the development and progression of cancer in different human tissues, including the breast [121–123]. PGE2 stimulates the expression of growth-promoting genes, such as *c-fos* and VEGF [124], and promotes COX-2 expression in colorectal cancer, breast cancer, and normal epithelial cells [124, 125]; this leads to a positive feedback effect on downstream growth-promoting signaling. PGE2 can functions in both autocrine and paracrine manner to stimulate aromatase expression in breast cancer and normal tissue [126]. Consequently, COX-2 upregulates the production of the most biologically active estrogen 17-β-estradiol (E2), and the subsequent stimulation of proliferative signaling pathways. cPLA2α can generate AA to produce PGEs and enhance tumorigenesis, but sPLA2 has tumor-suppressive functions [127–129]. Thus, the requirement to balance PLA2 activity with the metabolism of its products may be responsible for some inconsistencies in published data regarding whether PLA2 supports or suppresses breast carcinoma progression.

The PLA family may promote tumor progression via extracellular regulation of the tumor microenvironment, to trigger cell migration and invasion [130–132]. The lipid mediators of PLAs involved in tumor metastasis and angiogenesis are LPA, AA, leukotrienes, and prostaglandins [133–135]. Serum LPA is a well-established indicator of tumor initiation and progression in breast cancer [136], ovarian cancer [137] and multiple myeloma [138]. LPA receptors, which show deregulated expression in cancer cells and tissues [139–141], activate RHO family small GTPases to drive cell migration and invasion. Furthermore, AA induces the expression and surface exposure of GalT-1, which acts as a membrane receptor for ECM proteins and cell-to-cell interactions in MDA-MB-231 breast carcinoma cells, providing another mechanism by which PLA2 activity impacts the invasive capacity of breast carcinoma cells [142].

The altered metabolism of AA by COX and LOX in cancer cells has also been shown to play a role in cancer progression. In a mouse xenograft model, breast cancer cells overexpressing LPA1 has enhanced subcutaneous growth and bone metastasis [143]. Tumor cells stimulated LPA release from circulating platelets. The resulting pro-inflammatory PGs and leukotrienes are key mediators of intracellular crosstalk between tumor cells and stromal cells, and they induce the migration and proliferation of stromal cells such as immune cells, tumor-associated fibroblasts, and endothelial cells, which produce additional inflammatory cytokines and chemokines to establish the tumor microenvironment [144, 145]. The cooperation of phospholipases is important for angiogenesis because cell-cell communication must be tightly integrated and regulated. Malignant tumor cells express high levels of PLA2 and AA metabolic enzymes, resulting in the production of eicosanoid metabolites. These molecules mediate endothelial cell recruitment, proliferation, migration, and tube formation. Various studies have shown a correlation between COX2 overexpression and enhanced production of PGE2 by cancer cells. Through autocrine and paracrine pathways in tumor cells and stromal cells, PGE2 stimulates the production of VEGF and the chemokines CXCL1 to recruit endothelial cells. Moreover, cPLA2α-deficient endothelial cells are defective in tumor vascularization [134, 146, 147]. Therefore, the role of LOX signaling in proliferation, metastatic invasion and angiogenesis is emerging. The balance between COX and LOX activity in determining the nature of the AA metabolites produced is not only important establishing their respective and interacting roles in breast cancer progression, but also for potential novel therapeutic interventions.

2.3.4 A Multicellular Phospholipase Network

Invasion and metastasis is a multicellular and multistep process, and phospholipases contribute to this process by affecting both inter- and intracellular signal. First, overexpressed PLA2 and eicosanoid metabolic enzymes generate PGs and leukotrienes, which can activate stromal cells to migrate towards tumor cells. The recruited stromal cells secrete growth factors, cytokines, chemokines, and eicosanoids that coordinate the tumor microenvironment. Second, factors that are secreted from stromal cells probably go on to potentiate tumor cell migration and invasion by activating PLC and PLD (Fig. 2.3), as well as many other factors. This suggests that the phospholipase signal circuit could have crucial inter- and intracellular roles during metastasis.

Although many reports have suggested the functional association of phospholipases in physiological angiogenesis, the precise mechanism underlying tumor-associated angiogenesis remains unclear. The majority of such studies have used in vitro experiments, which do not consider the tumor microenvironment or cell-cell communication. As noted above, tumor microenvironments are complex and dynamically regulated by intracellular signaling evets. However, further investigation is needed to fully understand the roles of phospholipases in the context of tumor microenvironment.

2.3.5 *Phospholipases as Anticancer Drug Targets*

Despite strong evidence implicating phospholipases in tumorigenesis and progression, developing effective therapeutic strategies to inhibit phospholipases has been difficult for a number of reasons. In general, phospholipases are considered "undruggable" targets [148]. One of the major concerns that phospholipases regulates many key cellular processes, and therefore their inhibition would inevitably lead to severe side effects. Some phospholipases, such as iPLA2s, control normal brain and heart functions by remodeling phospholipids [149, 150]. On the other hand, abnormal hyperactivity, which is induced by the dysregulation of phospholipases, may be a potential therapeutic targets in cancer. Therefore, current challenges include developing therapeutics with optimal pharmacokinetic parameters that minimize side effects and maximize anticancer effects. In addition, isoform-specific inhibition of phospholipases has proven difficult. Historically, compounds that were structurally unrelated to PI(4,5)P2, such as aminosteroid U73122, were identified as potential candidates, but they showed great non-specificity. In fact, U73122 was suggested to have other targets, including calcium pumps and unrelated enzymes regulating lipid metabolism [151–153]. Furthermore, depending on the environmental stimulus, some phospholipase isozymes have oncogenic roles and others have tumor-suppressive roles. Therefore, the development of isozyme-specific inhibitors may improve our ability to target these enzymes. Second, although many reports have addressed the prognostic value of phospholipases in different tumor types, the number of studies has been small and detection methods have been limited. Additionally, breast cancer is a complex disease with very distinct clinical, morphological, and molecular entities. This heterogeneity cannot be explained only by clinical parameters like tumor size, histological grade, and ages. To evaluate the clinical and prognostic value of phospholipases as anticancer therapeutics, more careful clinical studies and integrated research approaches are needed [154]. Third, there are no reports on constitutively active mutations of the phospholipases in specific cancers, and few spontaneous animal models for cancer have been developed. In other words, phospholipases may be modulators of tumorigenesis and cancer progression by interacting each other. Finally, because lipid second messengers generated by phospholipases are quickly converted to the next metabolite, measuring the activation status of phospholipases in cancer tissue has proven impossible. Moreover, downstream targets of lipid mediators are not specific to phospholipase-mediated signaling. Therefore, identification of predictive biomarkers is crucial for drug development.

Although phospholipases themselves are not strong oncogenes or tumor suppressors, phospholipases and lipid mediators strongly interact with their binding partners, including oncogenes and tumor suppressors, in a complex tumor microenvironment. Furthermore, phospholipases can interact with other signaling pathways depending on the surrounding environment or cell type, implying that specific drugs could potentially be designed to target tumor-associated phospholipases. In this respect, blocking the eicosanoid signaling pathway through the deactivation of COX enzymes has been tested in clinical studies. The inhibition of COX enzymes using non-steroidal anti-inflammatory drugs (NSAIDs) had therapeutic effects on several tumors [155]. However, their therapeutic efficacy is insufficient because NSAIDs cannot block the generation of leukotrienes by PLA2. Therefore, the use of PLA2 inhibitors might be considered an attractive alternative. Varespladib, a sPLA2-specific inhibitor, was under clinical evaluation as an anti-inflammatory agent; unfortunately, this trial was halted in 2012 due to inadequate efficacy [156]. Thus, inhibitors of other PLA2 isozymes have to be developed as anticancer drugs, and their efficacy improved to reduce side effects [157]. Further development of isozyme-specific inhibitors of PLA2 may lead to novel therapeutic strategies.

Interest in targeting PLD isozymes with small-molecule inhibitors has grown steadily since PLD family members were implicated in a variety of human diseases, including cancer. The dual-PLD inhibitors FIPI and halopemide (more effective against PLD2) effectively block PA production and several biological processes that have been known to be mediated by PLD activation, such as cytoskeleton reorganization, cell spreading, and chemotaxis, in vitro [158]. Although isozyme selectivity remained elusive, this discovery represented an important advance. Recent advances in the development of isozyme-selective PLD inhibitors, and in molecular genetics, have suggested that PLD isozymes in mammalian cells and pathogenic organisms may be valuable targets for the treatment of several human disease. Isozyme-selective inhibitors of PLD have been generated that inhibit the migration of breast cancer cell lines [159, 160]. In different settings, it may be advantageous to use PLD1-specific or PLD2-specific inhibitors rather than a dual PLD1/2 inhibitor, depending on the extent of redundancy of the individual PLD isoforms in the process that is being inhibited. However, this remains an unexplored topic that will be important to address as therapeutic approaches are developed, in particular in the context of cancer.

Pharmacological inhibitors of PLC activity, selective small molecules, or other selective probes are crucial for elucidating physiological and aberrant functions of specific proteins in cells and whole organisms. Notably, however, PLCs not only lack potential drug molecules but also appear to lack even a reliable, direct small-molecule inhibitor. Based on structural insights and a detailed understanding of the catalytic mechanism of PIP2 hydrolysis, PLC proteins are not intrinsically intractable. The main limitations to inhibitor development have been related to a lack of suitable high-throughput screening, difficulties in generating chemical probes based on PIP2 substrate, and insufficient evidence linking changes in PLC function to disease development.

As mentioned above, several binding proteins of phospholipases and their lipid mediators may determine the role of phospholipases in cancer, and whether they act as cancer-promoting genes. For example, PLC-γ1 interacts with SOS1 to activate RAS, thereby increasing cell proliferation, and PLC-γ1 induces cell migration by interacting with the GUT1-Beta-Pix complex [161, 162]. These interactions are mediated by specific motifs and domains, suggesting that interaction blockers could be used as more specific anticancer therapies. However, no such blockers have developed to date. Therefore, understanding the mechanism of action of a specific domain-containing superfamily, as well as the roles of specific phospholipase isozymes in cellular signaling, metabolism, and cellular function, is paramount for the development of optimal therapeutic compounds.

Although some reagents that can block phospholipase signaling are available, we are far from developing anticancer therapies. By using integrated information (e.g., genomics, proteomics, and lipidomics) and animal experiments, the functional roles and regulatory mechanisms of phospholipases in tumorigenesis will be further defined. These efforts may lead to the generation of phospholipase-specific anticancer therapies.

2.4 Future Research Direction

Lipid signaling in pathology is an emerging field of investigation, and metabolite intermediates are a major lipid class involved in all of the crucial cell signaling pathways. Although phospholipases can regulate the pathways involved in tumorigenesis and cancer progression, and the signaling mechanisms of each phospholipase have been fairly well established, the functional roles of phospholipases in breast cancer are poorly understood. One of the major challenges to overcome this gap is to understand the complexity of the tumor microenvironment and intracellular signaling pathways. Tumor microenvironments generate various extracellular signals depending on the surrounding situation, which can trigger multiple signaling pathways, and different phospholipases can be simultaneously activated. Furthermore, phospholipases distributed throughout the signaling network can interact with one another and regulate each other's activities. Therefore, understanding the phospholipase-mediated signaling network within tumor microenvironments may be helpful for evaluating their functional importance in cancer. As shown in Fig. 2.3, phospholipases and their lipid mediators induce hierarchical pathways as well as complex networks that have feedback loops and crosstalk. For example, PLC is located in the immediately adjacent to the signaling receptors (e.g., RTKs and GPCRs) and generates two major second messengers (DAG and IP3) on activation. Thus, PLC serves as "generator" of second messengers and functions during the early stages of signaling transduction. Additionally, PA and PLD comprise a complex network with a variety of binding partners, and they have dynamic interrelationships with their binding partners that can, in turn, simultaneously or sequentially interact [31]. Hence, PLD act as a "signal mediator," which can finely regulate multiple signals as they pass downstream. PLAs generate LPA, an extracellular ligand for receptors, and AA, the intracellular precursor of extracellular PG and leukotriene ligands. On the basis of these characteristics, PLA2 is a "signal amplifier" that can transmit signals into the extracellular environment in an autocrine and/or paracrine manner. In this viewpoint, these signaling roles of phospholipases are supported by the localization of phospholipase binding partners, as well as the localization of the phospholipases themselves.

For the development of future therapeutic strategies, one of the main contributions of this breakthrough in cancer research is the integration of molecular studies into clinical trials. Despite evidence demonstrating the involvement of phospholipases in tumor-associated signaling in cells, there are few clinical studies presenting phospholipases as oncogenes or tumor suppressors. Recently, many bioinformatics data sets have been made available, including those derived from genomic and transcriptomic studies, as well as from the interactomes of phospholipases and their-associated signaling pathways. These combined analysis data can be used to assess the overall involvement of phospholipases in cancer. Interestingly, most experimental animal tumor models involving phospholipases were not established by single knockout or the overexpression of a single phospholipase molecule, but rather by a combination of knockouts or transgenic animals expressing different oncogenes or tumor suppressors. These results suggest that drugs that target phospholipases may be effective when combined with other drugs that target different cellular signaling pathways. It is possible that inhibitors of phospholipases could be developed to improve the efficacy of other targeted therapies, and to diminish toxicity arising from the inhibition of a physiologically important housekeeping enzyme. Thus, this integrated approach has provided valuable information on the nature of the disease, explaining in part the different responses to treatment and the disparate prognoses. Knowing the pathways regulating the processes involved in neoplastic development should help in the design of clinical trials aimed at patients with specific characteristics that are candidates to benefit from specific treatment.

Although many key questions remain regarding the development of isozyme-specific inhibitors and signal pathway blockers, phospholipases are considered as attractive targets for anticancer therapy. Targeting distinct phospholipases may have broad therapeutic potential, and it is likely that small molecule inhibitors of phospholipases will be tested for efficacy in diseases for which there is currently an unsatisfactory conventional therapy. The absence of toxic effects in animal models is highly encouraging. With current advances in mass spectrometry-based metabolomics, lipidomics, and phosphoproteomic analyses, new participants in established signaling and metabolic pathways are being revealed, which provide exciting opportunities for therapeutic targeting. The challenges for the future will be elucidating the complexity and variability of the phospholipase network in the tumor microenvironment, and understanding the tumor-specific roles of each phospholipase and its corresponding regulatory mechanisms.

2.5 Summary

- Phospholipases are essential mediators for many physiological processes; however, aberrant signaling is involved in carcinogenesis and cancer progression.
- Phospholipases are the link between two major pathways, HER2/HER3/PI3K and EGFR/HER2/PLC, and play an active role in breast cancer cell proliferation, migration, invasion, and angiogenesis.
- Phospholipases are not an easy target for therapy, so attention needs to be given to interacting partners, or cross-talk signaling pathways in tumor microenvironment.
- The integrated analyses of phospholipases are important for developing innovative therapeutic strategies or the comprehension of new molecular processes.

References

1. Siegel R, Naishadham D, Jemal A. Cancer statistics, 2013. CA Cancer J Clin. 2013;63(1):11–30.
2. Cianfrocca M, Goldstein LJ. Prognostic and predictive factors in early-stage breast cancer. Oncologist. 2004;9(6):606–16.
3. Jordan VC. Chemoprevention of breast cancer with selective oestrogen-receptor modulators. Nat Rev Cancer. 2007;7(1):46–53.
4. Rabindran SK. Antitumor activity of HER-2 inhibitors. Cancer Lett. 2005;227(1):9–23.
5. Linn SC, Van 't Veer LJ. Clinical relevance of the triple-negative breast cancer concept: genetic basis and clinical utility of the concept. Eur J Cancer. 2009;45(Suppl 1):11–26.
6. van Meer G, Voelker DR, Feigenson GW. Membrane lipids: where they are and how they behave. Nat Rev Mol Cell Biol. 2008;9(2):112–24.
7. Boesze-Battaglia K, Schimmel R. Cell membrane lipid composition and distribution: implications for cell function and lessons learned from photoreceptors and platelets. J Exp Biol. 1997;200(Pt 23):2927–36.
8. Eyster KM. The membrane and lipids as integral participants in signal transduction: lipid signal transduction for the non-lipid biochemist. Adv Physiol Educ. 2007;31(1):5–16.
9. Spiegel S, Foster D, Kolesnick R. Signal transduction through lipid second messengers. Curr Opin Cell Biol. 1996;8(2):159–67.
10. Wymann MP, Schneiter R. Lipid signalling in disease. Nat Rev Mol Cell Biol. 2008;9(2):162–76.
11. De Maria L, Vind J, Oxenboll KM, Svendsen A, Patkar S. Phospholipases and their industrial applications. Appl Microbiol Biotechnol. 2007;74(2):290–300.
12. Ramrakhiani L, Chand S. Recent progress on phospholipases: different sources, assay methods, industrial potential and pathogenicity. Appl Biochem Biotechnol. 2011;164(7):991–1022.
13. Alzayady KJ, Wang L, Chandrasekhar R, Wagner LE 2nd, Van Petegem F, Yule DI. Defining the stoichiometry of inositol 1,4,5-trisphosphate binding required to initiate Ca2+ release. Sci Signal. 2016;9(422):ra35.
14. Suh PG, Park JI, Manzoli L, Cocco L, Peak JC, Katan M, et al. Multiple roles of phosphoinositide-specific phospholipase C isozymes. BMB Rep. 2008;41(6):415–34.
15. Rhee SG. Regulation of phosphoinositide-specific phospholipase C. Annu Rev Biochem. 2001;70:281–312.
16. Yang YR, Follo MY, Cocco L, Suh PG. The physiological roles of primary phospholipase C. Adv Biol Regul. 2013;53(3):232–41.

17. Essen LO, Perisic O, Cheung R, Katan M, Williams RL. Crystal structure of a mammalian phosphoinositide-specific phospholipase C delta. Nature. 1996;380(6575):595–602.
18. Paterson HF, Savopoulos JW, Perisic O, Cheung R, Ellis MV, Williams RL, et al. Phospholipase C delta 1 requires a pleckstrin homology domain for interaction with the plasma membrane. Biochem J. 1995;312(Pt 3):661–6.
19. Wang T, Dowal L, El-Maghrabi MR, Rebecchi M, Scarlata S. The pleckstrin homology domain of phospholipase C-beta(2) links the binding of gbetagamma to activation of the catalytic core. J Biol Chem. 2000;275(11):7466–9.
20. Falasca M, Logan SK, Lehto VP, Baccante G, Lemmon MA, Schlessinger J. Activation of phospholipase C gamma by PI 3-kinase-induced PH domain-mediated membrane targeting. EMBO J. 1998;17(2):414–22.
21. Wen W, Yan J, Zhang M. Structural characterization of the split pleckstrin homology domain in phospholipase C-gamma1 and its interaction with TRPC3. J Biol Chem. 2006;281 (17):12060–8.
22. Nakashima S, Banno Y, Watanabe T, Nakamura Y, Mizutani T, Sakai H, et al. Deletion and site-directed mutagenesis of EF-hand domain of phospholipase C-delta 1: effects on its activity. Biochem Biophys Res Commun. 1995;211(2):365–9.
23. Otterhag L, Sommarin M, Pical C. N-terminal EF-hand-like domain is required for phosphoinositide-specific phospholipase C activity in Arabidopsis thaliana. FEBS Lett. 2001;497(2–3):165–70.
24. Rhee SG. Reflections on the days of phospholipase C. Adv Biol Regul. 2013;53(3):223–31.
25. Rebecchi MJ, Pentyala SN. Structure, function, and control of phosphoinositide-specific phospholipase C. Physiol Rev. 2000;80(4):1291–335.
26. Drin G, Scarlata S. Stimulation of phospholipase Cbeta by membrane interactions, interdomain movement, and G protein binding--how many ways can you activate an enzyme? Cell Signal. 2007;19(7):1383–92.
27. Kamat A, Carpenter G. Phospholipase C-gamma1: regulation of enzyme function and role in growth factor-dependent signal transduction. Cytokine Growth Factor Rev. 1997;8(2):109–17.
28. Smrcka AV, Brown JH, Holz GG. Role of phospholipase Cepsilon in physiological phosphoinositide signaling networks. Cell Signal. 2012;24(6):1333–43.
29. Jin TG, Satoh T, Liao Y, Song C, Gao X, Kariya K, et al. Role of the CDC25 homology domain of phospholipase Cepsilon in amplification of Rap1-dependent signaling. J Biol Chem. 2001;276(32):30301–7.
30. Thore S, Dyachok O, Tengholm A. Oscillations of phospholipase C activity triggered by depolarization and Ca2+ influx in insulin-secreting cells. J Biol Chem. 2004;279 (19):19396–400.
31. Young KW, Nash MS, Challiss RA, Nahorski SR. Role of Ca2+ feedback on single cell inositol 1,4,5-trisphosphate oscillations mediated by G-protein-coupled receptors. J Biol Chem. 2003;278(23):20753–60.
32. Kim JK, Choi JW, Lim S, Kwon O, Seo JK, Ryu SH, et al. Phospholipase C-eta1 is activated by intracellular Ca(2+) mobilization and enhances GPCRs/PLC/Ca(2+) signaling. Cell Signal. 2011;23(6):1022–9.
33. Peng X, Frohman MA. Mammalian phospholipase D physiological and pathological roles. Acta Physiol (Oxf). 2012;204(2):219–26.
34. Saito M, Kanfer J. Phosphatidohydrolase activity in a solubilized preparation from rat brain particulate fraction. Arch Biochem Biophys. 1975;169(1):318–23.
35. Osisami M, Ali W, Frohman MA. A role for phospholipase D3 in myotube formation. PLoS One. 2012;7(3):e33341.
36. Yoshikawa F, Banno Y, Otani Y, Yamaguchi Y, Nagakura-Takagi Y, Morita N, et al. Phospholipase D family member 4, a transmembrane glycoprotein with no phospholipase D activity, expression in spleen and early postnatal microglia. PLoS One. 2010;5(11):e13932.

37. Choi SY, Huang P, Jenkins GM, Chan DC, Schiller J, Frohman MA. A common lipid links Mfn-mediated mitochondrial fusion and SNARE-regulated exocytosis. Nat Cell Biol. 2006;8 (11):1255–62.
38. Ha EE, Frohman MA. Regulation of mitochondrial morphology by lipids. Biofactors. 2014;40 (4):419–24.
39. Song J, Jiang YW, Foster DA. Epidermal growth factor induces the production of biologically distinguishable diglyceride species from phosphatidylinositol and phosphatidylcholine via the independent activation of type C and type D phospholipases. Cell Growth Differ. 1994;5 (1):79–85.
40. Plevin R, Cook SJ, Palmer S, Wakelam MJ. Multiple sources of sn-1,2-diacylglycerol in platelet-derived-growth-factor-stimulated Swiss 3T3 fibroblasts. Evidence for activation of phosphoinositidase C and phosphatidylcholine-specific phospholipase D. Biochem J. 1991;279(Pt 2):559–65.
41. Motoike T, Bieger S, Wiegandt H, Unsicker K. Induction of phosphatidic acid by fibroblast growth factor in cultured baby hamster kidney fibroblasts. FEBS Lett. 1993;332(1–2):164–8.
42. Frohman MA, Sung TC, Morris AJ. Mammalian phospholipase D structure and regulation. Biochim Biophys Acta. 1999;1439(2):175–86.
43. Exton JH. Regulation of phospholipase D. FEBS Lett. 2002;531(1):58–61.
44. Brown FD, Thompson N, Saqib KM, Clark JM, Powner D, Thompson NT, et al. Phospholipase D1 localises to secretory granules and lysosomes and is plasma-membrane translocated on cellular stimulation. Curr Biol. 1998;8(14):835–8.
45. Freyberg Z, Sweeney D, Siddhanta A, Bourgoin S, Frohman M, Shields D. Intracellular localization of phospholipase D1 in mammalian cells. Mol Biol Cell. 2001;12(4):943–55.
46. Du G, Huang P, Liang BT, Frohman MA. Phospholipase D2 localizes to the plasma membrane and regulates angiotensin II receptor endocytosis. Mol Biol Cell. 2004;15(3):1024–30.
47. Park JB, Lee CS, Jang JH, Ghim J, Kim YJ, You S, et al. Phospholipase signalling networks in cancer. Nat Rev Cancer. 2012;12(11):782–92.
48. Ammar MR, Kassas N, Chasserot-Golaz S, Bader MF, Vitale N. Lipids in regulated exocytosis: what are they doing? Front Endocrinol (Lausanne). 2013;4:125.
49. Nishikimi A, Fukuhara H, Su W, Hongu T, Takasuga S, Mihara H, et al. Sequential regulation of DOCK2 dynamics by two phospholipids during neutrophil chemotaxis. Science. 2009;324 (5925):384–7.
50. Zhao C, Du G, Skowronek K, Frohman MA, Bar-Sagi D. Phospholipase D2-generated phosphatidic acid couples EGFR stimulation to Ras activation by Sos. Nat Cell Biol. 2007;9 (6):706–12.
51. Honda A, Nogami M, Yokozeki T, Yamazaki M, Nakamura H, Watanabe H, et al. Phosphatidylinositol 4-phosphate 5-kinase alpha is a downstream effector of the small G protein ARF6 in membrane ruffle formation. Cell. 1999;99(5):521–32.
52. Jang JH, Lee CS, Hwang D, Ryu SH. Understanding of the roles of phospholipase D and phosphatidic acid through their binding partners. Prog Lipid Res. 2012;51(2):71–81.
53. Aoki J. Mechanisms of lysophosphatidic acid production. Semin Cell Dev Biol. 2004;15 (5):477–89.
54. Csaki LS, Dwyer JR, Fong LG, Tontonoz P, Young SG, Reue K. Lipins, lipinopathies, and the modulation of cellular lipid storage and signaling. Prog Lipid Res. 2013;52(3):305–16.
55. Aoki J, Inoue A, Makide K, Saiki N, Arai H. Structure and function of extracellular phospholipase A1 belonging to the pancreatic lipase gene family. Biochimie. 2007;89(2):197–204.
56. Murakami M, Taketomi Y, Miki Y, Sato H, Hirabayashi T, Yamamoto K. Recent progress in phospholipase A(2) research: from cells to animals to humans. Prog Lipid Res. 2011;50 (2):152–92.
57. Kudo I, Murakami M. Phospholipase A2 enzymes. Prostaglandins Other Lipid Mediat. 2002;68–69:3–58.
58. Hirabayashi T, Murayama T, Shimizu T. Regulatory mechanism and physiological role of cytosolic phospholipase A2. Biol Pharm Bull. 2004;27(8):1168–73.

59. Nakanishi M, Rosenberg DW. Roles of cPLA2alpha and arachidonic acid in cancer. Biochim Biophys Acta. 2006;1761(11):1335–43.
60. Oude Weernink PA, Lopez de Jesus M, Schmidt M. Phospholipase D signaling: orchestration by PIP2 and small GTPases. Naunyn Schmiedeberg's Arch Pharmacol. 2007;374 (5–6):399–411.
61. Cho CH, Lee CS, Chang M, Jang IH, Kim SJ, Hwang I, et al. Localization of VEGFR-2 and PLD2 in endothelial caveolae is involved in VEGF-induced phosphorylation of MEK and ERK. Am J Physiol Heart Circ Physiol. 2004;286(5):H1881–8.
62. Alberghina M. Phospholipase A(2): new lessons from endothelial cells. Microvasc Res. 2010;80(2):280–5.
63. Lee CS, Kim KL, Jang JH, Choi YS, Suh PG, Ryu SH. The roles of phospholipase D in EGFR signaling. Biochim Biophys Acta. 2009;1791(9):862–8.
64. Wang X, Devaiah SP, Zhang W, Welti R. Signaling functions of phosphatidic acid. Prog Lipid Res. 2006;45(3):250–78.
65. Wen R, Chen Y, Bai L, Fu G, Schuman J, Dai X, et al. Essential role of phospholipase C gamma 2 in early B-cell development and Myc-mediated lymphomagenesis. Mol Cell Biol. 2006;26(24):9364–76.
66. Wakita M, Edamatsu H, Li M, Emi A, Kitazawa S, Kataoka T. Phospholipase C activates nuclear factor-kappaB signaling by causing cytoplasmic localization of ribosomal S6 kinase and facilitating its phosphorylation of inhibitor kappaB in Colon epithelial cells. J Biol Chem. 2016;291(24):12586–600.
67. Yoshida N, Amanai M, Fukui T, Kajikawa E, Brahmajosyula M, Iwahori A, et al. Broad, ectopic expression of the sperm protein PLCZ1 induces parthenogenesis and ovarian tumours in mice. Development. 2007;134(21):3941–52.
68. Bertagnolo V, Benedusi M, Querzoli P, Pedriali M, Magri E, Brugnoli F, et al. PLC-beta2 is highly expressed in breast cancer and is associated with a poor outcome: a study on tissue microarrays. Int J Oncol. 2006;28(4):863–72.
69. Bertagnolo V, Benedusi M, Brugnoli F, Lanuti P, Marchisio M, Querzoli P, et al. Phospholipase C-beta 2 promotes mitosis and migration of human breast cancer-derived cells. Carcinogenesis. 2007;28(8):1638–45.
70. Sengelaub CA, Navrazhina K, Ross JB, Halberg N, Tavazoie SF. PTPRN2 and PLCbeta1 promote metastatic breast cancer cell migration through PI(4,5)P2-dependent actin remodeling. EMBO J. 2016;35(1):62–76.
71. Cai S, Sun PH, Resaul J, Shi L, Jiang A, Satherley LK, et al. Expression of phospholipase C isozymes in human breast cancer and their clinical significance. Oncol Rep. 2017;37 (3):1707–15.
72. Arteaga CL, Johnson MD, Todderud G, Coffey RJ, Carpenter G, Page DL. Elevated content of the tyrosine kinase substrate phospholipase C-gamma 1 in primary human breast carcinomas. Proc Natl Acad Sci U S A. 1991;88(23):10435–9.
73. Noh DY, Lee YH, Kim SS, Kim YI, Ryu SH, Suh PG, et al. Elevated content of phospholipase C-gamma 1 in colorectal cancer tissues. Cancer. 1994;73(1):36–41.
74. Shepard CR, Kassis J, Whaley DL, Kim HG, Wells A. PLC gamma contributes to metastasis of in situ-occurring mammary and prostate tumors. Oncogene. 2007;26(21):3020–6.
75. Noh DY, Kang HS, Kim YC, Youn YK, Oh SK, Choe KJ, et al. Expression of phospholipase C-gamma 1 and its transcriptional regulators in breast cancer tissues. Anticancer Res. 1998;18 (4a):2643–8.
76. Balz LM, Bartkowiak K, Andreas A, Pantel K, Niggemann B, Zanker KS, et al. The interplay of HER2/HER3/PI3K and EGFR/HER2/PLC-gamma1 signalling in breast cancer cell migration and dissemination. J Pathol. 2012;227(2):234–44.
77. Shien T, Doihara H, Hara H, Takahashi H, Yoshitomi S, Taira N, et al. PLC and PI3K pathways are important in the inhibition of EGF-induced cell migration by gefitinib ('Iressa', ZD1839). Breast Cancer. 2004;11(4):367–73.

78. Piccolo E, Innominato PF, Mariggio MA, Maffucci T, Iacobelli S, Falasca M. The mechanism involved in the regulation of phospholipase Cgamma1 activity in cell migration. Oncogene. 2002;21(42):6520–9.
79. Sala G, Dituri F, Raimondi C, Previdi S, Maffucci T, Mazzoletti M, et al. Phospholipase Cgamma1 is required for metastasis development and progression. Cancer Res. 2008;68 (24):10187–96.
80. Uhlmann S, Zhang JD, Schwager A, Mannsperger H, Riazalhosseini Y, Burmester S, et al. miR-200bc/429 cluster targets PLCgamma1 and differentially regulates proliferation and EGF-driven invasion than miR-200a/141 in breast cancer. Oncogene. 2010;29(30):4297–306.
81. Gregory PA, Bert AG, Paterson EL, Barry SC, Tsykin A, Farshid G, et al. The miR-200 family and miR-205 regulate epithelial to mesenchymal transition by targeting ZEB1 and SIP1. Nat Cell Biol. 2008;10(5):593–601.
82. Lim YY, Wright JA, Attema JL, Gregory PA, Bert AG, Smith E, et al. Epigenetic modulation of the miR-200 family is associated with transition to a breast cancer stem-cell-like state. J Cell Sci. 2013;126(Pt 10):2256–66.
83. Leung DW, Tompkins C, Brewer J, Ball A, Coon M, Morris V, et al. Phospholipase C delta-4 overexpression upregulates ErbB1/2 expression, Erk signaling pathway, and proliferation in MCF-7 cells. Mol Cancer. 2004;3:15.
84. Nakamura Y, Fukami K, Yu H, Takenaka K, Kataoka Y, Shirakata Y, et al. Phospholipase Cdelta1 is required for skin stem cell lineage commitment. EMBO J. 2003;22(12):2981–91.
85. Bai Y, Edamatsu H, Maeda S, Saito H, Suzuki N, Satoh T, et al. Crucial role of phospholipase Cepsilon in chemical carcinogen-induced skin tumor development. Cancer Res. 2004;64 (24):8808–10.
86. Xiao W, Hong H, Kawakami Y, Kato Y, Wu D, Yasudo H, et al. Tumor suppression by phospholipase C-beta3 via SHP-1-mediated dephosphorylation of Stat5. Cancer Cell. 2009;16 (2):161–71.
87. Fu L, Qin YR, Xie D, Hu L, Kwong DL, Srivastava G, et al. Characterization of a novel tumor-suppressor gene PLC delta 1 at 3p22 in esophageal squamous cell carcinoma. Cancer Res. 2007;67(22):10720–6.
88. Rebecchi MJ, Raghubir A, Scarlata S, Hartenstine MJ, Brown T, Stallings JD. Expression and function of phospholipase C in breast carcinoma. Adv Enzym Regul. 2009;49(1):59–73.
89. Mu H, Wang N, Zhao L, Li S, Li Q, Chen L, et al. Methylation of PLCD1 and adenovirus-mediated PLCD1 overexpression elicits a gene therapy effect on human breast cancer. Exp Cell Res. 2015;332(2):179–89.
90. Uchida N, Okamura S, Nagamachi Y, Yamashita S. Increased phospholipase D activity in human breast cancer. J Cancer Res Clin Oncol. 1997;123(5):280–5.
91. Noh DY, Ahn SJ, Lee RA, Park IA, Kim JH, Suh PG, et al. Overexpression of phospholipase D1 in human breast cancer tissues. Cancer Lett. 2000;161(2):207–14.
92. Gozgit JM, Pentecost BT, Marconi SA, Ricketts-Loriaux RSJ, Otis CN, Arcaro KF. PLD1 is overexpressed in an ER-negative MCF-7 cell line variant and a subset of phospho-Akt-negative breast carcinomas. Br J Cancer. 2007;97(6):809–17.
93. Ye Q, Kantonen S, Henkels KM, Gomez-Cambronero J. A new signaling pathway (JAK-Fes-phospholipase D) that is enhanced in highly proliferative breast cancer cells. J Biol Chem. 2013;288(14):9881–91.
94. Chen Q, Hongu T, Sato T, Zhang Y, Ali W, Cavallo JA, et al. Key roles for the lipid signaling enzyme phospholipase d1 in the tumor microenvironment during tumor angiogenesis and metastasis. Sci Signal. 2012;5(249):ra79.
95. Wood LD, Parsons DW, Jones S, Lin J, Sjoblom T, Leary RJ, et al. The genomic landscapes of human breast and colorectal cancers. Science. 2007;318(5853):1108–13.
96. Hong KW, Jin HS, Lim JE, Cho YS, Go MJ, Jung J, et al. Non-synonymous single-nucleotide polymorphisms associated with blood pressure and hypertension. J Hum Hypertens. 2010;24 (11):763–74.

97. Carnero A, Cuadrado A, del Peso L, Lacal JC. Activation of type D phospholipase by serum stimulation and ras-induced transformation in NIH3T3 cells. Oncogene. 1994;9(5):1387–95.
98. Frankel P, Ramos M, Flom J, Bychenok S, Joseph T, Kerkhoff E, et al. Ral and Rho-dependent activation of phospholipase D in v-Raf-transformed cells. Biochem Biophys Res Commun. 1999;255(2):502–7.
99. Song JG, Pfeffer LM, Foster DA. v-Src increases diacylglycerol levels via a type D phospholipase-mediated hydrolysis of phosphatidylcholine. Mol Cell Biol. 1991;11 (10):4903–8.
100. Rizzo MA, Shome K, Vasudevan C, Stolz DB, Sung TC, Frohman MA, et al. Phospholipase D and its product, phosphatidic acid, mediate agonist-dependent raf-1 translocation to the plasma membrane and the activation of the mitogen-activated protein kinase pathway. J Biol Chem. 1999;274(2):1131–9.
101. Fang Y, Vilella-Bach M, Bachmann R, Flanigan A, Chen J. Phosphatidic acid-mediated mitogenic activation of mTOR signaling. Science. 2001;294(5548):1942–5.
102. Toschi A, Lee E, Xu L, Garcia A, Gadir N, Foster DA. Regulation of mTORC1 and mTORC2 complex assembly by phosphatidic acid: competition with rapamycin. Mol Cell Biol. 2009;29 (6):1411–20.
103. Hui L, Zheng Y, Yan Y, Bargonetti J, Foster DA. Mutant p53 in MDA-MB-231 breast cancer cells is stabilized by elevated phospholipase D activity and contributes to survival signals generated by phospholipase D. Oncogene. 2006;25(55):7305–10.
104. Zheng Y, Rodrik V, Toschi A, Shi M, Hui L, Shen Y, et al. Phospholipase D couples survival and migration signals in stress response of human cancer cells. J Biol Chem. 2006;281 (23):15862–8.
105. Thapa N, Anderson RA. PLD and PA take MT1-MMP for a metastatic ride. Dev Cell. 2017;43 (2):117–9.
106. Wang Z, Zhang F, He J, Wu P, Tay LWR, Cai M, et al. Binding of PLD2-generated Phosphatidic acid to KIF5B promotes MT1-MMP surface trafficking and lung metastasis of mouse breast Cancer cells. Dev Cell. 2017;43(2):186–97.e7.
107. Du G, Wang Z, Zhang F, Rog C, Lu M, Peng J, et al. Phospholipase D2 regulation of MT1-MMP membrane trafficking promotes breast cancer metastasis. FASEB J. 2015;29 (1_Suppl):715–24.
108. Henkels KM, Boivin GP, Dudley ES, Berberich SJ, Gomez-Cambronero J. Phospholipase D (PLD) drives cell invasion, tumor growth and metastasis in a human breast cancer xenograph model. Oncogene. 2013;32(49):5551–62.
109. Kang DW, Choi CY, Cho YH, Tian H, Di Paolo G, Choi KY, et al. Targeting phospholipase D1 attenuates intestinal tumorigenesis by controlling beta-catenin signaling in cancer-initiating cells. J Exp Med. 2015;212(8):1219–37.
110. Kang DW, Lee SW, Hwang WC, Lee BH, Choi YS, Suh YA, et al. Phospholipase D1 acts through Akt/TopBP1 and RB1 to regulate the E2F1-dependent apoptotic program in Cancer cells. Cancer Res. 2017;77(1):142–52.
111. Ghim J, Moon JS, Lee CS, Lee J, Song P, Lee A, et al. Endothelial deletion of phospholipase D2 reduces hypoxic response and pathological angiogenesis. Arterioscler Thromb Vasc Biol. 2014;34(8):1697–703.
112. Yamashita S, Yamashita J, Ogawa M. Overexpression of group II phospholipase A2 in human breast cancer tissues is closely associated with their malignant potency. Br J Cancer. 1994;69 (6):1166–70.
113. Caiazza F, McCarthy NS, Young L, Hill AD, Harvey BJ, Thomas W. Cytosolic phospholipase A2-alpha expression in breast cancer is associated with EGFR expression and correlates with an adverse prognosis in luminal tumours. Br J Cancer. 2011;104(2):338–44.
114. Caiazza F, Harvey BJ, Thomas W. Cytosolic phospholipase A2 activation correlates with HER2 overexpression and mediates estrogen-dependent breast cancer cell growth. Mol Endocrinol. 2010;24(5):953–68.

115. Chen L, Fu H, Luo Y, Chen L, Cheng R, Zhang N, et al. cPLA2alpha mediates TGF-beta-induced epithelial-mesenchymal transition in breast cancer through PI3k/Akt signaling. Cell Death Dis. 2017;8(4):e2728.
116. Brglez V, Pucer A, Pungercar J, Lambeau G, Petan T. Secreted phospholipases A(2)are differentially expressed and epigenetically silenced in human breast cancer cells. Biochem Biophys Res Commun. 2014;445(1):230–5.
117. Ilsley JN, Nakanishi M, Flynn C, Belinsky GS, De Guise S, Adib JN, et al. Cytoplasmic phospholipase A2 deletion enhances colon tumorigenesis. Cancer Res. 2005;65(7):2636–43.
118. Hong KH, Bonventre JC, O'Leary E, Bonventre JV, Lander ES. Deletion of cytosolic phospholipase A(2) suppresses Apc(Min)-induced tumorigenesis. Proc Natl Acad Sci U S A. 2001;98(7):3935–9.
119. Harizi H, Corcuff JB, Gualde N. Arachidonic-acid-derived eicosanoids: roles in biology and immunopathology. Trends Mol Med. 2008;14(10):461–9.
120. Buczynski MW, Dumlao DS, Dennis EA. Thematic review series: proteomics. An integrated omics analysis of eicosanoid biology. J Lipid Res. 2009;50(6):1015–38.
121. Funk CD. Prostaglandins and leukotrienes: advances in eicosanoid biology. Science. 2001;294 (5548):1871–5.
122. Stafforini DM, McIntyre TM, Carter ME, Prescott SM. Human plasma platelet-activating factor acetylhydrolase. Association with lipoprotein particles and role in the degradation of platelet-activating factor. J Biol Chem. 1987;262(9):4215–22.
123. Montrose DC, Nakanishi M, Murphy RC, Zarini S, McAleer JP, Vella AT, et al. The role of PGE2 in intestinal inflammation and tumorigenesis. Prostaglandins Other Lipid Mediat. 2015;116–117:26–36.
124. Mauritz I, Westermayer S, Marian B, Erlach N, Grusch M, Holzmann K. Prostaglandin E (2) stimulates progression-related gene expression in early colorectal adenoma cells. Br J Cancer. 2006;94(11):1718–25.
125. Rosch S, Ramer R, Brune K, Hinz B. Prostaglandin E2 induces cyclooxygenase-2 expression in human non-pigmented ciliary epithelial cells through activation of p38 and p42/44 mitogen-activated protein kinases. Biochem Biophys Res Commun. 2005;338(2):1171–8.
126. Richards JA, Petrel TA, Brueggemeier RW. Signaling pathways regulating aromatase and cyclooxygenases in normal and malignant breast cells. J Steroid Biochem Mol Biol. 2002;80 (2):203–12.
127. Meyer AM, Dwyer-Nield LD, Hurteau GJ, Keith RL, O'Leary E, You M, et al. Decreased lung tumorigenesis in mice genetically deficient in cytosolic phospholipase A2. Carcinogenesis. 2004;25(8):1517–24.
128. Cormier RT, Bilger A, Lillich AJ, Halberg RB, Hong KH, Gould KA, et al. The Mom1AKR intestinal tumor resistance region consists of Pla2g2a and a locus distal to D4Mit64. Oncogene. 2000;19(28):3182–92.
129. Papanikolaou A, Wang QS, Mulherkar R, Bolt A, Rosenberg DW. Expression analysis of the group IIA secretory phospholipase A(2) in mice with differential susceptibility to azoxymethane-induced colon tumorigenesis. Carcinogenesis. 2000;21(2):133–8.
130. Linkous AG, Yazlovitskaya EM, Hallahan DE. Cytosolic phospholipase A2 and lysophospholipids in tumor angiogenesis. J Natl Cancer Inst. 2010;102(18):1398–412.
131. MacPhee M, Chepenik KP, Liddell RA, Nelson KK, Siracusa LD, Buchberg AM. The secretory phospholipase A2 gene is a candidate for the Mom1 locus, a major modifier of ApcMin-induced intestinal neoplasia. Cell. 1995;81(6):957–66.
132. McHowat J, Gullickson G, Hoover RG, Sharma J, Turk J, Kornbluth J. Platelet-activating factor and metastasis: calcium-independent phospholipase A2beta deficiency protects against breast cancer metastasis to the lung. Am J Physiol Cell Physiol. 2011;300(4):C825–32.
133. Mills GB, Moolenaar WH. The emerging role of lysophosphatidic acid in cancer. Nat Rev Cancer. 2003;3(8):582–91.
134. Wang D, Wang H, Brown J, Daikoku T, Ning W, Shi Q, et al. CXCL1 induced by prostaglandin E2 promotes angiogenesis in colorectal cancer. J Exp Med. 2006;203(4):941–51.

135. Li H, Zhao Z, Wei G, Yan L, Wang D, Zhang H, et al. Group VIA phospholipase A2 in both host and tumor cells is involved in ovarian cancer development. FASEB J. 2010;24 (10):4103–16.
136. Xu Y, Fang XJ, Casey G, Mills GB. Lysophospholipids activate ovarian and breast cancer cells. Biochem J. 1995;309(Pt 3):933–40.
137. Fang X, Gaudette D, Furui T, Mao M, Estrella V, Eder A, et al. Lysophospholipid growth factors in the initiation, progression, metastases, and management of ovarian cancer. Ann N Y Acad Sci. 2000;905:188–208.
138. Sasagawa T, Okita M, Murakami J, Kato T, Watanabe A. Abnormal serum lysophospholipids in multiple myeloma patients. Lipids. 1999;34(1):17–21.
139. Goetzl EJ, Dolezalova H, Kong Y, Hu YL, Jaffe RB, Kalli KR, et al. Distinctive expression and functions of the type 4 endothelial differentiation gene-encoded G protein-coupled receptor for lysophosphatidic acid in ovarian cancer. Cancer Res. 1999;59(20):5370–5.
140. Pustilnik TB, Estrella V, Wiener JR, Mao M, Eder A, Watt MA, et al. Lysophosphatidic acid induces urokinase secretion by ovarian cancer cells. Clin Cancer Res. 1999;5(11):3704–10.
141. Schulte KM, Beyer A, Kohrer K, Oberhauser S, Roher HD. Lysophosphatidic acid, a novel lipid growth factor for human thyroid cells: over-expression of the high-affinity receptor edg4 in differentiated thyroid cancer. Int J Cancer. 2001;92(2):249–56.
142. Villegas-Comonfort S, Serna-Marquez N, Galindo-Hernandez O, Navarro-Tito N, Salazar EP. Arachidonic acid induces an increase of beta-1,4-galactosyltransferase I expression in MDA-MB-231 breast cancer cells. J Cell Biochem. 2012;113(11):3330–41.
143. Boucharaba A, Serre CM, Gres S, Saulnier-Blache JS, Bordet JC, Guglielmi J, et al. Platelet-derived lysophosphatidic acid supports the progression of osteolytic bone metastases in breast cancer. J Clin Invest. 2004;114(12):1714–25.
144. Wang D, DuBois RN. Eicosanoids and cancer. Nat Rev Cancer. 2010;10(3):181–93.
145. Poczobutt JM, Gijon M, Amin J, Hanson D, Li H, Walker D, et al. Eicosanoid profiling in an orthotopic model of lung cancer progression by mass spectrometry demonstrates selective production of leukotrienes by inflammatory cells of the microenvironment. PLoS One. 2013;8 (11):e79633.
146. Herbert SP, Ponnambalam S, Walker JH. Cytosolic phospholipase A2-alpha mediates endothelial cell proliferation and is inactivated by association with the Golgi apparatus. Mol Biol Cell. 2005;16(8):3800–9.
147. Herbert SP, Odell AF, Ponnambalam S, Walker JH. Activation of cytosolic phospholipase A2-{alpha} as a novel mechanism regulating endothelial cell cycle progression and angiogenesis. J Biol Chem. 2009;284(9):5784–96.
148. Park SY, Lee HE, Li H, Shipitsin M, Gelman R, Polyak K. Heterogeneity for stem cell-related markers according to tumor subtype and histologic stage in breast cancer. Clin Cancer Res. 2010;16(3):876–87.
149. Akiba S, Sato T. Cellular function of calcium-independent phospholipase A2. Biol Pharm Bull. 2004;27(8):1174–8.
150. Ong WY, Farooqui T, Farooqui AA. Involvement of cytosolic phospholipase A(2), calcium independent phospholipase A(2) and plasmalogen selective phospholipase A(2) in neurodegenerative and neuropsychiatric conditions. Curr Med Chem. 2010;17(25):2746–63.
151. Burgdorf C, Schafer U, Richardt G, Kurz T. U73122, an aminosteroid phospholipase C inhibitor, is a potent inhibitor of cardiac phospholipase D by a PIP2-dependent mechanism. J Cardiovasc Pharmacol. 2010;55(6):555–9.
152. Feisst C, Albert D, Steinhilber D, Werz O. The aminosteroid phospholipase C antagonist U-73122 (1-[6-[[17-beta-3-methoxyestra-1,3,5(10)-trien-17-yl]amino]hexyl]-1H-pyrrole-2,5-dione) potently inhibits human 5-lipoxygenase in vivo and in vitro. Mol Pharmacol. 2005;67 (5):1751–7.
153. Hollywood MA, Sergeant GP, Thornbury KD, McHale NG. The PI-PLC inhibitor U-73122 is a potent inhibitor of the SERCA pump in smooth muscle. Br J Pharmacol. 2010;160 (6):1293–4.

154. Eroles P, Bosch A, Perez-Fidalgo JA, Lluch A. Molecular biology in breast cancer: intrinsic subtypes and signaling pathways. Cancer Treat Rev. 2012;38(6):698–707.
155. Samoha S, Arber N. Cyclooxygenase-2 inhibition prevents colorectal cancer: from the bench to the bed side. Oncology. 2005;69(Suppl 1):33–7.
156. Chakraborti AK, Garg SK, Kumar R, Motiwala HF, Jadhavar PS. Progress in COX-2 inhibitors: a journey so far. Curr Med Chem. 2010;17(15):1563–93.
157. Fraser H, Hislop C, Christie RM, Rick HL, Reidy CA, Chouinard ML, et al. Varespladib (A-002), a secretory phospholipase A2 inhibitor, reduces atherosclerosis and aneurysm formation in ApoE−/− mice. J Cardiovasc Pharmacol. 2009;53(1):60–5.
158. Su W, Yeku O, Olepu S, Genna A, Park JS, Ren H, et al. 5-Fluoro-2-indolyl des-chlorohalopemide (FIPI), a phospholipase D pharmacological inhibitor that alters cell spreading and inhibits chemotaxis. Mol Pharmacol. 2009;75(3):437–46.
159. Scott SA, Selvy PE, Buck JR, Cho HP, Criswell TL, Thomas AL, et al. Design of isoform-selective phospholipase D inhibitors that modulate cancer cell invasiveness. Nat Chem Biol. 2009;5(2):108–17.
160. Brown HA, Thomas PG, Lindsley CW. Targeting phospholipase D in cancer, infection and neurodegenerative disorders. Nat Rev Drug Discov. 2017;16(5):351–67.
161. Kim MJ, Chang JS, Park SK, Hwang JI, Ryu SH, Suh PG. Direct interaction of SOS1 Ras exchange protein with the SH3 domain of phospholipase C-gamma1. Biochemistry. 2000;39(29):8674–82.
162. Jones NP, Katan M. Role of phospholipase Cgamma1 in cell spreading requires association with a beta-Pix/GIT1-containing complex, leading to activation of Cdc42 and Rac1. Mol Cell Biol. 2007;27(16):5790–805.

Chapter 3
HER2 Signaling in Breast Cancer

Incheol Shin

Abstract HER2 gene amplification occurs in many breast cancer patients and is associated with poor clinical prognosis. Trastuzumab is a therapeutic monoclonal antibody binding to HER2 and inhibits growth of HER2-positive breast cancer cells and used as a principal treatment for HER2-positive breast cancer. Unfortunately, some HER2-positive breast cancers eventually relapse after trastuzumab treatment. To investigate the molecular mechanism of trastuzumab resistance, we generated trastuzumab-resistant cells using a mouse model and found ECM1 protein is increased in trastuzumab-resistant cells. ECM1 was shown to increase EGFR signaling via upregulated matrix metalloproteinase 9/galectin-3/mucin pathway. To further find the novel mediators of HER2-driven signaling pathways in breast cancer, we investigated the upregulated proteins in HER2-overexpressing breast cancer cells using a proteomics approach and found that KRT19 is strongly upregulated in HER2-positive breast cancer cells and it activates HER2 signaling by binding to HER2 and stabilizes the receptor on the cell membrane. Moreover, we found that treatment of KRT19 antibody resulted in reduced cell viability of trastuzumab-resistant HER2-positive breast cancer cells as well as trastuzumab-sensitive cancer cells both in vitro and in vivo.

Keywords HER2 · Trastuzumab · ECM1 · KRT19 · EGFR

3.1 Introduction

Breast cancer can be classified into four well-established subtypes according to gene expression profiling and hierarchical clustering analysis: luminal A, luminal B, basal-like, and human epidermal growth factor receptor 2 (HER2) subtypes [1]. Luminal A breast cancer is estrogen receptor (ER) and/or progesterone receptor

I. Shin (✉)
Department of Life Science, Hanyang University, Seoul, South Korea

D.-Y. Noh et al. (eds.), *Translational Research in Breast Cancer*, Advances in Experimental Medicine and Biology 1187,
https://doi.org/10.1007/978-981-32-9620-6_3

(PR) positive and has low level of Ki-67, a cell proliferation marker. Luminal B is also ER and/or PR positive and HER2 negative or HER2 positive with high expression level of Ki-67 with worse prognosis than luminal A [2]. Basal-like breast cancer is ER, PR, and HER2 negative and hence often referred as triple-negative breast cancer with the most poorly characterized mechanism of pathogenesis [3]. HER2 subtype is ER and PR negative and HER2 positive and can have a worse clinical outcome than luminal subtypes. However, HER2 breast cancer patients are successfully treated by specific targeted therapies directed against HER2 [4].

HER2 belongs to the epidermal growth factor receptor (EGFR) family consisting of four receptor tyrosine kinases, EGFR (ErbB1 or HER1), HER2 (ErbB2, c-neu or CD340), HER3 (ErbB3), and HER4 (ErbB4) [5]. EGFR family receptors are expressed in various types of tissues and involved in the control of various biological processes including cell proliferation and differentiation. The receptors exert their effect via their tyrosine kinase activities upon ligand binding and subsequent dimerization with other family members [6]. Tyrosine residues on the intracellular domain of the receptors are transphosphorylated after dimerization and serve as docking sites for various signaling molecules [7].

By recruiting the docking molecules, EGFR family receptors can activate mitogen-activated protein kinase (MAPK) pathway [8]. In many cell types, activation of this pathway regulates cell proliferation, cell cycle progression, differentiation, migration, cell adhesion, and cell death [9]. The cytoplasmic tail domain of transphosphorylated EGFR family receptors recruit growth factor-bound protein 2 (GRB2), which then binds son of sevenless (SOS), the guanine nucleotide exchange factor [10]. The recruitment of SOS in turn activates membrane-bound Ras, which next leads to activation of Raf kinase [11, 12]. Raf kinase activates mitogen-activated protein kinase kinase (MAPKK) by phosphorylation and the activated MAPKK subsequently phosphorylates and activates MAPK [13]. The activation of MAPK can then activate various transcription factors such as Elk1, Myc, and Fos to regulate the expression of MAPK target genes [14–16].

EGFR family receptors can also activate phosphatidylinositol-3′ kinase (PI3K)/Akt pathway [6]. The Ser/Thr kinase Akt is a central signaling molecule acting by phosphorylating many downstream effector molecules [17]. Activation of Akt could promote cell survival by inhibition of proapoptotic pathways [18]. Akt can phosphorylate FOXO transcription factors resulting in the nuclear exclusion of the transcription factor culminating in downregulation of FOXO-dependent proapoptotic transcripts such as BH3-only protein B-cell lymphoma 2 interacting mediator of cell death (BIM) and Fas ligand [19, 20]. Akt can also phosphorylate Bcl-2 associated death promoter (BAD) and renders BAD separated from BCl-2 complex and loses proapoptotic function [21]. In addition to the inactivation of proapoptotic factors, Akt could also upregulate antiapoptotic genes such as Bcl-2, Bcl-X, and inhibitor of apoptosis (IAP) via regulation of IκB kinase (IKK)/NFκB signaling [22, 23]. Regulation of cell cycle can also be achieved by Akt signaling. Akt-mediated phosphorylation of p27 leads to cytosolic localization of the cyclin-dependent kinase inhibitor via binding to 14-3-3 proteins and this leads to cell cycle progression beyond G1/S checkpoint [24].

Akt is also involved in angiogenesis and control of cellular metabolism. Akt can activate endothelial nitric oxide synthase (eNOS) [25]. eNOS induces NO release which leads to vascular rearrangement and angiogenesis [26]. Akt/mammalian target of rapamycin complex 1 (mTORC1) can also induce hypoxia-inducible factor alpha (HIF-α)-dependent induction of glucose transporter (GLUT) gene expression leading to efficient transport of glucose to the cancer cells [26]. Akt/mTORC1-induced HIF-α increases secretion of vascular endothelial growth factor (VEGF) which in turn increases angiogenesis [27]. In addition to its effect on GLUT gene expression, Akt can also activate glycolysis rate-determining enzyme phosphofructokinase-1 (PFK-1) by activation of phosphofructokinase-2 (PFK-2) through phosphorylation [28]. Fructose-2,6-bisphosphate generated by PFK-2 acts as a potent allosteric activator of PFK-1, a key enzyme in glycolytic pathway [29]. FOXO-dependent suppression of glycolytic gene expression is also relieved by activation of Akt [30].

Given the plethora of EGFR family downstream signaling pathways involved in important biological phenomena such as cell proliferation, cell cycle regulation, tumorigenesis, angiogenesis, and control of metabolism as listed above, the deregulation of EGFR family receptors could lead to human diseases. Indeed, the abnormal activation and expression of these receptors have been reported to be associated with many different kinds of human cancers [31]. Among these receptors, HER2 gene amplification occurs in 25–30% of breast cancers and confers worse clinical and biological behaviors [32]. Among EGF family ligands, none has been previously reported to directly bind to HER2, suggesting that HER2 is an orphan receptor [33]. However, HER2 is a preferred dimerization partner for all other EGFR family members (EGFR or HER1, HER3 and HER4) rendering HER2 as a versatile co-receptor [34]. The structure of extracellular region of HER2 without bound ligand resembles a ligand-bound status of other EGFR family receptors, suggesting that the orphan receptor does not require ligand to release from an autoinhibited conformation [35]. Among HER2-containing homo- and heterodimers, HER2-HER3 heterodimer is the strongest stimulator of the receptor downstream pathways [36].

Direct targeting of HER2 was first challenged with trastuzumab (Herceptin), a humanized monoclonal antibody directed against extracellular subdomain IV of HER2 [37]. Upon binding to the orphan receptor, trastuzumab inhibits HER2 homo- and heterodimerization and HER2-downstream signaling pathways including MAPK pathway and PI3K/Akt pathway, blocking proliferation of the trastuzumab-treated cells [38]. HER2 can also be downregulated from the plasma membrane by trastuzumab-mediated internalization and subsequent degradation via ubiquitin ligase c-Cbl [39]. Trastuzumab also exhibits in vivo cytotoxicity by inducing an immune response of patients to cancer cells via antibody-dependent cellular cytotoxicity (ADCC) [40]. Xenograft study also revealed that natural killer cells target HER2-overexpressing cells by CD16-dependent ADCC [41]. These results suggest that ADCC is one of the possible in vivo action mechanism of trastuzumab.

3.2 Review of Past Studies

Although trastuzumab has been used as a therapeutic monoclonal antibody against HER2-positive breast cancer, significant portion of patients who initially respond to trastuzumab exhibited cancer relapse within 1 year of treatment [42, 43]. In addition, some of the metastatic HER2-positive breast cancer patients do not initially respond to trastuzumab treatment [44]. The elucidation of trastuzumab resistance mechanism has been difficult mainly due to obtained trastuzumab-resistant tumor samples but hyperactivation of HER2-downstream PI3K/Akt pathway was frequently observed in trastuzumab-resistant breast cancer biopsy samples [44]. Activation of PI3K/Akt is presumed to be resulted from reduced expression of PTEN, an antagonistic effector of PI3K, and activating mutations in PI3K [44]. The correlation between loss of PTEN tumor suppressor and lack of trastuzumab responsiveness is also implicated in cell culture and animal model systems [45, 46]. Trastuzumab resistance also shown to be associated with increased level of EGFR signaling [47] and heterotrimerization of HER2, HER3, and insulin-like growth factor receptor (IGFR) [48]. Co-expression of EGFR indeed attenuates the growth inhibitory effect of trastuzumab in HER2-overexpressing cell lines [49].

In addition to the activation of HER2-downstream signaling pathways and/or perturbation in other receptor tyrosine kinase signaling, trastuzumab resistance is also attributable to the reduced capacity of trastuzumab binding to HER2. In JIMT-1, a cell line derived from a trastuzumab-resistant HER2-amplified patient, MUC4, a membrane-associated mucin masks trastuzumab binding to HER2 rendering the cell line refractory to trastuzumab treatment [50]. Overexpression of MUC4 in breast cancer and melanoma cell line also reduces binding of series of antibodies against HER2 including trastuzumab [51]. Expression of p95HER2, a truncated form of HER2 retaining kinase activity, is strongly associated with trastuzumab resistance in patients because p95HER2 cannot bind to trastuzumab [52]. Shedding of HER2 extracellular domain in serum and culture media may also titrate trastuzumab away from HER2, resulting in resistance toward trastuzumab [53].

Due to the molecular heterogeneity of cancer cells and their surrounding microenvironment, there might be other molecular signatures associated with trastuzumab resistance in addition to the mechanisms listed above. To determine other signaling pathway that might be involved in conferring trastuzumab resistance, my colleagues generated trastuzumab-resistant BT-474 (BT-474 TR) cells using in vivo xenograft system from parental HER2-overexpressing BT-474 cells [54]. BT-474 TR clones exhibited in vitro resistance to trastuzumab (Fig. 3.1a).

To identify differentially expressed proteins in BT-474 TR and wild-type BT-474 cells (BT-474 WT), two-dimensional LC-MS/MS analyses were performed with the lysates obtained from the two cell lines. Several proteins were shown to be upregulated in BT-474 TR cells as compared to the parental cells (Table 3.1). Among these, ECM1, a glycosylated secretory protein was selected because high levels of ECM1 were previously reported in aggressive tumor cells and its expression is correlated with adverse patient outcome in some cancer types

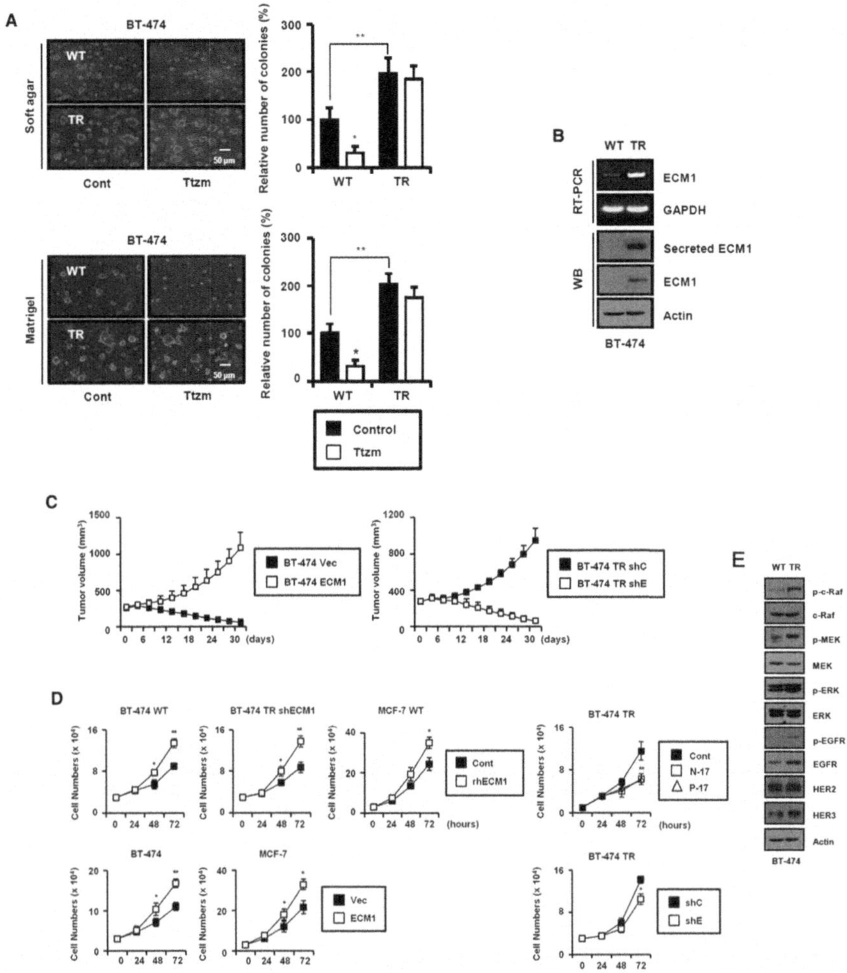

Fig. 3.1 ECM1 confers resistance toward trastuzumab. (**a**) 5×10^4 cells were plated on soft agar and Matrigel In Matrigel, trastuzumab (20 μg/mL) was treated every 3 days. The number of colonies (20 μm diameter) was counted at 12 days. The number of colonies is quantified in right panels. Error bars represent mean ± SD of triplicate experiments ($*P < 0.05$, $**P < 0.005$). (**b**) mRNAs were analyzed by RT-PCR using primers specific for ECM1 and GAPDH. Secreted ECM1 was obtained from trichloroacetic acid-precipitated cell supernatant medium. Each cell lysate was analyzed by western blotting using ECM1- and actin-specific antibodies. (**c**) BT-474 vector and ECM1 cells and BT-474 TR control (Cont) short-hairpin (shRNA; shC) and ECM1 shRNA (shE) cells were passaged by subcutaneous injection into the lower flank of each mouse. When the tumor size increased up to 250 mm^3, trastuzumab at 20 mg/kg was administered to each mouse by intraperitoneal injection twice per week ($n = 5$ or 6 for each group). (**d**) Each cell line was treated with 200 ng/mL recombinant human extracellular matrix protein 1 (rhECM1) or 5 μg/mL anti-ECM1 antibodies, and cells were counted with a hemocytometer over the course of 3 days ($*P < 0.05$, $**P < 0.005$). Cont, control; shC, control short-hairpin RNA; shE/shECM1, short-hairpin extracellular matrix protein 1 RNA; TR, trastuzumab-resistant; Vec, vector. (**e**) Cell lysates were analyzed by western blotting using indicated antibodies. Anti-actin antibody was applied as a loading control (Adapted from Lee et al., Breast Cancer Res. 2014)

Table 3.1 Liquid chromatography-tandem mass spectrometry identification of proteins differentially secreted by BT-474 WT and BT-474 TR cells[a] (Adapted from Lee et al., Breast Cancer Res. 2014)

UniProt accession number	Protein name	Gene name	SI $_{WT}$	SI $_{TR}$	Log $_2$(SI $_{TR}$/ SI $_{WT}$)
Q16610	Extracellular matrix protein 1	*ECM1*	0.0762	153.8420	8.94
P27797	Calreticulin	*CALR*	8.5510	32.8933	1.3853
P07339	Cathepsin D	*CTSD*	27.7801	168.2733	2.0520
P00338	L-lactate dehydrogenase A chain	*LDHA*	55.1457	171.2111	1.0651
P04626	Receptor tyrosine protein kinase erbB-2	*ERBB2*	12.7955	33.2680	0.7694
P17931	Galectin-3	*LGALS3*	0.4470	9.4270	3.7263

[a]*SI* spectral index, *TR* trastuzumab-resistant, *WT* wild type

[55, 56]. Overexpression of ECM1 in BT-474 TM cells was validated in the cell lines as well as in the conditioned medium, confirming that ECM1 is a secretory protein (Fig. 3.1b). Levels of ECM1 in serum from trastuzumab-resistant and trastuzumab-responsive breast cancer patients revealed that ECM1 is more abundant in trastuzumab-resistant patients' serum than serum from control patients (data not shown).

To further investigate the role of ECM1 in breast cancer cells, effects of recombinant human ECM1 (rhECM1) and ECM1 knockdown in BT-474 TR and BT-474 WT cells were monitored (Fig. 3.1a, b). Treatment with rhECM1 alleviated the antiproliferative effect of trastuzumab while ECM1 knockdown further increased the effect of trastuzumab. Xenograft studies also revealed the suppressive effect of ECM1 on trastuzumab effect (Fig. 3.1c).

Since it was previously confirmed that BT-474 TR cells grow faster than BT-474 WT cells in Matrigel (data not shown), it was tested whether ECM1 may promote cell proliferation per se. Treatment with rhECM1 or forced expression of ECM1 resulted in enhanced cell proliferation both in BT-474 WT and MCF-7 cells (Fig. 3.1d left panel), while treatment of anti-ECM1 antibodies (N-17 and P-27) and silencing of ECM1 resulted in a decreased cell proliferation rate (Fig. 3.1d right panel). In vivo xenograft experiments also indicated that ECM1-expressing tumors grow faster (data not shown), confirming the growth promoting effect of ECM1.

Then what is the mechanism by which ECM1 could potentiate proliferation rate of breast cancer cells? To answer this question, one of the HER2-downstream signaling pathways, MAPK pathway, was investigated. Interestingly, all the signaling molecules in MAPK pathway are activated in BT-474 TR cells compared to BT-474 WT cells and protein levels of EGFR and HER3 but not HER2 are also upregulated in BT-474 TR cells (Fig. 3.1e). Neutralizing ECM1 by ECM1 antibody treatment resulted in reduced EGFR and ERK phosphorylation (Fig. 3.2a) and co-treatment with EGF and ECM1 additively increased EGFR and ERK

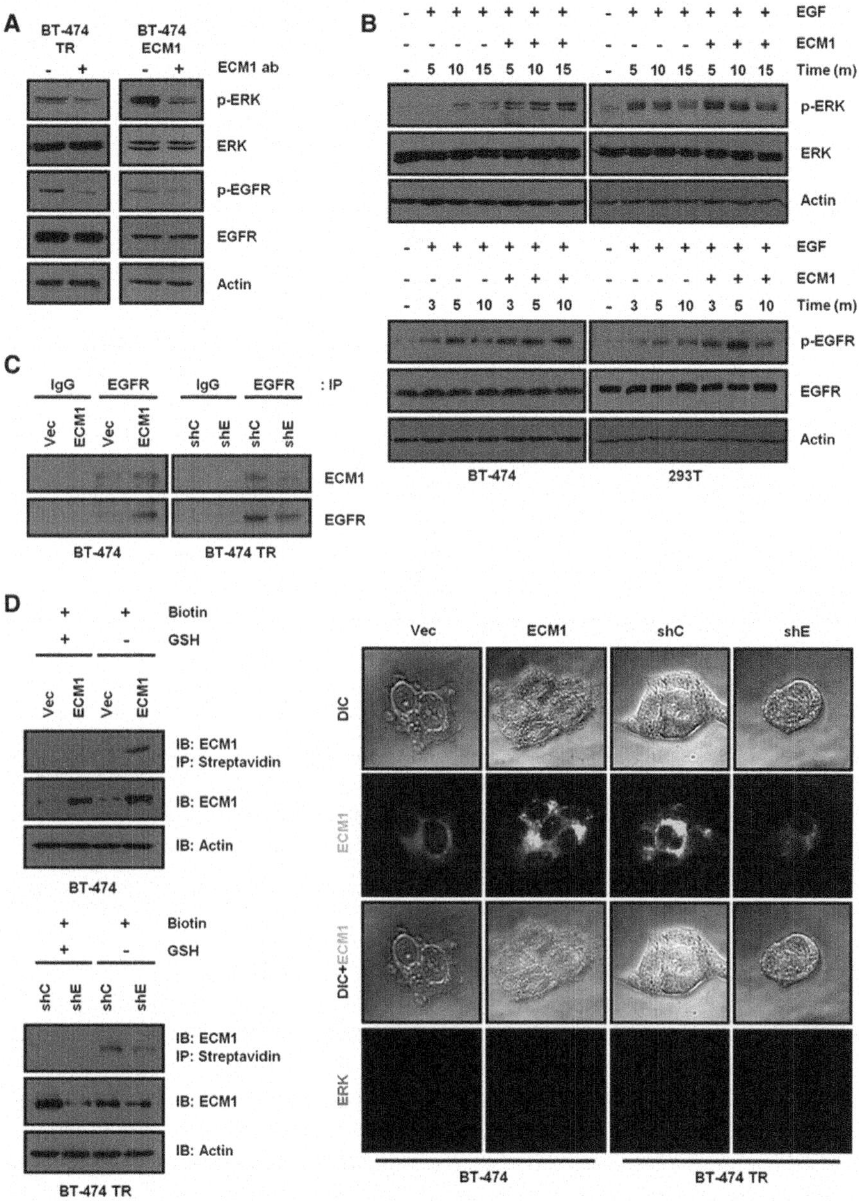

Fig. 3.2 ECM1 augments epidermal growth factor signaling. (**a**) At 24 h after seeding, BT-474 TR and BT-474 extracellular matrix protein 1 (ECM1)-expressing cells were treated with anti-ECM1 antibodies (ab; 5 μg/mL). Ten minutes later, cell lysates were analyzed on western blots. (**b**) After serum starvation for 24 h, cells were treated with recombinant human extracellular matrix protein 1 (rhECM1; 200 ng/mL) and epidermal growth factor (EGF; 10 ng/mL). Cell lysates were prepared at the indicated time points and analyzed on western blots. (**c**) Total cell lysates were incubated with epidermal growth factor receptor (EGFR) antibodies overnight, and immunoprecipitates (IP) were analyzed on western blots. IgG, immunoglobulin G; shC, control short-hairpin RNA; shE, extracellular matrix protein 1; Vec, vector. (**d**) Cells were incubated with 0.5 mg/mL EZ-Link NHS-SS-Biotin for 30 min at 4 °C. The biotinylated proteins were precipitated by streptavidin, and the

phosphorylation (Fig. 3.2b). These results suggest ECM1 may increase proliferation rate of breast cancer cells by enhancing EGFR/MAPK signaling.

Since ECM1 was previously known to modulate cellular signaling via association with cell surface receptors, the association between ECM1 and EGFR was checked (Fig. 3.2c, d). ECM1 was found to be physically associated with EGFR. Moreover, the addition of rhECM1 additively increased EGF-induced EGFR and downstream ERK phosphorylation (Fig. 3.2b). Since it was found that EGFR and HER3 levels were upregulated in BT-474 TR as compared to BT-474 WT, the effects of ECM1 antibody and rhECM1 on EGFR and HER2 levels were tested. Interestingly, ECM1 antibody treatment resulted in downregulation of EGFR, HER3, and ERK phosphorylation while rhECM1 increased EGFR, HER3, and ERK phosphorylation (Fig. 3.3a). Since it was found that ECM1 could not significantly modulate mRNA levels of EGFR and HER3 (data not shown), the possibility that ECM1 may modulate the protein stability of EGFR was tested. As indicated in Fig. 3.3b, expression of ECM1 was strongly correlated with increased protein stability of EGFR and HER3 as determined by cycloheximide decay assays.

It was previously reported that galectin-3 and mucin1 (MUC1) are associated with EGFR trafficking [57]. We found that galectin-3 level was increased in BT-474 TR cells (Table 3.1). We have also found that galectin-3 in the conditioned medium and cellular MUC1 levels were increased (data not shown). As expected, treatment with rhECM1 or overexpression of ECM1 both strongly upregulated secreted galectin-3 and MUC1 (Fig. 3.4a). Moreover, knockdown of galectin-3 or MUC1 in BT-474 TR cells resulted in decreased levels of EGFR, HER3, and downstream ERK phosphorylation (Fig. 3.4b). To test whether the effect of galectin-3/MUC1 on the receptor tyrosine kinases is attributable to the physical association of galectin-3/MUC1 on the receptors, series of co-immunoprecipitation experiments were performed (Fig. 3.4c, d). It was found that ECM1 overexpression and rhECM1 treatment increased the interaction between MUC1 and EGFR/HER3, while knockdown of ECM1 in BT-474 TR cells decreased the interaction between MUC1 and EGFR/HER3, suggesting that ECM1 promotes stabilization of EGFR and HER3 by inducing the interaction between galectin-3/MUC1 and EGFR/HER3.

To determine the mechanism of increased levels of secreted galectin-3 in BT-474 TR cells, the involvement of matrix metalloproteinase (MMP) on galectin-3 secretion was tested because some MMPs were known to proteolytically cleave galectin-3 [58]. It was found that ECM1 was also associated with increased MMP-9 activity in the cell lines tested (Fig. 3.5a) and the promoter activity of MMP-9 was also induced by ECM1 (Fig. 3.5b). Treatment with recombinant human MMP9 also resulted in increased levels of MUC1, EGFR, and HER3 (Fig. 3.5c). Taken all these results

---

Fig. 3.2 (continued) precipitates were analyzed on western blots (IB) using ECM1 antibody (left). Cell surface labeling of ECM1 was conducted by immunostaining without permeabilization (right). Extracellular signal-regulated kinase (ERK) was used as an endogenous negative control protein. *DIC* differential interference contrast, *GSH* glutathione (Adapted from Lee et al., Breast Cancer Res. 2014)

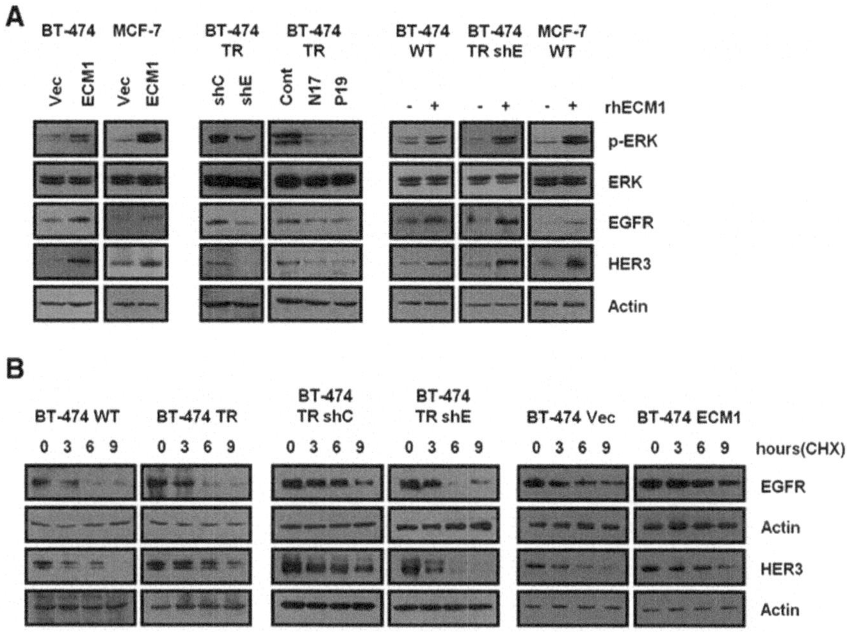

Fig. 3.3 ECM1 activates extracellular signal-regulated kinase signaling by upregulating epidermal growth factor receptor and HER3. (**a**) At 24 h after cell seeding, each cell line was treated with recombinant human extracellular matrix protein 1 (rhECM1; 200 ng/mL) or anti-ECM1 antibodies (5 μg/mL) and further incubated for 48 h. Cells lysates were then analyzed by western blotting. Cont, control; ERK, extracellular signal-regulated kinase; shC, control short-hairpin RNA; shE, extracellular matrix protein 1 short-hairpin RNA; TR, trastuzumab-resistant; Vec, vector; WT, wild type. (**b**) Each cell line was treated with 100 μg/mL cycloheximide (CHX). Cell lysates were prepared at the indicated time points and analyzed on western blots. Band intensities on the blots were quantified using 1DScan software (Scanalytics, Milwaukee, WI) and plotted versus time as the ratios of EGFR/actin and HER3/actin intensities (*$P < 0.05$) (Adapted from Lee et al., Breast Cancer Res. 2014)

together, ECM1 may increase EGFR/HER3 signaling by enhancing the stability of these receptors by inducing galectin-3/MUC association, which resulted from the ERK-downstream induction of MMP-9 and this ECM1-induced feedback activation of EGFR/HER3 signaling may contribute to trastuzumab resistance (Fig. 3.5d).

To further assess the role of ECM1 in breast cancer, my colleagues also investigated the role of ECM1 in regulating tumor metastasis and cancer stem cell (CSC)-like property [59]. It was found that ECM1 serum levels are upregulated in recurring patients after trastuzumab treatment (Fig. 3.6a) and ECM1 also contributes to the enhanced lung metastasis of MDA-MB-231 cells in mouse tail vein injection models (Fig. 3.6b). Similar to the ECM1-mediated stabilization of EGFR/HER3 in the previous set of experiments (Fig. 3.3a, b), ECM1 was also shown to be causally associated with the increase in β-catenin stabilization (Fig. 3.7a). Indeed, β-catenin was upregulated in both ECM1-expressing cells and BT-474 TR cells (Fig. 3.7b).

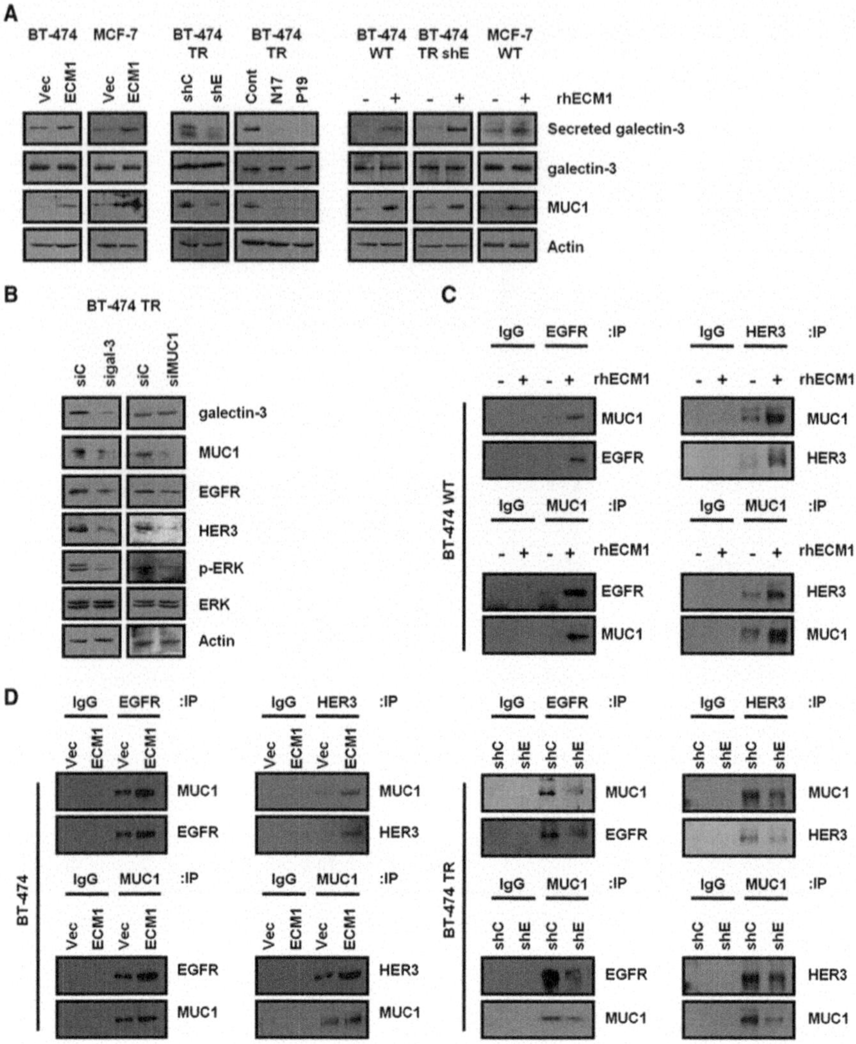

Fig. 3.4 ECM1 stabilizes epidermal growth factor receptor and HER3 proteins through galectin-3/mucin 1. (**a**) Lysates from each cell line were analyzed by western blotting. shC, control short-hairpin RNA; shE, ECM1 short-hairpin RNA; Vec, vector; WT, wild type. (**b**) At 24 h after seeding, BT-474 TR cells were transfected with each small interfering RNA (siRNA: siC, control; sigal-3, galectin-3; siMUC1, mucin 1), incubated further for 48 h and analyzed on western blots. (**c**) At 24 h after seeding, cells were treated with recombinant human ECM1 (rhECM1; 200 ng/mL) and incubated further for 48 h. Cell lysates were then incubated with mucin 1 (MUC1), epidermal growth factor receptor (EGFR) and HER3 antibodies overnight. Immunoprecipitates (IP) were analyzed on western blots. IgG, immunoglobulin G. (**d**) Total cell lysates were incubated with MUC1, EGFR and HER3 antibodies overnight, and immunoprecipitates were then analyzed on western blots (Adapted from Lee et al., Breast Cancer Res. 2014)

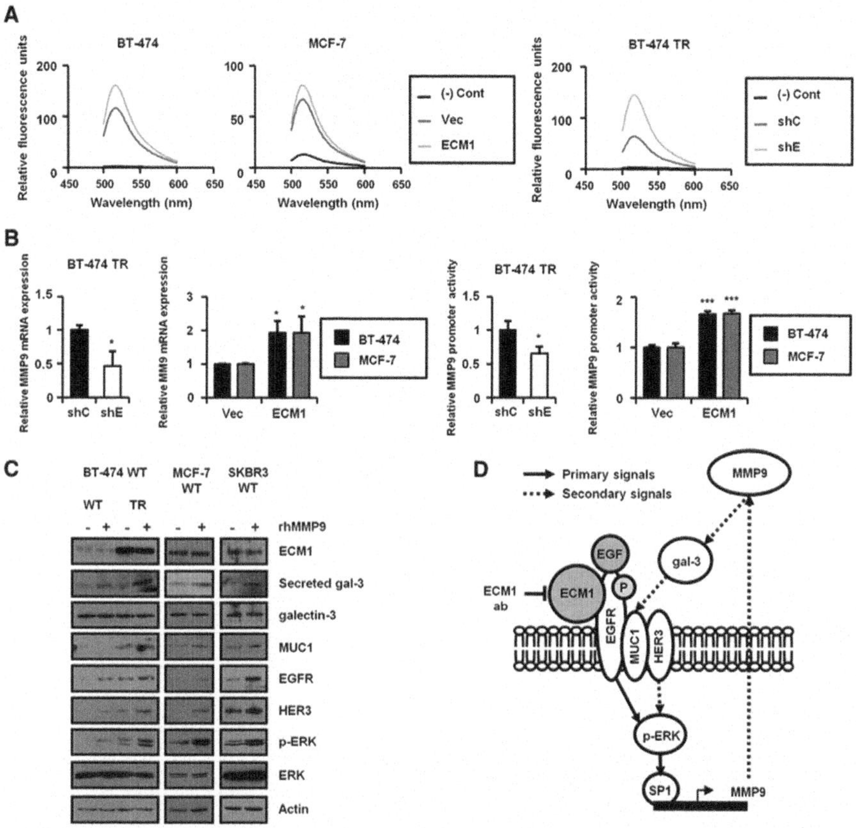

Fig. 3.5 ECM1 induces matrix metalloproteinase 9 transcription. (**a**) At 24 h after seeding, cells were incubated with serum-free medium for a further 24 h. Supernatant medium from each cell line was reacted with matrix metalloproteinase 9 (MMP9) substrate, and relative fluorescence units were determined at 480–620 nm. Cont, control; shC, control short-hairpin RNA; shE, extracellular matrix protein 1 short-hairpin RNA; TR, trastuzumab-resistant; Vec, vector. (**b**) MMP9 mRNA levels were determined by real-time PCR using primers specific for MMP9 (*$P < 0.05$). Each cell line was transfected with an MMP9 promoter luciferase reporter construct. After 48 h, cells were harvested, and the lysates were analyzed by dual-luciferase assay (*$P < 0.05$, ***$P < 0.0005$). (**c**) At 24 h after seeding, each cell line was treated with recombinant human MMP9 (rhMMP9; 20 ng/mL), incubated further for 48 h, and lysates from each cell were analyzed by western blotting. *EGFR* epidermal growth factor receptor, *ERK* extracellular signal-regulated kinase, *MUC1* mucin 1, *WT* wild type. (**d**) Schematic model showing the role of extracellular matrix protein 1 (ECM1) in cell signaling. *EGF* epidermal growth factor (Adapted from Lee et al., Breast Cancer Res. 2014)

Silencing of β-catenin in ECM1 overexpressing cells including BT-474 TR resulted in downregulation of epithelial to mesenchymal transition (EMT) as well as stemness-related transcripts, suggesting that ECM1-regulated β-catenin may be responsible for ECM1-induced modulation of EMT and CSC-like capacity (Fig. 3.8a-c). These results further indicate that trastuzumab resistance biomarker

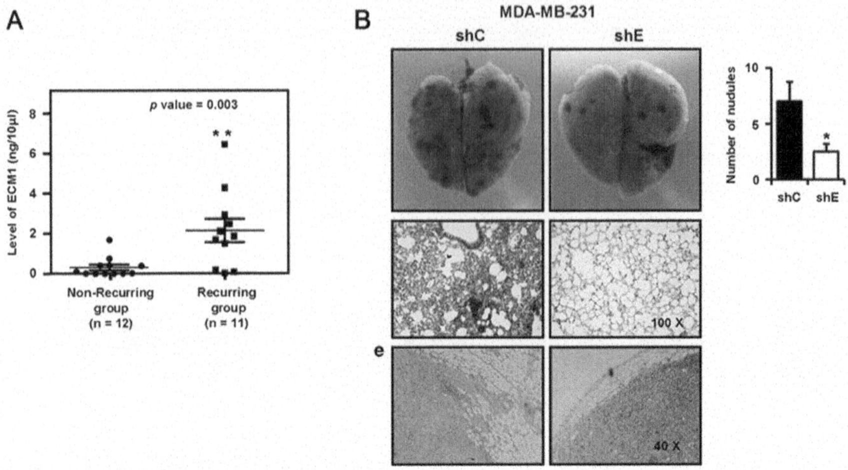

Fig. 3.6 Effect of ECM1 on cell migration and invasion in breast cancer cells. (**a**) ELISA showing circulating levels of ECM1 in plasma from breast cancer patients. (**b**) Lung metastatic nodules driven by tail vein injection of MDA-MB-231 control shRNA (shC, $n = 5$) and ECM1 shRNA (shE, $n = 4$) cells were counted with the naked eye. Bar graph represents the number of nodules on the lung surface. Error bars represent mean ± s.d. of all experiments (*$P < 0.05$) (Adapted from Lee et al., Oncogene 2015)

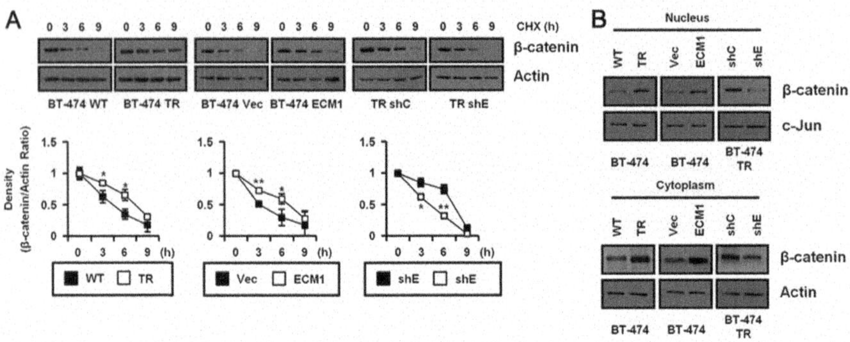

Fig. 3.7 ECM1 stabilizes β-catenin protein and induces the accumulation of nuclear β-catenin via MUC1. (**a**) Each cell was treated with CHX at 100 μg/mL. The cell lysates were obtained at the indicated time points and subjected to western blot analysis with the indicated antibodies. The intensities of the bands were quantified using 1DScan software and plotted as time versus the ratio of β-catenin/actin intensity. Error bars represent mean ± s.d. of triplicate experiments (*$P < 0.05$, **$P < 0.005$). (**b**) Each cell was fractionated into cytoplasmic and nuclear fractions. The lysates were analyzed by western blotting with the indicated antibodies (Adapted from Lee et al., Oncogene 2015)

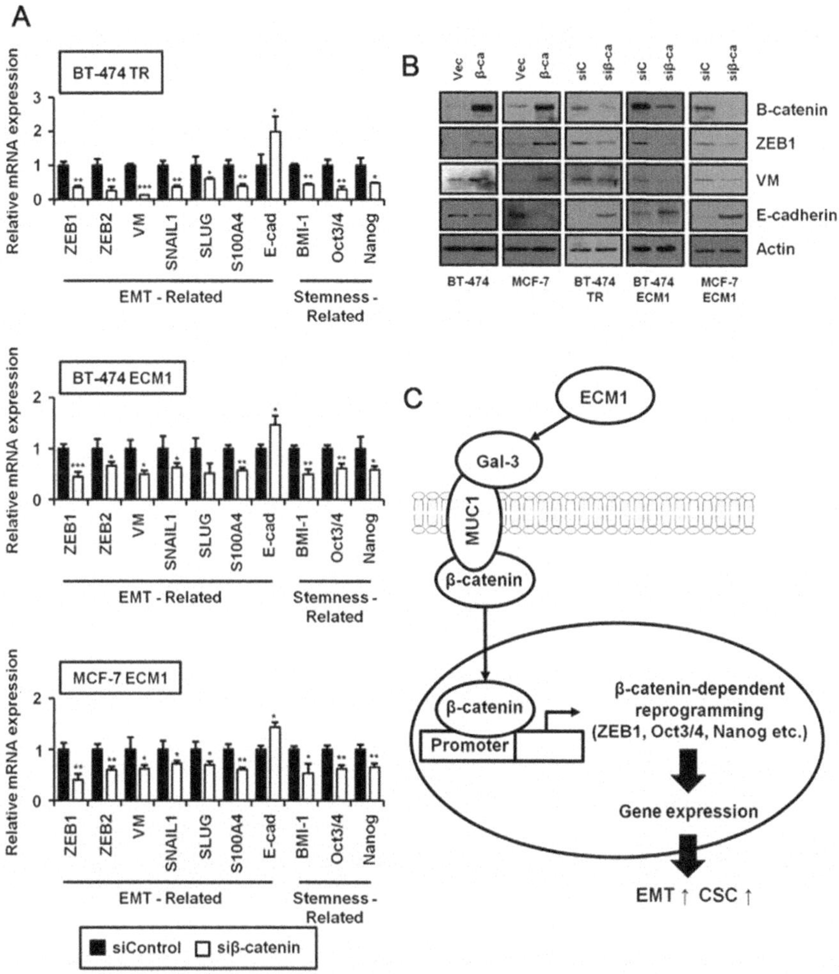

Fig. 3.8 Expression of β-catenin causes the modulation of gene expression toward EMT progression and CSC maintenance. (**a**) The cells were transfected with β-catenin siRNA and then mRNA levels of each gene were determined by real-time PCR using specific primers (VM = vimentin, E-cad = E-cadherin). Error bars represent mean ± s.d. of triplicate experiments ($*P < 0.05$, $**P < 0.005$, $***P < 0.0005$). (**b**) Each cell was transfected with pcDNA-β-catenin or β-catenin siRNA and then each cell lysate was subjected to western blot analysis using indicated antibodies. (**c**) Schematic model showing the role of ECM1 in regulation of EMT and CSC capacity (Adapted from Lee et al., Oncogene 2015)

ECM1 also contributes to EMT and CSC-like phenotype which may culminate in development of resistance toward cancer therapeutics including trastuzumab.

In another attempt to further find another cell surface targetable molecule in HER2-positive breast cancer, my colleagues used MCF-7 cells stably expressing HER2 (MCF-7 HER2) and vector control cells (MCF-7 vec) for differential proteomics analysis [60]. Expression levels of several keratin (KRT) proteins were significantly increased in MCF-7 HER2 cells as compared to MCF-7 vec cells as determined by LC-MS/MS analysis (data not shown). Among these KRT isoforms, my colleagues were particularly interested in KRT19, the smallest (40 kDa) among known intermediate filament protein [61], because KRT19 is used as a marker for RT-PCR-based detection of tumor cells in peripheral blood [62] and bone marrow [63].

By using breast cancer tissue samples from patients, cell lines and HER2-overexpressing MMTV-neu mouse models, we have confirmed a strong correlation between HER2 and KRT19 expression (Fig. 3.9). It was found that KRT19 overexpression is mediated by HER2-downstream ERK activity and ERK-mediated control is exerted at transcriptional level (Fig. 3.10a–e). HER2 expression increased KRT19 both at mRNA and protein levels and KRT19 promoter activity was also increased by HER2. Other KRT isoforms, which are also upregulated in MCF-7 HER2 cells, are not inhibited by kinase inhibitors of HER2 and downstream MEK (Fig. 3.10f), suggesting that upregulation of KRT19 by HER2/ERK is isoform-specific.

Another HER2-downstream kinase, Akt was also shown to regulate KRT19 protein posttranslationally. Sequence motif analyses (http://scansite.mit.edu) revealed two Akt phosphorylation sites, S10 and S35 in KRT19. It was found that S35 residue of KRT19 is efficiently phosphorylated by Akt (Fig. 3.11a-d). Interestingly, it was observed that KRT19 subcellular localization and appearance were varied dramatically different between MCF-7 HER2 and MCF-7 vec. In MCF-7 HER2 cells, KRT19 showed granulated morphology while KRT19 in MCF-7 vec cells appeared as filamentous (Fig. 3.11e, f). When HER2, or constitutively active Akt was co-expressed with KRT19 with functional Akt phosphorylation site on S35, KRT19 appeared as granules, suggesting that Akt-mediated phosphorylation of KRT19 on S35 is responsible for the granulated morphology of KRT19 (Fig. 3.11g).

In addition to having granulated morphology, S35 phosphorylated KRT19 also appeared to be co-localized on the cell membrane with HER2 (Fig. 3.12). Apparently, Akt-mediated phosphorylation on KRT9 resulted in depolymerization of KRT10 fibers into granules and transportation of KRT19 to cell membrane to be associated with HER2 or exported in exosomes (data not shown). Then what is the function of KRT19 bind to HER2 on cell membrane? It was found that KRT19 can increase the protein stability of HER2 as revealed by cycloheximide chase assays (Fig. 3.13a, b). KRT19 lacking Akt phosphorylation site, KRT19 S35A, failed to be localized in the membrane (data not shown) and could not stabilize HER2 on cell membrane. It was found that KRT19 blocks degradation of HER2 by inhibiting ubiquitin-mediated degradation of HER2 (data not shown).

My colleagues finally tested if KRT19 can be used as a therapeutic target for HER2-positive breast cancer. When HER2-overexpressing cells were treated with antibody raised against KRT19, HER2 was degraded by ubiquitin-mediated process (Fig. 3.14a, b). Treatment with KRT19 antibody to HER2-overexpressing cells resulted in dosage-dependent inhibition of cell proliferation, presumably due to downregulation of HER2 and its downstream signaling (Fig. 3.14c). Interestingly,

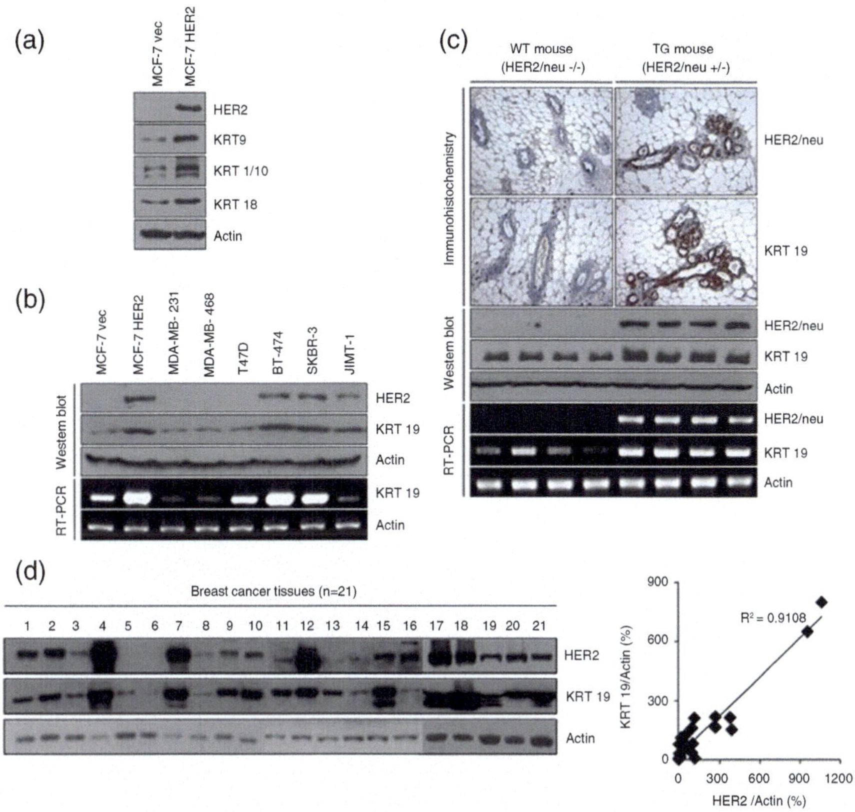

Fig. 3.9 Expression of KRT19 is strongly correlated with HER2 levels in cultured breast cancer cells, transgenic mouse tissues, and patient tumor samples. (**a**) Total cell lysates were prepared from MCF-7 vec and MCF-7 HER2 cells and subjected to the indicated western blot analyses with HER2, KRT9, KRT1/10, or KRT18 antibodies. Actin was used to verify equal loading. (**b**) Total cell lysates were prepared from human breast cancer cell lines. The samples were resolved by SDS-PAGE and subjected to western blot analyses with HER2 or KRT19 antibodies. RNA was extracted from human breast cancer cell lines and the samples were subsequently analyzed by RT-PCR using KRT19-specific primers. Actin primers were used as loading controls. (**c**) Paraffin-embedded sections from the #4 mammary gland tissues of MMTV-HER2/neu transgenic mice and wild-type littermates were subjected to immunohistochemistry with a KRT19 antibody. MMTV-HER2/neu transgenic mice and wild-type littermates (16 weeks, $n = 4$ each) #4 mammary gland tissues were analyzed by RT-PCR using mouse KRT19 primers, and western blot analyses with HER2 or KRT19 antibodies. (**d**) Western blot analysis showing expression levels of HER2 and KRT19 protein in primary tumor lysates from breast cancer patients ($n = 21$). The positive relationship between HER2 and KRT19 expression level is indicated (R2 = 0.9108) (Adapted from Ju et al., Cell Death Differ. 2014)

the growth of trastuzumab-resistant JIMT-1 cells was also decreased by KRT19 antibody treatment, suggesting that KRT19 antibody can be used as a novel therapeutic antibody for trastuzumab-resistant patients. When xenograft experiments were performed using HER2-positive KPL-4 cells, KRT19 could effectively inhibit

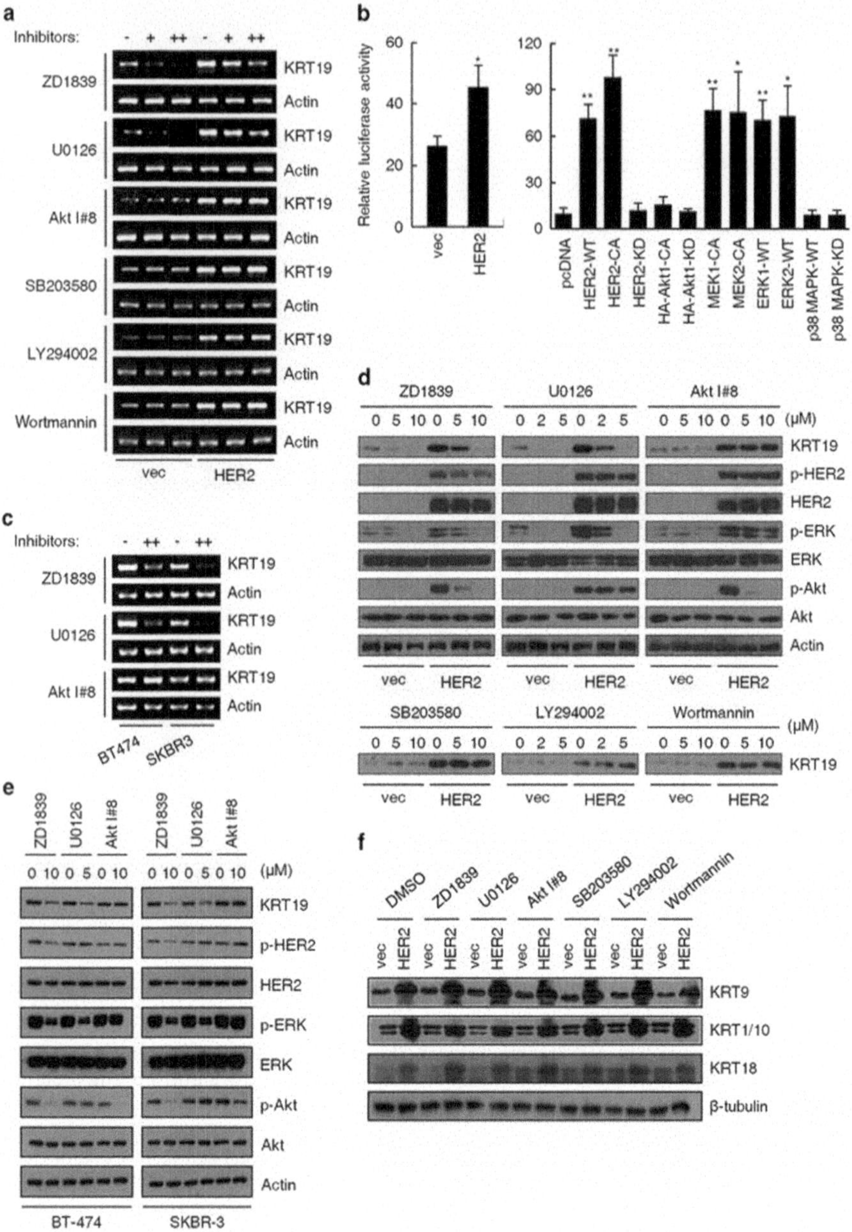

Fig. 3.10 Expression of KRT19 is mediated by HER2 downstream of ERK at the transcriptional level. (**a**) MCF-7 vec and MCF-7 HER2 cells were treated with kinase inhibitors (0, 5, 10 μM ZD1839; 0, 2, 5 μM U0126; 0, 5, 10 μM Akt inhibitor #8; 0, 5, 10 μM SB203580; 0, 5, 10 μM LY294002 or 0, 2, 5 μM Wortmannin) for 24 h. mRNA from samples were analyzed by RT-PCR. (**b**) MCF-7 vec and MCF-7 HER2 cells were transfected with pK19-1970-Luc reporter constructs, collected after 48 h and analyzed by dual luciferase assays. 293T cells were transfected with pK19-1970-Luc and pcDNA-vec, pcDNA-HER2-WT (wild type), pcDNA-HER2-CA (constitutive active), pcDNA-HER2-KD (kinase dead), pcDNA-HA-Akt1-CA, pcDNA-HA-Akt1-KD,

in vivo tumor formation (Fig. 3.14d). On the basis of these experimental findings, it was assumed that HER2-downstream ERK induces KRT19 expression and HER2-downstream Akt phosphorylates, disassembles, and translocates KRT19 to the cell membrane. Membrane-translocated KRT19 associates with HER2 to stabilize the receptor tyrosine kinase resulting in the formation of positive-feedback loop that amplifies HER2-induced cell proliferation and survival (Fig. 3.14e).

3.3 Current Evidence and Concepts

Although trastuzumab has been used as first-line therapy in HER2-positive metastatic breast cancer patients, other therapeutic drugs are currently used to target HER2 signaling. Lapatinib is a dual tyrosine kinase inhibitor (TKI) which inhibits tyrosine kinase activities of EGFR and HER2 [64]. Combined treatment of lapatinib and trastuzumab was reported to be effective in old metastatic breast cancer patients [65]. Hormone receptor and HER2-positive tumors were shown to be effectively treated with lapatinib and aromatase inhibitor [66].

Another humanized monoclonal antibody, pertuzumab binds to the extracellular domain II of HER2, while trastuzumab binds to extracellular domain IV [67]. Since domain II is essential for dimerization of HER family member receptor tyrosine kinases, pertuzumab preferentially inhibits ligand-induced HER2/HER3 heterodimerization while trastuzumab effectively inhibits ligand-independent dimerization of HER2 and has only marginal inhibitory effect on dimerization when ligands are present [67]. Since heregulin, a ligand for HER3, plays very important roles in tumorigenesis and metastasis [68], pertuzumab is shown to be superior to trastuzumab in inhibiting heregulin-induced cancer cell signaling [69]. These different mechanisms of action of two different antibodies may help to enhance treatment efficacies. Indeed, CLEOPATRA (Clinical Evaluation Of Pertuzumab And Trastuzumab), a phase III randomized double-blind study showed that combination of pertuzumab plus docetaxel plus trastuzumab significantly prolonged progression-free survival [70].

Trastuzumab derivative of maytanzine (trastuzumab emtansine, TDM-1) is the first drug conjugated antibody approved for HER2-positive breast cancer patients

Fig. 3.10 (continued) pcDNA-MEK1-CA, pcDNA-MEK2-CA, pcDNA-ERK1-WT, pcDNA-ERK2-WT, pcDNA-p38 MAPK-WT, or pcDNA-p38 MAPK-KD. After 48 h, cells were analyzed by dual luciferase assays (*$P < 0.05$, **$P < 0.005$). (**c**) BT-474 and SKBR-3 cells were treated with kinase inhibitors for 24 h. mRNA from samples were analyzed by RT-PCR. (**d**) MCF-7 vec and MCF-7 HER2 cells were treated with kinase inhibitors for 24 h, and the cell lysates were resolved by SDS-PAGE and subjected to western blot analyses with the indicated antibodies. (**e**) BT-474 and SKBR-3 cells were treated with kinase inhibitors for 24 h. The cell lysates were subjected to western blot analyses with the indicated antibodies. (**f**) MCF-7 vec and MCF-7 HER2 cells were treated with kinase inhibitors for 24 h. The cell lysates were subjected to western blot analyses with KRT9, KRT1/10, or KRT18 antibodies (Adapted from Ju et al., Cell Death Differ. 2014)

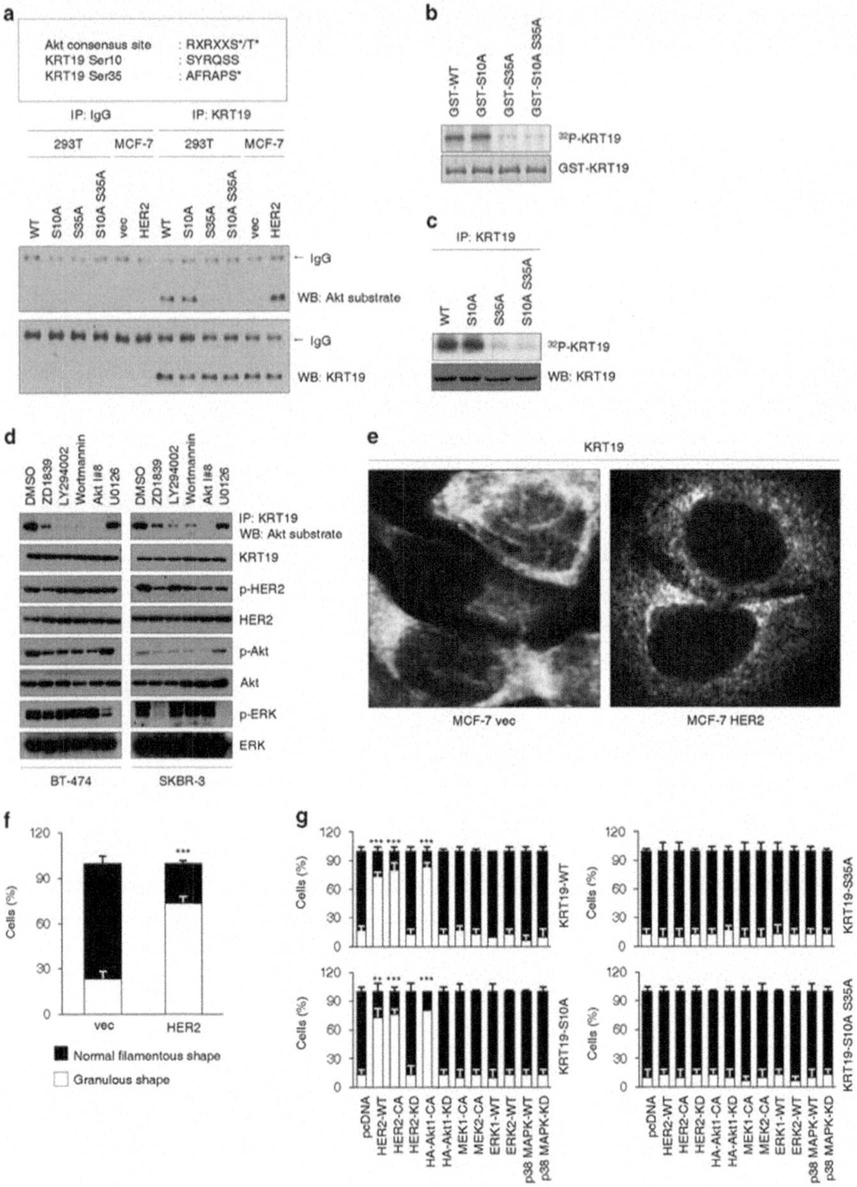

Fig. 3.11 KRT19 is phosphorylated by HER2 downstream of Akt at Ser35, resulting in remodeling of KRT19 from filamentous to granulous form. (**a**) Total cell lysates were incubated with KRT19 antibody overnight. Immunoprecipitates were subjected to western blot analysis with Akt substrate antibody or KRT19 antibody. (**b**) GST-KRT19 was prepared as described. HA-Akt precipitates were used as a kinase source for in vitro kinase assays. After the reaction, the samples were subjected to SDS-PAGE and subsequent autoradiography. Equal loading of KRT19 per reaction was confirmed by Coomassie brilliant blue staining. (**c**) In vivo phosphorylation of KRT19 was assessed by labeling 293 T cells transfected with KRT19 with 32P-orthophosphate. 32P-labeled KRT19 was precipitated with KRT19 antibody and analyzed by autoradiography. To normalize for transfection sufficiency, precipitates were subjected to KRT19 immunoblotting. (**d**) BT-474 and

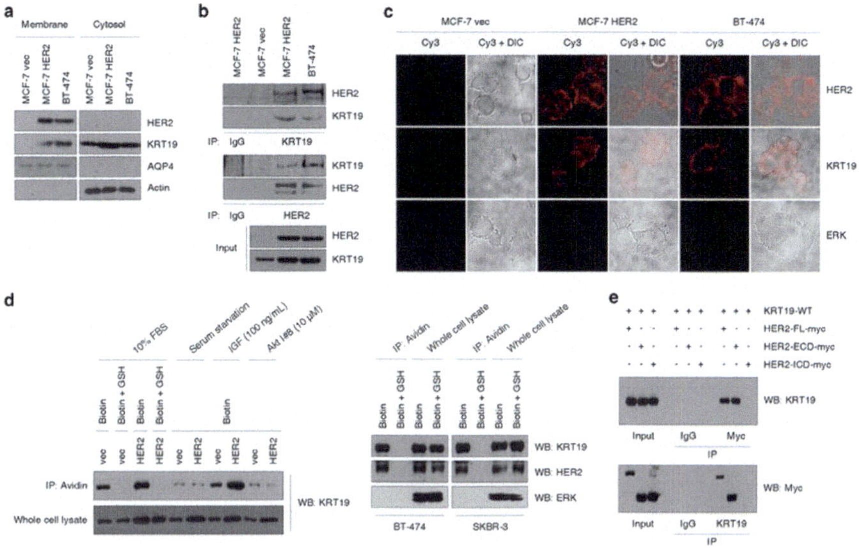

Fig. 3.12 KRT19 is physically associated with HER2 in the plasma membrane and HER2/Akt-induced phosphorylation of KRT19 at Ser35 can induce membrane localization of KRT19. (**a**) MCF-7 vec, MCF-7 HER2, and BT-474 cells were fractionated into membrane and cytosol fractions. The resulting fractions were subjected to western blot analysis with HER2, KRT19, AQP4 (aquaporin4) (as membrane marker) or actin (as cytosol marker) antibodies. (**b**) MCF-7 HER2 and BT-474 cell lysates were incubated with HER2 or KRT19 antibodies overnight. Immunoprecipitates were subjected to western blot analysis with KRT19 or HER2 antibodies. (**c**) Cell surface labeling of KRT19 was conducted by cell surface immunostaining. ERK was used as an endogenous negative control protein. (**d**) Cell surface labeling of KRT19 was conducted by the cell surface biotinylation assay. The labeled proteins were precipitated by streptavidin and analyzed by western blot with KRT19, HER2, and ERK antibodies. ERK was used as an endogenous negative control protein. (**e**) KRT19 constructs were co-transfected with HER2 full-length or truncated mutant constructs in 293T cells. After 48 h, cells were lysed and the supernatant was incubated with KRT19 or myc antibodies and protein A sepharose. The immunoprecipitates were analyzed by western blot with myc or KRT19 antibodies (Adapted from Ju et al., Cell Death Differ. 2014)

[71]. TDM-1 binds to HER2-positive cancer cells and active DM-1 is endocytosed into the cancer cell cytoplasm by receptor-mediated endocytosis, leading to cell death by microtubule toxicity [72]. Through some clinical trials, TDM-1 remains as

Fig. 3.11 (continued) SKBR-3 cells were treated with various kinase inhibitors. The cell lysates were then subjected to immunoprecipitation and western blotting. (**e**) KRT19 shape in MCF-7 cells was monitored by immunostaining. MCF-7 vec and MCF-7 HER2 cells were fixed and stained with KRT19 antibody. (**f**) Quantification of the results in (**e**). More than 100 cells per each independent microscopic field were observed and counted in triplicate (***$P < 0.0005$). (**g**) Quantification of the transient transfection results. More than 100 stained cells per each independent microscopic field were observed and counted in triplicate (**$P < 0.005$, ***$P < 0.0005$) (Adapted from Ju et al., Cell Death Differ. 2014)

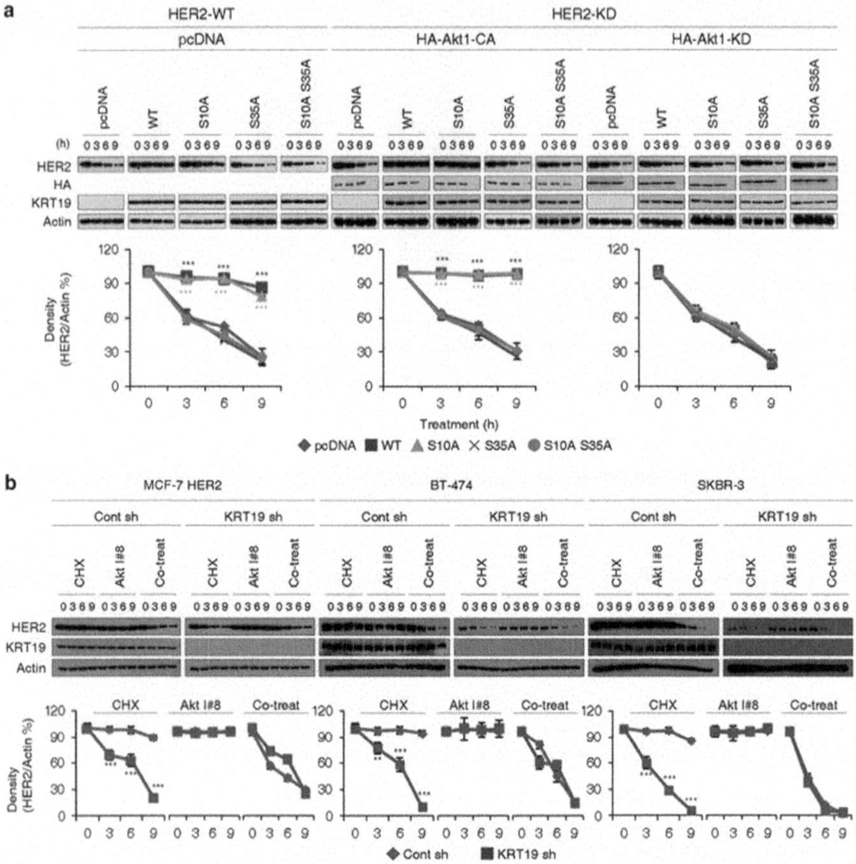

Fig. 3.13 HER2/Akt-induced phosphorylation of KRT19 at Ser35 is essential for maintaining HER2 stability at the membrane. (**a**) We transfected 293T cells with various combinations of HER2, Akt, and KRT19 as indicated. At 48 h post-transfection, 20 μg/mL CHX was treated to block further protein synthesis. Cells were collected at each of the indicated time points and subjected to western blot analysis. The intensity of the bands was quantified using 1DScan software (CSP Inc., Billerica, MA, USA) and plotted as time versus ratio of HER2/actin intensity (***$P < 0.0005$). (**b**) Control shRNA and KRT19 shRNA cells were treated with CHX at 100 μg/mL. The cell lysates were obtained at the indicated time points and prepared for western blot analysis. The intensity of the bands was quantified using 1DScan software and plotted as time versus the ratio of HER2/actin intensity for MCF-7 HER2 control shRNA and KRT19 shRNA cells (**$P < 0.005$, ***$P < 0.0005$) (Adapted from Ju et al., Cell Death Differ. 2014)

an optional therapeutics for older patients with advanced HER2-positive breast cancer who progressed after treatment with trastuzumab [65].

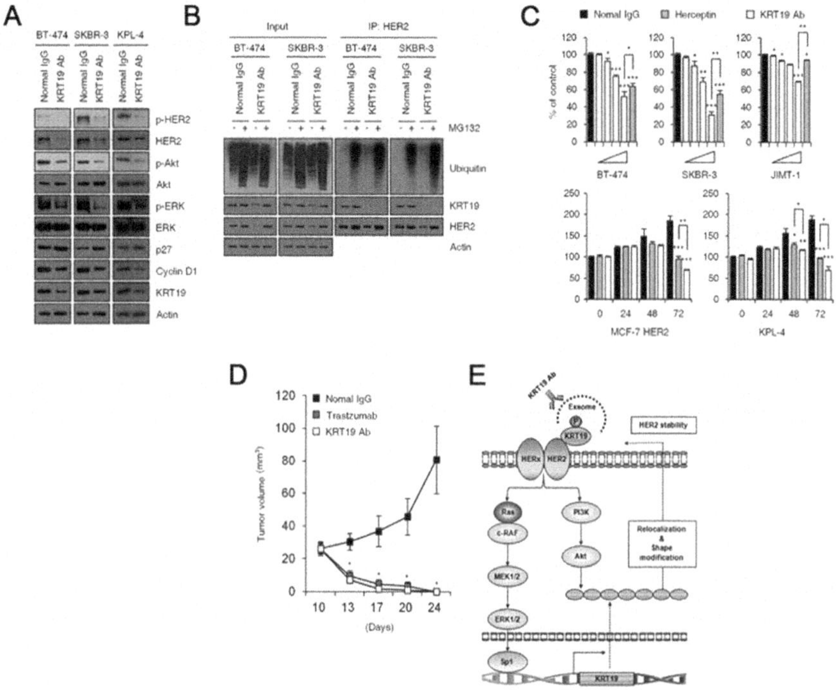

Fig. 3.14 KRT19 inhibits ubiquitin-mediated degradation of HER2, and treatment with KRT19 antibody induces a decrease in cell proliferation via HER2 downregulation. (**a**) BT-474, SKBR-3, and KPL-4 cells were treated with 20 μg/mL KRT19 antibodies for 24 h and lysed. The samples were resolved by SDS-PAGE and subjected to western blot analyses with indicated antibodies. (**b**) BT-474 and SKBR-3 cells were treated with 20 μg/mL KRT19 antibodies and 10 μM MG132 for 24 h and lysed. The supernatant was incubated with HER2 antibody and protein A sepharose. The immunoprecipitates were analyzed by western blot with each of the indicated antibodies. (**c**) BT-474, SKBR-3, JIMT-1 (0, 5, 10, 20 μg/mL), MCF-7 HER2 and KPL-4 cells (20 μg/mL) were treated with KRT19 antibody. Normal IgG and Trastzumab were treated at a dose of 20 μg/mL. After 72 h, cell viability was assessed by the proliferation assay. The value from normal IgG-treated cells was set to 100% and relative decreases in cell viability after KRT19 antibodies treatment were expressed as a percent of the control (*$P < 0.05$, **$P < 0.005$, ***$P < 0.0005$). (**d**) HER2-positive KPL-4 cells were injected in 8-week-old BALB/C nude mice by subcutaneous injection of 5 × 106 cells into both sides of the lower flank of mice ($n = 5$ per group). At day 10 after inoculation, normal IgG, Trastzumab or KRT19 antibodies were i.p. injected at the dose of 20 mg/kg (*$P < 0.05$). (**e**) A schematic model showing the mechanism of stabilization of HER2-induced KRT19 on the cell membrane. KRT19 binds HER2 via Akt-mediated phosphorylation in a Ser35-dependent manner and stabilizes HER2 on the cell membrane

3.4 Future Research Directions

Since the advent of trastuzumab, the development of targeted therapies for HER2-postive breast cancer evolved as a successful example of precision clinical oncology. Unfortunately, many patients eventually progress or relapse. The resistance mechanism(s) might be present in the HER2-positive cancer cells de novo, or induced by anti-HER2 therapeutics.

In addition to the HER family receptor tyrosine kinases that confer resistance to HER2-targeted therapies, other receptors like insulin-like growth factor 1 (IGF-1R) renders HER2-positive SKBR3 cells resistant to trastuzumab [73]. Tyrosine kinase c-Met is also reported to be overexpressed in HER2-positive breast cancer cell lines and a quarter of HER2-postivie breast cancer patient's samples [74]. Therefore, combined targeting of other receptors is currently under consideration to overcome trastuzumab resistance.

Moreover, the intracellular pathways are often selected as targets for combined therapeutic approaches. Everolimus, which inhibits PI3K/Akt/mTOR pathway, has been clinically tested for HER2-positive breast cancer patients [75]. PI3K inhibitors, IGF-1R inhibitors, and check point inhibitors are also currently under clinical trials to overcome resistance to HER2-targeted therapies [65].

Since HER2/HER3 is the most potent transducers of oncogenic signaling, several novel bispecific antibodies targeting HER2/HER3 heterodimer are under development. MM-111 is an antibody specifically targeting HER2/HER3 heterodimer [76]. Margetuximab is an Fc-engineered antibody made from a prototype of trastuzumab, a mouse monoclonal antibody 4D5 [77]. MCLA-128 is a HER2/HER targeting antibody with enhanced ADCC and currently under phase I/II clinical studies [65]. In addition to TDM-1, another novel drug-conjugated antibody is also considered. MM-302, a HER2-targeted antibody conjugated with doxorubicin, has been clinically tested in randomized phase II HERMIONE trial in anthracycline-naïve patients who progressed after treatment with pertuzumab and TDM-1 [78]. Regarding development of newer HER2-targeted therapies, further basic studies are urgently required to distinguish between de novo and acquired resistance. The information gathered will help in designing novel drugs and new combination therapeutics.

3.5 Summary

1. The bench.
   Novel proteomics approaches were employed to find a novel HER2-specific protein biomarkers and trastuzumab resistance protein biomarkers. These will help to find a new targetable proteins to overcome resistance to anti-HER2 therapeutics.
2. Translation.
   The newly found therapeutic targets will be validated for preclinical trials for HER2-positive patients.
3. The bedside.
   New studies are needed to establish a standard care protocols regarding the safety and tolerability for HER2-positive patients.

References

1. Parker JS, Mullins M, Cheang MC, Leung S, Voduc D, Vickery T, et al. Supervised risk predictor of breast cancer based on intrinsic subtypes. J Clin Oncol. 2009;27(8):1160–7.
2. Inic Z, Zegarac M, Inic M, Markovic I, Kozomara Z, Djurisic I, et al. Difference between luminal A and luminal B subtypes according to Ki-67, tumor size, and progesterone receptor negativity providing prognostic information. Clin Med Insights Oncol. 2014;8:107–11.
3. Toft DJ, Cryns VL. Minireview: basal-like breast cancer: from molecular profiles to targeted therapies. Mol Endocrinol. 2011;25(2):199–211.
4. Prat A, Pineda E, Adamo B, Galvan P, Fernandez A, Gaba L, et al. Clinical implications of the intrinsic molecular subtypes of breast cancer. Breast. 2015;24(Suppl 2):S26–35.
5. Navolanic PM, Steelman LS, McCubrey JA. EGFR family signaling and its association with breast cancer development and resistance to chemotherapy (review). Int J Oncol. 2003;22 (2):237–52.
6. Wieduwilt MJ, Moasser MM. The epidermal growth factor receptor family: biology driving targeted therapeutics. Cell Mol Life Sci. 2008;65(10):1566–84.
7. Moasser MM. The oncogene HER2: its signaling and transforming functions and its role in human cancer pathogenesis. Oncogene. 2007;26(45):6469–87.
8. Prenzel N, Fischer OM, Streit S, Hart S, Ullrich A. The epidermal growth factor receptor family as a central element for cellular signal transduction and diversification. Endocr Relat Cancer. 2001;8(1):11–31.
9. Yu Z, Ye S, Hu G, Lv M, Tu Z, Zhou K, et al. The RAF-MEK-ERK pathway: targeting ERK to overcome obstacles to effective cancer therapy. Future Med Chem. 2015;7(3):269–89.
10. Waters SB, Chen D, Kao AW, Okada S, Holt KH, Pessin JE. Insulin and epidermal growth factor receptors regulate distinct pools of Grb2-SOS in the control of Ras activation. J Biol Chem. 1996;271(30):18224–30.
11. Bowtell D, Fu P, Simon M, Senior P. Identification of murine homologues of the Drosophila son of sevenless gene: potential activators of ras. Proc Natl Acad Sci U S A. 1992;89 (14):6511–5.
12. Wood KW, Sarnecki C, Roberts TM, Blenis J. Ras mediates nerve growth factor receptor modulation of three signal-transducing protein kinases: MAP kinase, Raf-1, and RSK. Cell. 1992;68(6):1041–50.
13. Macdonald SG, Crews CM, Wu L, Driller J, Clark R, Erikson RL, et al. Reconstitution of the Raf-1-MEK-ERK signal transduction pathway in vitro. Mol Cell Biol. 1993;13(11):6615–20.
14. Gille H, Kortenjann M, Thomae O, Moomaw C, Slaughter C, Cobb MH, et al. ERK phosphorylation potentiates Elk-1-mediated ternary complex formation and transactivation. EMBO J. 1995;14(5):951–62.
15. Kerkhoff E, Houben R, Loffler S, Troppmair J, Lee JE, Rapp UR. Regulation of c-myc expression by Ras/Raf signalling. Oncogene. 1998;16(2):211–6.
16. Okazaki K, Sagata N. The Mos/MAP kinase pathway stabilizes c-Fos by phosphorylation and augments its transforming activity in NIH 3T3 cells. EMBO J. 1995;14(20):5048–59.
17. Manning BD, Cantley LC. AKT/PKB signaling: navigating downstream. Cell. 2007;129 (7):1261–74.
18. Dudek H, Datta SR, Franke TF, Birnbaum MJ, Yao R, Cooper GM, et al. Regulation of neuronal survival by the serine-threonine protein kinase Akt. Science. 1997;275(5300):661–5.
19. Sunters A, Fernandez de Mattos S, Stahl M, Brosens JJ, Zoumpoulidou G, Saunders CA, et al. FoxO3a transcriptional regulation of Bim controls apoptosis in paclitaxel-treated breast cancer cell lines. J Biol Chem. 2003;278(50):49795–805.
20. Marfe G, Tafani M, Fiorito F, Pagnini U, Iovane G, De Martino L. Involvement of FOXO transcription factors, TRAIL-FasL/Fas, and sirtuin proteins family in canine coronavirus type II-induced apoptosis. PLoS One. 2011;6(11):e27313.

21. Datta SR, Dudek H, Tao X, Masters S, Fu H, Gotoh Y, et al. Akt phosphorylation of BAD couples survival signals to the cell-intrinsic death machinery. Cell. 1997;91(2):231–41.
22. Salminen A, Kaarniranta K. Insulin/IGF-1 paradox of aging: regulation via AKT/IKK/NF-kappaB signaling. Cell Signal. 2010;22(4):573–7.
23. Radhakrishnan SK, Kamalakaran S. Pro-apoptotic role of NF-kappaB: implications for cancer therapy. Biochim Biophys Acta. 2006;1766(1):53–62.
24. Shin I, Yakes FM, Rojo F, Shin NY, Bakin AV, Baselga J, et al. PKB/Akt mediates cell-cycle progression by phosphorylation of p27(Kip1) at threonine 157 and modulation of its cellular localization. Nat Med. 2002;8(10):1145–52.
25. Fulton D, Gratton JP, McCabe TJ, Fontana J, Fujio Y, Walsh K, et al. Regulation of endothelium-derived nitric oxide production by the protein kinase Akt. Nature. 1999;399 (6736):597–601.
26. Kawasaki K, Smith RS Jr, Hsieh CM, Sun J, Chao J, Liao JK. Activation of the phosphatidylinositol 3-kinase/protein kinase Akt pathway mediates nitric oxide-induced endothelial cell migration and angiogenesis. Mol Cell Biol. 2003;23(16):5726–37.
27. Zhong H, Chiles K, Feldser D, Laughner E, Hanrahan C, Georgescu MM, et al. Modulation of hypoxia-inducible factor 1alpha expression by the epidermal growth factor/phosphatidylinositol 3-kinase/PTEN/AKT/FRAP pathway in human prostate cancer cells: implications for tumor angiogenesis and therapeutics. Cancer Res. 2000;60(6):1541–5.
28. Deprez J, Vertommen D, Alessi DR, Hue L, Rider MH. Phosphorylation and activation of heart 6-phosphofructo-2-kinase by protein kinase B and other protein kinases of the insulin signaling cascades. J Biol Chem. 1997;272(28):17269–75.
29. Robey RB, Hay N. Is Akt the "Warburg kinase"?-Akt-energy metabolism interactions and oncogenesis. Semin Cancer Biol. 2009;19(1):25–31.
30. Zhang W, Patil S, Chauhan B, Guo S, Powell DR, Le J, et al. FoxO1 regulates multiple metabolic pathways in the liver: effects on gluconeogenic, glycolytic, and lipogenic gene expression. J Biol Chem. 2006;281(15):10105–17.
31. Harari D, Yarden Y. Molecular mechanisms underlying ErbB2/HER2 action in breast cancer. Oncogene. 2000;19(53):6102–14.
32. Whenham N, D'Hondt V, Piccart MJ. HER2-positive breast cancer: from trastuzumab to innovatory anti-HER2 strategies. Clin Breast Cancer. 2008;8(1):38–49.
33. Tzahar E, Yarden Y. The ErbB-2/HER2 oncogenic receptor of adenocarcinomas: from orphanhood to multiple stromal ligands. Biochim Biophys Acta. 1998;1377(1):M25–37.
34. Karunagaran D, Tzahar E, Beerli RR, Chen X, Graus-Porta D, Ratzkin BJ, et al. ErbB-2 is a common auxiliary subunit of NDF and EGF receptors: implications for breast cancer. EMBO J. 1996;15(2):254–64.
35. Cho HS, Mason K, Ramyar KX, Stanley AM, Gabelli SB, Denney DW Jr, et al. Structure of the extracellular region of HER2 alone and in complex with the Herceptin fab. Nature. 2003;421 (6924):756–60.
36. Lee-Hoeflich ST, Crocker L, Yao E, Pham T, Munroe X, Hoeflich KP, et al. A central role for HER3 in HER2-amplified breast cancer: implications for targeted therapy. Cancer Res. 2008;68 (14):5878–87.
37. Carter P, Presta L, Gorman CM, Ridgway JB, Henner D, Wong WL, et al. Humanization of an anti-p185HER2 antibody for human cancer therapy. Proc Natl Acad Sci U S A. 1992;89 (10):4285–9.
38. Yakes FM, Chinratanalab W, Ritter CA, King W, Seelig S, Arteaga CL. Herceptin-induced inhibition of phosphatidylinositol-3 kinase and Akt is required for antibody-mediated effects on p27, cyclin D1, and antitumor action. Cancer Res. 2002;62(14):4132–41.
39. Klapper LN, Waterman H, Sela M, Yarden Y. Tumor-inhibitory antibodies to HER-2/ErbB-2 may act by recruiting c-Cbl and enhancing ubiquitination of HER-2. Cancer Res. 2000;60 (13):3384–8.

40. Arnould L, Gelly M, Penault-Llorca F, Benoit L, Bonnetain F, Migeon C, et al. Trastuzumab-based treatment of HER2-positive breast cancer: an antibody-dependent cellular cytotoxicity mechanism? Br J Cancer. 2006;94(2):259–67.
41. Clynes RA, Towers TL, Presta LG, Ravetch JV. Inhibitory Fc receptors modulate in vivo cytotoxicity against tumor targets. Nat Med. 2000;6(4):443–6.
42. Nahta R, Yu D, Hung MC, Hortobagyi GN, Esteva FJ. Mechanisms of disease: understanding resistance to HER2-targeted therapy in human breast cancer. Nat Clin Pract Oncol. 2006;3 (5):269–80.
43. Narayan M, Wilken JA, Harris LN, Baron AT, Kimbler KD, Maihle NJ. Trastuzumab-induced HER reprogramming in "resistant" breast carcinoma cells. Cancer Res. 2009;69(6):2191–4.
44. Chandarlapaty S, Sakr RA, Giri D, Patil S, Heguy A, Morrow M, et al. Frequent mutational activation of the PI3K-AKT pathway in trastuzumab-resistant breast cancer. Clin Cancer Res. 2012;18(24):6784–91.
45. Nagata Y, Lan KH, Zhou X, Tan M, Esteva FJ, Sahin AA, et al. PTEN activation contributes to tumor inhibition by trastuzumab, and loss of PTEN predicts trastuzumab resistance in patients. Cancer Cell. 2004;6(2):117–27.
46. Esteva FJ, Guo H, Zhang S, Santa-Maria C, Stone S, Lanchbury JS, et al. PTEN, PIK3CA, p-AKT, and p-p70S6K status: association with trastuzumab response and survival in patients with HER2-positive metastatic breast cancer. Am J Pathol. 2010;177(4):1647–56.
47. Ritter CA, Perez-Torres M, Rinehart C, Guix M, Dugger T, Engelman JA, et al. Human breast cancer cells selected for resistance to trastuzumab in vivo overexpress epidermal growth factor receptor and ErbB ligands and remain dependent on the ErbB receptor network. Clin Cancer Res. 2007;13(16):4909–19.
48. Huang X, Gao L, Wang S, McManaman JL, Thor AD, Yang X, et al. Heterotrimerization of the growth factor receptors erbB2, erbB3, and insulin-like growth factor-i receptor in breast cancer cells resistant to herceptin. Cancer Res. 2010;70(3):1204–14.
49. Diermeier S, Horvath G, Knuechel-Clarke R, Hofstaedter F, Szollosi J, Brockhoff G. Epidermal growth factor receptor coexpression modulates susceptibility to Herceptin in HER2/neu overexpressing breast cancer cells via specific erbB-receptor interaction and activation. Exp Cell Res. 2005;304(2):604–19.
50. Nagy P, Friedlander E, Tanner M, Kapanen AI, Carraway KL, Isola J, et al. Decreased accessibility and lack of activation of ErbB2 in JIMT-1, a herceptin-resistant, MUC4-expressing breast cancer cell line. Cancer Res. 2005;65(2):473–82.
51. Price-Schiavi SA, Jepson S, Li P, Arango M, Rudland PS, Yee L, et al. Rat Muc4 (sialomucin complex) reduces binding of anti-ErbB2 antibodies to tumor cell surfaces, a potential mechanism for herceptin resistance. Int J Cancer. 2002;99(6):783–91.
52. Scaltriti M, Rojo F, Ocana A, Anido J, Guzman M, Cortes J, et al. Expression of p95HER2, a truncated form of the HER2 receptor, and response to anti-HER2 therapies in breast cancer. J Natl Cancer Inst. 2007;99(8):628–38.
53. Todeschini P, Cocco E, Bellone S, Varughese J, Lin K, Carrara L, et al. Her2/neu extracellular domain shedding in uterine serous carcinoma: implications for immunotherapy with trastuzumab. Br J Cancer. 2011;105(8):1176–82.
54. Lee KM, Nam K, Oh S, Lim J, Kim YP, Lee JW, et al. Extracellular matrix protein 1 regulates cell proliferation and trastuzumab resistance through activation of epidermal growth factor signaling. Breast Cancer Res. 2014;16(6):479.
55. Han Z, Ni J, Smits P, Underhill CB, Xie B, Chen Y, et al. Extracellular matrix protein 1 (ECM1) has angiogenic properties and is expressed by breast tumor cells. FASEB J. 2001;15(6):988–94.
56. Wang L, Yu J, Ni J, Xu XM, Wang J, Ning H, et al. Extracellular matrix protein 1 (ECM1) is over-expressed in malignant epithelial tumors. Cancer Lett. 2003;200(1):57–67.
57. Merlin J, Stechly L, de Beauce S, Monte D, Leteurtre E, van Seuningen I, et al. Galectin-3 regulates MUC1 and EGFR cellular distribution and EGFR downstream pathways in pancreatic cancer cells. Oncogene. 2011;30(22):2514–25.

58. Ochieng J, Fridman R, Nangia-Makker P, Kleiner DE, Liotta LA, Stetler-Stevenson WG, et al. Galectin-3 is a novel substrate for human matrix metalloproteinases-2 and -9. Biochemistry. 1994;33(47):14109–14.
59. Lee KM, Nam K, Oh S, Lim J, Kim RK, Shim D, et al. ECM1 regulates tumor metastasis and CSC-like property through stabilization of beta-catenin. Oncogene. 2015;34(50):6055–65.
60. Ju JH, Oh S, Lee KM, Yang W, Nam KS, Moon HG, et al. Cytokeratin19 induced by HER2/ERK binds and stabilizes HER2 on cell membranes. Cell Death Differ. 2015;22(4):665–76.
61. Wu YJ, Rheinwald JG. A new small (40 Kd) keratin filament protein made by some cultured human squamous-cell carcinomas. Cell. 1981;25(3):627–35.
62. Xenidis N, Vlachonikolis I, Mavroudis D, Perraki M, Stathopoulou A, Malamos N, et al. Peripheral blood circulating cytokeratin-19 mRNA-positive cells after the completion of adjuvant chemotherapy in patients with operable breast cancer. Ann Oncol. 2003;14(6):849–55.
63. Bozionellou V, Mavroudis D, Perraki M, Papadopoulos S, Apostolaki S, Stathopoulos E, et al. Trastuzumab administration can effectively target chemotherapy-resistant cytokeratin-19 messenger RNA-positive tumor cells in the peripheral blood and bone marrow of patients with breast cancer. Clin Cancer Res. 2004;10(24):8185–94.
64. Bilancia D, Rosati G, Dinota A, Germano D, Romano R, Manzione L. Lapatinib in breast cancer. Ann Oncol. 2007;18(Suppl 6):vi26–30.
65. Soto-Perez-De-Celis E, Loh KP, Baldini C, Battisti NML, Chavarri-Guerra Y, De Glas NA, et al. Targeted agents for HER2-positive breast cancer in older adults: current and future perspectives. Expert Opin Investig Drugs. 2018;27(10):787–801.
66. Johnston S, Pippen J Jr, Pivot X, Lichinitser M, Sadeghi S, Dieras V, et al. Lapatinib combined with letrozole versus letrozole and placebo as first-line therapy for postmenopausal hormone receptor-positive metastatic breast cancer. J Clin Oncol. 2009;27(33):5538–46.
67. Capelan M, Pugliano L, De Azambuja E, Bozovic I, Saini KS, Sotiriou C, et al. Pertuzumab: new hope for patients with HER2-positive breast cancer. Ann Oncol. 2013;24(2):273–82.
68. Atlas E, Cardillo M, Mehmi I, Zahedkargaran H, Tang C, Lupu R. Heregulin is sufficient for the promotion of tumorigenicity and metastasis of breast cancer cells in vivo. Mol Cancer Res. 2003;1(3):165–75.
69. Agus DB, Akita RW, Fox WD, Lewis GD, Higgins B, Pisacane PI, et al. Targeting ligand-activated ErbB2 signaling inhibits breast and prostate tumor growth. Cancer Cell. 2002;2(2):127–37.
70. Baselga J, Cortes J, Kim SB, Im SA, Hegg R, Im YH, et al. Pertuzumabs plus trastuzumab plus docetaxel for metastatic breast cancer. N Engl J Med. 2012;366(2):109–19.
71. Lewis Phillips GD, Li G, Dugger DL, Crocker LM, Parsons KL, Mai E, et al. Targeting HER2-positive breast cancer with trastuzumab-DM1, an antibody-cytotoxic drug conjugate. Cancer Res. 2008;68(22):9280–90.
72. Erickson HK, Park PU, Widdison WC, Kovtun YV, Garrett LM, Hoffman K, et al. Antibody-maytansinoid conjugates are activated in targeted cancer cells by lysosomal degradation and linker-dependent intracellular processing. Cancer Res. 2006;66(8):4426–33.
73. Lu Y, Zi X, Zhao Y, Mascarenhas D, Pollak M. Insulin-like growth factor-I receptor signaling and resistance to trastuzumab (Herceptin). J Natl Cancer Inst. 2001;93(24):1852–7.
74. Lindemann K, Resau J, Nahrig J, Kort E, Leeser B, Annecke K, et al. Differential expression of c-met, its ligand HGF/SF and HER2/neu in DCIS and adjacent normal breast tissue. Histopathology. 2007;51(1):54–62.
75. Berns K, Horlings HM, Hennessy BT, Madiredjo M, Hijmans EM, Beelen K, et al. A functional genetic approach identifies the PI3K pathway as a major determinant of trastuzumab resistance in breast cancer. Cancer Cell. 2007;12(4):395–402.
76. Yu S, Liu Q, Han X, Qin S, Zhao W, Li A, et al. Development and clinical application of anti-HER2 monoclonal and bispecific antibodies for cancer treatment. Exp Hematol Oncol. 2017;6:31.

77. Bang YJ, Giaccone G, Im SA, Oh DY, Bauer TM, Nordstrom JL, et al. First-in-human phase 1 study of margetuximab (MGAH22), an Fc-modified chimeric monoclonal antibody, in patients with HER2-positive advanced solid tumors. Ann Oncol. 2017;28(4):855–61.
78. Miller K, Cortes J, Hurvitz SA, Krop IE, Tripathy D, Verma S, et al. HERMIONE: a randomized phase 2 trial of MM-302 plus trastuzumab versus chemotherapy of physician's choice plus trastuzumab in patients with previously treated, anthracycline-naive, HER2-positive, locally advanced/metastatic breast cancer. BMC Cancer. 2016;16:352.

Chapter 4
Ras Signaling in Breast Cancer

Aree Moon

Abstract Ras proteins mediate extracellular and cytoplasmic signaling networks via receptor tyrosine kinase. The Ras pathway induces activation of signaling molecules involved in cell proliferation and growth, cell survival and apoptosis, metabolism, and motility. Although Ras mutations in breast cancer are not frequently reported, hyperactivation of Ras signaling plays an important role in breast cancer growth and progression. Oncogenic Ras activation occurs via loss of Ras GTPase-activating proteins, overexpression of growth factor receptor, and stimulation by various cytokines. Effective control of oncogenic Ras is one of the therapeutic strategies in breast cancer. The mechanisms of intracellular localization, activation, and signaling pathway of Ras in cancer have been used to develop therapeutic candidates. Recent studies have reported an effective therapy for breast cancer by inhibition of enzymes involved in the posttranslational modification of Ras, such as farnesyltransferase and geranylgeranyltransferase 1, and anti-cancer therapies targeting the epidermal growth factor receptor (EGFR). Emerging targets involved in EGF-mediated Ras activity in breast cancer have shed new insight into Ras activation in breast cancer progression. These alternative mechanisms for Ras signaling pathway may suggest novel therapeutic approaches for targeting Ras in breast cancer. In spite of the difficulties in targeting Ras protein, important discoveries highlight the direct inhibition of Ras activity. Further studies may elucidate the effects of targeting Ras protein and the clinical relevance thereof.

Keywords Ras · Signaling · Breast cancer · Invasion · Metastasis

A. Moon (✉)
College of Pharmacy, Duksung Women's University, Seoul, South Korea
e-mail: armoon@duksung.ac.kr

D.-Y. Noh et al. (eds.), *Translational Research in Breast Cancer*, Advances in Experimental Medicine and Biology 1187,
https://doi.org/10.1007/978-981-32-9620-6_4

4.1 Introduction

The Ras family members including H-Ras, K-Ras (A and B), and N-Ras are small GTPases, and the first discovered human oncogenes that regulate a variety of biological responses [1]. Ras proteins relay extracellular signals to the cytoplasmic signaling network via receptor tyrosine kinase (RTK)/Ras pathway to the nucleus, inducing transcriptional activation of genes involved in cell proliferation, growth, metabolism, and motility. RTK activates the canonical Ras-Raf-MEK1/2-ERK1/2 mitogen-activated protein kinases (MAPK) signaling cascade, which is the best characterized Ras downstream pathway [2]. Noncanonical MAPK pathways, MKK4/7-JNKs, MKK3/6-p38, MEK5-ERK5, are also activated downstream of Ras [2]. Currently, more than 10 defined Ras effectors such as Raf, phosphoinositide 3-kinase (PI3K), RalGDS, and p120GAP trigger distinct signaling cascades [3].

Activated mutant forms of all three Ras genes are found in 27% of all human cancers [4]. The K-Ras mutation is the most frequent (85%), whereas N-Ras and H-Ras mutations constitute 11% and 4%, respectively, of all cancers [4]. Although the frequency of the mutant Ras gene is less than 2% of breast cancers [5, 6], mounting evidence suggests that hyperactive Ras signaling plays an important role in breast cancer growth and progression [7]. Ras oncogene is efficient not only for tumorigenicity but also for metastatic dissemination in breast cancer. Ras signaling correlates with reduced survival of patients with luminal breast cancer [8].

Epidermal growth factor receptor (EGFR) 1 and HER (human epidermal growth factor receptor) 2, responsible for Ras/MAPK signaling pathway, are largely overexpressed in human breast cancer [9]. The loss of Ras GTPase-activating proteins (RasGAPs), which are the negative regulators of Ras activation, is frequently observed in breast cancers [10–12]. Recently, a lipid raft protein, flotillin-1, has been reported for EGF-induced H-Ras activation and is associated with breast cancer aggressiveness [13]. These studies suggest that the hyperactive Ras pathway signaling contributes to breast cancer growth and progression.

Increasing experimental evidence shows the functional diversity of Ras isoforms in breast cancer [4, 14–16]. Both H-Ras and N-Ras promote phenotypic transformation of breast epithelial cells, while only H-Ras induces the invasive/migratory phenotype via Rac1-MKK3/6-p38 MAPK pathway [14–16]. In addition, H-Ras induced zinc finger E-box-binding homeobox 1 (ZEB1) and repressed discoidin domain receptor 1 (DDR1) in breast cells, leading to epithelial-to-mesenchymal transition (EMT) and invasion [17]. In this chapter, we will summarize the biological function of Ras isoform-specific pathway and emerging insights into Ras activation in breast cancer.

4.2 Review of Past Studies

4.2.1 Biological Function of Ras in Breast Cancer

4.2.1.1 Cell Proliferation and Growth

Ras proteins are well-known mediators of mitogenic stimuli. Overexpression of oncogenic H-Ras induces re-entry of cells in the G_0 phase into the cell cycle and initiates cell division without growth factor stimulation [18, 19]. Active Ras enhances the proliferative capacity of cells by inducing transcriptional upregulation of growth factors such as heparin-binding epidermal growth factor-like growth factor (HBEGF), transforming growth factor-α (TGFα), and amphiregulin (AREG) [20, 21]. In addition, it alters the expression of growth factor receptors and integrins, which promote cell proliferation [20–23].

Oncogenic Ras-induced proliferative signals result in overexpression of transcriptional factors, which are necessary for cell cycle entry and cell progression, such as c-Fos, c-Jun, ETS domain-containing protein ELK1, serum response factor (SRF), activating transcription factor (ATF) 2, and nuclear factor kappa-light-chain-enhancer of activated B cells (NF-κB) [24–27]. They affect the expression of cyclin D1, the cyclin protein in G_1 phase [28]. Oncogenic H-Ras^{G12V} mutant also influences the metabolic stability of cyclin D1 via inhibition of glycogen synthase kinase (GSK) 3β, which is associated with continuous ubiquitination and proteosomal degradation of cyclin D1, via phosphoinositide 3-kinase (PI3K)-dependent phosphorylation [29]. Oncogenic Ras promotes cell cycle progression by attenuating inhibition by anti-growth signaling pathways, which inhibit cyclin-dependent kinase inhibitors (CKIs) such as p27 and p21 ([30, 31], Fig. 4.1). In cells with defective DNA damage checkpoints, such as loss of p53, DNA replication induced by oncogenic Ras leads to abnormal chromosomal aberrations, resulting in inadequate chromosome segregation and subsequent cell division [32, 33]. Oncogenic H-Ras^{G12V} may contribute to gene instability observed in Ras-induced cancers via promotion of G_2/M phase transition, inhibition of the activation of G_2 DNA checkpoints, and induction of defects in mitotic spindle checkpoints, which may contribute to gene instability observed in Ras-induced cancers [33].

4.2.1.2 Cell Survival and Apoptosis

Apoptosis is a defense mechanism of cells against carcinogenesis. The collapse of the apoptotic mechanism is one of the characteristic features of cancer cells. Apoptosis is a balanced molecular behavior initiated by a wide range of signals and is regulated by positive or negative modulators. Apoptotic cell death occurs following the activation of death receptors by extracellular signals such as growth factor withdrawal or substrate separation, or by mitochondrial-mediated pathways activated by signals such as nutrient deficiency and DNA damage. Oncogenic Ras

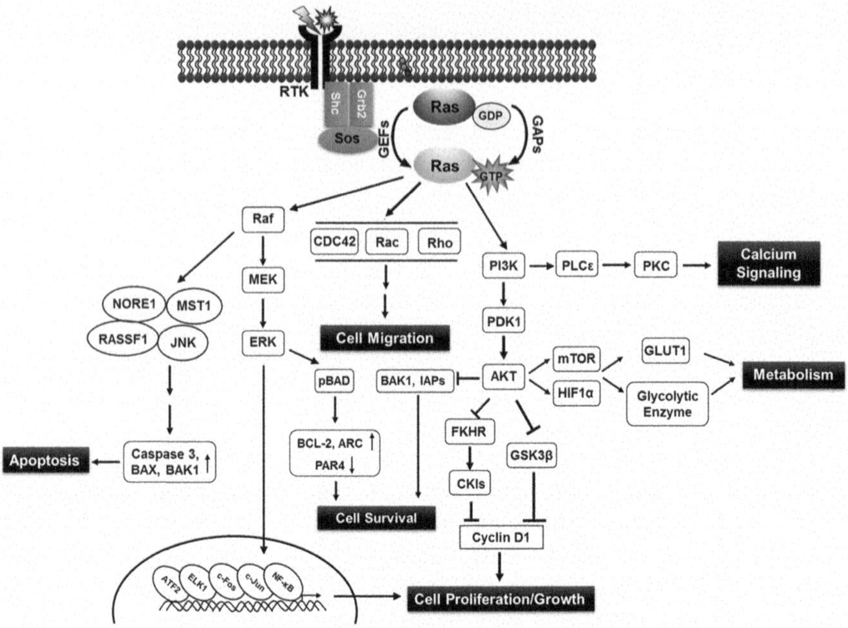

Fig. 4.1 Effects of oncogenic Ras signaling on breast cancer progression

mediates both proapoptotic and antiapoptotic functions depending on the status of Ras effector pathway or apoptotic machinery ([34], Fig. 4.1). Ras signaling in the MAPK/ERK pathway (also known as the Ras-Raf-MEK-ERK pathway) leads to apoptotic response via p53 and Ras effectors, such as Ras association domain-containing protein 1 (encoded by the RASSF1 gene), NORE1, MST (mammalian sterile 20–like kinase) 1, and JNK (c-Jun N-terminal kinase). It induces apoptotic cell death via activation of caspase 3 and proapoptotic proteins such as BAX (Bcl-2 associated X protein) and BAK (Bcl-2 homologous antagonist/killer) 1 [35, 36].

Phosphorylation of BAD, mediated via Ras-Raf pathway, leads to overexpression of antiapoptotic proteins BCL-2 and apoptosis repressor ARC and downregulation of proapoptotic transcriptional repressor prostate apoptosis response 4 (PAR4) [37, 38]. Ras-PI3K pathway induces antiapoptotic effects through downregulation of proapoptotic protein BAK1 and inhibitors of apoptosis proteins (IAPs) ([39, 40], Fig. 4.1). The survival or death of RAS-transformed cells depends on the shift in balance of the Ras signal toward prosurvival or proapoptotic outcomes. In cancer, the function of oncogenic Ras is biased towards prosurvival [41].

4.2.1.3 Metabolism

Cancer cells are highly dependent on the metabolic pathway to product building blocks necessary for the production of new cells via rapid proliferation [42]. As described by Warburg in the 1920s, cancer cells require increased glucose uptake to meet their energy needs [43].

Oncogenic Ras affects metabolic reprogramming of cancer cells through upregulation of hypoxia-inducible factor (HIF)1α (Fig. 4.1). Activation of MAPK and PI3K pathway, induced by oncogenic Ras, leads to accumulation of mammalian target of rapamycin (mTOR) activity and translation of HIF1α [44, 45]. Upregulation of HIF1α by Ras leads to an increase in the transport of glucose by transcription of GLUT1 (glucose transporter) and glycolytic capture by increasing the level of important glycolytic enzymes [46–48]. In addition, oncogenic Ras contributes to metabolic reactions favoring glucose as an anabolic substrate for direct production of substances for cell growth [42].

Autophagy is another mechanism of oncogenic Ras in intracellular metabolism. Although autophagy is known to affect both tumor-suppressive and tumor-promoting qualities, several studies have emphasized the role of oncogenic Ras in upregulation of autophagy such as maintenance of mitochondrial function and support for tumor growth in vivo [49, 50].

4.2.1.4 EMT, Invasion, and Metastasis

Many metastatic tumors, such as lung, pancreatic, and colorectal cancer, carry Ras mutations. The onset of metastatic cascade involves local tumor cell invasion and escape of the tumor cells from the primary tumor. Oncogenic Ras contributes to changes underlying cell–cell or cell–matrix interaction and acquisition of migratory phenotype. Changes in cell–cell contacts by oncogenic Ras ensure intercellular adhesion junctions via calcium-dependent E-cadherin receptor and related cytoplasmic protein, β-catenin [51–53]. Expression of oncogenic Ras reduces the expression of E-cadherin by increasing the expression of SNAIL and SLUG, which are transcriptional repressors of E-cadherin. Proteolytic degradation of E-cadherin and methylation of E-cadherin promoter suppress the levels of E-cadherin [54–56]. With the decrease in cell–cell interactions, oncogenic Ras expression decreases the interaction with extracellular matrix (ECM) by downregulating the integrin subunits that promote the formation and maintenance of stable adhesion complexes [57–59]. In addition, oncogenic Ras contributes directly to the motility of cancer cells by affecting the polymerization, organization and contraction of actin, the polymerization and stability of microtubules, and the transcriptional regulation of mitogenic gene products [60].

The progression of metastasis involves intravasation in which cancer cells enter the blood vessels or lymphatic vessels out of range of the primary tumor. The ability to invade the physical barrier, such as the basement membrane, is important in this process. The expression of oncogenic Ras regulates the invasive phenotype via ECM degradation. In particular, the downstream signaling pathways of activated RAS increase the expression and activity of various ECM proteases and reduce the expression of proteases inhibitors. It also prevents matrix deprivation-induced apoptosis when cancer cells are translocated through the circulatory system

[61, 62]. Ras-dependent signaling in metastasis occurs via Ras-MAPK, Ras-PI3K, Ras-Ral GTPase, Ras-Rho GTPase pathways [60]. For example, activation of Rho GTPases induces changes in cell adhesion and motility. Ras-dependent signals that promote metastasis induce changes in tissue morphology and genetic background ([63, 64], Fig. 4.1). Tumor metastasis may be induced as a result of interaction between oncogenic Ras and other metastasis-promoting pathways such as the transforming growth factor (TGF)-β pathway [54, 65].

4.2.2 *Ras-Specific Pathway*

4.2.2.1 Differential Signaling Between H-Ras and N-Ras

The varying effect of H-Ras and N-Ras in the induction of the invasive phenotype of human breast cells was investigated ([14, 16], Fig. 4.2). H-Ras, but not N-Ras, induced the invasive phenotype of MCF10A human breast epithelial cell line. H-Ras-induced invasive phenotype is associated closely with upregulation of matrix metalloproteinase (MMP)-2 via Rac-MKK3/6-p38 MAPK in MCF10A cells, rather than MMP-9 expression. In contrast, both H-Ras and N-Ras activate Raf-MEK-ERK and PI3K-Akt pathways [14]. P38 kinase is a key signaling molecule that is differentially regulated by H-Ras and N-Ras [14, 15]. In human breast epithelial cells, p38 MAPK upregulates MMP-2 through the transcription factor ATF2,

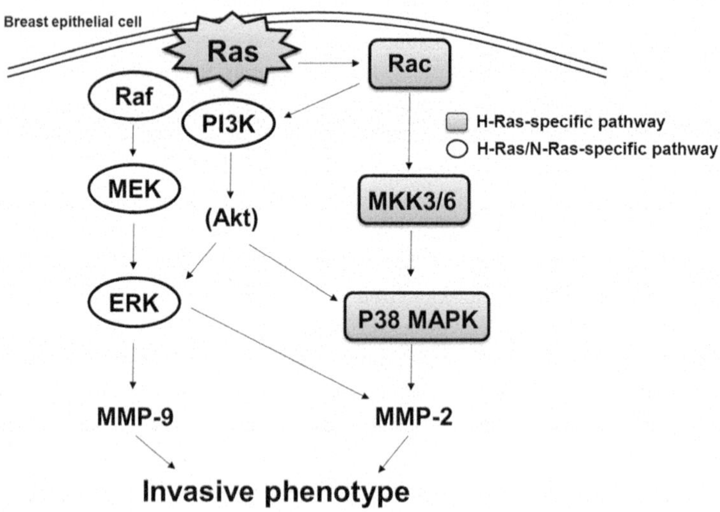

Fig. 4.2 Differential signaling between H-Ras and N-Ras in breast cells

indicating the crucial role of ATF2 in malignant phenotypic changes occurring in human breast epithelial cells [66]. In a study identifying the major regions of the H-Ras-specific invasive phenotype, two consecutive proline residues Pro 173 and Pro 174 in the hypervariable region (HVR) consisting of amino acids 166 to 189 of H-Ras were found to be important in the H-Ras-induced invasive phenotype of breast cells [67]. The wild-type N-Ras was overexpressed in basal-like breast cancers (BLBC), but not in other breast cancer subtypes. Inhibition of N-Ras prevents transformation and tumor growth, whereas its overexpression enhances this process in preinvasive BLBC cells. In addition, most of the genes that react with N-Ras encode chemokines such as IL8 acting on both cancer cells and interstitial fibroblasts. Expression levels of these chemokines and N-Ras in tumors appear to correlate with the outcome. Thus, BLBC progression is involved in the autocrine/paracrine signaling of chemokines that affects both cancer and stromal cells. The process is promoted by increased activity of wild-type N-Ras [68].

4.2.2.2 K-Ras Signaling

K-Ras is a member of the cellular signaling pathway, such as the EGFR/Ras/MAPK, and is involved in physiological and pathological processes. Increased expression of K-Ras is associated with various cancer progression including breast cancer. Most of K-Ras mutations are located on codon 12 and rarely on codon 61 in breast cancer. Oncogenic K-Ras (G12V) or PI3K (H1047R) in MCF10A breast epithelial cells induces de novo lipogenesis via downstream signaling target of rapamycin complex 1 (mTORC1) [69]. The expression of K-Ras (V12) using retrovirus induced autophagic vacuole formation and malignant transformation in human breast epithelial cells [70]. Galectin-3 (Gal-3), a β-galactoside-binding protein, selectively binds activated K-Ras-GTP and activates wild-type K-Ras. Overexpression of Gal in breast cancer increases oncogenic subversion of cell membrane nanostructure by increasing the K-Ras signal output [71]. A preferential activation of K-Ras occurs in basal-like breast cancer cells compared with luminal type, and requires K-Ras for maintenance of mesenchymal phenotype and metastasis. Therefore, K-Ras plays an important role in the mesenchymal characteristics and metastatic behavior of breast cancer cells, suggesting K-Ras as an important therapeutic target in breast cancer [72].

4.2.2.3 Ras Isoform-Induced EMT

EMT is a process in which epithelial cells lose differentiation of cellular polarity and dissociate from each other, resulting in invasion, intravasation, and metastatic spread of breast cancer cells [73]. Accumulating evidence suggests that Ras/MAPK pathway induces metastasis via EMT. Recent studies including our group showed that oncogenic H-Ras induces EMT leading to breast cell invasion [17, 74, 75]. H-Ras-induced EMT involves upregulation of ZEB1, a transcription factor [17]. ZEB1 is a transcription factor that initiates EMT by directly suppressing the transcription of a key epithelial gene, E-cadherin [76]. Interestingly, H-Ras represses the expression of DDR1, a unique RTK, which interacts with E-cadherin in breast epithelial cells. ZEB1 acts as a transcriptional repressor of DDR1, and ectopic expression of DDR1 decreases the invasive phenotype of triple-negative breast cancer (TNBC) cells [17]. Consistently, induction of active H-Ras mutant leads to EMT by increasing vimentin, a mesenchymal marker [74]. Recently, it has been found that the activated form of the H-Ras and phosphatidylinositol-4,5-bisphosphate 3-kinase catalytic subunit alpha (PIK3CA) oncogenes induces EMT of breast cells through inhibition of p53-related transcription factor p63 [75].

4.2.2.4 Regulation of Ras Isoform-Specific Signaling by Cytokines

Various cytokines contribute to increase the H-Ras-induced invasive phenotype of breast cells. TGF-β affects various intracellular processes including cell proliferation, differentiation, and death [77, 78]. TGF-β is a potent inhibitor of the growth of normal epithelial cells and stimulates tumor invasion in advanced cancer cells. TGF-β signaling pathway enhances the invasive and migratory properties of H-Ras MCF10A cells via p38-mediated upregulation of MMP-2 and MMP-9 [79]. The downstream signaling molecule of TGF-β, a Smad2, cooperates with H-Ras signaling to regulate EMT and tumor metastasis [80]. In particular, activation of H-Ras in mammary epithelial cells induces EMT through autocrine production of TGF-β and leukotriene B4 receptor-2-linked signaling [81, 82]. The transcription factor NF-kB is a major factor in TGF-β-induced EMT regulation of Ras oncogene overexpression in mammary epithelial cells [82]. Increased TGF-β signaling promotes p21-dependent premature senescence and promotes oncogenic Ras-mediated metastatic transformation in human mammary epithelial cells [83]. Ras and TGF-β signaling enhances cancer progression by promoting the transcriptional activation of p63 isoform ΔNp63 [84].

EGF and its receptor EGFR exert important roles in the abnormal growth of various tumor cell types including breast, lung, and colorectal cancers [85]. EGF signaling is involved in tumor invasion and metastasis via activation of the Ras downstream pathway, with the Ras-MEK1/2-ERK and Ras-Cdc42-Rac signaling pathways playing a predominant role in EGF-induced invasion and motility [86, 87]. EGF-induced Grb7 activation recruits and activates Ras-GTPases and promotes tumor growth through phosphorylation of ERK1/2 in Sk-Br3 breast cancer cells [88]. EGF-promoted oncogenesis occurs via tissue transglutaminase-dependent signaling leading to Src activation in SKBR3 and BT20 breast cancer cell lines [89]. Differential activation of Ras isoforms by EGF has been studied in breast cancer models [90]. EGF treatment significantly increased the active form of H-Ras in Hs578T cells, in which H-Ras was initially activated, whereas K-Ras and N-Ras were not activated by treatment of EGF. In MDA-MB-231 cells originally containing an active mutant of K-Ras, EGF treatment markedly increased activation of H-Ras as well as activation of K-Ras and N-Ras. Although EGF activated all of the Ras isoforms, only H-Ras and K-Ras were involved in EGF-induced invasion of breast cells [90]. It was suggested that NgBR, a Nogo-B specific receptor, was a unique receptor that promoted prenylated H-Ras accumulation in the cell membrane, activating EGF pathway [91].

Granulocyte-colony stimulating factor (G-CSF) is an extracellular regulator of hemopoiesis required for the proliferation and differentiation of granulocytic progenitor cells and mature neutrophils [92]. G-CSF plays a crucial role in H-Ras-induced invasive and migratory phenotypes of MCF10A cell [92]. H-Ras, but not N-Ras, specifically increases the expression of G-CSF, and the increased G-CSF enhances the invasiveness of H-Ras via upregulation of MMP-2 in the Rac-MKK3/3-p38 pathway [93]. In human breast tissues and serum derived from breast cancer patients, the expression of G-CSF is strongly correlated with pathologically diagnosed breast cancer. These data provide a molecular basis supporting the crucial role of G-CSF in promoting invasiveness of human breast epithelial cells. The RAS/RAF/MEK pathway is constitutively active in many cancer cells with elevated G-CSF expression. Treatment with a Ras signaling inhibitor, a MEK inhibitor, reduced G-CSF production in a mouse model of pancreatic adenocarcinoma [94].

4.2.3 Inhibition of Ras Signaling Pathway

4.2.3.1 EGFR Inhibitor

Anticancer therapy targeting EGFR is popular in clinical oncology. EGFR is a member of the HER/ErbB family of transmembrane growth factor receptors with tyrosine kinase activity. Activation of EGFR induces phosphorylation of downstream signaling molecules of Ras signaling pathway. Anti-EGFR monoclonal antibodies (mAbs) are frequently used in chemotherapy. The most widely used mAbs are cetuximab and panitumumab [96]. The K-Ras mutation is strongly correlated with EGFR and is resistant to cetuximab and panitumumab [97]. EGFR-TKIs (tyrosine kinase inhibitors), such as erlotinib and gefitinib, are chemotherapeutic agents approved in clinical trials [98, 99]. They prolong survival or show prominent anticancer activity in patients with non-small cell lung cancer (NSCLC) and solid tumors following treatment with single agent and with monoclonal antibody (bevacizumab), respectively [99, 100].

4.2.3.2 Farnesyltransferase Inhibitors (FTIs)

Oncogenic Ras, which is a frequent target in cancer, is a significant molecule of interest in anticancer therapy. The most effective way to control oncogenic Ras is to inhibit enzymes involved in the posttranslational modification of Ras proteins. The most commonly targeted enzymes include farnesyltransferase and geranylgeranyltransferase 1, which are involved in the prenylation of Ras proteins

[95]. FTIs are anticancer drugs acting as prominent inhibitors of CAAX processing of Ras proteins [101–103]. FTIs exhibit anti-H-Ras and antitumor activity in preclinical cell culture [104, 105] and mouse models of H-Ras-driven mammary tumor [106]. FTI-277 inhibits proliferation and invasiveness of H-Ras-MCF10A cells, and Hs578T breast cancer cells expressing an active mutant of H-Ras. FTI-277 treatment reduced H-Ras activation and increased invasiveness following exposure to EGF, indicating that FTI-277 inhibits the invasion and migration of breast cells by blocking H-Ras activation [107]. FTIs show a tumor suppressor effect in TNBC cells. FTIs inhibit the aggressive phenotype of TNBC by inhibiting the HIF-1α-Snail pathway in MDA-MB-231 cells [108]. The combination of farnesyltransferase and Akt inhibitor shows synergy in MDA-MB-231 cells and a significant tumor suppression in ErbB2 transgenic mice [109]. FTI-R115777 (tipifarnib) in combination with tamoxifen shows synergistic effects on the suppression of MCF-7 breast cancer cells and cell cycle progression [110]. Several studies of FTI in clinical trials have shown a noticeable effect on the active Ras-MAPK pathway. For example, FTI SCH66336 (Lonafarnib) is active against metastatic breast cancer following treatment with a single agent [111].

FTIs are effective against H-Ras and N-Ras, but do not affect activated K-Ras mutations that do not undergo CAAX processing. Chemotherapy for K-Ras-induced malignancy is still a challenge clinically. Since K-Ras4B isoform represents essentially geranylgeranylation, the use of geranylgeranyltransferase 1 inhibitors (GGTIs) can inhibit K-Ras4B isoform very effectively. Antisense K-Ras therapy using oligonucleotide inhibitor may be another solution [112].

A few FTIs are ineffective because of their nonspecificity and target closely related molecules in the Ras-MAPK pathway. In order to overcome these limitations, combinational therapies have been proposed and are under investigation in clinical trials. Farnesyl thiosalicylic acid (FTS, Salirasib) inhibits Ras-mediated signaling, which acts to dissociate Ras from the cell membrane and inhibits the action of Ras via a counter-mechanism to FTI [113, 114]. Combinations of FTS and glycolysis inhibitors or FTS and VEGF receptor inhibitors have been used as combination therapies [115].

4.2.3.3 Statins

Isoprenylation of Ras involves the activity of 3-hydroxy 3-methylglutaryl (HMG)-CoA reductase, a major enzyme in the synthesis of mevalonate, which is the precursor for the production of farnesylpyrophosphate and geranylgeranylpyrophosphate. The HMG-CoA reductase inhibitors, simvastatin and lovastatin, are statins used to lower cholesterol in patients with hypercholesterolemia to reduce the risk of cardiovascular disease [116]. Simvastatin and/or lovastatin exhibit antimetastatic and antitumorigenic effects in breast [117, 118], pancreatic [119], and colorectal cancer [120]. Simvastatin and lovastatin reduce the amount of isoprenylated H-Ras in the cell membrane and increase the amount of unprenylated H-Ras in the cytosol. These drugs inhibit cellular invasiveness by inhibiting the level of MMP-9 in H-Ras MCF10A cells [121]. Recently, a combination of statins and anticancer drugs including NF-κB inhibitor [122], atorvastatin [123], exemestane [124], and metformin [125] has shown synergistic antitumor effects.

4.2.3.4 Natural Compounds Inhibiting Ras Signaling Pathway

Curcumin

Curcumin is an edible pigment found in turmeric, and exhibits anticarcinogenic and antimetastatic properties [126] in prostate [127] and breast [128] cells. Curcumin induces apoptosis of H-Ras MCF10A cells through redox signaling and caspase-3 activation [129]. Curcumin induces paraptosis by promoting vacuolation due to swelling and fusion of mitochondria and/or endoplasmic reticulum in Hs578T cells carrying a mutated Ras gene (Q61L HRAS) with constitutively active H-Ras [130, 131]. In particular, paraptotic events following exposure to curcumin did not occur in MCF10A normal breast epithelial cells. Curcumin-induced paraptosis provides novel insights into the anticancer mechanisms of curcumin in malignant cancer cells [132]. Curcumin decreased anchorage-independent growth as well as increased the percentage of cells from G_0/G_1, and decreased Rho-A and RasGRF1 expression in transformed breast cancer cells [133]. A novel curcumin derivative, RL91, exhibits a synergistic effect with raloxifene, a member of the class of selective estrogen receptor modulators (SERM), in inducing apoptosis of Hs578T and MDA-MB-231 cells [134].

Capsaicin

Capsaicin, an active component of red pepper, exhibits antitumorigenic and chemopreventive properties [135, 136]. Capsaicin has been known to suppress the growth of several tumor cells [137, 138], including leukemic [139], gastric [140], hepatic [141], glioma [142], and prostate cells in humans [143]. Treatment of capsaicin markedly activated c-Jun-1 and p38 MAPK and deactivated ERKs in H-Ras MCF10A cells. The use of kinase inhibitors and overexpression of dominant-negative forms of MAPKs demonstrated the role of JNK-1 and p38, but not that of ERKs, in capsaicin-induced apoptosis of H-Ras-transformed MCF10A cells [144]. Capsaicin also induced apoptosis by inhibition of H-Ras-induced reactive oxygen species (ROS) and Rac activation in breast cells. Pretreatment of H-Ras MCF10A cells with an antioxidant N-acetylcysteine markedly reversed capsaicin-induced growth inhibition, suggesting that ROS may mediate the apoptosis of H-Ras-transformed cells induced by capsaicin [145].

4.2.3.5 Other Inhibitors

Competitive inhibitors targeting Ras downstream signaling molecules represent another strategy to treat Ras-induced oncogenesis. The most potent targets include Raf kinase, MEK, and PI3K [146]. PI3K inhibitors target PI3K in the PI3K/AKT/mTOR pathway that induces apoptosis [147]. Anthrapyrazolone inhibitors such as SP600125 inhibit JNK [148].

4.3 Current Evidence and Concepts

4.3.1 Genetic Aspects of Ras Activity in Breast Cancer

Active mutations in the canonical Ras/MAPK pathway are very rare in breast cancer. Next-generation sequencing reveals that the frequency of mutations in the Ras and Raf families is less than 2% of all primary breast tumors [5, 6]. Instead, PI3K/Akt pathway is frequently associated with breast cancer, mainly in ER+ subtype [5, 6, 149]. Overexpression of RTKs such as EGFR and HER2 in the hyperactive Ras/MAPK signaling pathway explains the clinical significance of Ras activation in breast cancer [9].

Recent reports of novel mechanisms for activation of Ras pathway in breast cancer demonstrated that mutations/deletions of RasGAPs such as NF1, RASAL2, DAB2IP, and RASA1 act as negative regulators of Ras pathway in breast cancer [10–12, 150, 151]. Loss of NF1 gene occurs in 28–31% of invasive BC, increasing to 40–62% of triple-negative and HER2-enriched subtypes [10]. The RasGAP genes, RASAL2 and DAB2IP, are mutated or suppressed in breast cancer and suggest poor prognosis of luminal B type [11, 151]. Allelic loss of RASA1, another RasGAP, is frequent in triple-negative and ER-negative subtypes, supporting the loss of negative regulators of RAS in breast cancer [11]. RASAL2 ablation promotes breast tumor development and metastasis of luminal mouse tumors [151]. Further, RASAL2 promotes Rac1 signaling independent of its RAS-GAP catalytic activity in TNBC, resulting in invasion and metastasis of breast cancer [150].

4.3.2 Emerging Strategies Targeting Ras

Numerous studies have elucidated molecular mechanisms for intracellular localization, activation, and signaling pathway of Ras in cancer. Efforts to develop therapeutic drugs targeting Ras signaling include direct and indirect approaches. Druggable targets include the membrane association and activation of Ras, farnesyltransferase, kinases, which is crucial for membrane association and activity of H-Ras [152]. However, FTIs did not increase the survival of patients with K-Ras-mutated pancreatic cancer in clinical trials. The alternative prenylation for membrane association of K-Ras abrogates anticancer effects of FTIs [153, 154]. In clinical trials associated with metastatic breast cancer, tipifarnib, another FTI, demonstrated clinical activity, which warrants further study [155]. Novel regulatory enzymes such as Rce1, Icmt, and Pdeδ involved in membrane association of Ras suggest a promising strategy for targeting Ras in breast cancer [4].

Recent attempts to develop small molecules targeted Ras protein. Although the challenges relate to difficulties in identifying druggable pockets on the surface of Ras protein, recent studies represent important breakthroughs and discoveries [156–158]. A specific inhibitor to active mutant RasG12C was identified [156]. A small molecule, rigosertib, interacts with the Ras-binding domains of RAF kinase and disrupts Ras-RAF-MEK pathway [157]. Another group reported a human IgG_1 antibody targeting oncogenic Ras mutants, resulting in inhibition of in vivo tumor growth in xenograft models [158].

Novel emerging targets involving EGF-mediated Ras signaling pathway in breast cancer include flotillin-1, a lipid raft protein, upregulated in human breast cancer tissues and inversely correlated with disease-free survival [13]. Flotillin-1 is an important regulator of H-Ras activation and breast cell invasion. Flotillin-1 is required for EGF-induced activation of H-Ras, cell invasion and migration in TNBC cells. In mouse tumor models with TNBC xenografts, knockdown of flotillin-1 significantly inhibited the tumor growth, suggesting that targeting flotillin-1 may be a novel strategy for breast cancer treatment [13]. Nogo-B receptor interacts with prenylated H-Ras, promoting Ras plasma membrane association and activation. Knockdown of Nogo-B receptor inhibits EGF-stimulated Ras signaling and tumor growth of breast cancer in vivo [91].

4.4 Future Research Directions

In this chapter, we review important aspects of Ras activity and its impact on breast cancer. Recent studies show genetic and epigenetic mechanisms of Ras activation in breast cancer, where RAS mutations are rarely reported. The loss of RasGAPs, negative regulators for Ras activation, plays an important role in the development, progression, and metastasis of breast cancer and is associated with poor survival of patients. The tumor microenvironment including IL-4 and reduced tumor-infiltrating lymphocytes promotes tumor growth of breast cancer. Emerging targets including flotillin-1 regulate EGF-mediated Ras activity in breast cancer, shedding new insight into Ras activation in breast cancer progression. These alternative mechanisms in the Ras signaling pathway may suggest novel therapeutic approaches for targeting Ras in breast cancer. In spite of the difficulties of targeting Ras, recent breakthroughs and discoveries have directly inhibited Ras activity. Further studies may elucidate the effects of targeting Ras protein for clinical relevance.

4.5 Summary

Oncogenic Ras plays an important role in the proliferation, survival, metabolism, and motility of breast cancer cells through hyperactivation of downstream signaling molecules in canonical or noncanonical MAPK signaling pathways. H-, N-, and K-Ras-specific signaling pathways contribute to breast cancer progression through overlapping or differential signaling regulation. Cytokines activate Ras signaling in breast cells to enhance cellular invasion and oncogenic signaling pathways. Novel mechanisms for Ras activity, genetic alterations of RasGAPs, and emerging targets for Ras activation are unveiled, informing new strategies to inhibit Ras signaling in breast cancer.

References

1. Fernández-Medarde A, Santos E. Ras in cancer and developmental diseases. Genes Cancer. 2011;2(3):344–58.
2. Zhao Y, Adjei AA. The clinical development of MEK inhibitors. Nat Rev Clin Oncol. 2014;11 (7):385–400.
3. Rajalingam K, Schreck R, Rapp UR, Albert S. Ras oncogenes and their downstream targets. Biochim Biophys Acta. 2007;1773(8):1177–95.
4. Hobbs GA, Der CJ, Rossman KL. RAS isoforms and mutations in cancer at a glance. J Cell Sci. 2016;129(7):1287–92.
5. Cerami E, Gao J, Dogrusoz U, et al. The cBio cancer genomics portal: an open platform for exploring multidimensional cancer genomics data. Cancer Discov. 2012;2(5):401–4.
6. CGAN (Cancer Genome Atlas Network). Comprehensive molecular portraits of human breast tumours. Nature. 2012;490(7418):61–70.
7. Giltnane JM, Balko JM. Rationale for targeting the Ras/MAPK pathway in triple-negative breast cancer. Discov Med. 2014;17(95):275–83.
8. Wright KL, Adams JR, Liu JC, et al. Ras signaling is a key determinant for metastatic dissemination and poor survival of luminal breast Cancer patients. Cancer Res. 2015;75 (22):4960–72.
9. Park K, Han S, Shin E, Kim HJ, Kim JY. EGFR gene and protein expression in breast cancers. Eur J Surg Oncol. 2007;33(8):956–60.
10. Howell SJ, Hockenhull K, Salih Z, Evans DG. Increased risk of breast cancer in neurofibromatosis type 1: current insights. Breast Cancer (Dove Med Press). 2017;9:531–6.
11. Suárez-Cabrera C, Quintana RM, Bravo A, et al. A transposon-based analysis reveals RASA1 is involved in triple-negative breast cancer. Cancer Res. 2017;77(6):1357–68.
12. Olsen SN, Wronski A, Castaño Z, et al. Loss of RasGAP tumor suppressors underlies the aggressive nature of luminal B breast cancers. Cancer Discov. 2017;7(2):202–17.
13. Koh M, Yong HY, Kim ES, Son H, Jeon YR, Hwang JS, et al. A novel role for flotillin-1 in H-Ras-regulated breast cancer aggressiveness. Int J Cancer. 2016;138(5):1232–45.
14. Shin I, Kim S, Song H, Kim HR, Moon A. H-Ras-specific activation of Rac-MKK3/6-p38 pathway: its critical role in invasion and migration of breast epithelial cells. J Biol Chem. 2005;280(15):14675–83.
15. Kim MS, Lee EJ, Kim HR, Moon A. p38 kinase is a key signaling molecule for H-Ras-induced cell motility and invasive phenotype in human breast epithelial cells. Cancer Res. 2003;63 (17):5454–61.

16. Moon A, Kim MS, Kim TG, et al. H-ras, but not N-ras, induces an invasive phenotype in human breast epithelial cells: a role for MMP-2 in the H-ras-induced invasive phenotype. Int J Cancer. 2000;85(2):176–81.
17. Koh M, Woo Y, Valiathan RR, et al. Discoidin domain receptor 1 is a novel transcriptional target of ZEB1 in breast epithelial cells undergoing H-Ras-induced epithelial to mesenchymal transition. Int J Cancer. 2015;136(6):E508–20.
18. Stacey DW, Kung HF. Transformation of NIH 3T3 cells by microinjection of Ha-ras p21 protein. Nature. 1984;310(5977):508–11.
19. Feramisco JR, Gross M, Kamata T, Rosenberg M, Sweet RW. Microinjection of the oncogene form of the human H-ras (T-24) protein results in rapid proliferation of quiescent cells. Cell. 1984;38(1):109–17.
20. McCarthy SA, Samuels ML, Pritchard CA, Abraham JA, McMahon M. Rapid induction of heparin-binding epidermal growth factor/diphtheria toxin receptor expression by Raf and Ras oncogenes. Genes Dev. 1995;9(16):1953–64.
21. Gangarosa LM, Sizemore N, Graves-Deal R, Oldham SM, Der CJ, Coffey RJ. A raf-independent epidermal growth factor receptor autocrine loop is necessary for Ras transformation of rat intestinal epithelial cells. J Biol Chem. 1997;272(30):18926–31.
22. Woods D, Cherwinski H, Venetsanakos E. Induction of β3-integrin gene expression by sustained activation of the Ras-regulated Raf-MEK-extracellular signal-regulated kinase signaling pathway. Mol Cell Biol. 2001;21(9):3192–205.
23. Dajee M, Tarutani M, Deng H, Cai T, Khavari PA. Epidermal Ras blockade demonstrates spatially localized Ras promotion of proliferation and inhibition of differentiation. Oncogene. 2002;21(10):1527–38.
24. Gutman A, Wasylyk C, Wasylyk B. Cell-specific regulation of oncogene-responsive sequences of the C-fos promoter. Mol Cell Biol. 1991;11(10):5381–7.
25. Urich M, Senften M, Shaw PE, Ballmer-Hofer K. A role for the small GTPase Rac in polyomavirus middle-T antigen-mediated activation of the serum response element and in cell transformation. Oncogene. 1997;14(10):1235–41.
26. Westwick JK, Cox AD, Der CJ, et al. Oncogenic Ras activates c-Jun via a separate pathway from the activation of extracellular signal-regulated kinases. Proc Natl Acad Sci U S A. 1994;91(13):6030–4.
27. Finco TS, Westwick JK, Norris JL, Beg AA, Der CJ, Baldwin AS Jr. Oncogenic Ha-Ras-induced signaling activates NF-κB transcriptional activity, which is required for cellular transformation. J Biol Chem. 1997;272(39):24113–6.
28. Filmus J, Robles AI, Shi W, Wong MJ, Colombo LL, Conti CJ. Induction of cyclin D1 overexpression by activated ras. Oncogene. 1994;9(12):3627–33.
29. Diehl JA, Cheng M, Roussel MF, Sherr CJ. Glycogen synthase kinase-3β regulates cyclin D1 proteolysis and subcellular localization. Genes Dev. 1998;12(22):3499–511.
30. Kfir S, Ehrlich M, Goldshmid A, Liu X, Kloog Y, Henis YI. Pathway- and expression level-dependent effects of oncogenic N-Ras: p27(Kip1) mislocalization by the Ral-GEF pathway and Erk-mediated interference with Smad signaling. Mol Cell Biol. 2005;25(18):8239–50.
31. Sa G, Stacey DW. P27 expression is regulated by separate signaling pathways, downstream of Ras, in each cell cycle phase. Exp Cell Res. 2004;300(2):427–39.
32. Denko N, Stringer J, Wani M, Stambrook P. Mitotic and post mitotic consequences of genomic instability induced by oncogenic Ha-ras. Somat Cell Mol Genet. 1995;21(4):241–53.
33. Knauf JA, Ouyang B, Knudsen ES, Fukasawa K, Babcock G, Fagin JA. Oncogenic RAS induces accelerated transition through G2/M and promotes defects in the G2 DNA damage and mitotic spindle checkpoints. J Biol Chem. 2006;281(7):3800–9.
34. Cox AD, Der CJ. The dark side of Ras: regulation of apoptosis. Oncogene. 2003;22 (56):8999–9006.
35. Vos MD, Ellis CA, Bell A, Birrer MJ, Clark GJ. Ras uses the novel tumor suppressor RASSF1 as an effector to mediate apoptosis. J Biol Chem. 2000;275(46):35669–72.

36. Khokhlatchev A, Rabizadeh S, Xavier R, et al. Identification of a novel Ras-regulated proapoptotic pathway. Curr Biol. 2002;12(4):253–65.
37. Ahmed MM, Sheldon D, Fruitwala MA, et al. Downregulation of PAR-4, a pro-apoptotic gene, in pancreatic tumors harboring K-ras mutation. Int J Cancer. 2008;122(1):63–70.
38. Wu L, Nam YJ, Kung G, Crow MT, Kitsis RN. Induction of the apoptosis inhibitor ARC by Ras in human cancers. J Biol Chem. 2010;285(25):19235–45.
39. Kennedy NJ, Sluss HK, Jones SN, Bar-Sagi D, Flavell RA, Davis RJ. Suppression of Ras-stimulated transformation by the JNK signal transduction pathway. Genes Dev. 2003;17(5):629–37.
40. Lei K, Nimnual A, Zong WX, et al. The Bax subfamily of Bcl2-related proteins is essential for apoptotic signal transduction by c-Jun NH(2)-terminal kinase. Mol Cell Biol. 2002;22(13):4929–42.
41. Pylayeva-Gupta Y, Grabocka E, Bar-Sagi D. RAS oncogenes: weaving a tumorigenic web. Nat Rev Cancer. 2011;11(11):761–74.
42. Jones RG, Thompson CB. Tumor suppressors and cell metabolism: a recipe for cancer growth. Genes Dev. 2009;23(5):537–48.
43. Mathupala SP, Heese C, Pedersen PL. Glucose catabolism in cancer cells. The type II hexokinase promoter contains functionally active response elements for the tumor suppressor p53. J Biol Chem. 1997;272(36):22776–80.
44. Johannessen CM, Reczek EE, James MF, Brems H, Legius E, Cichowski K. The NF1 tumor suppressor critically regulates TSC2 and mTOR. Proc Natl Acad Sci U S A. 2005;102(24):8573–8.
45. Foster KG, Fingar DC. Mammalian target of rapamycin (mTOR): conducting the cellular signaling symphony. J Biol Chem. 2010;285(19):14071–7.
46. Flier JS, Mueckler MM, Usher P, Lodish HF. Elevated levels of glucose transport and transporter messenger RNA are induced by ras or src oncogenes. Science. 1987;235(4795):1492–5.
47. Dang CV, Semenza GL. Oncogenic alterations of metabolism. Trends Biochem Sci. 1999;24(2):68–72.
48. Chen C, Pore N, Behrooz A, Ismail-Beigi F, Maity A. Regulation of glut1 mRNA by hypoxia-inducible factor-1. Interaction between H-ras and hypoxia. J Biol Chem. 2001;276(12):9519–25.
49. Guo JY, Chen HY, Mathew R, et al. Activated Ras requires autophagy to maintain oxidative metabolism and tumorigenesis. Genes Dev. 2011;25(5):460–70.
50. Lock R, Roy S, Kenific CM, et al. Autophagy facilitates glycolysis during Ras-mediated oncogenic transformation. Mol Biol Cell. 2010;22(2):165–78.
51. Grunert S, Jechlinger M, Beug H. Diverse cellular and molecular mechanisms contribute to epithelial plasticity and metastasis. Nat Rev Mol Cell Biol. 2003;4(8):657–65.
52. Smakman N, Borel Rinkes IH, Voest EE, Kranenburg O. Control of colorectal metastasis formation by K-Ras. Biochim Biophys Acta. 2005;1756(2):103–14.
53. Bondy GP, Wilson S, Chambers AF. Experimental metastatic ability of H-ras-transformed NIH3T3 cells. Cancer Res. 1985;45(12 Pt 2):6005–9.
54. Huber MA, Kraut N, Beug H. Molecular requirements for epithelial-mesenchymal transition during tumor progression. Curr Opin Cell Biol. 2005;17(5):548–58.
55. Schmidt CR, Gi YJ, Patel TA, Coffey RJ, Beauchamp RD, Pearson AS. E-cadherin is regulated by the transcriptional repressor SLUG during Ras-mediated transformation of intestinal epithelial cells. Surgery. 2005;138(2):306–12.
56. Horiguchi K, Shirakihara T, Nakano A, Imamura T, Miyazono K, Saitoh M. Role of Ras signaling in the induction of snail by transforming growth factor-β. J Biol Chem. 2009;284(1):245–53.
57. Plantefaber LC, Hynes RO. Changes in integrin receptors on oncogenically transformed cells. Cell. 1989;56(2):281–90.

58. Danen EH, Yamada KM. Fibronectin, integrins, and growth control. J Cell Physiol. 2001;189 (1):1–13.
59. Pollock CB, Shirasawa S, Sasazuki T, Kolch W, Dhillon AS. Oncogenic K-RAS is required to maintain changes in cytoskeletal organization, adhesion, and motility in colon cancer cells. Cancer Res. 2005;65(4):1244–50.
60. Campbell PM, Der CJ. Oncogenic Ras and its role in tumor cell invasion and metastasis. Semin Cancer Biol. 2004;14(2):105–14.
61. Frisch SM, Francis H. Disruption of epithelial cell-matrix interactions induces apoptosis. J Cell Biol. 1994;124(4):619–26.
62. Rosen K, Rak J, Leung T, Dean NM, Kerbel RS, Filmus J. Activated Ras prevents downregulation of Bcl-X(L) triggered by detachment from the extracellular matrix. A mechanism of Ras-induced resistance to anoikis in intestinal epithelial cells. J Cell Biol. 2000;149 (2):447–56.
63. Zondag GC, Evers EE, ten Klooster JP, Janssen L, van der Kammen RA, Collard JG. Oncogenic Ras downregulates Rac activity, which leads to increased Rho activity and epithelial-mesenchymal transition. J Cell Biol. 2000;149(4):775–82.
64. Braga VM, Betson M, Li X, Lamarche-Vane N. Activation of the small GTPase Rac is sufficient to disrupt cadherin-dependent cell-cell adhesion in normal human keratinocytes. Mol Biol Cell. 2000;11(11):3703–21.
65. Turley EA, Veiseh M, Radisky DC, Bissell MJ. Mechanisms of disease: epithelial-mesenchymal transition--does cellular plasticity fuel neoplastic progression? Nat Clin Pract Oncol. 2008;5(5):280–90.
66. Song H, Ki SH, Kim SG, Moon A. Activating transcription factor 2 mediates matrix metalloproteinase-2 transcriptional activation induced by p38 in breast epithelial cells. Cancer Res. 2006;66(21):10487–96.
67. Yong HY, Hwang JS, Son H, et al. Identification of H-Ras-specific motif for the activation of invasive signaling program in human breast epithelial cells. Neoplasia. 2011;13(2):98–107.
68. Zheng ZY, Tian L, Bu W, et al. Wild-type N-Ras, overexpressed in basal-like breast cancer, promotes tumor formation by inducing IL-8 secretion via JAK2 activation. Cell Rep. 2015;12 (3):511–24.
69. Ricoult SJ, Yecies JL, Ben-Sahra I, Manning BD. Oncogenic PI3K and K-Ras stimulate de novo lipid synthesis through mTORC1 and SREBP. Oncogene. 2016;35(10):1250–60.
70. Kim MJ, Woo SJ, Yoon CH, et al. Involvement of autophagy in oncogenic K-Ras-induced malignant cell transformation. J Biol Chem. 2011;286(15):12924–32.
71. Shalom-Feuerstein R, Plowman SJ, Rotblat B, et al. K-ras nanoclustering is subverted by overexpression of the scaffold protein galectin-3. Cancer Res. 2008;68(16):6608–16.
72. Kim RK, Suh Y, Yoo KC, et al. Activation of KRAS promotes the mesenchymal features of basal-type breast cancer. Exp Mol Med. 2015;47(1):e137.
73. Thiery JP. Epithelial-mesenchymal transitions in tumour progression. Nat Rev Cancer. 2002;2 (6):442–54.
74. Vuoriluoto K, Haugen H, Kiviluoto S, et al. Vimentin regulates EMT induction by Slug and oncogenic H-Ras and migration by governing Axl expression in breast cancer. Oncogene. 2011;30(12):1436–48.
75. Yoh KE, Regunath K, Guzman A, et al. Repression of p63 and induction of EMT by mutant Ras in mammary epithelial cells. Proc Natl Acad Sci U S A. 2016;113(41):E6107–16.
76. Remacle JE, Kraft H, Lerchner W, et al. New mode of DNA binding of multi-zinc finger transcription factors: deltaEF1 family members bind with two hands to two target sites. EMBO J. 1999;18(18):5073–84.
77. Massague J. TGF-beta signal transduction. Annu Rev Biochem. 1998;67:753–91.
78. Whitman M. Smads and early developmental signaling by the TGFbeta superfamily. Genes Dev. 1998;12:2445–62.

79. Kim ES, Kim MS, Moon A. Transforming growth factor (TGF)-beta in conjunction with H-ras activation promotes malignant progression of MCF10A breast epithelial cells. Cytokine. 2005;29(2):84–91.
80. Oft M, Akhurst RJ, Balmain A. Metastasis is driven by sequential elevation of H-ras and Smad2 levels. Nat Cell Biol. 2002;4:487–94.
81. Lehmann K, Janda E, Pierreux CE, et al. Beug H and downward J. Raf induces TGFbeta production while blocking its apoptotic but not invasive responses: a mechanism leading to increased malignancy in epithelial cells. Genes Dev. 2000;14:2610–22.
82. Kim H, Choi JA, Kim JH. Ras promotes transforming growth factor-β (TGF-β)-induced epithelial-mesenchymal transition via a leukotriene B4 receptor-2-linked cascade in mammary epithelial cells. J Biol Chem. 2014;289(32):22151–60.
83. Lin S, Yang J, Elkahloun AG, et al. Attenuation of TGF-β signaling suppresses premature senescence in a p21-dependent manner and promotes oncogenic Ras-mediated metastatic transformation in human mammary epithelial cells. Mol Biol Cell. 2012;23(8):1569–81.
84. Vasilaki E, Morikawa M, Koinuma D, et al. Ras and TGF-β signaling enhance cancer progression by promoting the ΔNp63 transcriptional program. Sci Signal. 2016;9(442):ra84.
85. Khazaie K, Schirrmacher V, Lichtner RB. EGF receptor in neoplasia and metastasis. Cancer Metastasis Rev. 1993;12(3–4):255–74.
86. Hunter T. Oncoprotein networks. Cell. 1997;88(3):333–46.
87. Blume-Jensen P, Hunter T. Oncogenic kinase signalling. Nature. 2001;411(6835):355–65.
88. Chu PY, Li TK, Ding ST, Lai IR, Shen TL. EGF-induced Grb7 recruits and promotes Ras activity essential for the tumorigenicity of Sk-Br3 breast cancer cells. J Biol Chem. 2010;285 (38):29279–85.
89. Li B, Antonyak MA, Druso JE, et al. EGF potentiated oncogenesis requires a tissue transglutaminase-dependent signaling pathway leading to Src activation. Proc Natl Acad Sci U S A. 2010;107(4):1408–13.
90. Koh MS, Moon A. Activation of H-Ras and Rac1 correlates with epidermal growth factor-induced invasion in Hs578T and MDA-MB-231 breast carcinoma cells. Biochem Biophys Res Commun. 2011;406(1):25–9.
91. Zhao B, Hu W, Kumar S, et al. The Nogo-B receptor promotes Ras plasma membrane localization and activation. Oncogene. 2017;36(24):3406–16.
92. Demetri GD, Griffin JD. Granulocyte colony-stimulating factor and its receptor. Blood. 1991;78:2791–808.
93. Park S, Kim ES, Noh DY, Hwang KT, Moon A. H-Ras-specific upregulation of granulocyte colony-stimulating factor promotes human breast cell invasion via matrix metalloproteinase-2. Cytokine. 2011;55(1):126–33.
94. Phan VT, Wu X, Cheng JH, et al. Oncogenic RAS pathway activation promotes resistance to anti-VEGF therapy through G-CSF-induced neutrophil recruitment. Proc Natl Acad Sci U S A. 2013;110(15):6079–84.
95. Rajasekharan SK, Ramen T. Ras and Ras mutations in cancer. Cent Eur J Biol. 2013;8 (7):609–24.
96. Martinelli E, De Palma R, Orditura M, De Vita F, Ciardiello F. Anti-epidermal growth factor receptor monoclonal antibodies in cancer therapy. Clin Exp Immunol. 2009;158(1):1–9.
97. Heinemann V, Stintzing S, Kirchner T, Boeck S, Jung A. Clinical relevance of EGFR- and KRAS-status in colorectal cancer patients treated with monoclonal antibodies directed against the EGFR. Cancer Treat Rev. 2009;35(3):262–71.
98. Giaccone G, Herbst RS, Manegold C, et al. Gefitinib in combination with gemcitabine and cisplatin in advanced non-small-cell lung cancer: a phase III trial–INTACT 1. J Clin Oncol. 2004;22(5):777–84.
99. Perez-Soler R, Chachoua A, Hammond LA, et al. Determinants of tumor response and survival with erlotinib in patients with non-small-cell lung cancer. J Clin Oncol. 2004;22(16):3238–47.
100. Herbst RS, Johnson DH, Mininberg E, et al. Phase I/II trial evaluating the anti-vascular endothelial growth factor monoclonal antibody bevacizumab in combination with the

HER-1/epidermal growth factor receptor tyrosine kinase inhibitor erlotinib for patients with recurrent non-small-cell lung cancer. J Clin Oncol. 2005;23(11):2544–55.
101. Cox AD, Der CJ. Farnesyltransferase inhibitors and cancer treatment: targeting simply Ras. Biochim Biophys Acta. 1997;1333(1):F51–71.
102. Reuter CW, Morgan MA, Bergmann L. Targeting the Ras signaling pathway: a rational, mechanism-based treatment for hematologic malignancies? Blood. 2000;96(5):1655–69.
103. Alsina M, Fonseca R, Wilson EF, et al. Farnesyltransferase inhibitor tipifarnib is well tolerated, induces stabilization of disease, and inhibits farnesylation and oncogenic/tumor survival pathways in patients with advanced multiple myeloma. Blood. 2004;103(9):3271–7.
104. James GL, Goldstein JL, Brown MS, et al. Benzodiazepine peptidomimetics: potent inhibitors of Ras farnesylation in animal cells. Science. 1993;260(5116):1937–42.
105. Kohl NE, Mosser SD, deSolms SJ, et al. Selective inhibition of ras-dependent transformation by a farnesyltransferase inhibitor. Science. 1993;260(5116):1934–7.
106. Kohl NE, Omer CA, Conner MW, et al. Inhibition of farnesyltransferase induces regression of mammary and salivary carcinomas in ras transgenic mice. Nat Med. 1995;1(8):792–7.
107. Lee KH, Koh M, Moon A. Farnesyl transferase inhibitor FTI-277 inhibits breast cell invasion and migration by blocking H-Ras activation. Oncol Lett. 2016;12(3):2222–6.
108. Tanaka T, Ikegami Y, Nakazawa H, et al. Low-dose Farnesyltransferase inhibitor suppresses HIF-1α and snail expression in triple-negative breast cancer MDA-MB-231 cells in vitro. J Cell Physiol. 2017;232(1):192–201.
109. Balasis ME, Forinash KD, Chen YA, et al. Combination of farnesyltransferase and Akt inhibitors is synergistic in breast cancer cells and causes significant breast tumor regression in ErbB2 transgenic mice. Clin Cancer Res. 2011;17(9):2852–62.
110. Martin LA, Head JE, Pancholi S, et al. The farnesyltransferase inhibitor R115777 (tipifarnib) in combination with tamoxifen acts synergistically to inhibit MCF-7 breast cancer cell proliferation and cell cycle progression in vitro and in vivo. Mol Cancer Ther. 2007;6 (9):2458–67.
111. Johnston SR, Hickish T, Ellis P, et al. Phase II study of the efficacy and tolerability of two dosing regimens of the farnesyl transferase inhibitor, R115777, in advanced breast cancer. J Clin Oncol. 2003;21(13):2492–9.
112. Aoki K, Ohnami S, Yoshida T. Suppression of pancreatic and colon cancer cells by antisense K-ras RNA expression vectors. Methods Mol Med. 2005;106:193–204.
113. Rotblat B, Ehrlich M, Haklai R, Kloog Y. The Ras inhibitor farnesyl thio salicylic acid (Salirasib) disrupts the spatiotemporal localization of active Ras: a potential treatment for cancer. Methods Enzymol. 2008;439:467–89.
114. Barkan B, Starinsky S, Friedman E, Stein R, Kloog Y. The Ras inhibitor farnesyl thio salicylic acid as a potential therapy for neurofibromatosis type 1. Clin Cancer Res. 2006;12 (18):5533–42.
115. Moore M, Hirte HW, Siu L, et al. Phase I study to determine the safety and pharmacokinetics of the novel Raf kinase and VEGFR inhibitor BAY 43-9006, administered for 28 days on/7 days off in patients with advanced, refractory solid tumors. Ann Oncol. 2005;16(10):1688–94.
116. Endres M, Laufs U, Huang Z, et al. Stroke protection by 3-hydroxy-3-methylglutaryl (HMG)-CoA reductase inhibitors mediated by endothelial nitric oxide synthase. Proc Natl Acad Sci U S A. 1998;95:8880–5.
117. Mc Menamin ÚC, Murray LJ, Hughes CM, Cardwell CR. Statin use and breast cancer survival: a nationwide cohort study in Scotland. BMC Cancer. 2016;16:600.
118. Wolfe AR, Debeb BG, Lacerda L, et al. Simvastatin prevents triple-negative breast cancer metastasis in pre-clinical models through regulation of FOXO3a. Breast Cancer Res Treat. 2015;154(3):495–508.
119. Lee HS, Lee SH, Lee HJ, et al. Statin use and its impact on survival in pancreatic cancer patients. Medicine (Baltimore). 2016;95(19):e3607.
120. Li G, Zheng J, Xu B, Ling J, Qiu W, Wang Y. Simvastatin inhibits tumor angiogenesis in HER2-overexpressing human colorectal cancer. Biomed Pharmacother. 2017;85:418–24.

121. Kang S, Kim ES, Moon A. Simvastatin and lovastatin inhibit breast cell invasion induced by H-Ras. Oncol Rep. 2009;21(5):1317–22.
122. Kang M, Lee KH, Lee HS, et al. Concurrent treatment with simvastatin and NF-κB inhibitor in human castration-resistant prostate cancer cells exerts synergistic anti-cancer effects via control of the NF-κB/LIN28/let-7 miRNA signaling pathway. PLoS One. 2017;12(9): e0184644.
123. Buranrat B, Senggunprai L, Prawan A, Kukongviriyapan V. Simvastatin and atorvastatin as inhibitors of proliferation and inducers of apoptosis in human cholangiocarcinoma cells. Life Sci. 2016;153:41–9.
124. Shen Y, Du Y, Zhang Y, Pan Y. Synergistic effects of combined treatment with simvastatin and exemestane on MCF-7 human breast cancer cells. Mol Med Rep. 2015;12(1):456–62.
125. Babcook MA, Sramkoski RM, Fujioka H, et al. Combination simvastatin and metformin induces G1-phase cell cycle arrest and Ripk1- and Ripk3-dependent necrosis in C4-2B osseous metastatic castration-resistant prostate cancer cells. Cell Death Dis. 2014;5:e1536.
126. Wattenberg LW. Inhibition of carcinogenesis by minor anutrient constituents of the diet. Proc Natl Acad Sci. 1990;49:173–83.
127. Dorai T, Cao YC, Dorai B, Buttyan R, Katz AE. Therapeutic potential of curcumin in human prostate cancer. Ill. Curcumin inhibits proliferation, induces apoptosis, and inhibits angiogenesis of LNCaP prostate cancer cells in vivo. Prostate. 2001;47:293–303.
128. Ramachandran C, You W. Differential sensitivity of human mammary epithelial and breast carcinoma cell lines to curcumin. Breast Cancer Res Treat. 1999;54:269–78.
129. Kim MS, Kang HJ, Moon A. Inhibition of invasion and induction of apoptosis by curcumin in H-ras-transformed MCF10A human breast epithelial cells. Arch Pharm Res. 2001;24 (4):349–54.
130. Sepp-Lorenzino L, Rosen N. A farnesyl-protein transferase inhibitor induces p21 expression and G1 block in p53 wild type tumor cells. J Biol Chem. 1998;273:20243–51.
131. Eckert LB, Repasky GA, Ulkü AS, et al. Involvement of Ras activation in human breast cancer cell signaling, invasion, and anoikis. Cancer Res. 2004;64:4585–92.
132. Yoon MJ, Kim EH, Lim JH, Kwon TK, Choi KS. Superoxide anion and proteasomal dysfunction contribute to curcumin-induced paraptosis of malignant breast cancer cells. Free Radic Biol Med. 2010;48(5):713–26.
133. Calaf GM, Echiburú-Chau C, Wen G, Balajee AS, Roy D. Effect of curcumin on irradiated and estrogen-transformed human breast cell lines. Int J Oncol. 2012;40(2):436–42.
134. Taurin S, Nimick M, Larsen L, Rosengren RJ. A novel curcumin derivative increases the cytotoxicity of raloxifene in estrogen receptor-negative breast cancer cell lines. Int J Oncol. 2016;48(1):385–98.
135. Iwai K, Suzuki T, Fujiwake H. Formation and accumulation of pungent principle of hot pepper fruits, capsaicin and its analogues, in Capsicum annuum var. annuum cv. Karayatsubusa at different growth stages after flowering. Agric Biol Chem. 1979;43:2493–8.
136. Tj S, Iwai K. Constitution of red pepper species: chemistry, biochemistry, pharmacology, and food science of the pungent principle of capsicum species. In: Brosi A, editor. The alkaloides. New York: Academic Press; 1984. p. 227–99.
137. Morre DJ, Chueh PJ, Morre DM. Capsaicin inhibits preferentially the NADH oxidase and growth of transformed cells in culture. Proc Natl Acad Sci U S A. 1995;92:1831–5.
138. Morre DJ, Sun E, Geilen C, et al. Capsaicin inhibits plasma membrane NADH oxidase and growth of human and mouse melanoma lines. Eur J Cancer. 1996;32A:1995–2003.
139. Kang SN, Chung SW, Kim TS. Capsaicin potentiates 1,25-dihydroxyvitamin D3- and all-trans retinoic acid-induced differentiation of human promyelocytic leukemia HL-60 cells. Eur J Pharmacol. 2001;420:83–90.
140. Kim JD, Kim JM, Pyo JO, et al. Capsaicin can alter the expression of tumor forming-related genes which might be followed by induction of apoptosis of a Korean stomach cancer cell line, SNU-1. Cancer Lett. 1997;120:235–41.

141. Jung MY, Kang HJ, Moon A. Capsaicin-induced apoptosis in SK-Hep-1hepatocarcinoma cells involves Bcl-2 downregulation and caspase-3 activation. Cancer Lett. 2001;165:139–45.
142. Qiao S, Li W, Tsubouchi R, Haneda M, Murakami K, Yoshino M. Involvement of peroxynitrite in capsaicin-induced apoptosis of C6 glioma cells. Neurosci Res. 2005;51:175–83.
143. Mori A, Lehmann S, O'Kelly J, et al. Capsaicin, a component of red peppers, inhibits the growth of androgen- independent, p53 mutant prostate cancer cells. Cancer Res. 2006;66:3222–9.
144. Kang HJ, Soh Y, Kim MS, et al. Roles of JNK-1 and p38 in selective induction of apoptosis by capsaicin in ras-transformed human breast epithelial cells. Int J Cancer. 2003;103(4):475–82.
145. Kim S, Moon A. Capsaicin-induced apoptosis of H-ras-transformed human breast epithelial cells is Rac-dependent via ROS generation. Arch Pharm Res. 2004;27(8):845–9.
146. Gysin S, Salt M, Young A, McCormick F. Therapeutic strategies for targeting Ras proteins. Gen Canc. 2011;2(3):359–72.
147. Wu P, Liu T, Hu Y. PI3K inhibitors for cancer therapy: what has been achieved so far? Curr Med Chem. 2009;16(8):916–30.
148. Bennett BL, Sasaki DT, Murray BW, et al. SP600125, an anthrapyrazolone inhibitor of Jun N-terminal kinase. Proc Natl Acad Sci U S A. 2001;98(24):13681–6.
149. Bachman KE, Argani P, Samuels Y, et al. The PIK3CA gene is mutated with high frequency in human breast cancers. Cancer Biol Ther. 2004;3(8):772–5.
150. Feng M, Bao Y, Li Z, et al. RASAL2 activates RAC1 to promote triple-negative breast cancer progression. J Clin Invest. 2014;124(12):5291–304.
151. McLaughlin SK, Olsen SN, Dake B, et al. The RasGAP gene, RASAL2, is a tumor and metastasis suppressor. Cancer Cell. 2013;24(3):365–78.
152. Liu M, Bryant MS, Chen J, et al. Antitumor activity of SCH 66336, an orally bioavailable tricyclic inhibitor of farnesyl protein transferase, in human tumor xenograft models and wap-ras transgenic mice. Cancer Res. 1998;58(21):4947–56.
153. Van Cutsem E, van de Velde H, Karasek P, et al. Phase III trial of gemcitabine plus tipifarnib compared with gemcitabine plus placebo in advanced pancreatic cancer. J Clin Oncol. 2004;22 (8):1430–8.
154. Cox AD, Fesik SW, Kimmelman AC, Luo J, Der CJ. Drugging the undruggable RAS: mission possible? Nat Rev Drug Discov. 2014;13(11):828–51.
155. Head J, Johnston SR. New targets for therapy in breast cancer: farnesyltransferase inhibitors. Breast Cancer Res. 2004;6(6):262–8.
156. Ostrem JM, Peters U, Sos ML, Wells JA, Shokat KM. K-Ras(G12C) inhibitors allosterically control GTP affinity and effector interactions. Nature. 2013;503(7477):548–51.
157. Athuluri-Divakar SK, Vasquez-Del Carpio R, Dutta K, et al. A small molecule RAS-mimetic disrupts RAS association with effector proteins to block signaling. Cell. 2016;165(3):643–55.
158. Shin SM, Choi DK, Jung K, et al. Antibody targeting intracellular oncogenic Ras mutants exerts anti-tumour effects after systemic administration. Nat Commun. 2017;8:15090.

Chapter 5
Epigenetic Regulation in Breast Cancer

Hye Jin Nam and Sung Hee Baek

Abstract Aberrant epigenetic alteration has been associated with development of various cancers, including breast cancer. Since epigenetic modifications such as DNA methylation and histone modification are reversible, epigenetic enzymes, including histone modifying enzymes and DNA methyltransferases, emerge as attractive targets for cancer therapy. Although epi-drugs targeting histone deacetylation or DNA methylation have received FDA approval for cancer therapy, a very modest anti-tumor activity has been observed with monotherapy in clinical studies of breast cancer. To improve efficacy of epi-drugs in breast cancer, combination of epi-drugs with other therapies currently has been investigated. Additionally, basic researches to elucidate molecular causes of cancer should be extensively and intensively conducted in order to find novel epigenetic druggable targets. In this chapter, we summarize how epigenetic regulation affects the development of breast cancer and how to control cancer phenotype by modulating abnormal epigenetic modifications, and then suggest future research directions in epigenetics for breast cancer treatment.

Keywords Epigenetics · Post-translational modification (PTM) · Reptin · Pontin · RORα · LSD1 · Epigenetic drug

---

H. J. Nam
Korea Research Institute of Chemical Technology, Daejeon, Republic of Korea

S. H. Baek (✉)
Seoul National University, Seoul, Republic of Korea
e-mail: sbaek@snu.ac.kr

D.-Y. Noh et al. (eds.), *Translational Research in Breast Cancer*, Advances in Experimental Medicine and Biology 1187,
https://doi.org/10.1007/978-981-32-9620-6_5

5.1 Introduction

Epigenetics refers to heritable changes in gene expression without altering DNA sequence. DNA methylation, one of the well-characterized modifications in epigenetic regulation, is written by DNA methyltransferases (DNMTs) and leads to gene silencing. Since DNA methylation patterns are different in cancer compared to normal counterpart, many researchers have studied how DNA methylation patterns in cancer can be restored to those in normal counterpart in order to treat cancer. Especially in breast cancer cells, DNA methylation levels are high in the loci of proapoptotic genes (HOXA5, TMS1), cell cycle inhibitor genes (p16, RASSF1A), and DNA repair genes (BRCA1), which are related to inappropriate gene silencing [1–3].

Post-translational modification of histones also affects chromatin structure and function, leading to altered gene expression. Since DNA is packaged with histone H2A, H2B, H3, H4 octamer to form chromatin, post-translational modifications of histone tails alter chromatin structure and induce recruitment of coactivators or corepressors complex [4]. For example, histone lysine acetylation reduces the binding affinity between histone and DNA by neutralizing the positive charge on histones, thereby creating more open and accessible chromatin structure. In addition to acetylation, gene expression is controlled by various post-translational modifications such as methylation, ubiquitination, phosphorylation, and SUMOylation [5]. Among them, histone methylation has emerged as an important mechanism that regulates chromatin structure and function. Unlike acetylation, histone methylation can either activate or repress transcription, depending on the locations and degrees (mono-, di-, and tri-methylation). For instance, methylation on H3K4 is associated with transcriptional activation, whereas H3K9 methylation is associated with transcriptional repression [4]. Epigenetic enzymes also control gene expression by modulating post-translational modifications of non-histone proteins as well as histones. How post-translational modifications of non-histone proteins control gene expression and ultimately regulate cancer phenotype are summarized and discussed in this review. Since transcriptional dysregulations and altered epigenetic functions are observed in many types of cancers, including breast cancer, modulating abnormal enzymatic activity of epigenetic enzymes in cancer is expected to be an effective cancer therapy.

5.2 Review of Roles of Epigenetic Enzymes in Cancer

Among various post-translational modifications, we have focused on how lysine methylation or ubiquitination of proteins regulates breast cancer progression or suppression depending on various signals. In this section, we describe how epigenetic regulation affects breast cancer progression or suppression.

5.2.1 Methylation of Chromatin Remodeling Factors in Breast Cancer

Reptin and Pontin are chromatin remodeling factors that possess both AAA+ ATPase and DNA helicase activities [6]. Reptin and Pontin perform a variety of functions, including transcriptional regulation, chromatin remodeling, DNA damage signaling, and telomerase biogenesis processes [7–10]. Since Reptin and Pontin form a complex and usually work together, comparing how Reptin and Pontin are differentially regulated by upstream signal is helpful to understand their roles in breast cancer.

5.2.2 Methylation of Reptin Chromatin Remodeling Factor

Reptin is methylated on lysine 67 site by G9a, a histone H3K9 methyltransferase [11]. Hypoxic signal induces Reptin methylation by G9a in breast cancer. Hypoxia (a state of low oxygen) occurs under several physiological and pathological conditions, such as ischemia and solid tumors [12, 13]. Many hypoxic responses are mediated by hypoxia-inducible factor 1 (HIF-1), a heterodimeric transcription factor that is comprised of an oxygen-regulated α subunit (HIF-1α or HIF-2α) and a constitutively expressed β subunit (HIF-1β) [14]. Under low oxygen conditions, stabilized HIF-1α translocates to the nucleus and activates target gene expression through binding to hypoxia response element (HRE, RCGTG DNA sequence). HIF-1 regulates numerous downstream target genes involved in tumor angiogenesis, glycolysis, invasion, metabolism, and survival [15, 16]. Since hypoxia is induced in many types of solid tumors, Reptin methylation by hypoxic conditions turns out to affect tumor progression. Using genome-wide analysis from RNAs isolated in breast cancer cells, Reptin methylation-dependent target genes that are involved in regulating tumor growth properties are identified having HIF-1 as a major transcription factor of these genes. At early time in hypoxia, methylated Reptin fails to be recruited to the target promoters, whereas at late time in hypoxia, methylated Reptin recruitment with concurrent reduction in RNA polymerase II recruitment and induction in HDAC1 recruitment is observed, indicating that Reptin methylation is crucial for negative regulation of hypoxic responsive genes via binding to HDAC1. In vitro cell migration assay and in vivo xenograft assay using human breast cancer cells reveal that Reptin methylation is crucial for negative regulation of tumorigenic properties, such as proliferation and migration. These findings identify an important signaling axis by which HIF-1 transcription activity can be repressed by Reptin methylation, thereby affecting metabolic, cell death, and survival pathways that are important for the development and progression of breast cancer. Although previous studies by many other researchers have extended lysine methylation of histone to that of non-histone proteins, underlying molecular mechanisms of how upstream signal induces lysine methylation and modulates downstream target genes have not been extensively elucidated. This study uncovers not only molecular mechanism but also in vivo functions of hypoxia-dependent Reptin methylation in breast cancer, and is recognized as a milestone study revealing the biological roles of methylation of non-histone proteins induced by upstream signal.

5.2.3 Methylation of Pontin Chromatin Remodeling Factor

To identify methyltransferase that causes Pontin methylation, in vitro methylation assay using various methyltransferases is conducted, and G9a and GLP turned out to induce Pontin methylation [17]. Since G9a protein levels are increased by hypoxia [11], protein levels of GLP are induced as in the case of G9a under hypoxic conditions, and increased expression levels of G9a and GLP cause Pontin methylation. In contrast to Reptin methylation, Pontin methylation is responsible for transcriptional activation of a subset of hypoxia-responsive genes by recruiting p300 acetyltransferase to the target promoters. In addition, Pontin methylation enhances proliferative and invasive potential of breast cancer cells, and *Ets1* gene is important for exerting cell motility upon hypoxia. These findings shed light on a potential therapeutic targeting of Pontin methylation in tumor progression and metastasis upon hypoxia.

Although Pontin and Reptin share high structural homology, they have distinct functions in regulating their specific target genes as a coactivator and as a corepressor, respectively [8, 9, 18]. Hypoxia-induced G9a methylates both Reptin and Pontin, but the outcome for cancer cell mobility and growth is in the opposite direction. The overall data suggest that Pontin methylation is induced at an early time point in hypoxia to promote HIF-1α-dependent transcriptional activation, whereas Reptin methylation is induced at a later time point for negative regulation (Fig. 5.1).

5.2.4 Methylation-Dependent Degradation of Transcription Factors in Breast Cancer

5.2.4.1 Methylation-Dependent Degradation of Retinoic Acid-Related Orphan Nuclear Receptor α (RORα).

RORα is a member of the orphan nuclear receptor family for which no cognate ligands have been identified thus far [19]. RORα inhibits colon cancer growth, enhances p53 stability, and reduces the migration and invasiveness of androgen-independent prostate cancer [20–22]. These findings suggest that RORα plays a critical role in tumor suppression. Enhancer of zeste homolog 2 (EZH2), a SET domain-containing protein is responsible for histone H3K27 methylation and forms a polycomb group repressive complex 2 (PRC2) with EED and SUZ12 [23–

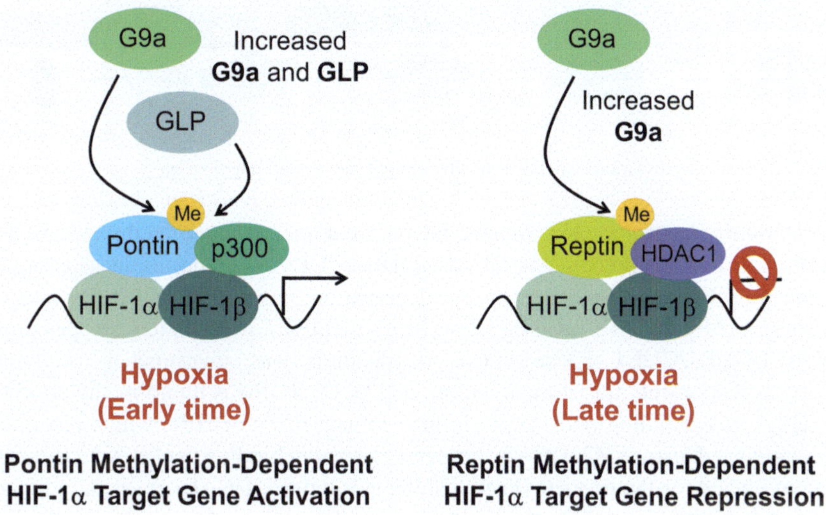

Fig. 5.1 Distinct roles of Reptin and Pontin methylation in hypoxia

25]. EZH2 plays an important role not only in stem cell development but also in cancer cell proliferation. It is reported that overexpression of EZH2 in breast and prostate cancers correlates with poor prognosis [26, 27]. Since upregulation of EZH2 in cancer induces abnormal epigenetic changes in histone, it is predicted that abnormal methylation could be induced on non-histone substrates of EZH2 and finally affect cancer phenotype. To find non-histone substrates of EZH2, the substrate specificity of EZH2 for histones was compared to non-histone proteins. Through in silico screening of proteins having similar amino acid sequence to histone H3K27 that is methylated by EZH2 (R-K-S sequence), RORα was selected for further study. RORα is mono-methylated on K38 site by EZH2 [28]. To identify the functional consequence of the EZH2-mediated RORα methylation, RORα protein and mRNA levels in WT and EZH2-deficient ($Ezh2^{-/-}$) mouse embryonic fibroblasts (MEFs) were compared. The mRNA levels of RORα were not affected by EZH2, whereas the protein levels of RORα in $Ezh2^{-/-}$ MEFs were significantly higher than those in WT MEFs. Additionally, reconstitution of EZH2 WT in $Ezh2^{-/-}$ MEFs reduced RORα protein expression levels, whereas EZH2 enzymatic inactive mutant failed to do so, indicating that RORα methylation by EZH2 induces its proteasomal degradation. RORα-interacting proteins were identified in the presence of MG132, an inhibitor of proteasomal degradation. DDB1 and DCAF1 were identified, which were previously reported to be components of a CUL4 E3 ligase-containing complex, as binding partners of RORα. Knockdown of DDB1 or DCAF1 induced ubiquitin-dependent RORα degradation, indicating that these CUL4-binding proteins are highly involved in RORα methylation-dependent degradation. Since DCAF1 has putative chromo domain which can recognize methylated proteins, it is hypothesized that methylated RORα is degraded by DCAF1/DDB1/CUL4

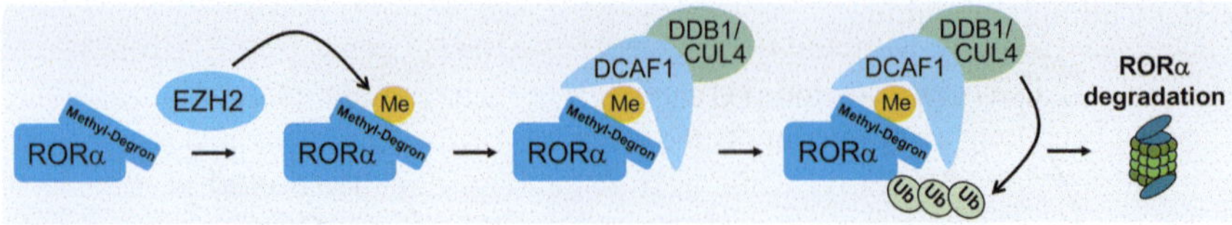

Fig. 5.2 Mono-methylation-dependent RORα ubiquitination and degradation

E3 ubiquitin ligase complex. Indeed, DCAF1 recognized mono-methylated RORα through its chromo domain and DCAF1/DDB1/CUL4 E3 ubiquitin ligase complex induced RORα methylation-dependent degradation. Given that RORα degradation is triggered by DCAF1 binding, how histone H3K27 methylation escapes from DCAF1/DDB1/CUL4 E3-dependent degradation was investigated. Although EZH2 is responsible for tri-methylation in H3K27, RORα is mono-methylation by EZH2. Unlike binding pockets of chromo domain of Pc or HP1, which recognize tri-methylated histone H3, DCAF1 possesses a smaller binding pocket, which cannot accommodate for the tri-methylated histone H3. Indeed, DCAF1 reads only mono-methylated RORα peptide but not H3K27 tri-methylated peptide despite their R-K-S sequence similarity. As it has been reported that EZH2 is overexpressed and oncogenic in breast cancer [26], whether there is an inverse correlation between EZH2 and RORα in breast cancer and whether introduction of RORα to breast cancer ultimately inhibits cancer cell growth are explored. The inverse correlation between EZH2 and RORα expression was found in breast tumor tissue specimens compared to the normal counterpart. RORα protein levels are very low in tumors with high levels of EZH2, strongly supporting the idea that elevated levels of EZH2 in tumors might facilitate RORα methylation-dependent degradation. Furthermore, overexpression of RORα, knockdown of DCAF1, or treatment with DZNep, an inhibitor of EZH2, in breast cancer cells diminish anchorage-independent cancer cell growth.

Although phosphorylation-dependent ubiquitination is well known for the regulation of protein stability, methylation-triggering ubiquitination is not fully understood. DCAF1 has a chromo domain with a restricted pocket size such that only mono-methylated substrate can bind (Fig. 5.2). By understanding the mechanism by which mono-methylation of substrate can serve as a mark for protein degradation, it has been proposed that a post-translational modification can modulate protein turnover, gene expression, and ultimately cancer progression.

5.2.4.2 Dynamic Regulation of HIF-1α Stability by Methylation and Demethylation

In order to prompt adaption to hypoxia, HIF-1α protein level is tightly regulated by post-translational modification. The primary post-translational modification of HIF-1α is hydroxylation in the cytoplasm by prolyl hydroxylase domain (PHD)-containing protein 1/2/3, which is recognized and degraded by von Hippel-Lindau

(VHL)-Culllin2 ubiquitin E3 ligase complex under normoxic conditions [29–33]. Since PHDs use oxygen as a cofactor, low oxygen levels reduce enzymatic activity of PHDs, leading to HIF-1α stabilization. Besides, HIF-1α protein stability is controlled by other means of regulation such as SUMOylation, acetylation, and phosphorylation [34–36]. Near the lysine 32 site in HIF-1α amino acids sequences, a SET7/9 methyltransferase recognition motif designated by [K/R]-[S/T/A]-K (methylated lysine site is underlined) is found. Indeed, HIF-1α methylation occurs on lysine 32 site in the nucleus by SET7/9 and leads to HIF-1α degradation, which is independent of the VHL-dependent cytosolic destabilization of HIF-1α [37]. Lysine-specific demethylase 1 (LSD1) is identified as a HIF-1α binding protein in the presence of MG132. HIF-1α protein levels are significantly decreased in *Lsd1*-deficient MEFs compared to WT MEFs in hypoxia. Reconstitution of LSD1 WT, but not enzymatic inactive LSD1 mutant, in *Lsd1*-deficient MEFs restores HIF-1α protein levels, suggesting that LSD1 demethylase activity is required for regulating HIF-1α stability. The physiological significance of this mechanism was evaluated with a $Hif1a^{KA/KA}$ methylation-defective knock-in mouse model. These mice are normal from birth until adulthood and largely indistinguishable from their WT littermates in viability, growth, and fertility. The distinct phenotype was observed after DMOG injection to eliminate the hydroxylation effects or mimic hypoxic conditions. $Hif1a^{KA/KA}$ knock-in mouse display increases hematocrit, red blood cell count, and hemoglobin levels. HIF-1α target genes involved in angiogenesis, glucose metabolism, and erythrocytosis are upregulated in $Hif1a^{KA/KA}$ knock-in mouse by elevated protein expression levels of HIF-1α. Both renal and tumor-associated angiogenesis are significantly increased in $Hif1a^{KA/KA}$ knock-in mouse along with elevated expression level of VEGF. Another intriguing characteristic of $Hif1a^{KA/KA}$ knock-in cells and mice is an increased tendency for tumorigenesis. Cell migration and colony formation ability of $Hif1a^{KA/KA}$ MEFs are enhanced due to higher expression levels of HIF-1α protein. To identify in vivo function of HIF-1α methylation in human breast cancer, MDA-MB231 cells stably expressing either HIF-1α WT or K32A mutant were injected subcutaneously into athymic nude mice. Methylation-resistant HIF-1α K32A mutant-expressing cells result in the increased tumor formation, weight, and volume. To determine whether the identified mechanism has any relevance to human cancers, HIF-1α somatic mutations in human cancers are examined. Although a mutation of HIF-1α at the methylation site is not detected in the database, mutations near the K32 methylation site such as S28Y and R30Q HIF-1α mutants in human cancers are found. Indeed, S28Y and R30Q are highly resistant to methylation by SET7/9 and following methylation-dependent degradation. How HIF-1α is regulated in physiological and pathological conditions by its methylation using in vitro cell-based assay, in vivo mouse model, and database of cancer patient mutations is summarized (Fig. 5.3).

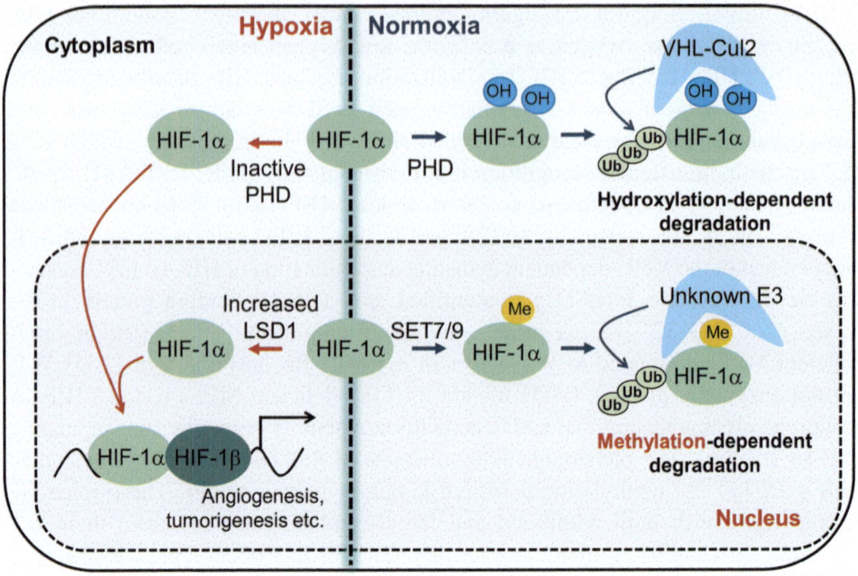

Fig. 5.3 Schematic model of regulation of HIF-1α stability by post-translational modification

5.2.4.3 Ubiquitination of Important Modulators in Breast Cancer

Many proteins implicated in tumorigenesis and metastasis show high or low expression levels in breast cancer. Therefore, properties of cancer cell can be changed by modulating the expression of these tumor promoting proteins, that are good candidate targets for cancer therapy. In this section, how stability of proteins involved in tumorigenesis or metastasis of breast cancer are regulated is summarized.

5.2.4.4 Ubiquitination of Brest Cancer Metastasis Suppressor 1 (BRMS1)

BRMS1 functions as an inhibitor of metastasis without affecting tumorigenesis in breast cancer, bladder cancer, and melanomas [38, 39]. However, the detailed mechanism on how BRMS1 protein stability is controlled remained unclear. To elucidate the regulatory mechanism of BRMS1, BRMS1 complex purification was conducted. As complex components, Cul3 and SPOP were identified [40]. SPOP, Speckle-type POZ protein acts as an adaptor which recruits several substrates to Cul3 for degradation [41, 42]. Indeed, SPOP overexpression increased the binding between BRMS1 and Cul3, suggesting that SPOP mediates interaction between Cul3 and BRMS1. To clarify, three different mutants of Cul3, SPOP, and BRMS1 were generated. Cul3 Y62G mutant loses its binding affinity to SPOP. SPOP D130A mutant failed to bind substrates. Since putative SPOP binding consensus sequences

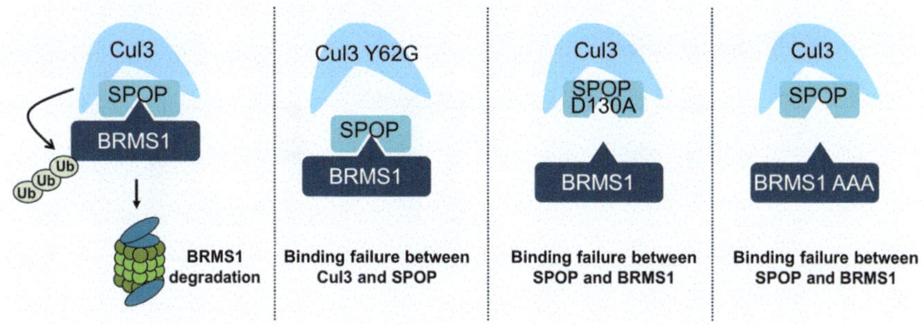

Fig. 5.4 SPOP-Cul3 E3 ligase complex for BRMS1 degradation

in BRMS1 (residues 189-193, GSSRS amino acids sequences) were reported, SPOP binding consensus sequences were changed to GSAAA to block binding to SPOP. SPOP mediates interaction between Cul3 and BRMS1 and regulates ubiquitin-dependent degradation of BRMS1 (Fig. 5.4). Normal breast cells show high expression levels of BRMS1 protein but low expression levels of Cul3-SPOP protein, whereas breast cancer cell lines display opposite expression patterns between them. This suggests that downregulation of BRMS1 by Cul3-SPOP has biological significances in breast cancer. Furthermore, SPOP-mediated BRMS1 protein stability altered gene expression patterns associated with metastasis. Therefore, blocking Cul3-SPOP-mediated degradation of BRMS1 could be a new therapeutic strategy for the treatment of metastatic breast cancer.

5.2.4.5 Bcl3-Dependent Stabilization of CtBP1 for Breast Cancer Progression

Bcl3 is a proto-oncogene as a member of IκB family, and its expression levels are elevated in many cancers, including breast cancer [43, 44]. Bcl3 confers a survival advantage to cancer cells due to its anti-apoptotic functions [45]. Since Bcl3 is critical for cancer cell survival, Bcl3-interacting partners that contribute to the proto-oncogenic function of Bcl3 were searched for. Through Bcl3-complex purification and LC-MS/MS analysis, CtBP1 exerting anti-apoptotic effects was identified as a binding molecule. Intriguingly, both Bcl3 and CtBP1 protein expression levels were higher in various breast cancer cell lines and breast cancer patient samples, but lower in normal breast cell and normal breast tissue counterparts, suggesting the biological significance of their positive correlations in breast cancer [46]. As a molecular mechanism for how mutual Bcl3 and CtBP1 expression is regulated, Bcl3 blocks CtBP1 ubiquitination through binding between Bcl3 and CtBP1, resulting in CtBP1 stabilization (Fig. 5.5). Since Bcl3 possesses a PXDLS/R sequence, a consensus motif that allows to associate with CtBP1, a Bcl3 binding mutant, in which PVDLR sequence is substituted with PVASR sequence to clarify the importance of mutual binding was generated. Although the E3 ligase complex to mediate Bcl3 degradation

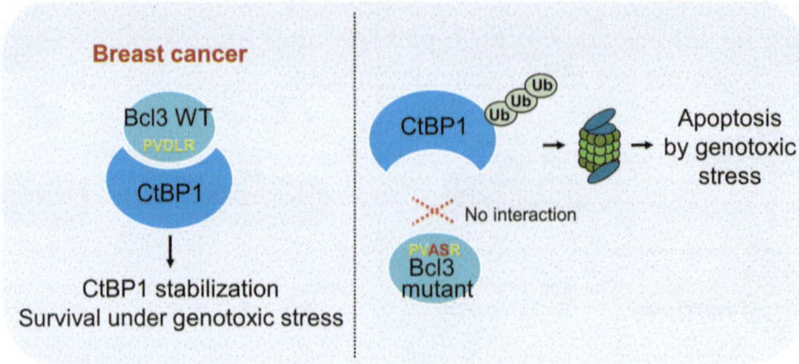

Fig. 5.5 Stabilization of CtBP1 through interaction with Bcl3

was not found, binding between Bcl3 and CtBP1 turns out to contribute CtBP1 stabilization. In addition, apoptotic genes which are dependent on Bcl3-CtBP1 binding were determined by comparing the effects of Bcl3 WT or mutant form under genotoxic stress. Introduction of Bcl3 WT to the cell escapes from apoptosis, whereas Bcl3 binding mutant-expressing cells failed to do it due to unstable CtBP1. These findings provide a novel link between two anti-apoptotic molecules, Bcl3 and CtBP1, and their biological significance in breast cancer. Given that elevated levels of Bcl3 have been reported in other human cancers [47, 48], it is tempting to speculate that combinatorial proto-oncogenic role of Bcl3 and CtBP1 might be applied to other types of cancers.

5.2.4.6 Transcriptional Regulation by Histone Demethylase in Breast Cancer

RORα has four different isoforms in human by alternative splicing. These isoforms have common DNA binding domain, but have different N-terminal domains (NTD) which confers different DNA binding specificities and transcriptional activities [49]. Among isoforms of RORα, only RORα2 interacts with LSD1 demethylase through NTD of RORα2 [50]. LSD1 activates RORα2-mediated transcription through its demethylase activity. Since RORα2 binds to a distinct DNA sequence (RORα2E:WWAWNTAGGTCA) as compared to other RORα isoforms, genes harboring RORα2E in the promoter were searched from the whole genome of human and mouse to identify RORα2-dependent target genes. Nineteen genes were found to be the common genes harboring RORα2E both in human and mouse. Among them, it was validated that CTNND1 gene was activated by cooperation of RORα2 and LSD1. Since CTNND1 induces cell migration and invasion, regulating RORα2 levels in breast cancer affects cell migration or invasion mediated by CTNND1. Indeed, knockdown of RORα2 reduced the migration potential of breast cancer cells, while overexpression of RORα2 increased cell migration. Protein levels of RORα2 and LSD1 are significantly elevated in human breast cancer patients and many breast cancer cell lines. This study suggests that RORα2 and LSD1 may be powerful therapeutic targets for human breast cancer.

5.3 Current Evidence and Concepts

Dysregulation of epigenetic enzymes and the subsequent aberrant epigenetic modifications are highly associated with cancer progression and development. In addition, the reversibility of epigenetic modifications makes epigenetic enzymes more attractive therapeutic targets of cancer. Therapeutic strategies for restoring the abnormal epigenetic modifications in cancers are currently under preclinical and clinical investigations. Although methylation of histone and non-histone proteins has emerged as attractive epigenetic drug targets for cancer treatment, these inhibitors of methylation-related enzymes are currently under development. In the near future, epi-drugs targeting histone methylation–related enzymes are expected to be preclinical or clinical trials to treat breast cancer. Epi-drugs, targeting DNA methylation (DNMT inhibitors) or histone acetylation (HDAC inhibitors), are currently in clinical trials or United States Food and Drug Administration (FDA)-approved. In this section, the efficacy and mechanism of action of several DNMT inhibitors and HDAC inhibitors for cancer treatment will be discussed.

5.3.1 DNA Methyltransferase Inhibitors

The best-studied epigenetic alterations in cancer are the changes in DNA methylation that occur within CpG islands. Abnormal methylation in CpG island is observed in various cancers. Besides, recurrent mutations in DNMT3A, which functions as a de novo DNA methyltransferase, are observed in about 25% of patients with acute myeloid leukemia [51]. Two well-known DNMT inhibitors are azacitidine (5azaC, marketed as Vidaza) and decitabine (5azadC, marketed as Dacogen), which are chemical analogs of cytidine, a nucleotide in DNA [52]. Azacitidine is a ribonucleoside that can be incorporated into both DNA and RNA. In contrast, decitabine is a deoxyribonucleoside, which can only be incorporated into DNA. In animal experiments, treatment with azacitidine results in tumor size reduction in xenograft mice transplanted with breast cancer cells or patient-derived tumors [53]. Decitabine treatment also reduces tumor size in animals with orthotopically implanted breast cancer cells [54]. Both are approved by FDA for the treatment of myelodysplastic syndrome.

5.3.2 *HDAC Inhibitors*

HDACs are subdivided into four major classes, depending on sequence homology: class I (HDAC1-3 and HDAC8), class II (HDAC4-7 and HDAC9-10), class III (sirtuin 1-7), class VI (HDAC11) [4]. Since class I, II and IV HDACs require a zinc metal ion, HDAC inhibitors chelate the zinc ion to block HDACs catalytic activity. Among several HDAC inhibitors, vorinostat and romidepsin were granted FDA approval for clinical use in patients with cutaneous T cell lymphoma [55, 56]. Since treatment with HDAC inhibitors showed antitumor effects on various cancer both in vivo and in vitro [57, 58], HDAC inhibitors could be used clinically in a broad range of tumors including breast cancer.

5.3.3 *Efficacy of DNMT Inhibitors or HDAC Inhibitors in Breast Cancer*

The efficacy of DNMT inhibitors and HDAC inhibitors in breast cancer was evaluated in clinical phase I and II studies [59]. Treatment with epi-drugs in breast cancer shows very limited anti-tumor efficacy. Epi-drugs monotherapy is effective in only 10% of breast cancer patients, suggesting that monotherapy is not suitable for breast cancer treatment. However, a combination of epi-drug with cytotoxic therapies or targeted therapies, such as ER-targeted therapy, improved progression-free survival and overall survival in phase I and II studies [59]. Therefore, current clinical trials mainly focus on the combination of epi-drugs with conventional therapies.

5.4 Future Research Direction

Our understanding of epigenetics has dramatically expanded over the last few years with the advancement of global proteomics and whole genome sequencing technologies. Next generation sequencing (NGS) technologies such as chromatin immunoprecipitation-sequencing (ChIP-seq), RNA-seq, and GRO-seq have revealed a new insight of the epigenome and transcriptome [60]. These quantitative methods have allowed us to generate comprehensive epigenetic maps with gene expression patterns including histone modifications, DNA modifications, RNA modifications, and recruitment of transcription factors/cofactors and chromatin modifiers. In addition, recent technological advances in labeling methods of mass spectrometry (MS) such as Stable Isotope Labeling by Amino acids in Cell culture (SILAC), Isobaric Tags for Relative and Absolute Quantification (ITRAQ), Isotope-Coded Affinity Tag (ICAT), and Tandem Mass Tag (TMT) have enabled quantitative measurement of proteins expression and modifications [61]. Deep sequencing of epigenome and quantitative measurement of proteome would reveal the fundamental causes of epigenetic abnormalities in cancer and enable the development of novel potent epigenetic drugs.

Recently, small molecules targeting the BET family (BRD2, BRD3, BRD4, and testis-specific BRDT) have emerged as new epigenetic drugs. BET family recognizes and binds acetylated lysine through bromodomain and plays important roles in transcriptional elongation and cell cycle progression. The efficacy of BET inhibitors was initially explored in NUT-midline carcinoma [62] and hepatological malignancies [63–66]. Later on, the anti-tumor activity of BET inhibitors in other solid tumors like prostate, non-small cell lung cancer, pancreatic, and breast cancer was evaluated [67–70] in preclinical research. In breast cancer, BET inhibitors show the efficacy in triple negative breast cancer (TNBC) alone, in combination with chemotherapies or PLK1 inhibitors, or in resistance to conventional therapies [71]. However, since these researches are currently pre-clinical, the efficacy of BET inhibitors in breast cancer should be confirmed in clinical settings.

Nowadays, cancer immunotherapy has been actively and intensively investigated to cure various cancers. Although cancer immunotherapy is a very powerful and effective method to cure cancers, the efficacy of this therapy is limited in some types of cancer. For instance, about 15–20% of advanced non-small cell lung cancer (NSCLC) patients, 30–40% of advanced melanoma patients, 20–30% renal cell carcinoma patients, 30% bladder urothelial carcinoma patients, and 80–90% Hodgkin's lymphoma patients showed effective responses to PD-1 blockade monotherapy [72]. Therefore, applying and expanding cancer immunotherapy in more types of cancer is considered to be an important breakthrough in cancer treatment. Recently, remarkable two studies were reported that T cell exhaustion, a state of impaired effector function, is highly associated with extensive changes in chromatin, especially enhancer and transcription factor binding regions [73, 74]. Since T cell exhaustion occurs in cancer by persistent antigen stimulation, reinvigoration of exhausted T cell contributes to treatment of cancer through improving its effector functions [75]. Although blocking immune checkpoint molecules (PD-L1, PD-1) can reinvigorate exhausted T cell, reinvigorated T cell became reexhausted if antigen concentration remains high due to distinct epigenetic profile [73]. Since successful cancer immunotherapies might be determined by the degree of epigenetic changes in T cells, combination treatment with epigenetic drug is expected to enable the application of a broad spectrum of immunotherapies. In the near future, more interesting and attractive targets for epigenetic drugs to improve cancer immunotherapies would be provided by intensive biological studies and clinical trials.

5.5 Summary

Extensive studies on how epigenetic modifications occur during breast cancer progression will help to understand the cause of breast cancer and lead to the development of powerful epi-drugs to treat cancer.

References

1. Esteller M. CpG island hypermethylation and tumor suppressor genes: a booming present, a brighter future. Oncogene. 2002;21(35):5427–40.
2. Jones PA, Baylin SB. The fundamental role of epigenetic events in cancer. Nat Rev Genet. 2002;3(6):415–28.
3. Radpour R, Barekati Z, Kohler C, Schumacher MM, Grussenmeyer T, Jenoe P, et al. Integrated epigenetics of human breast cancer: synoptic investigation of targeted genes, microRNAs and proteins upon demethylation treatment. PLoS One. 2011;6(11):e27355.
4. Dawson MA, Kouzarides T. Cancer epigenetics: from mechanism to therapy. Cell. 2012;150 (1):12–27.
5. Jenuwein T, Allis CD. Translating the histone code. Science. 2001;293(5532):1074–80.
6. Venteicher AS, Meng Z, Mason PJ, Veenstra TD, Artandi SE. Identification of ATPases pontin and reptin as telomerase components essential for holoenzyme assembly. Cell. 2008;132 (6):945–57.
7. Bauer A, Chauvet S, Huber O, Usseglio F, Rothbacher U, Aragnol D, et al. Pontin52 and reptin52 function as antagonistic regulators of beta-catenin signalling activity. EMBO J. 2000;19(22):6121–30.
8. Kim JH, Choi HJ, Kim B, Kim MH, Lee JM, Kim IS, et al. Roles of sumoylation of a reptin chromatin-remodelling complex in cancer metastasis. Nat Cell Biol. 2006;8(6):631–9.
9. Kim JH, Lee JM, Nam HJ, Choi HJ, Yang JW, Lee JS, et al. SUMOylation of pontin chromatin-remodeling complex reveals a signal integration code in prostate cancer cells. Proc Natl Acad Sci U S A. 2007;104(52):20793–8.
10. Shen X, Mizuguchi G, Hamiche A, Wu C. A chromatin remodelling complex involved in transcription and DNA processing. Nature. 2000;406(6795):541–4.
11. Lee JS, Kim Y, Kim IS, Kim B, Choi HJ, Lee JM, et al. Negative regulation of hypoxic responses via induced Reptin methylation. Mol Cell. 2010;39(1):71–85.
12. Graeber TG, Osmanian C, Jacks T, Housman DE, Koch CJ, Lowe SW, et al. Hypoxia-mediated selection of cells with diminished apoptotic potential in solid tumours. Nature. 1996;379 (6560):88–91.
13. Semenza GL. HIF-1 and tumor progression: pathophysiology and therapeutics. Trends Mol Med. 2002;8(4 Suppl):S62–7.
14. Bruick RK. Oxygen sensing in the hypoxic response pathway: regulation of the hypoxia-inducible transcription factor. Genes Dev. 2003;17(21):2614–23.
15. Eales KL, Hollinshead KE, Tennant DA. Hypoxia and metabolic adaptation of cancer cells. Oncogenesis. 2016;5:e190.
16. Rankin EB, Giaccia AJ. The role of hypoxia-inducible factors in tumorigenesis. Cell Death Differ. 2008;15(4):678–85.
17. Lee JS, Kim Y, Bhin J, Shin HJ, Nam HJ, Lee SH, et al. Hypoxia-induced methylation of a pontin chromatin remodeling factor. Proc Natl Acad Sci U S A. 2011;108(33):13510–5.
18. Kim JH, Kim B, Cai L, Choi HJ, Ohgi KA, Tran C, et al. Transcriptional regulation of a metastasis suppressor gene by Tip60 and beta-catenin complexes. Nature. 2005;434 (7035):921–6.
19. Giguere V. Orphan nuclear receptors: from gene to function. Endocr Rev. 1999;20(5):689–725.
20. Kim H, Lee JM, Lee G, Bhin J, Oh SK, Kim K, et al. DNA damage-induced RORalpha is crucial for p53 stabilization and increased apoptosis. Mol Cell. 2011;44(5):797–810.
21. Lee JM, Kim IS, Kim H, Lee JS, Kim K, Yim HY, et al. RORalpha attenuates Wnt/beta-catenin signaling by PKCalpha-dependent phosphorylation in colon cancer. Mol Cell. 2010;37 (2):183–95.
22. Moretti RM, Montagnani Marelli M, Motta M, Limonta P. Role of the orphan nuclear receptor ROR alpha in the control of the metastatic behavior of androgen-independent prostate cancer cells. Oncol Rep. 2002;9(5):1139–43.

23. Cao R, Wang L, Wang H, Xia L, Erdjument-Bromage H, Tempst P, et al. Role of histone H3 lysine 27 methylation in Polycomb-group silencing. Science. 2002;298(5595):1039–43.
24. Jones CA, Ng J, Peterson AJ, Morgan K, Simon J, Jones RS. The Drosophila esc and E (z) proteins are direct partners in polycomb group-mediated repression. Mol Cell Biol. 1998;18(5):2825–34.
25. Kuzmichev A, Jenuwein T, Tempst P, Reinberg D. Different EZH2-containing complexes target methylation of histone H1 or nucleosomal histone H3. Mol Cell. 2004;14(2):183–93.
26. Kleer CG, Cao Q, Varambally S, Shen R, Ota I, Tomlins SA, et al. EZH2 is a marker of aggressive breast cancer and promotes neoplastic transformation of breast epithelial cells. Proc Natl Acad Sci U S A. 2003;100(20):11606–11.
27. Varambally S, Dhanasekaran SM, Zhou M, Barrette TR, Kumar-Sinha C, Sanda MG, et al. The polycomb group protein EZH2 is involved in progression of prostate cancer. Nature. 2002;419 (6907):624–9.
28. Lee JM, Lee JS, Kim H, Kim K, Park H, Kim JY, et al. EZH2 generates a methyl degron that is recognized by the DCAF1/DDB1/CUL4 E3 ubiquitin ligase complex. Mol Cell. 2012;48 (4):572–86.
29. Bruick RK, McKnight SL. A conserved family of prolyl-4-hydroxylases that modify HIF. Science. 2001;294(5545):1337–40.
30. Epstein AC, Gleadle JM, McNeill LA, Hewitson KS, O'Rourke J, Mole DR, et al. C. elegans EGL-9 and mammalian homologs define a family of dioxygenases that regulate HIF by prolyl hydroxylation. Cell. 2001;107(1):43–54.
31. Huang LE, Gu J, Schau M, Bunn HF. Regulation of hypoxia-inducible factor 1alpha is mediated by an O2-dependent degradation domain via the ubiquitin-proteasome pathway. Proc Natl Acad Sci U S A. 1998;95(14):7987–92.
32. Maxwell PH, Wiesener MS, Chang GW, Clifford SC, Vaux EC, Cockman ME, et al. The tumour suppressor protein VHL targets hypoxia-inducible factors for oxygen-dependent proteolysis. Nature. 1999;399(6733):271–5.
33. Ohh M, Park CW, Ivan M, Hoffman MA, Kim TY, Huang LE, et al. Ubiquitination of hypoxia-inducible factor requires direct binding to the beta-domain of the von Hippel-Lindau protein. Nat Cell Biol. 2000;2(7):423–7.
34. Cheng J, Kang X, Zhang S, Yeh ET. SUMO-specific protease 1 is essential for stabilization of HIF1alpha during hypoxia. Cell. 2007;131(3):584–95.
35. Duyndam MC, Hulscher ST, van der Wall E, Pinedo HM, Boven E. Evidence for a role of p38 kinase in hypoxia-inducible factor 1-independent induction of vascular endothelial growth factor expression by sodium arsenite. J Biol Chem. 2003;278(9):6885–95.
36. Jeong JW, Bae MK, Ahn MY, Kim SH, Sohn TK, Bae MH, et al. Regulation and destabilization of HIF-1alpha by ARD1-mediated acetylation. Cell. 2002;111(5):709–20.
37. Kim Y, Nam HJ, Lee J, Park DY, Kim C, Yu YS, et al. Methylation-dependent regulation of HIF-1alpha stability restricts retinal and tumour angiogenesis. Nat Commun. 2016;7:10347.
38. Phadke PA, Vaidya KS, Nash KT, Hurst DR, Welch DR. BRMS1 suppresses breast cancer experimental metastasis to multiple organs by inhibiting several steps of the metastatic process. Am J Pathol. 2008;172(3):809–17.
39. Seraj MJ, Samant RS, Verderame MF, Welch DR. Functional evidence for a novel human breast carcinoma metastasis suppressor, BRMS1, encoded at chromosome 11q13. Cancer Res. 2000;60(11):2764–9.
40. Kim B, Nam HJ, Pyo KE, Jang MJ, Kim IS, Kim D, et al. Breast cancer metastasis suppressor 1 (BRMS1) is destabilized by the Cul3-SPOP E3 ubiquitin ligase complex. Biochem Biophys Res Commun. 2011;415(4):720–6.
41. Hernandez-Munoz I, Lund AH, van der Stoop P, Boutsma E, Muijrers I, Verhoeven E, et al. Stable X chromosome inactivation involves the PRC1 Polycomb complex and requires histone MACROH2A1 and the CULLIN3/SPOP ubiquitin E3 ligase. Proc Natl Acad Sci U S A. 2005;102(21):7635–40.

42. Kwon JE, La M, Oh KH, Oh YM, Kim GR, Seol JH, et al. BTB domain-containing speckle-type POZ protein (SPOP) serves as an adaptor of Daxx for ubiquitination by Cul3-based ubiquitin ligase. J Biol Chem. 2006;281(18):12664–72.
43. Cogswell PC, Guttridge DC, Funkhouser WK, Baldwin AS Jr. Selective activation of NF-kappa B subunits in human breast cancer: potential roles for NF-kappa B2/p52 and for Bcl-3. Oncogene. 2000;19(9):1123–31.
44. Ohno H, Takimoto G, McKeithan TW. The candidate proto-oncogene bcl-3 is related to genes implicated in cell lineage determination and cell cycle control. Cell. 1990;60(6):991–7.
45. Ahmed SU, Milner J. Basal cancer cell survival involves JNK2 suppression of a novel JNK1/c-Jun/Bcl-3 apoptotic network. PLoS One. 2009;4(10):e7305.
46. Choi HJ, Lee JM, Kim H, Nam HJ, Shin HJ, Kim D, et al. Bcl3-dependent stabilization of CtBP1 is crucial for the inhibition of apoptosis and tumor progression in breast cancer. Biochem Biophys Res Commun. 2010;400(3):396–402.
47. O'Neil BH, Buzkova P, Farrah H, Kashatus D, Sanoff H, Goldberg RM, et al. Expression of nuclear factor-kappaB family proteins in hepatocellular carcinomas. Oncology. 2007;72 (1-2):97–104.
48. Thornburg NJ, Pathmanathan R, Raab-Traub N. Activation of nuclear factor-kappaB p50 homodimer/Bcl-3 complexes in nasopharyngeal carcinoma. Cancer Res. 2003;63 (23):8293–301.
49. Giguere V, Tini M, Flock G, Ong E, Evans RM, Otulakowski G. Isoform-specific amino-terminal domains dictate DNA-binding properties of ROR alpha, a novel family of orphan hormone nuclear receptors. Genes Dev. 1994;8(5):538–53.
50. Kim K, Lee JM, Yu YS, Kim H, Nam HJ, Moon HG, et al. RORalpha2 requires LSD1 to enhance tumor progression in breast cancer. Sci Rep. 2017;7(1):11994.
51. Ley TJ, Ding L, Walter MJ, McLellan MD, Lamprecht T, Larson DE, et al. DNMT3A mutations in acute myeloid leukemia. N Engl J Med. 2010;363(25):2424–33.
52. Derissen EJ, Beijnen JH, Schellens JH. Concise drug review: azacitidine and decitabine. Oncologist. 2013;18(5):619–24.
53. Tsai HC, Li H, Van Neste L, Cai Y, Robert C, Rassool FV, et al. Transient low doses of DNA-demethylating agents exert durable antitumor effects on hematological and epithelial tumor cells. Cancer Cell. 2012;21(3):430–46.
54. Borges S, Doppler H, Perez EA, Andorfer CA, Sun Z, Anastasiadis PZ, et al. Pharmacologic reversion of epigenetic silencing of the PRKD1 promoter blocks breast tumor cell invasion and metastasis. Breast Cancer Res. 2013;15(2):R66.
55. Olsen EA, Kim YH, Kuzel TM, Pacheco TR, Foss FM, Parker S, et al. Phase IIb multicenter trial of vorinostat in patients with persistent, progressive, or treatment refractory cutaneous T-cell lymphoma. J Clin Oncol. 2007;25(21):3109–15.
56. Piekarz RL, Frye R, Turner M, Wright JJ, Allen SL, Kirschbaum MH, et al. Phase II multi-institutional trial of the histone deacetylase inhibitor romidepsin as monotherapy for patients with cutaneous T-cell lymphoma. J Clin Oncol. 2009;27(32):5410–7.
57. Beckers T, Burkhardt C, Wieland H, Gimmnich P, Ciossek T, Maier T, et al. Distinct pharmacological properties of second generation HDAC inhibitors with the benzamide or hydroxamate head group. Int J Cancer. 2007;121(5):1138–48.
58. Kim YJ, Greer CB, Cecchini KR, Harris LN, Tuck DP, Kim TH. HDAC inhibitors induce transcriptional repression of high copy number genes in breast cancer through elongation blockade. Oncogene. 2013;32(23):2828–35.
59. Falahi F, van Kruchten M, Martinet N, Hospers GA, Rots MG. Current and upcoming approaches to exploit the reversibility of epigenetic mutations in breast cancer. Breast Cancer Res. 2014;16(4):412.
60. Park PJ. ChIP-seq: advantages and challenges of a maturing technology. Nat Rev Genet. 2009;10(10):669–80.

61. Stunnenberg HG, Vermeulen M. Towards cracking the epigenetic code using a combination of high-throughput epigenomics and quantitative mass spectrometry-based proteomics. BioEssays. 2011;33(7):547–51.
62. Filippakopoulos P, Qi J, Picaud S, Shen Y, Smith WB, Fedorov O, et al. Selective inhibition of BET bromodomains. Nature. 2010;468(7327):1067–73.
63. Dawson MA, Prinjha RK, Dittmann A, Giotopoulos G, Bantscheff M, Chan WI, et al. Inhibition of BET recruitment to chromatin as an effective treatment for MLL-fusion leukaemia. Nature. 2011;478(7370):529–33.
64. Delmore JE, Issa GC, Lemieux ME, Rahl PB, Shi J, Jacobs HM, et al. BET bromodomain inhibition as a therapeutic strategy to target c-Myc. Cell. 2011;146(6):904–17.
65. Mertz JA, Conery AR, Bryant BM, Sandy P, Balasubramanian S, Mele DA, et al. Targeting MYC dependence in cancer by inhibiting BET bromodomains. Proc Natl Acad Sci U S A. 2011;108(40):16669–74.
66. Zuber J, Rappaport AR, Luo W, Wang E, Chen C, Vaseva AV, et al. An integrated approach to dissecting oncogene addiction implicates a Myb-coordinated self-renewal program as essential for leukemia maintenance. Genes Dev. 2011;25(15):1628–40.
67. Asangani IA, Dommeti VL, Wang X, Malik R, Cieslik M, Yang R, et al. Therapeutic targeting of BET bromodomain proteins in castration-resistant prostate cancer. Nature. 2014;510 (7504):278–82.
68. Garcia PL, Miller AL, Kreitzburg KM, Council LN, Gamblin TL, Christein JD, et al. The BET bromodomain inhibitor JQ1 suppresses growth of pancreatic ductal adenocarcinoma in patient-derived xenograft models. Oncogene. 2016;35(7):833–45.
69. Ocana A, Nieto-Jimenez C, Pandiella A. BET inhibitors as novel therapeutic agents in breast cancer. Oncotarget. 2017;8(41):71285–91.
70. Shimamura T, Chen Z, Soucheray M, Carretero J, Kikuchi E, Tchaicha JH, et al. Efficacy of BET bromodomain inhibition in Kras-mutant non-small cell lung cancer. Clin Cancer Res. 2013;19(22):6183–92.
71. Nieto-Jimenez C, Alcaraz-Sanabria A, Perez-Pena J, Corrales-Sanchez V, Serrano-Heras G, Galan-Moya EM, et al. Targeting basal-like breast tumors with bromodomain and extraterminal domain (BET) and polo-like kinase inhibitors. Oncotarget. 2017;8(12):19478–90.
72. Johnson DB, Estrada MV, Salgado R, Sanchez V, Doxie DB, Opalenik SR, et al. Melanoma-specific MHC-II expression represents a tumour-autonomous phenotype and predicts response to anti-PD-1/PD-L1 therapy. Nat Commun. 2016;7:10582.
73. Pauken KE, Sammons MA, Odorizzi PM, Manne S, Godec J, Khan O, et al. Epigenetic stability of exhausted T cells limits durability of reinvigoration by PD-1 blockade. Science. 2016;354 (6316):1160–5.
74. Sen DR, Kaminski J, Barnitz RA, Kurachi M, Gerdemann U, Yates KB, et al. The epigenetic landscape of T cell exhaustion. Science. 2016;354(6316):1165–9.
75. Wherry EJ, Kurachi M. Molecular and cellular insights into T cell exhaustion. Nat Rev Immunol. 2015;15(8):486–99.

Chapter 6
Role of tRNAs in Breast Cancer Regulation

Nam Hoon Kwon, Jin Young Lee, and Sunghoon Kim

Abstract Increased proliferation and protein synthesis are characteristics of transformed and tumor cells. Although the components of the translation machinery are often dysregulated in cancer, the role of tRNAs in cancer cells has not been well studied. Nevertheless, the number of related studies has recently started increasing. With the development of high throughput technologies such as next-generation sequencing, genome-wide differential tRNA expression patterns in breast cancer–derived cell lines and breast tumors have been investigated. The genome-wide transcriptomics analyses have been linked with many studies for functional and phenotypic characterization, whereby tRNAs or tRNA-related fragments have been shown to play important roles in breast cancer regulation and as promising prognostic biomarkers. Here, we review their expression patterns, functions, prognostic value, and potential therapeutic use as well as related technologies.

Keywords tRNA · tRNA-derived fragments · tRFs · tRNA modifications · miRNAs · piRNAs

N. H. Kwon
Medicinal Bioconvergence Research Center, Institute for Artificial Intelligence and Biomedical Research, Yonsei University, Incheon, South Korea

J. Y. Lee
Buck Institute for Research on Aging, Novato, CA, USA

S. Kim (✉)
Medicinal Bioconvergence Research Center, Institute for Artificial Intelligence and Biomedical Research, College of Pharmacy & College of Medicine, Gangnam Severance Hospital, Yonsei University, Incheon, South Korea
e-mail: sunghoonkim@yonsei.ac.kr

D.-Y. Noh et al. (eds.), *Translational Research in Breast Cancer*, Advances in Experimental Medicine and Biology 1187,
https://doi.org/10.1007/978-981-32-9620-6_6

6.1 Introduction

Transfer RNAs (tRNAs), aminoacyl-tRNA synthetases (ARSs), and amino acids are essential elements for protein synthesis. ARSs ligate tRNAs with cognate amino acids, after which aminoacyl-tRNAs participate in translation by transporting precursor amino acids to the ribosome [1]. Although a tRNA is usually charged with only one of the 20 different amino acids, the human tRNAome is very complicated and consists of >500 interspersed tRNA genes and 51 anticodon families, constituting 4–10% of total cellular RNA (Fig. 6.1) [2, 3]. According to the nomenclature of tRNAs, $tRNA^{Leu}$ refers to the tRNA type to be charged with Leucine (Leu). When $tRNA^{Leu}$ is aminoacylated with Leu, it is represented as Leu-$tRNA^{Leu}$. Most tRNA types incorporate isoacceptors that are charged with the same type of amino acid but have different anti-codons. For example, $tRNA^{Leu}$(CAG) and $tRNA^{Leu}$(UAG) are isoacceptors of each other, which recognize CTG and CTA codons in a messenger RNA (mRNA) and incorporate Leu into the growing polypeptides, respectively, during translation. In addition, functional equivalence or expression patterns of tRNAs have been revealed to be irrespective of their sequence similarity [4, 5].

For a long time, tRNAs had been considered as mere house-keeping RNAs; however, recent studies have suggested that tRNAs and their fragments may have diverse roles. For example, Mey et al. reported that several tRNAs can bind to cytochrome C, inhibiting caspase activation and apoptosis upon apoptotic stimuli [6]. Initiator tRNA ($tRNA_i^{Met}$) is unique in the sense that it can initiate translation; overexpression of $tRNA_i^{Met}$ has been reported to change the translational efficiency of specific genes and alter the global tRNA expression, resulting in various cellular responses such as proliferation, enhanced invasion, and metastasis [7, 8]. Various stimuli have been reported to cause digestion of tRNAs, generating small tRNA-derived fragments (tRFs) [9]. These fragments can be derived from precursor tRNAs (pre-tRNAs) or mature tRNAs and are similar in size to microRNAs. Our

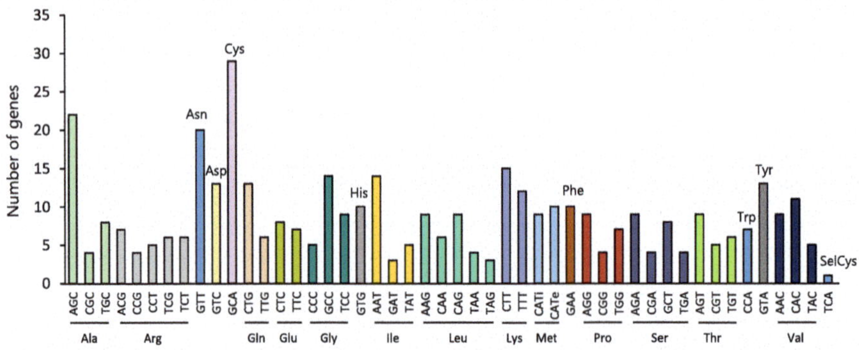

Fig. 6.1 Number of tRNA (transfer RNA) genes in the human genome. Numbers of tRNA genes per amino acid are presented. Different anticodons per amino acid mean isoacceptors of tRNA. Data were based on the high confident set of *Homo sapiens* (GRCh37/hg19) chromosome, in tRNA database (http://gtrnadb.ucsc.edu/) with a total of 416 tRNAs with a selenocysteine (SelCys) tRNA

understanding of the diverse functions of tRFs has recently improved. They are now known to participate in translational regulation, neuroprotection, cell proliferation, tumorigenesis, and RNA silencing like microRNAs [10–14].

In addition, overexpression of tRNAs has been observed in various cancer cell lines and tissues, although their biogenesis and translational requirements remain obscure [5, 15, 16]. Given that tRNA abundance is correlated with protein synthesis [17], it has been hypothesized that tRNA content may affect the rate of translation globally or for a subset of proteins based on codon usage [18]. A recent study has revealed that breast cancer metastasis is promoted by $tRNA^{Glu}$(UUC) and $tRNA^{Arg}$(CCG) (Table 6.1) [5]. This study has demonstrated that overexpression of specific tRNAs can modulate protein expression in a codon-dependent manner, resulting in metastatic behavior. It has also shed light on the importance of quantitative changes in tRNAs. However, it is still debated whether tRNA abundance and codon usage are under concerted regulation of translation rate and efficiency [19–21]. In fact, several studies have suggested that preferentially used codons are not translated faster, and that tRNA variation might play an adaptive role in coping with environmental changes. Analyses of human tRNA expression patterns using microarrays have revealed that tRNA expression is modulated according to the cell cycle, such as during proliferation and differentiation [21, 22]. Taken together, these observations suggest that more studies are required for understanding the relationship between tRNAs and the translational need.

Even with this uncertainty, many reports have suggested important roles of tRNAs and tRFs in cancer as translational and signaling modulators as well as possible biomarkers. Here, we review tRNAs and tRFs reported in breast cancer and their potential as biomarkers, and discuss the future prospects.

6.2 Review of Past Studies

6.2.1 Expressional Analysis of tRNAs and tRFs

6.2.1.1 Generation of tRNAs and tRFs

In eukaryotic cells, tRNA genes are transcribed by RNA polymerase III (RNA Pol III), and pre-tRNAs undergo further processing to generate mature tRNAs. During this process, RNase P and RNase Z remove the 5′ leader and 3′ trailer sequences, respectively, and then CCA trinucleotide is added to the 3′ end of the tRNA for maturation (Fig. 6.2) [23].

tRFs can be generated from pre-tRNAs as well as mature tRNAs (Fig. 6.2). While 3′ trailer of pre-tRNAs is called tRF-1 and identified in itself, 5′ leader is not observed as an independent tRF. Two groups of tRNA halves, namely 5′ and 3′ halves, can be created by digestion of the anticodon loop by RNase T2 or RNase A superfamily, which is released by stress stimuli [24, 25]. It is known that endogenous 5’ tRNA halves generally inhibit translation via diverse mechanisms. In addition,

Table 6.1 Functions of representative tRNAs and tRFs in breast cancer

tRNA	Type	Function or characteristics	Naming in the original article	References
tRNA^{Leu}	Mature tRNA	Association between estrogen receptor alpha (ERα) and Brf1 in ER-positive breast cancer	–	[53]
tRNA^{Leu}, tRNA^{Tyr}	Pre-transcript	Positive correlation with the expression of telomerase reverse transcriptase (TERT)	–	[50, 51]
tRNA^{Leu}	Mature tRNA	Enhanced proliferation of ErbB2-positive breast cancer	–	[54]
tRNA^{Arg}(UCU), tRNA^{Arg}(CCU), tRNA^{Thr}(CGU), tRNA^{Ser}(CGA), tRNA^{Tyr}(GUA)	Mature tRNA	Overexpression in breast cancer	–	[15]
tRNA^{Ser}, tRNA^{Arg}, tRNA^{Glu}, tRNA^{Gly}	Mature tRNA	Differential expression in breast cancer and correlation with overall or recurrence-free survival	–	[34]
tRNA^{Glu}(UUC), tRNA^{Arg}(CCG)	Mature tRNA	Enhanced ribosome occupancy and stability of transcripts enriched with their cognate codons for Glu and Arg to enhance metastasis	–	[5]
tRNA^{Val}(CAC), tRNA^{Val}(ACC), tRNA^{Gly}(GCC), tRNA^{Gly}(CCC), tRNA^{Glu}(CUC), tRNA^{Lys}(CUU), tRNA^{His}(GUG)	Mature tRNA	High expression in triple-negative breast cancer cells	–	[52]
tRNA^{Ser}	Mature tRNA	Less expression in basal-like 1 subtype of triple-negative breast cancer cells	–	[52]
tRNAi^{Met}(CAU)	Precursor tRNA	Target of tumor suppressive miR-34a	–	[48]
tRNA^{Glu}(Y*UC), tRNA^{Asp}(GUC), tRNA^{Gly}(UCC)	i-tRF	Suppression of cell proliferation and cancer metastasis via destabilization of YBX-1-bound oncogenic transcripts	tRF^{GluYTC}, tRF^{AspGTC}, tRF^{GlyTCC}	[27, 62]
tRNA^{Tyr}(GUA)	Intron region		tRF^{TyrGTA}	[27, 62]
tRNA^{Asp}(GUC), tRNA^{His}(GUG), tRNA^{Lys}(CUU)	tRF-5	Promotion of cell proliferation via sex hormone-dependent induction	5'-SHOT-RNA^{AspGUC}, 5'-SHOT-	[12, 62]

(continued)

Table 6.1 (continued)

tRNA	Type	Function or characteristics	Naming in the original article	References
			RNA^{HisGUG}, 5'-SHOT-RNA^{LysCUU}	
tRNA^{Asp}(GUC)	i-tRF	High expression in cancer	i-tRF from the AspGTC anticodon	[62, 84]
tRNA^{His}(GUG), tRNA^{Arg}(UCG)	tRF-1	Upregulation by mutations in the oncogenic KRAS, or PIK3CA	Ts-46, and ts-47	[62, 63]
mtRNA^{Asp}		Alteration of mtRNA metabolism by the mutation of T7581C in mtRNA^{Asp}	Mt-tRNA^{Asp}	[42]
tRNA^{Thr}, tRNA^{Lys}, tRNA^{Lys}, tRNA^{Leu}		High level in extracellular vesicles of breast cancer cells	miR-720, miR-1274a, miR-1274b, and miR-1260	[58, 59]
tRNA^{Thr}, tRNA^{Leu}	tRF-3	High level in the blood from patients of ER+/HER2—Breast cancer	miR-720, miR-1260 and miR-1280	[61]
tRNA^{Cys}(GCA)	i-tRF	Significant increase in trastuzumab-resistant breast cancer	tRF-30-JZOYJE22RR33, tRF-27-ZDXPHO53KSN	[81]

*Y in tRNA^{Glu}(YUC) represents C or U, that is, tRNA^{Glu}(CUC) and tRNA^{Glu}(UUC)

many tRFs are induced by sex hormones in breast cancer [12]. To date, 3 types of tRFs originating from mature tRNAs have been identified: tRF-5s, tRF-3s, and i-tRFs, which correspond to 5′, 3′, and internal fragments of tRNAs, respectively. tRF-5 s and tRF-3 s are generated by cleavage of tRNAs by Dicer and/or members of the RNase A superfamily. The anticodon loop is usually contained in i-tRFs, which were first identified in breast cancer cells, but biogenesis of i-tRFs is not entirely clear [26]. While the mechanism of tRF-mediated regulation of gene expression remains elusive, involvement of tRFs in the regulation of transcript stability and signaling pathways has been suggested. These assumptions are supported by the fact that tRFs have been shown to associate with Argonautes as siRNAs and miRNAs do, and tRFs interact with several transcription-regulating and RNA-binding proteins [27].

6.2.1.2 Detection of tRNAs and tRFs

The size of a tRNA and tRF ranges from 76 to 90 nucleotides and 14 to 50 nucleotides, respectively. The most conventional detection method for tRNAs and tRFs is

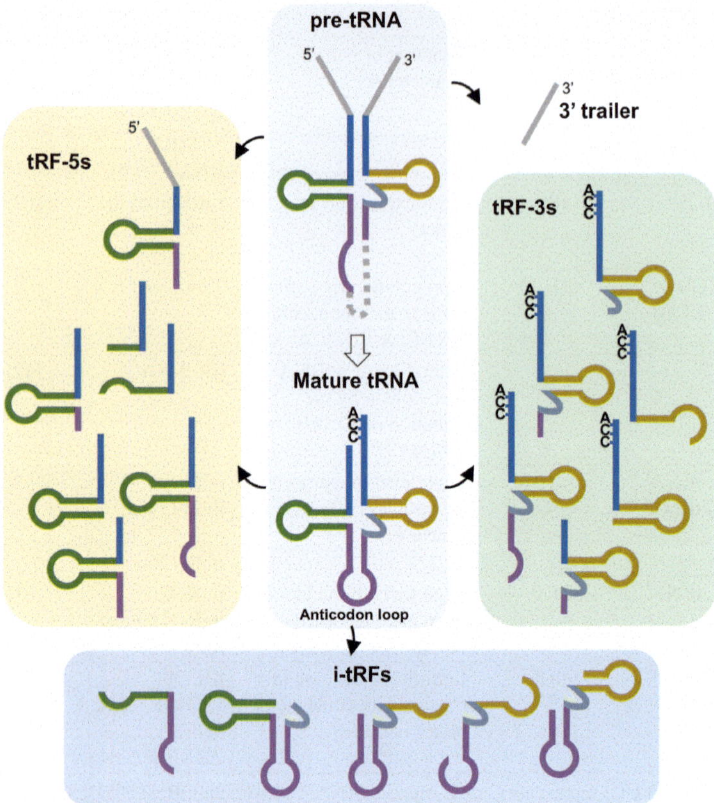

Fig. 6.2 tRNA processing and generation of tRFs (tRNA-derived fragments). Mature tRNAs are generated from precursor tRNA (pre-tRNA) transcripts by digestion of the 5′ leader and 3′ trailer, and then CCA is added to the 3′-end by CCA enzymes. Several kinds of tRFs, tRF-1 (*3′ trailer* of tRNA*)*, tRF-5 (5′ fragment of tRNA), tRF-3 (3′ fragment of tRNA), and i-tRF (internal fragment of tRNA) can be generated by cleavage of pre-mature or mature tRNAs under stimuli such as stress response. Intronic sequences, depicted as the dotted gray line in the pre-tRNA, exist in several tRNAs such as $tRNA^{Tyr}$, $tRNA^{Leu}$, $tRNA^{Ile}$, $tRNA^{Pro}$, and $tRNA^{Arg}$, and part of them are also identified as tRFs

northern blotting. By using specific nucleotide probes labeled radioactively or non-radioactively [28], the size of tRNAs and tRFs can be identified, and even tRNAs loaded with an amino-acid can be distinguished from the unloaded tRNAs based on size [29]. However, northern blotting is a labor-intensive and quantitatively imperfect procedure, which makes northern blotting be considered inadequate to analyze huge amount of samples. To overcome these limitations, Pavon-Eternod et al., for the first time, developed a microarray platform to profile tRNAs in breast cancer [15]. This microarray platform enabled simultaneous analysis of tRNAs in multiplex conditions, but it is still labor-intensive and difficult to be generalized because it is still based on specialized probing techniques. Owing to the revolutionary development of next-generation sequencing (NGS) techniques, numerous small non-coding RNAs, including tRNAs and tRFs, can be massively analyzed in large and complex datasets at single nucleotide resolution in a rather unbiased way [30]. Recently, several NGS methodologies have been developed to find the optimal conditions for the analysis of mature tRNAs and/or tRFs [31]. Consequently, the sequences of numerous tRFs detected in human samples in various contexts are currently available in several databases [9, 32, 33]. For example, tRFinCancer shows the expression patterns of tRFs in multiple cancer types [32], tRFdb is a relational database of tRFs and other tRNA-related RNA fragments [9], and MINTbase is a database for tRFs of mitochondrial or nuclear origin [33].

6.2.1.3 tRNA Overexpression in Breast Cancer

Pavon-Eternod et al. analyzed the expression levels of individual tRNAs in breast cancer cells using a microarray platform and revealed an unexpected selectivity that is based on cognate amino acid properties and isoacceptor identities [15]. Each breast cancer cell line generates unique tRNA profiles that are markedly different from that of non-cancer breast epithelial cell lines. Overall, the results of Pavon-Eternod et al. highlight the potential of using both genomic DNA- and mitochondrial DNA-encoded tRNAs as biomarkers for malignancy, tumor type, or tumor progression. Remarkably, $tRNA^{Arg}$(CCU), $tRNA^{Ser}$(GCU), $tRNA^{Thr}$(CGU), and $tRNA^{Tyr}$(GUA) are among the most overexpressed tRNAs in the breast cancer cell lines and breast tumors analyzed (Table 6.1). Since the amino acid residues Ser, Thr, and Tyr are targets for protein kinases and phosphatases, this observation suggests that these tRNAs might be part of a potential mechanism for potentiating post-translational regulation of proteins involved in signal transduction. Significant differences in the relative expression levels of tRNA isoacceptors have also been observed. For example, $tRNA^{Arg}$(CCU) and $tRNA^{Lys}$(UUU) were more overexpressed than $tRNA^{Arg}$(ICG) and $tRNA^{Lys}$(CUU). Differential expression of tRNA isoacceptors may provide an additional level of translational regulation for key genes involved in tumorigenesis. Initiator $tRNA^{Met}$ has been found overexpressed in all cancer-derived breast cell lines compared with the healthy controls. However, $tRNA_i^{Met}$ is not overexpressed as much as a few other tRNAs, such as $tRNA^{Ser}$, $tRNA^{Thr}$, and $tRNA^{Tyr}$ in the breast cancer cells. Therefore, further studies are needed to elucidate the regulatory relationship between tRNA expression and cancer.

Krishnan et al., for the first time, investigated the differential expression patterns of tRNAs in breast tumor tissues using NGS to determine if these patterns had any prognostic significance for breast cancer [34]. They profiled 571 tRNAs from 11 normal breast and 104 breast tumor tissues and found that 76 tRNAs were differentially expressed, among which several tRNAs, including $tRNA^{Ser}$, $tRNA^{Arg}$, $tRNA^{Glu}$, and $tRNA^{Gly}$, showed a positive correlation with the overall or recurrence-free survival (Table 6.1). Although the analysis results were dependent on the controls used, this observation suggests the global tRNA upregulation and differentially expressed tRNAs as potential novel prognostic markers in breast cancer.

6.2.1.4 tRF Detection in Breast Cancer

It is known that 321 tRNA genes out of 625 total human tRNA genes generate diverse forms of tRFs, and the most common form is tRF-3, which consists of the C-terminal half of a tRNA (http://genome.bioch.virginia.edu/trfdb/statistics.php). Various kinds of tRFs have been identified in breast cancer cells and tissues, and they seem to be involved in breast cancer regulation and progression. An interesting report has indicated that levels of several tRFs may be associated with racial disparities in triple negative breast cancer, which is characterized by marked differences between white and black/African-American women [35]. These tRFs include nuclear $tRNA^{Gly}$ and $tRNA^{Leu}$, and mitochondrial $tRNA^{Val}$ and $tRNA^{Pro}$. The functions of tRFs identified in breast cancer will be discussed later.

Small noncoding RNAs circulating in the blood may serve as signaling molecules because of their ability to carry out a variety of cellular functions. Dhahbi et al. have previously described tRFs and other small RNAs circulating as components of larger complexes in the blood of humans and mice, implying that these small RNAs may specifically be processed, secreted, and regulated [36]. Recently, deep sequencing and informatics analysis revealed that 5′ tRNA halves were abundant and significantly different in the serum of clinicopathologic breast cancer patients, showing the potentials of 5′ tRNA halves as circulating biomarkers of breast cancer. Larger studies with multiple types of cancer are needed to adequately evaluate their potential use for the development of noninvasive cancer screening.

6.2.2 Modifications of tRNAs in Breast Cancer

6.2.2.1 Genetic Alterations of tRNAs

In addition to genomic 625 tRNA genes, mitochondrial DNA encodes its own 22 mitochondrial tRNA (mtRNA) genes. mtDNAs are known to be more vulnerable to mutation than their genomic counterparts due to the lack of protective histones, introns, and efficient DNA repair mechanisms [37]. Polymorphism or mutations of mtRNAs, therefore, are more frequently reported to be associated with various diseases than those in genomic tRNAs. There have been indications that mitochondrial function and polymorphisms are involved in the carcinogenic process and increased risk of cancer [38].

tRNA genes do not appear to be hot spots in breast cancer given that trials to find any changes in chromosomal tRNA genes have not revealed any mutations [38, 39]. However, depletion and mutation of mtRNA have been reported in the increased tumorigenic and invasive phenotype [40–42]. An example would be the case of mtRNA^{Asp} mutation which has been shown to be involved in the carcinogenesis of breast cancer (Table 6.1) [42]. The mutation of T7581C in mtRNA^{Asp} gene creates a new conserved base-pairing (G4-C69), which presumably causes a failure in mtRNA^{Asp} metabolism. It implies that mutations may cause alterations in the tertiary structure of mtRNAs resulting in impairment of mitochondrial protein synthesis.

Other polymorphisms in mtRNAs have also been identified in breast cancer patients [38]. The authors have analyzed all the 22 genes encoding mtRNAs in breast cancer carcinoma as well as blood. Polymorphism of mtRNA^{Asp}, mtRNA^{Lys}, mtRNA^{Gly}, mtRNA^{Arg}, mtRNA^{Leu}, and mtRNA^{Thr} have been found in 6–12% of patients. Distinguishing the polymorphisms or mutations in mt-tRNA genes is still puzzling for the clinicians and geneticists when confronted with breast cancer. Although it is unclear whether these polymorphisms are connected with the pathology or not, it cannot be excluded that mutations in tRNA genes in breast cancer may impact the cell physiology, and cause its dysfunction.

6.2.2.2 tRNA Modifications in Breast Cancer

On average, 13 bases in a tRNA molecule are modified after transcription (Fig. 6.3) [43]. These modifications play multifaceted roles in decoding genetic information as well as in other cellular processes. Abundance, modification, and aminoacylation levels of tRNAs contribute to the translation and differ in different cell types and/or cellular environment [44]. To date, a complete compilation of tRNA modifications and the corresponding modification enzymes have not been determined. Among the predicted and known human tRNA modification enzymes, those linked to breast cancer are listed in Table 6.2 [44].

In fact, base modification itself and the enzymes in charge of tRNA modifications play an important role in the pathogenesis of breast cancer [26, 40]. Studies have indicated that increased tRNA modifications in anticodon swinging bases enhance the translational efficiency due to the increased decoding power of the tRNA [45]. Methyltransferase Misu (NSUN2) and tRNA methyltransferase homolog 12 (TRMT12) have been shown to be significantly increased in breast cancer cell lines and tissues, and they are presumably involved in the proliferation of cancer cells [26, 46]. In human breast cancer, the elevated expression of U34-modifying enzymes directly promotes the translation of oncoprotein DEK, which in turn increases the translation of the oncogenic LEF-1 (lymphoid enhancer binding factor 1) mRNA, promoting the invasion and metastasis of breast cancer cells [47]. Given that extensive base modifications in tRNAs are crucial for their function, future studies should address the potential role of tRNA modifications in breast cancer.

Recent studies suggest that tRNA modifications can increase the stability of tRNAs. Wang et al. observed that miRNA-34a targets pre-tRNA$_i^{Met}$ and induces Argonaute 2 (AGO2)-mediated degradation resulting in reduction of mature tRNA$_i^{Met}$ [48]. Overexpression of tRNA$_i^{Met}$ promotes proliferation and cell cycle transition. Given that mature tRNA$_i^{Met}$ is not a substrate for miRNA-34a-mediated degradation, modification of mature tRNA$_i^{Met}$ may protect it from AGO2-mediated

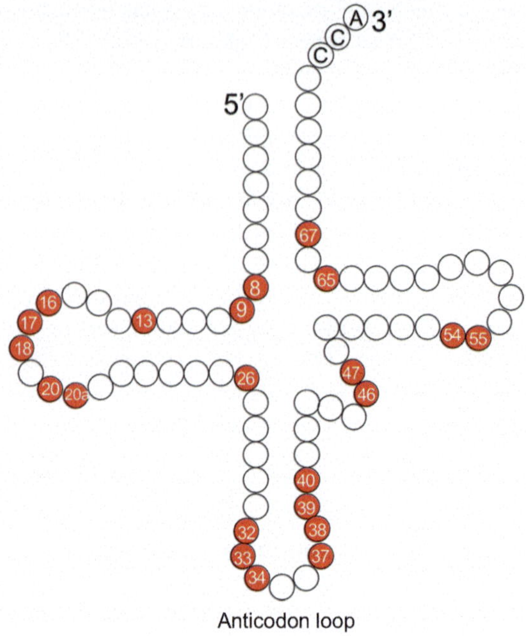

Fig. 6.3 Modification site of tRNAs. Representative modification sites and the number of bases in tRNAs are depicted in red. Base modifications usually happen after the removal of the 5′- and 3′-ends from pre-tRNAs and before the splicing

Table 6.2 tRNA modification genes known or predicted to be linked with breast cancer

Enzyme	Modification	References
THUMPD1 (THUMP domain containing 1)	ac^{4}C	[85]
METTL6 (methyltransferase like 6)	m^{3}C	[86]
NSUN2 (NOP2/Sun RNA methyltransferase 2)	m^{5}C	[46, 87, 88]
ELP3 (elongator complex protein 3)	cm^{5}U, ncm^{5}U, mcm^{5}U, mcm^{5}s^{2}U	[47]
CTU1 (cytosolic thiouridylase subunit 1)	s^{2}U, mcm^{5}s^{2}U	[47]
CTU2 (cytosolic thiouridylase subunit 2)	s^{2}U, mcm^{5}s^{2}U	[47]
TRMT12 (tRNA methyltransferase 12 homolog)	o_2yW, yW	[89]
CDKAL1 (CDK5 regulatory subunit associated protein 1 like 1)	ms^{2}t^{6}A	[90]
TRMT2A (tRNA methyltransferase 2 homolog A)	m^{5}U	[91]
MTO1 (mitochondrial tRNA translation optimization 1)	tm^{5}U	[92]
TRIT1 (tRNA isopentenyltransferase, mitochondrial)	i^{6}A	[93]
TRMT61B (tRNA methyltransferase 61B)	m^{1}A	[94]

Most enzymes are expressed in the cytotosol. TRIT1 and TRMT61 are in mitochondria. Ac^{4}C, N4-acetylcytidine; m^{3}C, 3-methylcytosine; m^{5}C, 5-methylcytosine; cm^{5}U, 5-carboxymethyluridine; ncm^{5}U, 5-carbamoylmethyluridine; mcm^{5}U, 5-methoxycarbonylmethyluridine; mcm^{5}s^{2}U, 5-methoxycarbonylmethyl-2-thiouridine; s^{2}U, 2-thiouridine; o_2yW, peroxywybutosine; yW, wybutosine; ms^{2}t^{6}A, 2-methylthio-N6-threonyl carbamoyladenosine; m^{5}U, 5-methyluridine; tm^{5}U, 5-taurinomethyluridine; i^{6}A, N6-isopentenyladenosine; and m^{1}A, 1-methyladenosine degradation. It has also been reported that BCDIN3D (bicoid interacting 3 domain containing RNA methyltransferase) monomethylated 5′ monophosphate of cytoplasmic $tRNA^{His}$ in vivo and in vitro [49]. BCDIN3D is highly overexpressed in breast cancer and is associated with poor prognosis. BCDIN3D specifically modified cytoplasmic $tRNA^{His}$, without affecting the aminoacylation of $tRNA^{His}$ by histidyl-tRNA synthetase. The exact function of $tRNA^{His}$ in breast cancer was not investigated in this study, but it suggests another link between tRNA modifications with the tumorigenic phenotype of breast cancer beyond translation.

6.2.3 *Functions of tRNAs in Breast Cancer*

Since tRNAs are principally involved in protein synthesis, their abundance, modification, and mutation are all closely related to protein expression. Synthesis of tRNA is controlled by many oncogenes and tumor suppressors, such as Ras, c-myc, Rb, and p53, all of which affect RNA Pol III-mediated transcription, causing serious dysregulation of tRNA levels [40]. Due to this relation, the alteration of proteins regulating RNA Pol III-mediated transcription also affects the level of tRNAs. In addition, tRNAs can bind to other proteins containing RNA-binding domains and control the function of these proteins they bind to. Accumulating evidence has identified that certain tRNAs and tRFs are involved in the control of proliferation, metastasis, and angiogenesis in human cancers, including breast cancer.

6.2.3.1 tRNA Over-expression in the Subtypes of Breast Cancer

It seems that there are specific tRNA expression patterns, depending on the subtype of breast cancer. In triple-negative breast cancer (TNBC), there is a positive correlation between the expression of telomerase reverse transcriptase (TERT) and pre-transcripts of $tRNA^{Leu}$ and $tRNA^{Tyr}$ in the aggressiveness of cancer (Table 6.1) [50, 51]. In another report, 7 tRNAs, $tRNA^{Val}$(CAC), $tRNA^{Val}$(ACC), $tRNA^{Gly}$(GCC), $tRNA^{Gly}$(CCC) $tRNA^{Glu}$(CUC), $tRNA^{Lys}$(CUU), and $tRNA^{His}$(GUG), have been found to be highly expressed in 26 TNBC cells [52]. All these tRNA types are equally proportional in all the TNBC subtypes, while $tRNA^{Ser}$ is significantly less expressed in the basal-like 1 subtype. It has been reported that $tRNA^{Leu}$ is regulated by the interaction between estrogen receptor alpha (ERα) and Brf1 in estrogen receptor (ER)-positive breast cancer (Table 6.1) [53]. Additionally, it has been suggested that $tRNA^{Leu}$ plays a role in the proliferation of erythroblastic oncogene B (ERBB2)-positive breast cancer (Table 6.1) [54]. Kwon et al. showed that overexpressed $tRNA^{Leu}$ interacted with EBP1 (ERBB3-binding protein 1), reinforcing ERBB2/ERBB3 signaling pathway and enhancing phosphorylation of RSK1 (ribosomal S6 kinase 1) and MSK2 (mitogen-and stress-activated protein kinase 2) [54]. These results suggest that overexpression of any type of $tRNA^{Leu}$ isoacceptors can improve cell proliferation and apoptotic resistance, showing the possible link between $tRNA^{Leu}$ overexpression and several signaling pathways, such as the RSK1, MSK2, and ERBB2/ERBB3 pathways. All these results suggest that tRNA expression patterns differ in different contexts of breast cancer.

It has been reported that increased $tRNA_i^{Met}$(CAU) levels in carcinoma-associated fibroblasts promote tumor growth and angiogenesis [40, 55]. According to Clarke et al., increased levels of $tRNA_i^{Met}$(CAU) promote growth and angiogenesis of melanoma and lung cancer allografts. They used a mouse model that expressed additional copies of the $tRNA_i^{Met}$(CAU) gene and observed that growth and vascularization of subcutaneous tumor allografts were enhanced in the mice compared with wild-type littermate controls. Elevated expression of $tRNA_i^{Met}$(CAU) was also investigated in the breast cancer–associated fibroblasts obtained from patients; however, due to the small number of samples, the high expression of $tRNA_i^{Met}$(CAU) level was not validated in the breast cancer–associated fibroblasts. The function of $tRNA_i^{Met}$(CAU) in the stroma of breast cancer needs to be studied further. Although the link between upregulation of $tRNA_i^{Met}$(CAU) and breast cancer is obscure at this point, this research shows that $tRNA_i^{Met}$(CAU) may have the ability to generate pro-migratory extracellular matrix for cancer growth and invasion.

6.2.3.2 tRNA Over-expression Promotes Breast Cancer Metastasis

Goodarzi et al. found that specific tRNAs were upregulated in human breast cancer cells resulting in increased metastasis [5]. They found that $tRNA^{Glu}$(UUC) and $tRNA^{Arg}$(CCG) were promoters of breast cancer metastasis, and this observation was corroborated by loss-of-function and gain-of-function analyses as well as clinical-association studies (Table 6.1). Upregulation of these tRNAs enhances the ribosome occupancy and stability of transcripts enriched with the cognate codons of these tRNAs for Glu and Arg. Expression of $tRNA^{Glu}$(UUC) directly upregulates EXOSC2 (exosome component 2) and GRIPAP1 (glutamate receptor-interacting protein 1-associated protein 1), which have high Glu contents. Reduced levels of $tRNA^{Glu}$(UUC) and $tRNA^{Arg}$(CCG) exhibited significantly reduced colonization in the lungs in mice. Consistently, higher levels of these tRNAs were detected in patients with metastatic breast cancer compared with that in the patients without metastasis. These observations suggest that specific tRNAs can induce specific pathways where proteins enriched for their cognate codons are actively involved. Such target transcripts become stabilized in the context of their favored tRNAs and can be more effectively translated, resulting in a greater protein output. Thus, it appears that tRNAs can dynamically regulate gene expression, and the tRNA codon landscape can specifically affect disease progression.

6.2.4 *Functions of tRFs in Breast Cancer*

6.2.4.1 Tumor Suppressive Roles of tRFs

While overexpression of tRNAs usually shows a positive correlation with poor prognosis of breast cancer [5, 50, 51, 53, 54], tRFs show more diverse effects than tRNAs in many cases. It may be due to the characteristics of full-length tRNA, which support translation and are required under nutritious conditions. Fragmentation of tRNAs can be induced in periods of cellular stress, such as when cells cannot be supported for global translation anymore. Under such conditions, cells should sense the status of their environment, and tRFs may work as regulators to suppress the cell growth since there are already plenty full-length tRNAs that can be processed to generate additional regulators. Of course, there are several clues that tRFs may modulate cancer progression via inhibition of global translation. Thomson and Parker have proposed several possible roles of tRNA halves [56]: [1] translation inhibition via GCN2-mediated stress response activated by nicked tRNAs, [2] formation of a repression complex with other unknown binding partners that should be investigated further, [3] guiding small RNA-mediated translational repression or mRNA destabilization by interacting with Argonaute or PIWI proteins, resulting in silencing of specific transcripts, and [4] guiding mRNA destabilization by interacting with tRNA processing enzymes, such as RNase Z or RNase P [56]. These functions may be linked to breast cancer regulation.

tRFs can also control cancer independently of translation. Upon exposure to stress, tRNAs are enzymatically degraded, yielding distinct classes of tRFs. A novel class of tRFs, derived from $tRNA^{Glu}$, $tRNA^{Asp}$, $tRNA^{Gly}$, and $tRNA^{Tyr}$, shares a common motif that matches the oncogenic RNA-binding protein YBX1 (Y-box binding protein 1) recognition sequence (Table 6.1) [27]. YBX1 is expressed in various kinds of cancers and stabilizes diverse oncogenic transcripts. The fragments derived from $tRNA^{Glu}$, $tRNA^{Asp}$, and $tRNA^{Gly}$ appear to be i-tRFs since they map to the anticodon loops, whereas the $tRNA^{Tyr}$-derived fragment matches to the intronic region (Fig. 6.2). Association of these tRFs with YBX1 displaces the 3′ UTRs of oncogenic transcripts, such as HMGA1 (high mobility group AT-hook 1), CD151 (cluster of differentiation 151), CD97, and TIMP3 (tissue inhibitor of metalloproteinases-3) from YBX1, destabilizing multiple oncogenic transcripts in breast cancer cells. These tRFs are upregulated under hypoxic conditions suppressing breast cancer metastasis. Loss-of-function and gain-of-function studies by using antisense locked nucleic acids (LNAs) and synthetic RNA mimics, respectively, have revealed that these fragments suppress cell growth under serum-starvation, cancer cell invasion, and metastasis of breast cancer cells in vivo. Interestingly, highly metastatic breast cancer cells do not show significant overexpression of these tRFs, implying that a mechanism to attenuate induction of these tRFs exists to evade the tRF-mediated modulation of cancer metastasis. These findings have revealed a tumor-suppressive role of specific tRFs, which can be expanded to other tRFs, non-coding RNAs, or small RNAs.

6.2.4.2 Tumor Proliferative Roles of tRFs

There are also several tRFs which are positively involved in tumorigenesis. Honda et al. reported that a novel type of tRFs that was responsive to sex hormones [12]. These tRFs are specifically and abundantly expressed in ER-positive breast cancer as well as androgen receptor (AR)-positive prostate cancer cell lines. The authors also observed that these tRFs are abundant in human patient tissues, designating these tRFs as sex-hormone-dependent tRNA-derived RNAs (SHOT-RNAs). As expected, SHOT-RNAs are not abundant in other hormone-insensitive cancers, including ER-negative breast cancer and AR-negative prostate cancer, among many others. These SHOT-RNAs are largely identified as the 5′ halves of mature tRNAs by a sort of specific RNA sequencing method. These 5′ halves are generated by angiogenin, a type of RNase A family enzyme, and they increase cell proliferation, strongly suggesting a novel pathway that engages tRNA halves in the development and growth of sex hormone-dependent cancers.

6.2.4.3 MicroRNA (miRNA)-like Role of tRFs

Due to the rapid release of new data from NGS sequencing, numerous novel small non-coding RNAs have been identified expanding our understanding of their characteristics and functions. Yet, experimental data to verify this information are still scarce, causing mis-annotation of some small non-coding RNAs. In fact, there are several small non-coding RNAs that were first recognized as miRNAs but finally proven to be tRFs [57]. Some examples of these RNAs are listed in Table 6.3 (Table 6.3). Among these mis-annotated miRNAs, several of them have been reported to be linked to breast cancer.

Extracellular vesicles (EV), such as exosomes and membrane-shed vesicles, have been implicated in inter-cellular communication. Additionally, their possible use as biomarkers has been being pursued. Guzman et al. investigated the small RNAs in the EVs derived from the breast cancer cell line MCF7 and non-cancerous cell line MCF10A and observed unique miRNA profiles in these secreted vesicles [58]. There was a high abundance of "miRNA-like" tRFs specifically in the EVs of MCF7 but not in the EVs of MCF10A. Whereas the cellular levels of miR-125b, miR-100, and let-7a were correlatively mirrored in the EVs, several small RNAs were only detected in the MCF7 EVs. Interestingly these small RNAs comprised 65% of the total number of small RNAs in MCF7 EVs. The authors reported the four most abundant MCF7 EV miRNAs, such as miR-720, miR-1274a, miR-1274b, and miR-1260 (also known as miR-1260a), which share high sequence homology with $tRNA^{Thr}$, $tRNA^{Lys}$, $tRNA^{Lys}$, and $tRNA^{Leu}$, respectively (Tables 6.1 and 6.3) [58, 59]. Among them, miR-720, miR-1274a, and miR-1274b have been withdrawn from the miRNA database (miRBase) since they are now regarded to originate from the corresponding tRNAs (Table 6.3). It has been reported that tRFs can be induced and secreted under starvation conditions [60], but the small RNA-containing EVs mentioned above were identified under nutritious conditions [58]. Therefore, the

Table 6.3 Probable mis-annotation of human miRNA genes and the corresponding tRNAs

miRNA	Sequence	tRNA	tRF	References
miR-720	UCUCGCUGGGGCCUCCA	Human $tRNA^{Thr}$(UGU)	tRF-3	[57]
miR-1260	AUCCCACCUCU*GCCACCA	Human $tRNA^{Leu}$(AAG)	tRF-3	[95]
miR-1260b	AUCCCACCACUGCCACCAU**	Human $tRNA^{Leu}$(UAG)	tRF-3	[95]
miR-1274a	GUCCCUGUUCAGGCGCCA	Human $tRNA^{Lys}$(UUU)	tRF-3	[57]
miR-1274b	UCCCUGUUCGGGCGCCA	Human $tRNA^{Lys}$(UUU)	tRF-3	[57]
miR-1280	UCCCACCGCUGCCACCC	Human $tRNA^{Leu}$(AAG)	tRF-3	[57]
miR-1308	GCAUGGGUGGUUCAGUGG	Human $tRNA^{Gly}$(GCC)	tRF-5	[57]
miR-3182	GCUUCUGUAGUGUAGUC*	Human $tRNA^{Val}$(CAC)	tRF-5	[96]
miR-4286	ACCCCACUCCUGGUACC	Human $tRNA^{Leu}$(UAA)	tRF-3	
miR-4284	GGGCUCACAUCACCCCAU	Human $mtRNA^{Phe}$	tRF-3	[96]

miR-1260 is also known as miR-1260a. *There are single-base mismatches. Both U and C in miR-1260 and miR-3182 are G in the corresponding tRNA sequences, **U in the miR-1260b does not exist in the corresponding tRNA sequence

mechanisms underlying induction and secretion of the miRNA-derived tRFs detected in this study [58] may be different than those in the study of Lee et al. [60]. These observations imply that high tRF content of tumor-derived EVs alongside the tumor-specific miRNA signatures in them can be used to distinguish these EVs from those of other sources in the circulation.

Another study has also observed that miR-720, miR-1260, and miR-1280 are upregulated in the blood of patients with ER-positive/HER2-negative breast cancer [61]. As mentioned above, miR-720 and miR-1260 are tRF-3s processed from $tRNA^{Thr}$ and $tRNA^{Leu}$, respectively. Additionally, miR-1280 is also a mis-annotated miRNA, and it is actually a tRF-3 derived from $tRNA^{Leu}$ (Table 6.3). In particular, the miR-1280 level is significantly elevated in breast cancer patients, and it is positively correlated with the severity of the disease; the level is the highest in metastatic breast cancer, reduced after systemic treatment. These observations suggest that circulating tRFs, such as miR-1280, may serve as biomarkers for ER-positive breast cancer.

6.2.4.4 Mutations of tRFs in Breast Cancer

Several tRF mutations and their roles have been identified in other cancers. For example, ts-53 and ts-101 are often found to be mutated in chronic lymphocytic leukemia and lung cancer samples suggesting a key role of these tRFs in tumorigenesis [62]. They are derived from $tRNA^{Thr}$(AGU) and $tRNA^{Ser}$(GCU) but mis-annotated as miR-3676 and miR-4521, respectively. These tRFs associate with PIWI-2 protein to form PIWI-ribonucleoprotein complexes, but the mutations hamper this association. Additionally, these mutations are located in a region required for the interaction of the tRFs with the promoter of ZAP-70 (Zeta-chain–associated protein kinase 70). Consequently, these mutations impair targeting of ZAP-70 promoter by PIWI like protein 2 [63, 64].

It seems that there are no tRFs whose mutations have been identified in breast cancer. However, it has been suggested that tRFs can be key effectors in the pathways regulated by oncogenic mutations. In the MCF7 and MDA-MB-231 breast cancer cells carrying oncogenic mutants of *HRAS*, *KRAS*, or *PIK3CA* genes, the $tRNA^{Arg}$(UCG)-derived tRF, ts-47, is upregulated in *KRAS* mutant cells, and the $tRNA^{His}$(GUG)-derived tRF, ts-46, is upregulated in *PIK3CA* mutant cells (Table 6.1) [63]. Since mutations of *KRAS* and *PIK3CA* have pivotal roles in carcinogenesis, [65–67], tRFs might also function as key effectors in these pathways. Future research is expected to reveal the types and functions of tRF mutants in breast cancer.

6.3 Current Evidence and Concepts

6.3.1 Global Upregulation of tRNA Levels in Cancer

Recently, Zhang et al. have analyzed expression of tRNAs in the uniquely comprehensive data resource from The Cancer Genome Atlas [68]. According to the analysis, almost all cancers express similar overall average expression levels and patterns of tRNAs, while the expression levels of tRNA for each amino acid varies greatly. Among the tRNAs, $tRNA^{His}$ is the most highly expressed, and $tRNA^{Trp}$, $tRNA^{Leu}$, $tRNA^{Phe}$, $tRNA^{Asn}$, or $tRNA^{Sec}$ are not included in the high-expression cluster. Breast cancer is among the 9 cancers that show predominant upregulation of tRNAs across the 31 cancer types analyzed. This study suggests that tRNA overexpression in tumors might increase the translational efficiency in favor of cancer development. They also analyzed other molecules related to tRNAs including ARSs, tRNA-modifying enzymes, and translation factors, including ribosomes. It seems that overexpressed tRNAs may be stabilized by overexpressed tRNA-modifying enzymes, and the increased level of ARSs and translational factors may accelerate the translation in cancers. The merit of this study is that it provides the groundwork for an integrated functional interpretation by covering a broad set of various cancers. By doing so, the authors found that $tRNA^{Arg}$ was overexpressed in multiple cancer types in addition to breast cancer, where $tRNA^{Arg}$ had been reported to promote breast cancer metastasis [5].

6.3.2 Function of tRFs as miRNAs or piRNAs (PIWI-Interacting RNAs)

Since tRFs were first detected in the urine and serum of patients with cancers in the 1970s [62, 69–71], various tRFs have been identified, expanding the roles of tRFs as regulators but not as mere by-products of tRNA degradation. Many reports have suggested the involvement of tRNAs and tRFs in the regulation of transcription, translation, proliferation, cell cycle, apoptosis, and cell signaling. Breast cancer is one of the major cancers where the important implication of tRFs in the regulation of cancer has been shown. As mentioned before, several tRFs have been mis-annotated as miRNAs, suggesting that tRFs may work like miRNAs. However, this relationship between tRFs and miRNAs has not conclusively been clarified. A recent study has shown the interaction of tRFs with the miRNA- and piRNA-related proteins via meta-analysis [72]. Kumar et al. analyzed 50 small RNA datasets and found that tRFs might play a major role in RNA silencing via a microRNA-like mechanism. It is worth noting that tRFs appear to be an abundant class of small RNAs with a distinct biogenesis mechanism different from that of miRNAs. Similarly, several studies have demonstrated that tRFs can also function as piRNAs [64, 73]. A few tRFs have been found in the complexes containing Argonaute proteins, such as AGO1 and AGO2, as well as in complexes containing PIWI proteins. Unlike tRFs, miRNAs are only loaded onto protein complexes containing AGO1 and AGO2. This finding supports that some tRFs could act as piRNAs involved in the epigenetic and post-transcriptional control, such as histone methylation. More evidence, supporting the role of tRFs as an independent group of small non-coding RNAs may come from the breast cancer field with deep mechanistic analyses of the biogenesis and function of tRFs.

6.3.3 tRNAs as Substrates of miRNAs

While tRFs may work as miRNAs or piRNAs do, an interesting report has suggested that pre-tRNAs can be substrates of miRNAs. Wang et al. demonstrated that a tumor-suppressive miRNA, miR-34a, degraded the precursor of $tRNA_i^{Met}$ through AGO2-mediated destabilization [48]. The reduced level of $tRNA_i^{Met}$ inhibited proliferation of breast cancer cells and induced cell cycle arrest resulting in apoptosis. The expression level of miR-34a shows an inverse correlation with that of $tRNA_i^{Met}$ in breast cancer cells, and the cell phenotypes induced by miR-34a are restored by overexpression of $tRNA_i^{Met}$. These observations suggest that $tRNA_i^{Met}$ precursor is a functional target of miR-34a. Accordingly, this study supports the pro-oncogenic role of $tRNA_i^{Met}$ as reported elsewhere [55] and also suggests the protective role of $tRNA_i^{Met}$ modification against cleavage by reducing the interaction of mature $tRNA_i^{Met}$ with miR-34a and AGO2.

6.3.4 Progress in the Detection Methods for tRNAs and tRFs

As mentioned before, recent studies have used NGS to detect small RNAs including tRNAs and tRFs, rather than conventional methods such as northern blotting. However, tRNAs and tRFs have their own characteristics which make their detection more challenging. First, tRNAs and tRFs are post-translationally modified (Fig. 6.3) making the mapping of their deep sequencing reads more challenging [74, 75]. Second, their strong folding characteristics decrease their hybridization onto DNA chips. Overcoming these features can increase the curative and correct detection and interpretation of tRNAs and related fragments. Currently, one of the most reliable approaches for measuring tRNA levels is by DNA chips designed specifically for this purpose by Prof. Tao Pan [15, 76]. Recent studies have utilized the sequencing methods specialized for tRNAs. Several methods have been suggested to overcome the strong self-hybridization tendency of tRNAs via employing novel ligation strategies. For example, a two-step ligation strategy [77], addition of a poly-A tail to the deacylated 3′-ends of mature tRNAs for RT-PCR (real-time-PCR) amplification of tRNAs [78], and Y-shaped adapter application [31]. Furthermore, a DM-tRNA-seq (demethylase tRNA-seq) is intended to reduce the sequence bias from tRNA post-transcriptional methylations by treating tRNAs with AlkB demethylase, followed by a template-switching reaction of thermostable group II intron reverse transcriptase for adapter attachment to tRNAs [79]. There are other methods available for measuring tRNA levels, such as liquid chromatography-mass spectrometry and signature digestion products [80].

6.3.5 The Diagnostic Potential of tRNAs

There is increasing evidence that the expression levels of tRNAs and tRFs may be implicated in disease progression including cancer since their expression is changed or dysregulated in the specific context of diseases.

Recently, several papers have suggested tRFs as predictive markers for breast cancer. Sun et al. investigated tRF profiles in trastuzumab-sensitive and trastuzumab-resistant breast cancer cells via high-throughput sequencing and qRT-PCR and found that two tRFs originated from $tRNA^{Cys}$(GCA) were significantly upregulated in trastuzumab-resistant patients with a positive correlation of ROC (receiver operating characteristic) curve with trastuzumab resistance (Table 6.1) [81].

There are still several challenging points to be considered for the development of tRNAs and tRFs as diagnostic markers. First, robust and efficient approaches to measure tRNA and tRF levels are required. Recent developments in the tools to detect them may shed a light on this field. It is worth noting that tRNAs are relatively stable than other RNAs owing to their self-folding characteristics. This feature protects tRNAs from being digested by RNA-degrading enzymes and can be advantageous considering that sample-processing time is usually the limiting factor.

Second, there are >500 interspersed tRNA genes, and some of them share the same mature tRNA sequence despite the difference in pre-tRNA sequence. If a tRNA transcribed from a specific locus of a chromosome is to be used as a diagnostic marker, there should be a strategy to differentiate it from the other copies. In addition, a diagnostic tool should consider the adaptation of the mutations or single nucleotide polymorphisms to the human tRNA pool [75].

6.4 Future Research Direction

Based on the reports that have been published in the field of cancer and tRNAs, major studies have focused on the expression levels of these RNA molecules in a specific context of cancer, showing their positive correlations. Deeper and more thoroughly done studies are required to solve the biogenesis and functions of tRNAs and tRFs in breast cancer. It should not be fragmental but comprehensive to give a concrete understanding of tRNAs and tRFs to be used for therapeutic or diagnostic uses. tRNAs and their derivatives are abundant in human body fluids, including serum [62, 69–71, 82]. Therefore, detection of tRNAs and tRFs from EVs in body fluids from cancer patients can be performed via minimally invasive methods. Since they can work as regulatory molecules, widely involved in the pathogenesis of cancers, application of tRNAs and tRF-based non-invasive biomarkers in tumor diagnosis is expected to have broad prospects [83].

There are several things to be solved in basic research. First, the nomenclature of tRFs is still inconsistent. There are >500 tRNA genes in the human genome, and theoretically, all the tRNAs could be cleaved by different types of ribonucleases to produce various tRFs. However, these tRFs have not been categorized with a unified name yet. Many factors should be considered for the unification: the origins and types of tRFs, their chromosomal locations, and inclusion of intron sequences. Li et al. proposed a naming scheme in the form of X-tsRNA$^{\text{AA-NNN}}$, where tsRNA represents the species; X represents the subtypes of tsRNAs based on the mapped location of tRNAs; superscript AA represents the abbreviation of amino acid carried by the mapped tRNAs; superscript NNN represents the anticodon of the mapped tRNAs. For example, 5'-tiRNA and 3a-tRF derived from tRNA$^{\text{Glu-CTC}}$ can be named as 5'-tiRNA$^{\text{Glu-CTC}}$ and 3a-tRF$^{\text{Glu-CTC}}$, respectively [3]. This proposal can be considered as an option before a consensus among the researchers is reached.

Second, the biogenesis process of tRFs is not clearly understood. RNase families and Dicer are known to be involved in the biogenesis of tRFs [3, 26]; however, the understanding of ribonucleases is not very comprehensive. Therefore, the exact biogenesis mechanism of many tRFs remains elusive.

Third, animal models focusing on tRNAs or tRFs would aid to understand the function of tRNAs and tRFs as well as to investigate the phenotypic significance of these RNAs [83]. Animal models are promising tools for analyzing the function and effect of targets on diseases; therefore, animal model studies with specific tRNAs and tRFs can decrease the gap between in vitro and in vivo studies. Transgenic mice expressing additional copies of $tRNA_i^{Met}$(CAU) will be a good example showing the importance of the animal models [55], where the pro-oncogenic function of $tRNA_i^{Met}$(CAU) for the tumor growth and angiogenesis can be successfully validated.

6.5 Summary

6.5.1 The Bench

An increasing number of reports have revealed that tRNAs and tRFs are involved in various biological processes, such as transcription, translation, proliferation, apoptosis, and metastasis. tRFs are small RNAs working as miRNA and piRNAs do, but they have different biogenesis mechanisms as an independent pool of cell-regulating small RNAs. However, information regarding their expression profiles is fragmented, and the molecular basis behind their biogenesis and function remains still elusive. In accordance with the informatics-based studies, more mechanistic studies will be required to understand the diverse role of tRNAs and tRFs.

6.5.2 Translation and the Bedside

There is growing evidence that tRNAs and tRFs may work as diagnostic markers. The involvement of tRFs and tRNAs in cancers provides fresh perspectives for the exploration and development of new biomarkers and novel therapeutic strategies. The stage of tRNA-based translational research is just at the conceptual step; therefore, active translational research will be on full track in future in accordance with deeper studies.

Acknowledgments This work was supported by NRF-M3A6A4-2010-0029785 (SK) and NRF-2015M3A6A4065724 (NHK) from the National Research Foundation, MSIT of Korea.

References

1. Kim S, You S, Hwang D. Aminoacyl-tRNA synthetases and tumorigenesis: more than housekeeping. Nat Rev Cancer. 2011;11(10):708–18.
2. Iben JR, Maraia RJ. tRNA gene copy number variation in humans. Gene. 2014;536(2):376–84.
3. Li S, Xu Z, Sheng J. tRNA-derived small RNA: A novel regulatory small non-coding RNA. Genes. 2018;9(5):246.

4. Goodenbour JM, Pan T. Diversity of tRNA genes in eukaryotes. Nucleic Acids Res. 2006;34 (21):6137–46.
5. Goodarzi H, Nguyen HC, Zhang S, Dill BD, Molina H, Tavazoie SF. Modulated expression of specific tRNAs drives gene expression and cancer progression. Cell. 2016;165(6):1416–27.
6. Mei Y, Yong J, Liu H, Shi Y, Meinkoth J, Dreyfuss G, et al. tRNA binds to cytochrome c and inhibits caspase activation. Mol Cell. 2010;37(5):668–78.
7. Birch J, Clarke CJ, Campbell AD, Campbell K, Mitchell L, Liko D, et al. The initiator methionine tRNA drives cell migration and invasion leading to increased metastatic potential in melanoma. Biol Open. 2016;5(10):1371–9.
8. Pavon-Eternod M, Gomes S, Rosner MR, Pan T. Overexpression of initiator methionine tRNA leads to global reprogramming of tRNA expression and increased proliferation in human epithelial cells. RNA. 2013;19(4):461–6.
9. Kumar P, Mudunuri SB, Anaya J, Dutta A. tRFdb: a database for transfer RNA fragments. Nucleic Acids Res. 2015;43:D141–5.
10. Ivanov P, Emara MM, Villen J, Gygi SP, Anderson P. Angiogenin-induced tRNA fragments inhibit translation initiation. Mol Cell. 2011;43(4):613–23.
11. Ivanov P, O'Day E, Emara MM, Wagner G, Lieberman J, Anderson P. G-quadruplex structures contribute to the neuroprotective effects of angiogenin-induced tRNA fragments. Proc Natl Acad Sci U S A. 2014;111(51):18201–6.
12. Honda S, Loher P, Shigematsu M, Palazzo JP, Suzuki R, Imoto I, et al. Sex hormone-dependent tRNA halves enhance cell proliferation in breast and prostate cancers. Proc Natl Acad Sci U S A. 2015;112(29):E3816–25.
13. Cole C, Sobala A, Lu C, Thatcher SR, Bowman A, Brown JW, et al. Filtering of deep sequencing data reveals the existence of abundant dicer-dependent small RNAs derived from tRNAs. RNA. 2009;15(12):2147–60.
14. Haussecker D, Huang Y, Lau A, Parameswaran P, Fire AZ, Kay MA. Human tRNA-derived small RNAs in the global regulation of RNA silencing. RNA. 2010;16(4):673–95.
15. Pavon-Eternod M, Gomes S, Geslain R, Dai Q, Rosner MR, Pan T. tRNA over-expression in breast cancer and functional consequences. Nucleic Acids Res. 2009;37(21):7268–80.
16. Marshall L, White RJ. Non-coding RNA production by RNA polymerase III is implicated in cancer. Nat Rev Cancer. 2008;8(12):911–4.
17. Zouridis H, Hatzimanikatis V. Effects of codon distributions and tRNA competition on protein translation. Biophys J. 2008;95(3):1018–33.
18. Gustafsson C, Govindarajan S, Minshull J. Codon bias and heterologous protein expression. Trends Biotechnol. 2004;22(7):346–53.
19. dos Reis M, Savva R, Wernisch L. Solving the riddle of codon usage preferences: a test for translational selection. Nucleic Acids Res. 2004;32(17):5036–44.
20. Qian W, Yang JR, Pearson NM, Maclean C, Zhang J. Balanced codon usage optimizes eukaryotic translational efficiency. PLoS Genet. 2012;8(3):e1002603.
21. Subramaniam AR, Pan T, Cluzel P. Environmental perturbations lift the degeneracy of the genetic code to regulate protein levels in bacteria. Proc Natl Acad Sci U S A. 2013;110 (6):2419–24.
22. Gingold H, Tehler D, Christoffersen NR, Nielsen MM, Asmar F, Kooistra SM, et al. A dual program for translation regulation in cellular proliferation and differentiation. Cell. 2014;158 (6):1281–92.
23. Xu WL, Yang Y, Wang YD, Qu LH, Zheng LL. Computational approaches to tRNA-derived small RNAs. Noncoding RNA. 2017;3(1):2.
24. MacIntosh GC, Bariola PA, Newbigin E, Green PJ. Characterization of Rny1, the Saccharomyces cerevisiae member of thc T2 RNase family of RNases: unexpected functions for ancient enzymes? Proc Natl Acad Sci U S A. 2001;98(3):1018–23.
25. Thompson DM, Lu C, Green PJ, Parker R. tRNA cleavage is a conserved response to oxidative stress in eukaryotes. RNA. 2008;14(10):2095–103.

26. Towns WL, Begley TJ. Transfer RNA methytransferases and their corresponding modifications in budding yeast and humans: activities, predications, and potential roles in human health. DNA Cell Biol. 2012;31(4):434–54.
27. Goodarzi H, Liu X, Nguyen HC, Zhang S, Fish L, Tavazoie SF. Endogenous tRNA-derived fragments suppress breast cancer progression via YBX1 displacement. Cell. 2015;161 (4):790–802.
28. DMM A. In: Walker JM, editor. Probe Design, Production, and Applications. Totowa, NJ: Humana Press; 2005.
29. Kohrer C, Rajbhandary UL. The many applications of acid urea polyacrylamide gel electrophoresis to studies of tRNAs and aminoacyl-tRNA synthetases. Methods. 2008;44(2):129–38.
30. Han Y, Gao S, Muegge K, Zhang W, Zhou B. Advanced applications of RNA sequencing and challenges. Bioinform Biol Insights. 2015;9(Suppl 1):29–46.
31. Shigematsu M, Honda S, Loher P, Telonis AG, Rigoutsos I, Kirino Y. YAMAT-seq: an efficient method for high-throughput sequencing of mature transfer RNAs. Nucleic Acids Res. 2017;45(9):e70.
32. Zheng LL, Xu WL, Liu S, Sun WJ, Li JH, Wu J, et al. tRF2Cancer: a web server to detect tRNA-derived small RNA fragments (tRFs) and their expression in multiple cancers. Nucleic Acids Res. 2016;44(W1):W185–93.
33. Pliatsika V, Loher P, Magee R, Telonis AG, Londin E, Shigematsu M, et al. MINTbase v2.0: a comprehensive database for tRNA-derived fragments that includes nuclear and mitochondrial fragments from all the Cancer genome atlas projects. Nucleic Acids Res. 2018;46(D1):D152–D9.
34. Krishnan P, Ghosh S, Wang B, Heyns M, Li D, Mackey JR, et al. Genome-wide profiling of transfer RNAs and their role as novel prognostic markers for breast cancer. Sci Rep. 2016;6:32843.
35. Telonis AG, Rigoutsos I. Race disparities in the contribution of miRNA isoforms and tRNA-derived fragments to triple-negative breast cancer. Cancer Res. 2018;78(5):1140–54.
36. Dhahbi JM, Spindler SR, Atamna H, Boffelli D, Martin DI. Deep sequencing of serum small RNAs identifies patterns of 5' tRNA half and YRNA fragment expression associated with breast cancer. Biomark Cancer. 2014;6:37–47.
37. Wallace DC. Mitochondrial DNA variation in human radiation and disease. Cell. 2015;163 (1):33–8.
38. Grzybowska-Szatkowska L, Slaska B. Polymorphisms in genes encoding mt-tRNA in female breast cancer in Poland. Mitochondrial DNA. 2012;23(2):106–11.
39. Tan DJ, Bai RK, Wong LJ. Comprehensive scanning of somatic mitochondrial DNA mutations in breast cancer. Cancer Res. 2002;62(4):972–6.
40. Huang SQ, Sun B, Xiong ZP, Shu Y, Zhou HH, Zhang W, et al. The dysregulation of tRNAs and tRNA derivatives in cancer. J Exp Clin Cancer Res. 2018;37(1):101.
41. Lu J, Sharma LK, Bai Y. Implications of mitochondrial DNA mutations and mitochondrial dysfunction in tumorigenesis. Cell Res. 2009;19(7):802–15.
42. Meng XL, Meng H, Zhang W, Qin YH, Zhao NM. The role of mitochondrial tRNA variants in female breast cancer. Mitochondrial DNA A DNA Mapp Seq Anal. 2016;27(5):3199–201.
43. Pan T. Modifications and functional genomics of human transfer RNA. Cell Res. 2018;28 (4):395–404.
44. de Crecy-Lagard V, Boccaletto P, Mangleburg CG, Sharma P, Lowe TM, Leidel SA, et al. Matching tRNA modifications in humans to their known and predicted enzymes. Nucleic Acids Res. 2019;47(5):2143–59.
45. Novoa EM, Pavon-Eternod M, Pan T. Ribas de Pouplana L. a role for tRNA modifications in genome structure and codon usage. Cell. 2012;149(1):202–13.
46. Frye M, Watt FM. The RNA methyltransferase Misu (NSun2) mediates Myc-induced proliferation and is upregulated in tumors. Curr Biol. 2006;16(10):971–81.

47. Delaunay S, Rapino F, Tharun L, Zhou Z, Heukamp L, Termathe M, et al. Elp3 links tRNA modification to IRES-dependent translation of LEF1 to sustain metastasis in breast cancer. J Exp Med. 2016;213(11):2503–23.
48. Wang B, Li D, Kovalchuk I, Apel IJ, Chinnaiyan AM, Woycicki RK, et al. miR-34a directly targets tRNAi(met) precursors and affects cellular proliferation, cell cycle, and apoptosis. Proc Natl Acad Sci U S A. 2018;115(28):7392–7.
49. Tomita K, Liu Y. Human BCDIN3D is a cytoplasmic tRNA(his)-specific 5′-monophosphate methyltransferase. Front Genet. 2018;9:305.
50. Khattar E, Kumar P, Liu CY, Akincilar SC, Raju A, Lakshmanan M, et al. Telomerase reverse transcriptase promotes cancer cell proliferation by augmenting tRNA expression. J Clin Invest. 2016;126(10):4045–60.
51. Fornier M, Fumoleau P. The paradox of triple negative breast cancer: novel approaches to treatment. Breast J. 2012;18(1):41–51.
52. Guo Y, Yu H, Wang J, Sheng Q, Zhao S, Zhao YY, et al. The landscape of small non-coding RNAs in triple-negative breast cancer. Genes. 2018;9(1):29.
53. Fang Z, Yi Y, Shi G, Li S, Chen S, Lin Y, et al. Role of Brf1 interaction with ERalpha, and significance of its overexpression, in human breast cancer. Mol Oncol. 2017;11(12):1752–67.
54. Kwon NH, Lee MR, Kong J, Park SK, Hwang BJ, Kim BG, et al. Transfer-RNA-mediated enhancement of ribosomal proteins S6 kinases signalling for cell proliferation. RNA Biol. 2017;15(4–5):635–48.
55. Clarke CJ, Berg TJ, Birch J, Ennis D, Mitchell L, Cloix C, et al. The initiator methionine tRNA drives secretion of type II collagen from stromal fibroblasts to promote tumor growth and angiogenesis. Curr Biol. 2016;26(6):755–65.
56. Thompson DM, Parker R. Stressing out over tRNA cleavage. Cell. 2009;138(2):215–9.
57. Schopman NC, Heynen S, Haasnoot J, Berkhout B. A miRNA-tRNA mix-up: tRNA origin of proposed miRNA. RNA Biol. 2010;7(5):573–6.
58. Guzman N, Agarwal K, Asthagiri D, Yu L, Saji M, Ringel MD, et al. Breast cancer-specific miR signature unique to extracellular vesicles includes "microRNA-like" tRNA fragments. Mol Cancer Res. 2015;13(5):891–901.
59. Keam SP, Hutvagner G. tRNA-derived fragments (tRFs): emerging new roles for an ancient RNA in the regulation of gene expression. Life. 2015;5(4):1638–51.
60. Lee SR, Collins K. Starvation-induced cleavage of the tRNA anticodon loop in Tetrahymena thermophila. J Biol Chem. 2005;280(52):42744–9.
61. Park IH, Kang JH, Lee KS, Nam S, Ro J, Kim JH. Identification and clinical implications of circulating microRNAs for estrogen receptor-positive breast cancer. Tumour Biol. 2014;35 (12):12173–80.
62. Sun C, Fu Z, Wang S, Li J, Li Y, Zhang Y, et al. Roles of tRNA-derived fragments in human cancers. Cancer Lett. 2018;414:16–25.
63. Balatti V, Nigita G, Veneziano D, Drusco A, Stein GS, Messier TL, et al. tsRNA signatures in cancer. Proc Natl Acad Sci U S A. 2017;114(30):8071–6.
64. Pekarsky Y, Balatti V, Palamarchuk A, Rizzotto L, Veneziano D, Nigita G, et al. Dysregulation of a family of short noncoding RNAs, tsRNAs, in human cancer. Proc Natl Acad Sci U S A. 2016;113(18):5071–6.
65. Zardavas D, Phillips WA, Loi S. PIK3CA mutations in breast cancer: reconciling findings from preclinical and clinical data. Breast Cancer Res. 2014;16(1):201.
66. Mei ZB, Duan CY, Li CB, Cui L, Ogino S. Prognostic role of tumor PIK3CA mutation in colorectal cancer: a systematic review and meta-analysis. Ann Oncol. 2016;27(10):1836–48.
67. Kawada K, Toda K, Sakai Y. Targeting metabolic reprogramming in KRAS-driven cancers. Int J Clin Oncol. 2017;22(4):651–9.
68. Zhang Z, Ye Y, Gong J, Ruan H, Liu CJ, Xiang Y, et al. Global analysis of tRNA and translation factor expression reveals a dynamic landscape of translational regulation in human cancers. Commun Biol. 2018;1:234.

69. Speer J, Gehrke CW, Kuo KC, Waalkes TP, Borek E. tRNA breakdown products as markers for cancer. Cancer. 1979;44(6):2120–3.
70. Waalkes TP, Gehrke CW, Tormey DC, Zumwalt RW, Hueser JN, Kuo KC, et al. Urinary excretion of polyamines by patients with advanced malignancy. Cancer Chemother Rep. 1975;59(6):1103–16.
71. Borek E, Baliga BS, Gehrke CW, Kuo CW, Belman S, Troll W, et al. High turnover rate of transfer RNA in tumor tissue. Cancer Res. 1977;37(9):3362–6.
72. Kumar P, Anaya J, Mudunuri SB, Dutta A. Meta-analysis of tRNA derived RNA fragments reveals that they are evolutionarily conserved and associate with AGO proteins to recognize specific RNA targets. BMC Biol. 2014;12:78.
73. Zhang X, He X, Liu C, Liu J, Hu Q, Pan T, et al. IL-4 inhibits the biogenesis of an epigenetically suppressive PIWI-interacting RNA to upregulate CD1a molecules on monocytes/dendritic cells. J Immunol. 2016;196(4):1591–603.
74. Gustilo EM, Vendeix FA, Agris PF. tRNA's modifications bring order to gene expression. Curr Opin Microbiol. 2008;11(2):134–40.
75. Mahlab S, Tuller T, Linial M. Conservation of the relative tRNA composition in healthy and cancerous tissues. RNA. 2012;18(4):640–52.
76. Dittmar KA, Goodenbour JM, Pan T. Tissue-specific differences in human transfer RNA expression. PLoS Genet. 2006;2(12):e221.
77. Pang YL, Abo R, Levine SS, Dedon PC. Diverse cell stresses induce unique patterns of tRNA up- and down-regulation: tRNA-seq for quantifying changes in tRNA copy number. Nucleic Acids Res. 2014;42(22):e170.
78. Zhong J, Xiao C, Gu W, Du G, Sun X, He QY, et al. Transfer RNAs mediate the rapid adaptation of Escherichia coli to oxidative stress. PLoS Genet. 2015;11(6):e1005302.
79. Zheng G, Qin Y, Clark WC, Dai Q, Yi C, He C, et al. Efficient and quantitative high-throughput tRNA sequencing. Nat Methods. 2015;12(9):835–7.
80. Castleberry CM, Limbach PA. Relative quantitation of transfer RNAs using liquid chromatography mass spectrometry and signature digestion products. Nucleic Acids Res. 2010;38(16): e162.
81. Sun C, Yang F, Zhang Y, Chu J, Wang J, Wang Y, et al. tRNA-derived fragments as novel predictive biomarkers for trastuzumab-resistant breast cancer. Cell Physiol Biochem. 2018;49 (2):419–31.
82. Dhahbi JM, Spindler SR, Atamna H, Yamakawa A, Boffelli D, Mote P, et al. 5' tRNA halves are present as abundant complexes in serum, concentrated in blood cells, and modulated by aging and calorie restriction. BMC Genomics. 2013;14:298.
83. Zhu L, Ge J, Li T, Shen Y, Guo J. tRNA-derived fragments and tRNA halves: the new players in cancers. Cancer Lett. 2019;452:31–7.
84. Telonis AG, Loher P, Honda S, Jing Y, Palazzo J, Kirino Y, et al. Dissecting tRNA-derived fragment complexities using personalized transcriptomes reveals novel fragment classes and unexpected dependencies. Oncotarget. 2015;6(28):24797–822.
85. Zhang X, Jiang G, Sun M, Zhou H, Miao Y, Liang M, et al. Cytosolic THUMPD1 promotes breast cancer cells invasion and metastasis via the AKT-GSK3-snail pathway. Oncotarget. 2017;8(8):13357–66.
86. Gatza ML, Silva GO, Parker JS, Fan C, Perou CM. An integrated genomics approach identifies drivers of proliferation in luminal-subtype human breast cancer. Nat Genet. 2014;46 (10):1051–9.
87. Okamoto M, Hirata S, Sato S, Koga S, Fujii M, Qi G, et al. Frequent increased gene copy number and high protein expression of tRNA (cytosine-5-)-methyltransferase (NSUN2) in human cancers. DNA Cell Biol. 2012;31(5):660–71.
88. Yi J, Gao R, Chen Y, Yang Z, Han P, Zhang H, et al. Overexpression of NSUN2 by DNA hypomethylation is associated with metastatic progression in human breast cancer. Oncotarget. 2017;8(13):20751–65.

89. Rodriguez V, Chen Y, Elkahloun A, Dutra A, Pak E, Chandrasekharappa S. Chromosome 8 BAC array comparative genomic hybridization and expression analysis identify amplification and overexpression of TRMT12 in breast cancer. Genes Chromosomes Cancer. 2007;46 (7):694–707.
90. Cheng TY, Shankar J, Zirpoli G, Roberts MR, Hong CC, Bandera EV, et al. Genetic variants in the mTOR pathway and interaction with body size and weight gain on breast cancer risk in African-American and European American women. Cancer Causes Control. 2016;27 (8):965–76.
91. Hicks DG, Janarthanan BR, Vardarajan R, Kulkarni SA, Khoury T, Dim D, et al. The expression of TRMT2A, a novel cell cycle regulated protein, identifies a subset of breast cancer patients with HER2 over-expression that are at an increased risk of recurrence. BMC Cancer. 2010;10:108.
92. Kim TW, Kim B, Kim JH, Kang S, Park SB, Jeong G, et al. Nuclear-encoded mitochondrial MTO1 and MRPL41 are regulated in an opposite epigenetic mode based on estrogen receptor status in breast cancer. BMC Cancer. 2013;13:502.
93. Yue Z, Li HT, Yang Y, Hussain S, Zheng CH, Xia J, et al. Identification of breast cancer candidate genes using gene co-expression and protein-protein interaction information. Oncotarget. 2016;7(24):36092–100.
94. Couch FJ, Kuchenbaecker KB, Michailidou K, Mendoza-Fandino GA, Nord S, Lilyquist J, et al. Identification of four novel susceptibility loci for oestrogen receptor negative breast cancer. Nat Commun. 2016;7:11375.
95. Venkatesh T, Suresh PS, Tsutsumi R. tRFs: miRNAs in disguise. Gene. 2016;579(2):133–8.
96. Guo L, Liang T, Gu W, Xu Y, Bai Y, Lu Z. Cross-mapping events in miRNAs reveal potential miRNA-mimics and evolutionary implications. PLoS One. 2011;6(5):e20517.

Chapter 7
Fusion Genes in Breast Cancer

Jisun Kim and Wonshik Han

Abstract Fusion gene is a hybrid form of two distinct genes resulting in broad spectrum of downstream pathway alterations. Gene fusion events are mostly from genomic rearrangements though diverse mechanisms have now been identified from in-depth analyses of next generation sequencing data. While profound level of genomic, transcriptomic driver alterations have been identified, till now, not many gene fusions are found to be the 'driver' of cancer development nor progression.

ESR1 gene is a protein coding gene, encoding estrogen receptor, a transcription factor which is a key pathway in hormone sensitive breast cancers. Several hotspot mutations of this *ESR1* gene have recently been associated with resistance to endocrine therapy. *ESR1* gene fusion with diverse partner genes have also been identified recently, and are suggested to be acquired during previous endocrine therapy. Recurrent *ESR1* gene fusions are indicative of ligand-independent hyper-activity according to 3′ partner gene found among 1%~ of metastatic hormone sensitive metastatic breast cancers.

Keywords Gene fusion · Fusion transcript · RNA sequencing · *ESR1* · Endocrine resistance · Breast cancer

J. Kim
Department of Surgery, Asan Medical Center, Seoul, South Korea

W. Han (✉)
Department of Surgery, Seoul National University College of Medicine, Seoul, South Korea

Biomedical Research Institute, Seoul National University Hospital, Seoul, South Korea

Cancer Research Institute, Seoul National University, Seoul, South Korea
e-mail: hanw@snu.ac.kr

D.-Y. Noh et al. (eds.), *Translational Research in Breast Cancer*, Advances in Experimental Medicine and Biology 1187,
https://doi.org/10.1007/978-981-32-9620-6_7

7.1 Introduction

Gene fusions have long been recognized among hematologic malignancies and sarcomas. Philadelphia chromosome, a reciprocal translocation of chromosomes 9 and 22 creating *BCR-ABL1* fusion gene, serves as both diagnostic marker and therapeutic target for chronic myeloid leukemia [1]. *EWSR1-FLI1* fusion gene is a characteristic translocation of Ewing sarcoma. In breast carcinomas, gene fusions have been reported among rare histologic types of tumors, e.g., *ETV6-NTRK3* in salivary carcinoma by in situ hybridization. While not commonly found among normal tissues, profound level of gene fusion events is observed among cancers. Recently reported recurrent fusions among epithelial tumors, *TMPRSS2-ERG* fusion was found in 50% of prostate tumors and *EML4-ALK* fusion was observed in 6.7% of nonsmall cell lung cancer (NSCLC) [2, 3].

7.2 Review of Past Studies

7.2.1 Mechanism of Gene Fusions

Advances in sequencing technology have enabled illustrating an overview of genomic, transcriptomic repertoire in cancers. While single nucleotide variants, insertion/deletions, and copy number variations comprise large fraction of somatic alterations, analyses of RNA-sequencing data revealed a number of fusions across cancer types. Fusion genes commonly arise from a genomic rearrangement, or during transcription, or through a cellular catastrophe called 'chromothripsis'. Though most are known to be passengers, fusion genes may lead to downstream pathway alterations, thereby potentially be oncogenic.

Genomic rearrangements do not occur randomly across the genome; however, up to 50% are found in chromosomes 17, 8, 1, 20, 6, and 11. Fusions were rarely found in chromosome 15 or 18. Hotspots for fusions were found at 17q21, 17q12, 17q11.2, 17q23, 8q24, and 20q13. Previous studies have shown that fusion breakpoints colocalize with copy number aberration site [4]. These fusions have been noted as 'amplicon-associated gene fusions,' which are predominantly a by-product meaning passenger aberrations. Fimereli et al. have recently reported that 26% percent of fusions had at least one copy number breakpoint located within 100 Kb from fusion breakpoint [5]. Similarly, the number of fusions positively correlated with the number of amplifications, while not associated with the number of deletions especially with when analyzed separately.

Fusion genes can be categorized according to the type of genomic rearrangement, whether it is located at the amplicon, if not, whether it is interchromosomal translocation or intrachromosomal fusions. Within intrachromosomal fusions, whether it results in tandem duplication, deletion, or inversion [6]. Intrachromosomal fusion genes outnumbered interchromosomal fusion genes among breast cancers, and tandem duplication was most commonly observed. Interestingly, a majority of fusion junctions were found at coding regions and more likely to be seen at 5′-UTR than 3′-UTR. This may be due to 5′-UTR having more open chromatin though 3′-UTR is generally longer.

7.2.2 Fusion Detecting Algorithms

As substantial portion of detected fusions results from false positive calls, discriminating true positive fusions from false positive calls has long been great interest. In an effort to increase accuracy of detecting fusion genes, many bioinformatics algorithms have been introduced and been applied, yet with substantial level of disagreement. Fusion detecting tools are available in the OMICtools portal (www.omictools.com). More than 20 fusion detecting tools utilizing whole genome, RNA sequencing have been introduced [7]. Each tool varies in performance depending on quality of dataset, e.g., number of reads and read length, suggesting that fusion detecting tool should be decided upon those factors, especially given that no single method showed best performance across multiple datasets [6, 8–12].

7.2.3 Number of Fusion Genes

Initial studies have focused on a number of fusion genes with the understanding that genomic rearrangement represents genomic instability and in part contributes to have greater mutational burden. The total number of fusions within each sample varies for different types of cancers. For tumors arising in kidney (clear cell carcinoma and papillary cell carcinoma), low-grade gliomas, pheochromocytoma, paraganglioma, and thyroid carcinoma displayed a least number of fusion genes. Other types of carcinomas including breast cancers showed a range between 0 and 5 fusions in each sample. Regardless of the number of fusions detected, for most of the tumors, if any, only one in-frame oncogenic fusion was found. From our previous study of primary breast cancers, *HER2*-enriched tumors harbored a greater number of fusion genes compared to other subtypes and *HER2* negative breast cancers [13]. Similar observation was recently reported from an analysis of 55 primary breast cancer samples [5]. With a median of 6.7 fusions, *HER2*-enriched tumors displayed a greater number of fusions, 12.6/sample followed by triple negative, luminal A and B tumors (7.1, 1.8, and 5.8 per sample, respectively). This could be in part with the previously described colocalization of fusion and copy number breakpoint, and therefore, hotspot of fusion location exists, among which *HER2* gene is located.

7.2.4 Mechanisms of How it Drives Tumor Progression

Gene fusion can result in downstream pathway alteration depending on the involved genes, and thus, its breakage junction is of importance. Recently, from a comprehensive systematic review of large-scale public data, Gao and colleagues analyzed the expression of the fusion genes in regard to its known function of involved genes [1]. Samples with fusions involving kinases and/or oncogenes, e.g., *EGFR*, *RET*, and *ERBB2*, displayed oncogene overexpression, while samples with fusions involving tumor suppressor genes displayed decreased expression. (Fig. 7.1) Of note, *TP53*, the master tumor suppressor gene commonly mutated in solid tumors, fusions involving this gene were rarely found (TCGA). Fusions involving kinase genes or oncogenes should be in-frame fusions to be driver alteration, while tumor suppressor gene fusion could be either in-frame or out-of-frame. Yoshihara et al. have analyzed 1019 breast cancers and found 3.7% harboring in-frame fusions involving chromatin modifier genes, some of which encode histone demethylase [14]. As chromatin remodeling has been revealed to have tumor suppressor role, these subsets of fusions, resulting in loss of function, may induce tumorigenesis or tumor progression. A comprehensive review of currently reported gene fusions across breast

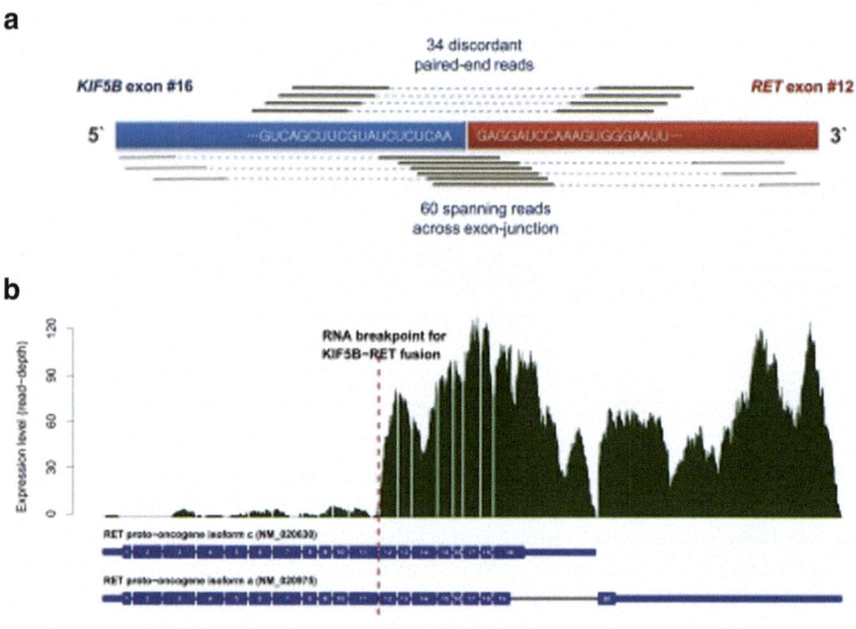

Fig. 7.1 (**a**) KIF5B-RET fusion gene, B. Overexpression of 3' fusion partner gene, RET kinase. Mechanisms of how gene fusions promote, drive tumorigenesis and/or tumor progression. A, A oncogene, RET fusion in lung cancer is driven by overexpression of 3' RET gene and its' downstream pathway. (**b**) PMID: 22194472 KIF5B-RET lung Figure 2B, 2E https://www.ncbi.nlm.nih.gov/core/lw/2.0/html/tileshop_pmc/tileshop_pmc_inline.html?title=Click%20on%20image%20to%20zoom&p=PMC3&id=3290779_436fig2.jpg

cancers was done by Kim and colleagues [15]. Diverse gene fusions across breast cancers have also been revealed. Though with growing amount of accumulated data, it has not been long since the oncogenic functions of specific fusion genes came into our understanding. Similarly, while next generation sequencing method has generated millions of fusion genes throughout cancers, not many are found to be recurrent among breast cancers.

7.2.5 *Rare Recurrent Fusions in Breast Cancers; Fusion Gene Confers Genotypic-Phenotypic Correlation*

Breast cancer displays a profound level of inter- and intratumor heterogeneity. Understandings of genomic and transcriptomic repertoire have revealed diverse spectrum of mutations including fusion genes. As mentioned previously, while a great number of fusion genes were identified, not many are found to be recurrent. Recent analyses of 560 breast cancer genome revealed rare recurrent fusions among breast cancers [16]. Robinson et al. have reported fusions with MAST kinase family genes, and although not '*recurrent*', this adds to the previous notions that individual fusion partner gene may play critical role as oncogenic driver [17]. Rather, recurrent fusions were represented in rare subset of breast cancers. While most breast cancers are, ductal/lobular carcinoma of no special type (IDC-NSTs), there are subsets of rare histologic types of breast cancers. Among these rare types of breast cancers, characteristic fusion genes have been recognized. *ETV6-NTRK3* fusion has known to be a causative alteration found in 90% of secretory breast carcinoma since the 1990s [13]. This in-frame fusion encodes a dimerization domain of the transcription factor *ETV6* joined with kinase domain of *NTRK3* enabling ligand-independent activation, thus causing oncogenic transformation [18]. Therapeutic benefit of NTRK inhibitors for solid tumors harboring this fusion is being evaluated in phase II clinical trials [19].

Adenoid cystic carcinoma (AdCC) of the breast is also a rare type of triple negative breast cancers displaying a distinct phenotype of dual luminal and basaloid ductal linings. Unlike typical triple negative breast cancers (TNBCs), it shows favorable clinical outcome. At molecular level, genomic repertoire is relatively quiescent, with less mutational burden, absence of *TP53, PIK3CA* mutation, 5q losses, and 8q, which are commonly observed alterations found in TNBC-NSTs. Rather, AdCCs are known to be driven by MYB pathway activation mostly underpinned by *MYB-NFIB* fusion gene [20, 21]. Recent in-depth analyses performed in a series of breast AdCCs revealed *MYB-NFIB* fusion in 83%, if not, *MYBL1* fusions or *MYB* amplification also converging into MYB family activation [20, 21]. These observations demonstrated that at molecular level, breast AdCCs are similar to salivary gland AdCCs distinct from TNBC-NSTs, illustrating a clear example of genotypic-phenotypic correlation, typical histological characteristics even across different anatomic site.

7.3 Current Evidence and Concepts

There are emerging evidences of fusion genes as ‘driver alteration’ in breast cancers. Though not many, some are found recurrently across several datasets. *ESR1* fusion gene has now come into our understanding as one of the alterations that drive endocrine resistance among hormone receptor positive breast cancers. *ESR1* gene encodes estrogen receptor protein, a transcription factor that serves as a key molecule in hormone receptor breast cancers. *ESR1* gene mutation is a known driver mutation in advanced hormone receptor (HR) positive breast cancers. It is found approximately in 20% of advanced HR positive breast cancers, while observed in only <1% of endocrine therapy naïve primary tumors [22]. *ESR1* gene mutation mostly occurs at ligand-binding domain (LBD), resulting in estrogen-independent tumor growth mostly acquired during endocrine therapy by clonal selection. Well-known hotspot mutations are illustrated in Fig. 7.2.

Genomic rearrangements involving *ESR1* gene and *ESR1-YAP1* fusion were first identified by Li and colleagues from patient-derived xenograft [22, 23]. In both *ESR1-YAP1* fusion positive and subsequently identified *ESR1-CCDC170* fusion-harboring tumors, ligand binding domain (LBD) is absent, leading to ligand-independent tumor growth and endocrine resistance in similar manner found in *ESR1* hotspot mutations [24]. Recently, other *ESR1* gene rearrangements have been reported with multiple partner genes [25]. Though 3′ partner genes differ, the break junctions were all between exon 6.7, leading to loss of ligand binding domain (LBD), which drives estrogen-independent tumor growth and resistance to endocrine therapy. (Figure 7.3a) Most cases exhibited co-occurrence of *ESR1* missense

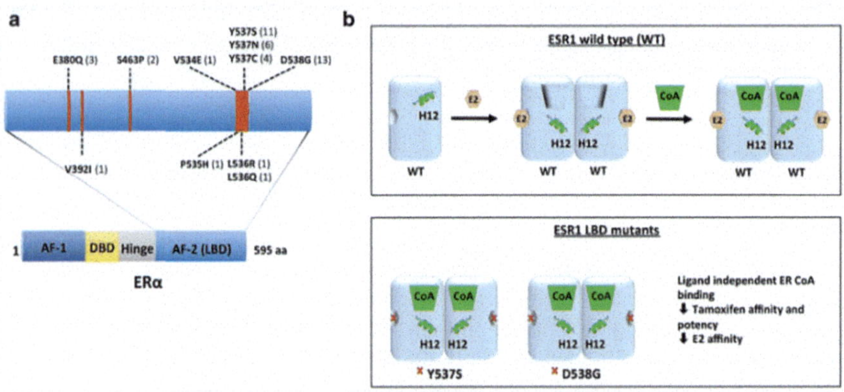

Fig. 7.2 (**a**) *ESR1* gene hotspot mutation, (**b**) Functional alteration of the ESR1 mutant protein. PMID: 28374222 Jeselsohn R, Curr Oncol Rep 2017 https://media.springernature.com/original/springer-static/image/art%3A10.1007%2Fs11912-017-0591-8/MediaObjects/11912_2017_591_Fig1_HTML.gif Estrogen receptor α (ER) structural/functional domains and the distribution of the somatic ESR1 ligand-binding domain (LBD) point mutations identified in tissue specimens of ER-positive breast tumors

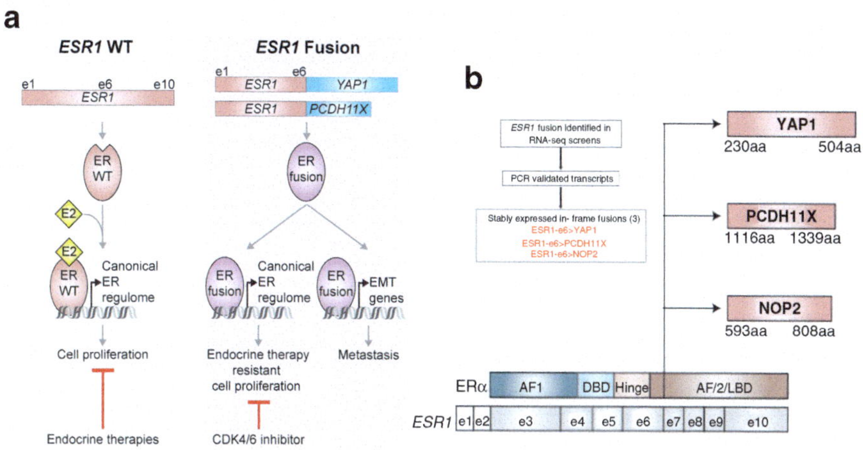

Fig. 7.3 *ESR1* fusion genes with multiple partner genes found in advanced hormone receptor positive breast cancers. PMID: 30089255, https://www.sciencedirect.com/science/article/pii/S2211124718310866?via%3Dihub. (**a**) *ESR1* fusion genes resulting in loss of ligand binding domain results in endocrine resistance, (**b**) *ESR1* fusion genes with different 3' partner genes

mutations suggesting the polyclonal resistance. *ESR1* fusion genes with different partner genes are illustrated in Fig. 7.3b.

Matissek et al. have recently applied a new methodology, anchored multiplex PCR (AMP), and identified driver fusion genes among 14% (24/173) of advanced HR positive BCs [26]. Among fusion positive cases, fusions were observed exclusively in 75% (18/24), while six cases were found to have *PIK3CA* mutation. (Fig. 7.4a) One third of these fusions were *ESR1* fusions, and others included known driver genes, e.g., *PIK3CA, AKT3*, and *RAF1*.(Figure 7.4b) Genomic rearrangements were confirmed by in situ hybridization method, and these kinase fusions promoted oncogenic phenotype when induced in mammary epithelium. *AKT3* fusions induced increased activity of downstream PIK3/mTORC1 pathway along with estrogen-independent proliferation. In the same context, patients harboring these fusions displayed worse outcome than fusion-negative patients and conferred resistance to AKT inhibitor. In vivo experiments have demonstrated the benefit of adding CDK4/6 inhibitor, Palbociclib for this *AKT3* fusion-expressing tumors [26]. These findings demonstrate that fusion genes in breast cancer can also be predictive to therapy or potentiate resistance to therapy.

More recently, for metastatic breast cancers, *ESR1* rearrangements were found in plasma DNA. Chung et al. have performed MPS for 254 metastatic HR positive patients and three were found to have *ESR1* rearrangement resulting in loss of ligand binding domain [27]. All three cases exhibited co-occurrence with *ESR1* missense mutations. By applying copyshift method, MPS of rearrangement could be identified with increased sensitivity for analyzing circulating tumor DNA. Genomic profiling of ctDNA has proven to provide a complementary and possibly alternative approach to tissue-based genomic testing. High sensitivity of detecting fusions in ctDNA may

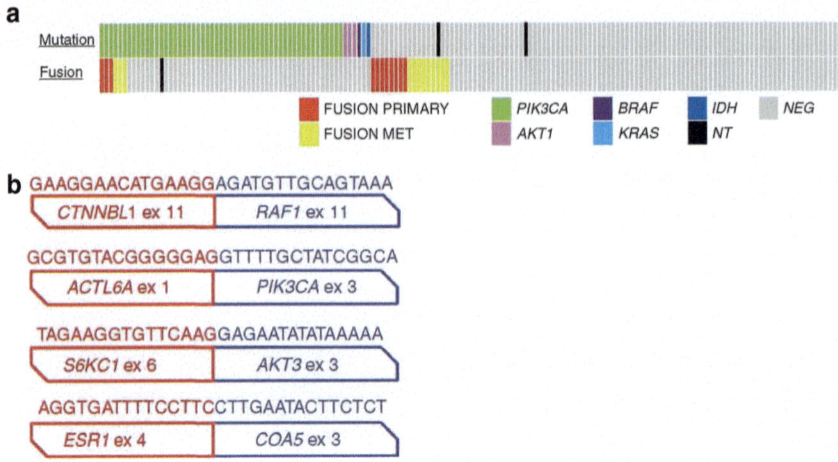

Fig. 7.4 Novel fusion genes found in advanced hormone receptor positive breast cancers. PMID: 29242214. http://cancerdiscovery.aacrjournals.org/content/8/3/336.long (**a**) Summary of mutations and fusions identified in primary and metastatic hormone receptor positive breast cancers, (**b**) Novel fusions, other than ESR1 fusions

even lead to greater opportunity for clinical application especially for patients with estrogen receptor-positive metastatic breast cancer.

7.4 Future Research Direction

Large-scale sequencing data revealed numerous fusion genes among breast cancers. As most are assumed to be passenger alterations, further studies incorporating both whole genome and transcriptome are required to discriminate true driver alteration and fully understand its' biologic nature and role in oncogenesis, especially given that RNA sequencing doesn't necessarily cover fusions involving promoters or enhancers. Validation using RT-PCR or other methods, e.g., Whole-genome sequencing, is critical due to high false positivity. Also intervalidation of various fusion calling algorithms achieve higher accuracy along with concordance between each algorithm. For fusions with known functional impact, e.g., *ESR1* fusion genes, as noninvasive, most commonly circulating tumor DNA is becoming a promising tool.

7.5 Summary

7.5.1 The Bench

Numerous fusion genes have been identified from thousands of breast cancer samples, and yet not much has been accomplished in understanding its oncogenic functions. In order to achieve clinical relevance of these numerously identified fusion genes, the ultimate downstream pathway alterations should deeply be investigated. Also as outputs of fusion gene detecting tools vary substantially, effort for standardization aiming to minimize false positivity and to choose fusions with higher impact should be accompanied.

7.5.2 Translation

While a number of recurrent driver fusion genes were found among other solid cancers, e.g., *ALK* fusion in lung adenocarcinoma, most fusion genes are thought to be passengers in breast cancers. Recently, along with hotspot mutations, *ESR1* gene fusions were found in advanced hormone receptor positive breast cancers. These fusions were demonstrated to be drivers of endocrine resistance, and yet polyclonal, display ligand-independent estrogen pathway activation as fusion event leads to loss of ligand binding domain. The presence of the *ESR1* fusions represents resistant to endocrine therapy, especially aromatase inhibitors, and could guide in making decisions for patient management. Similarly, with newly developed methods, fusions of *PIK3CA*, *AKT3*, and *RAF1* genes were found among advanced hormone receptor positive BCs. These fusions, along with *ESR1* fusion genes, were found in 14% of displaying worse outcome than fusion negative cases; yet, validations in larger cohorts should be preceded to achieve evidence for clinical trials.

7.5.3 The Bedside

Several fusion genes have demonstrated their role as oncogenic driver, mainly among hormone receptor positive breast cancers, and data suggest that the subset of patients harboring these fusion genes may benefit from additional combination therapy, e.g., CDK4/6 inhibitors with estrogen deprivation. The fusions were also found in patients' plasma, exemplifying the possibility to overcome spatial and temporal heterogeneity of the tumor during treatment. While data seem promising to take part in the ultimate goal of precision medicine, many steps are ahead to achieve clinical application in real world. First, analytical validity should be obtained across samples of tumors, and plasma DNA that is sensitive in detection of fusion genes should be reproducible throughout methods and institutes. Establishment of evidences by randomized trials should be preceded whether it is beneficial to guide therapy depending on the presence of fusion genes, along with consideration of socioeconomic issues to confirm its' clinical utility.

References

1. Gao Q, Liang WW, Foltz SM, Mutharasu G, Jayasinghe RG, Cao S, et al. Driver fusions and their implications in the development and treatment of human cancers. Cell Rep. 2018;23 (1):227–38.
2. Soda M, Choi YL, Enomoto M, Takada S, Yamashita Y, Ishikawa S, et al. Identification of the transforming EML4-ALK fusion gene in non-small-cell lung cancer. Nature. 2007;448 (7153):561–6.
3. Tomlins SA, Rhodes DR, Perner S, Dhanasekaran SM, Mehra R, Sun XW, et al. Recurrent fusion of TMPRSS2 and ETS transcription factor genes in prostate cancer. Science. 2005;310 (5748):644–8.
4. Campbell PJ, Stephens PJ, Pleasance ED, O'Meara S, Li H, Santarius T, et al. Identification of somatically acquired rearrangements in cancer using genome-wide massively parallel paired-end sequencing. Nat Genet. 2008;40(6):722–9.
5. Fimereli D, Fumagalli D, Brown D, Gacquer D, Rothe F, Salgado R, et al. Genomic hotspots but few recurrent fusion genes in breast cancer. Genes Chromosomes Cancer. 2018;57 (7):331–8.
6. Stephens PJ, McBride DJ, Lin ML, Varela I, Pleasance ED, Simpson JT, et al. Complex landscapes of somatic rearrangement in human breast cancer genomes. Nature. 2009;462 (7276):1005–10.
7. Latysheva NS, Babu MM. Discovering and understanding oncogenic gene fusions through data intensive computational approaches. Nucleic Acids Res. 2016;44(10):4487–503.
8. Liu S, Tsai WH, Ding Y, Chen R, Fang Z, Huo Z, et al. Comprehensive evaluation of fusion transcript detection algorithms and a meta-caller to combine top performing methods in paired-end RNA-seq data. Nucleic Acids Res. 2016;44(5):e47.
9. Wang XS, Prensner JR, Chen G, Cao Q, Han B, Dhanasekaran SM, et al. An integrative approach to reveal driver gene fusions from paired-end sequencing data in cancer. Nat Biotechnol. 2009;27(11):1005–11.
10. Zhang J, White NM, Schmidt HK, Fulton RS, Tomlinson C, Warren WC, et al. INTEGRATE: gene fusion discovery using whole genome and transcriptome data. Genome Res. 2016;26 (1):108–18.
11. Jia W, Qiu K, He M, Song P, Zhou Q, Zhou F, et al. SOAPfuse: an algorithm for identifying fusion transcripts from paired-end RNA-Seq data. Genome Biol. 2013;14(2):R12.
12. Chen K, Navin NE, Wang Y, Schmidt HK, Wallis JW, Niu B, et al. BreakTrans: uncovering the genomic architecture of gene fusions. Genome Biol. 2013;14(8):R87.
13. Kim J, Kim S, Ko S, In YH, Moon HG, Ahn SK, et al. Recurrent fusion transcripts detected by whole-transcriptome sequencing of 120 primary breast cancer samples. Genes Chromosomes Cancer. 2015;54(11):681–91.
14. Yoshihara K, Wang Q, Torres-Garcia W, Zheng S, Vegesna R, Kim H, et al. The landscape and therapeutic relevance of cancer-associated transcript fusions. Oncogene. 2015;34(37):4845–54.
15. Kim RN, Moon HG, Han W, Noh DY. Perspective insight into future potential fusion gene transcript biomarker candidates in breast Cancer. Int J Mol Sci. 2018;19(2):502.
16. Nik-Zainal S, Davies H, Staaf J, Ramakrishna M, Glodzik D, Zou X, et al. Landscape of somatic mutations in 560 breast cancer whole-genome sequences. Nature. 2016;534(7605):47–54.
17. Robinson DR, Kalyana-Sundaram S, Wu YM, Shankar S, Cao X, Ateeq B, et al. Functionally recurrent rearrangements of the MAST kinase and notch gene families in breast cancer. Nat Med. 2011;17(12):1646–51.
18. Tognon C, Knezevich SR, Huntsman D, Roskelley CD, Melnyk N, Mathers JA, et al. Expression of the ETV6-NTRK3 gene fusion as a primary event in human secretory breast carcinoma. Cancer Cell. 2002;2(5):367–76.
19. Doebele RC, Davis LE, Vaishnavi A, Le AT, Estrada-Bernal A, Keysar S, et al. An oncogenic NTRK fusion in a patient with soft-tissue sarcoma with response to the tropomyosin-related kinase inhibitor LOXO-101. Cancer Discov. 2015;5(10):1049–57.

20. Martelotto LG, De Filippo MR, Ng CK, Natrajan R, Fuhrmann L, Cyrta J, et al. Genomic landscape of adenoid cystic carcinoma of the breast. J Pathol. 2015;237(2):179–89.
21. Kim J, Geyer FC, Martelotto LG, Ng CK, Lim RS, Selenica P, et al. MYBL1 rearrangements and MYB amplification in breast adenoid cystic carcinomas lacking the MYB-NFIB fusion gene. J Pathol. 2018;244(2):143–50.
22. Jeselsohn R, Buchwalter G, De Angelis C, Brown M, Schiff R. ESR1 mutations-a mechanism for acquired endocrine resistance in breast cancer. Nat Rev Clin Oncol. 2015;12(10):573–83.
23. Li S, Shen D, Shao J, Crowder R, Liu W, Prat A, et al. Endocrine-therapy-resistant ESR1 variants revealed by genomic characterization of breast-cancer-derived xenografts. Cell Rep. 2013;4(6):1116–30.
24. Veeraraghavan J, Tan Y, Cao XX, Kim JA, Wang X, Chamness GC, et al. Recurrent ESR1-CCDC170 rearrangements in an aggressive subset of oestrogen receptor-positive breast cancers. Nat Commun. 2014;5:4577.
25. Hartmaier RJ, Trabucco SE, Priedigkeit N, Chung JH, Parachoniak CA, Vanden Borre P, et al. Recurrent hyperactive ESR1 fusion proteins in endocrine therapy-resistant breast cancer. Ann Oncol. 2018;29(4):872–80.
26. Matissek KJ, Onozato ML, Sun S, Zheng Z, Schultz A, Lee J, et al. Expressed gene fusions as frequent drivers of poor outcomes in hormone receptor-positive breast Cancer. Cancer Discov. 2018;8(3):336–53.
27. Chung JH, Pavlick D, Hartmaier R, Schrock AB, Young L, Forcier B, et al. Hybrid capture-based genomic profiling of circulating tumor DNA from patients with estrogen receptor-positive metastatic breast cancer. Ann Oncol. 2017;28(11):2866–73.

Chapter 8
DNA Damage Repair Inhibitor for Breast Cancer Treatment

Ahrum Min, Kyung-Hun Lee, and Seock-Ah Im

Abstract Cancer has been defined as a genetic disorder caused by the accumulation of genetic alterations, which result from various internal and external DNA damage that is left unrepaired. One of the main characteristics of cancer is a partial loss of DNA damage repair (DDR) pathway, resulting in increased DNA damage levels and replication stress. DDR inhibitors have been suggested as a new anticancer strategy, under the concept of synthetic lethality. The poly-(ADP-ribose) polymerase (PARP) inhibitor is the first DDR inhibitor to be used in clinical practice. PARP inhibitors have been tested in patients with *BRCA1/2* germline mutations (gBRCA1/2mt) and shown robust clinical benefits in breast cancer with gBRCA1/2mt and serous ovarian cancer patients. The concept of synthetic lethality is not limited to gBRCAmt for PARP inhibitor, and discovering homologous recombination deficiency (HRD) markers beyond *BRCA1/2* and identifying best candidates for DDR inhibitors are the active research areas. At the same time, various combinations of DDR inhibitors and other anticancer drugs are being tested in both preclinical and clinical studies. In addition, based on recent evidence of the immune-modulatory effect of PARP inhibitors, the combination of DDR inhibitors and immune checkpoint inhibitors is being actively investigated. Acquired resistance mechanism of DDR inhibitors, as well as defining best candidates and best combinations, would be future research topics for DDR inhibitors. Furthermore, it would also be crucial to establish a clinically relevant standardized method to detect HRD for future clinical use.

A. Min
Cancer Research Institute, Seoul National University, Biomedical Research Institute, Seoul National University Hospital, Seoul, South Korea

K.-H. Lee
Department of Internal Medicine, Seoul National University Hospital, Cancer Research Institute, Seoul National University, Seoul, South Korea

S.-A. Im (✉)
Department of Internal Medicine, Seoul National University Hospital, Cancer Research Institute, Seoul National University College of Medicine, Seoul National University, Seoul, South Korea
e-mail: moisa@snu.ac.kr

D.-Y. Noh et al. (eds.), *Translational Research in Breast Cancer*, Advances in Experimental Medicine and Biology 1187,
https://doi.org/10.1007/978-981-32-9620-6_8

Keywords DNA damage repair · Homologous recombination deficiency · PARP inhibitor · Synthetic lethality · BRCAness

8.1 DNA Damage Repair Pathway

Every cell undergoes more than tens of thousands of events everyday that damage DNA in various ways, including single-base mismatches, bulky adducts on DNA bases, intra- and interstrand DNA crosslinks, single-strand breaks (SSBs), and double-strand breaks (DSBs). Increased levels of DNA damage cause genomic instability, which is an underlying hallmark of cancer [1, 2]. The DNA damage response (DDR) refers to the overall cellular signaling pathways that aim to detect and reverse various types of DNA damage in cells, and it can be broadly classified into four mechanisms [3]. First, DNA lesions can be repaired by delaying or stopping the cell cycle after DNA damage or unstable DNA replication by activating a cell cycle checkpoint pathway. Second, the transcription of repair molecules or proapoptotic molecules can be activated to induce overexpression of the relevant molecules. Third, chromatid instability can be induced by severe DNA damage, which in turn leads to apoptosis to remove the damaged cell [4]. Finally, DNA damage can be repaired by three different types of DNA repair pathways that are independently activated depending on the type of DNA damage (Fig. 8.1).

First, when a base is damaged by radiation, oxidation, or hydrolysis, the damage is repaired by a direct reversal mechanism. When irradiation induces the formation of thymidine dimers, the dimer is typically removed by photolyase. When guanine is methylated, the MGMT enzyme removes the methyl-guanine directly, and when adenine or cytosine is methylated, the dealkylating protein removes the methylated base [1, 2].

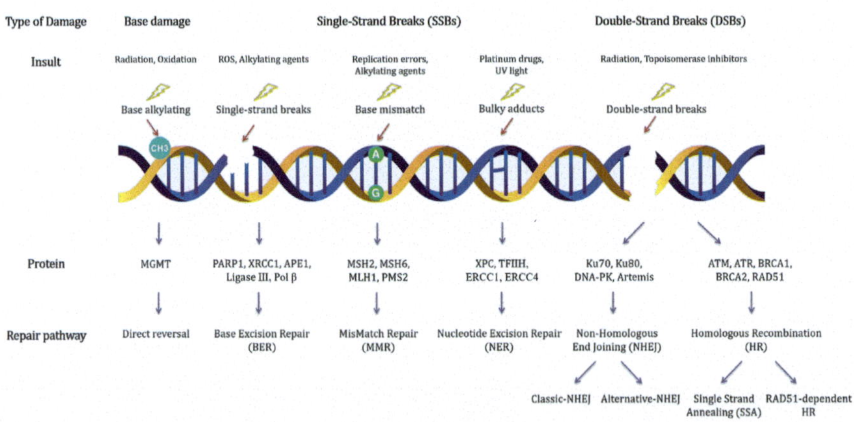

Fig. 8.1 DNA damage and DNA damage repair pathways

Second, when a base mismatch occurs between two completely replicated DNA strands, MSH2 and MSH6 detect the mismatched bases and activate mismatch repair (MMR) by MLH1 (an endonuclease), PMS2, a DNA helicase, and an exonuclease [5, 6]. If a base mismatch is caused by a single-base excision, DNA glycosylase recognizes the mismatch and hydrolyzes the bond by flipping the incorrect base. Base excision repair (BER) can also occur, which involves the excision of the abasic site by AP endonuclease, removal of deoxyribose phosphate by DNA phosphodiesterase, and repair by DNA polymerase and ligase [7, 8]. Nucleotide excision repair (NER) is activated in response to the presence of a bulky base: XPC recognizes the damage, while TFIIH and XPD/B/G/F cut the damaged DNA strand and repair according to the complementary strand [9].

Third, DSBs are repaired via the nonhomologous end joining (NHEJ) and homologous recombination (HR) repair pathways [3, 10]. NHEJ is well known as an error-prone repair mechanism in which repair occurs without regard to the sequence of the original chromatin structure. For sticky ended DSBs, Ku70/80 molecules bind to the DSB, and the Ku-DNA complex recruits the DNA-PK catalytic subunit. The sticky ends are cleaned by nucleases, such as Artemis and Metnase, followed by direct ligation of the exposed blunt ends of DNA [11]. On the other hand, HR is a process of repairing DSBs that depends on an intact sister chromatid sequence template. During HR, the Mre11/Rad50/Nbs1 (MRN) complex recognizes the damage and repairs it by activating kinases such as ATR and ATM and forming RAD51 filaments. During HR, DNA synthesis typically occurs using the sister chromatid as a template, and so it can only occur after DNA replication, that is, only in the S/G2/M cell cycle phases; on the other hand, NHEJ frequently occurs in the G0/G1 phase [3, 10, 12]. The NHEJ pathway is further classified into classic and alternative NHEJ. This has been reported to be mainly determined by 53BP1 expression. Alternative NHEJ induces large deletions or translocations compared to classic NHEJ because a greater amount of free DNA ends is resected before ligation to search for microhomology between the complementary DNA strand sequences. In such cases, PARP1 is bound to the free DNA ends instead of the Ku complex, leading to ligation by ligase III and XRCC1, and 53BP1 suppresses this process [11, 13]. HR is also divided into two subpathways. The first pathway is RAD51-dependent HR, which is also known as accurate HR. In this pathway, single-strand ends are exposed through end resection, to which RPA then binds and is replaced with RAD51 by BRCA2. This forms a RAD51 nucleoprotein filament, which searches for a homologous template and mediates strand invasion to synthesize new DNA [14, 15]. The second pathway is single strand annealing (SSA), which is also known as inaccurate HR. SSA is activated when a DSB occurs between two repeated sequences oriented in the same direction. The single-stranded region exposed by RAD52 through end resection is annealed to the other sequence in the complementary strand of repeated sequence, after which the remaining part is synthesized. This process is an inaccurate pathway because the sequence of one of the repeats may be deleted or a chromosomal translocation may occur if separate DSBs have occurred in repeated sequences on different chromosomes [16].

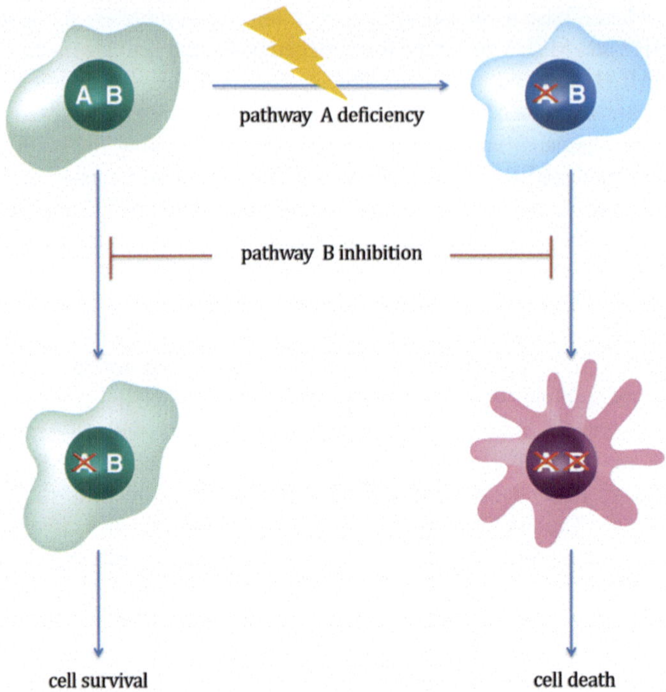

Fig. 8.2 The concept of synthetic lethality

Diverse DNA damage responses occur by different mechanisms, which also vary in relation to the type of damage, their cell-cycle dependence, and DDR molecule activity. However, evidence supporting the presence of significant functional overlap among these DDR pathways has emerged as studies continue to investigate DDR [12, 17]. Furthermore, normal DDR activation is highly important in maintaining genomic stability. Aberrant DDR induces an accumulation of mutations, and an accumulation of unrepaired DNA damage ultimately induces mitotic catastrophe or cell death [1, 18]. What is interesting is that cancer oftentimes involves a defect in the accurate DDR pathway, and thus, cancer is associated with a tolerance for unrepaired, under-replicated DNA caused by the inaccurate DDR pathway and with elevated genomic instability caused by increased mutations. Thus, paradoxically, making the inaccurate DDR pathway defective to induce cell death caused by an accumulation of unrepaired DNA damage has been introduced as an attractive cancer therapeutic strategy, as cancer cells have defective accurate DDR and are only capable of initiating the inaccurate DDR pathway [19–21].

The concept of synthetic lethality was first introduced 20 years ago in order to identify a novel anticancer drug [22–24]. A synthetic lethal interaction is identified when cell death is induced by a genetic alteration in the presence of another genetic alteration (Fig. 8.2). For example, cell death increases as a result of an accumulation of unrepaired damage when the poly (ADP-ribose) polymerase (PARP)-dependent pathway is inhibited by PARP inhibitors, which inhibit an enzyme that recognizes various types of DNA damage (e.g., NER and SSBs) and are recruited to the damage site to induce recruitment of DDR molecules in other DDR pathway defective cells. Synthetic lethality is thought to be the explanation for the anticancer effects of DDR inhibitors and has become a promising new cancer treatment strategy [25–27].

8.2 HR Deficiency (HRD) in Breast Cancer (BC)

Olaparib, a PARP inhibitor, has been proven to be more effective than conventional anticancer agents for breast cancer (BC) patients who have a germline mutation in the *BRCA1* or *BRCA2* gene, which is known to be key molecules in the HR pathway. Therefore, PARP inhibitors, which inhibit DDR, have become standard treatment for patients with a *BRCA1/2* germline mutation (gBRCAmt) [28–31]. In other words, when PARP is inhibited, the endogenous SSB repair pathway is inhibited; furthermore, as a result of a *BRCA1* or *BRCA2* defect, when unrepaired SSBs are converted to DSBs by the passage of the replication fork, the resulting DSBs cannot be repaired by the HR repair pathway for DSBs and instead are repaired by the inaccurate DDR pathway, which increases cell death due to elevated genomic stability and the accumulation of DSBs [25, 27]. The inactivation of the HR repair pathway caused by germline or somatic alterations in genes involved in the HR pathway, such as *BRCA1/2*, is called HR deficiency (HRD), and there is evidence suggesting that HRD may respond favorably to DDR targeting therapy.

Hereditary *BRCA1/2* mutation occurs in about 7% of all BC cases and in about 11–15% of triple-negative breast cancer (TNBC) subtypes. When somatic alterations were included, 10% of BC patients were reported to have a *BRCA1* or *BRCA2* mutation [32]. A tumor that lacks a *BRCA* mutation but results in HRD with similar responses to DNA damaging agents and clinicopathologic features is referred to as having “BRCAness”. The classic genetic alterations that induce BRCAness are mutations in *RAD51C, PALB2, BARD1, RAD51D,* and *CHEK2*, with recent reports suggesting that germline mutations such as *ATM, BAP1, CDK12*, and *FANCM* also cause HRD [33]. In our previous study, we used immunohistochemistry (IHC) to assess the level of HR protein expression in BC tissues from 419 Korean patients who underwent a mastectomy. The results showed that loss of BRCA1, BRCA2, or ATM was high, at about 33.7%, 89.9%, and 30.8%, respectively. From 399 cases that were evaluated for these three genes plus p53 and NBS1, at least one of the molecules was lost in 258 cases (64.7%). When DDR gene expression was suppressed, the 5-year disease-free survival was markedly lower by 10.8%, confirming that a deficiency of DDR genes other than *BRCA* affects the prognosis of BC (unpublished data). In addition, recent reports have presented evidence suggesting that biallelic alterations of HR genes cause HRD [32, 34, 35]. As the importance of HRD in cancer treatment has become highlighted, various efforts have been made to identify the phenotype of HRD, and the mutational signature in general cancers has been analyzed using a large-scale cancer genome dataset [36]. The results confirmed that a mutation signature with a particular pattern, defined as signature 3, is highly correlated with breast, pancreatic, and ovarian cancer with *BRCA* mutation. Signature 3, characterized by large insertions and deletions at breakpoint junctions, was strongly associated with biallelic inactivation of *BRCA1, BRCA2,* and *PALB2.* Serena Nik-Zainal *et al.* analyzed the Cancer Genome Atlas (TCGA) dataset of 560 BC patients and reported that less than 50% of cases showed signature 3 with *BRCA* mutation, signifying that the remaining 50% of cases involve another HRD marker and that developing a method to detect HRD is crucial, as it enables the prediction of response to platinum drug or DDR inhibitor therapies in cancer treatment [37]. In fact, Myriad's BRACAnalysis™ CDx and FoundationFocus™ CDx_{BRCA} are used to predict the response to drugs that target PARP and HRD, and these FDA-approved drugs are currently used in clinics for patients with gBRCAmt. In addition to these methods, various other methods have been developed to detect HRD.

Methods to detect tumors with HRD can be broadly divided into several categories, including identification of genomic instability through integrated genomic analysis, evaluation of tumor genome loss of heterozygosity (LOH), telomeric allelic imbalance (TAI) and large-scale state transition, analysis of recombination proficiency score using gene expression profiles, and ex vivo examination of RAD51 foci formation to confirm HR function. The most common method by genomics approach is BROCA gene panel, which performs 320-1000x targeted sequencing for about 70 HRD-related genes, and the Foundation medicine T5 NGS assay, a targeted sequencing method with a depth of greater than 500x. Although these assays are limited to identifying known pathogenic variants in germline *BRCA1/2* and a limited number of known relevant genes, they can be used for patient selection, as they can identify good candidates with HRD for platinum drugs and others [33]. Seoul National University Hospital (SNUH) also developed a targeted panel sequencing tool with prognostic and predictive purposes. Using this panel, SNUH strives to predict response to platinum drugs and DDR inhibitors, including multiple HR genes, and to apply this information into clinical care for patients. In addition to the methods of screening HRD tumors by identifying the genetic alterations of HR genes as shown above, the Sanger Institute group suggested that 'mutational signatures 3 and 8', which were presented based on the analysis of the deletion or substitution patterns through microhomology, can best predict HRD [38]. Using this method, there were biallelic losses of *BRCA1* or *BRCA2* in 88 out of 247 cases within the top quartile for signature 3 features among 992 patients with breast cancer, whereas the remaining 159 cases exhibited BRCA-like features so-called 'BRCAness' [32]. Moreover, Connor AA *et al.* analyzed 249 pancreatic ductal adenocarcinoma (PDCA) cases and reported that 11 tumors out of 27 tumors exhibiting signature 3 had a biallelic loss of *BRCA1, BRCA2,* or *PALB2* and 12 cases showed BRCAness [39]. These results suggest that signature 3 successfully predicts HRD, and some argue that this method is more effective than the conventional targeted gene panel sequencing methods. Furthermore, Myriad HRD analysis to analyze LOH and TAI and large-scale state transitions (also known as HRD scores), allele-specific copy number analysis from SNP microarray analysis, and array comparative genomic hybridization (aCGH) have also been suggested to detect HRD in TNBC and serous ovarian cancer. However, both LOH-based HRD score computation method and Foundation Medicine T5 NGS assay failed to predict PARP inhibitor response in a large phase III clinical trial, and the binary cutoffs failed to distinguish PARP inhibitor responders in both methods, necessitating incorporation of multiple genomic features between structural alteration and germline or somatic alterations [40]. In addition to these methods, using gene expression profiles was suggested to be useful for predicting PARP inhibitor responses in vitro, and a functional analysis that could assess HRD by observing the nuclear localization of RAD51, an essential component of HR response (HRR), was presented [41, 42]. The accurate detection of HRD would play a crucial role in accurate treatment strategy by enabling the prediction of interactions between DNA damage agents, such as platinum drugs, and DDR inhibitors, such as PARP inhibitors, and would provide a tool for tailored therapy. Hence, the appropriate methodology needs to be developed and implemented for the treatment of cancer.

8.3 Clinical Development of DDR Inhibitors for Breast Cancer and Ovarian Cancer

Cancer cells with DDR deficiency are dependent on a particular DDR pathway, and when that pathway is disrupted, cell death is increased as described by the concept of 'synthetic lethality'. Based on this concept, several PARP inhibitors have been developed and recently approved for use in serious ovarian cancer and BC [30, 43, 44]. PARP is a crucial protein for DNA repair that recognizes SSBs, recruits repair proteins through PARylation, and then dissociates to enable normal repair. When PARP is inhibited, SSBs cannot be recognized, and unrepaired SSBs progress to DSBs during the replication process. When this occurs, DSBs in tumors with HRD cannot be repaired, resulting in cell death (Fig. 8.3). In addition, by blocking the PARylation enzymatic activity of PARP, the PARP protein is trapped at SSBs due to an inhibition of PARP dissociation. This stalls or collapses the replication fork, blocking cellular replication and ultimately inducing more deleterious DSBs [26].

The most well-defined HRD tumors are ovarian, breast, pancreatic, and prostate cancers with gBRCAmt. Olaparib, a PARP inhibitor, has been reported to induce cell death caused by synthetic lethality in *BRCA*-deficient ovarian, breast, and prostate cancers. Olaparib is currently approved for clinical use in ovarian cancer. In a phase II trial for olaparib in platinum-sensitive relapsed ovarian cancer, maintenance olaparib had an improved median progression-free survival (PFS) at 8.4 *vs* 4.8 months in the placebo group (HR = 0.35; 95% CI: 0.25–0.49; $P < 0.001$), with a longer time to progression [45]. This led to the approval of olaparib in Europe by the EMA as maintenance treatment in patients with platinum-sensitive, relapsed, germline, or somatic *BRCA1/2* mutation-associated ovarian cancer, who have received 2 or more platinum-based regimens with a response in the last regimen

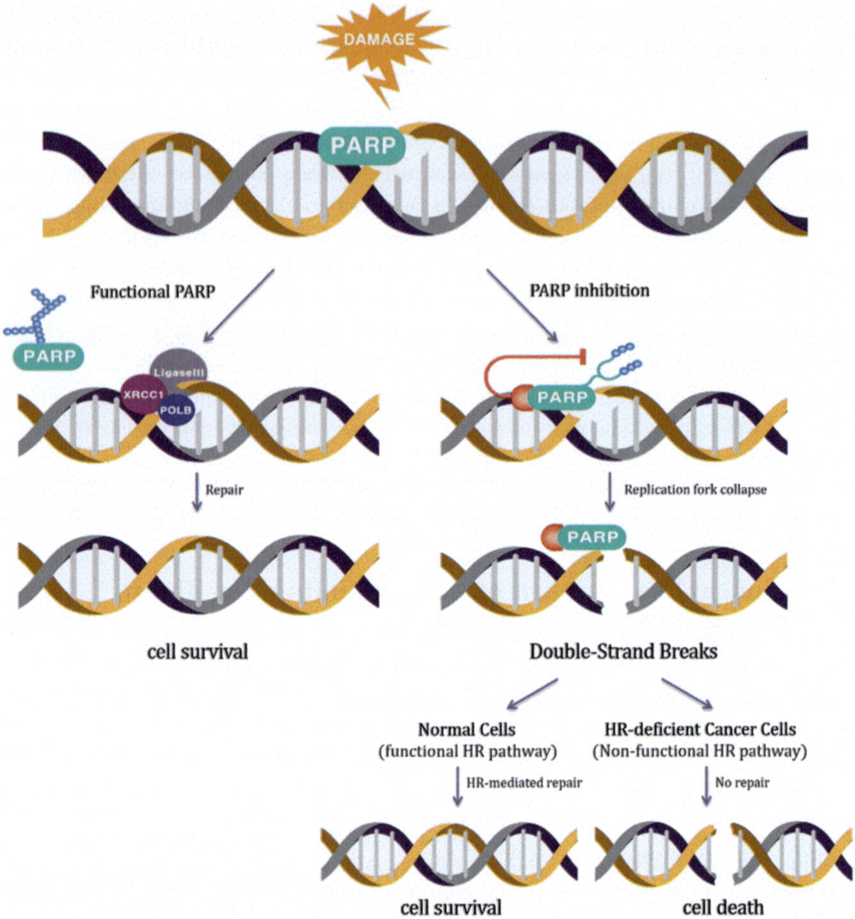

Fig. 8.3 Synthetic lethality of PARP inhibition in cancer cells

[46]. In the United States, the FDA approved olaparib as a single agent for the treatment of patients with germline *BRCA1/2*-mutated advanced ovarian cancer who have received three or more prior lines of chemotherapy [46]. This was based on a phase II study in 298 patients with germline *BRCA1* or *BRCA2* mutations. Of the patients, 193 patients with ovarian cancer showed a response rate of 31.1% (95% CI: 24.6–38.1) and PFS of 7 months [47]. Moreover, olaparib was additionally approved by United States FDA as a maintenance treatment for patients with recurrent, epithelial ovarian, fallopian tube, or primary peritoneal adult cancer who are in response to platinum-based chemotherapy, regardless of *BRCA* status. This was based on both phase III SOLO-2 trial [31] and Study 19, which showed 65–70% reduced risk of disease progression or death in this setting [48].

In addition to olaparib, other PARP inhibitors, such as rucaparib and niraparib, were approved for clinical use. Rucaparib has proven efficacy in relapsed platinum-sensitive ovarian cancers, after at least two prior lines of platinum-based chemotherapy in a phase II study, and was approved by FDA for this indication [49]. Recently, FDA also approved rucaparib for the maintenance treatment of patients with recurrent epithelial ovarian, fallopian tube, or primary peritoneal cancer who are in a complete or partial response to platinum-based chemotherapy, based on a phase III trial [50]. Niraparib was approved by FDA for the maintenance treatment of adult patients with recurrent epithelial ovarian, fallopian tube, or primary peritoneal cancer who are in complete or partial response to platinum-based chemotherapy, based on a phase III trial [40].

Olaparib is the first PARP inhibitor that proved efficacy in breast cancer in phase III randomized trial. In the OlympiAD study in 302 patients with germline *BRCA1* or *BRCA2* mutant, HER2-negative metastatic breast cancer patients were randomized in a 2:1 ratio to receive olaparib tablets (300 mg twice daily) or standard therapy with single-agent chemotherapy of the physician's choice (capecitabine, eribulin, or vinorelbine in 21-day cycles) [30]. Median progression-free survival (7.0 months *vs* 4.2 months; hazard ratio 0.58; $P < 0.001$) and the response rate (59.9% *vs* 28.8%) were significantly better in the olaparib group. The rate of grade three or higher adverse events was lower in the olaparib group (36.6% *vs* 50.5%). The most common adverse reactions reported in at least 20% of patients taking olaparib in clinical trials were anemia, nausea, fatigue (including asthenia), vomiting, neutropenia, leukopenia, nasopharyngitis/upper respiratory tract infection/influenza, respiratory tract infection, diarrhea, arthralgia/myalgia, dysgeusia, headache, dyspepsia, decreased appetite, constipation, and stomatitis. This led to the first approval of PARP inhibitor by FDA in breast cancer. FDA also granted marketing authorization for the BRACAnalysis CDx® test (Myriad Genetic Laboratories, Inc.) for use as an aid in identifying patients with breast cancer with deleterious or suspected deleterious gBRCAm who may be eligible for olaparib.

Talazoparib, the most potent PARP inhibitor, also proved efficacy in patients with germline *BRCA1* or *BRCA2* mutant, HER2-negative metastatic breast cancer. In phase III EMBRACA trial, talazoparib was compared to physician's choice standard of care chemotherapy in a 2:1 ratio [51]. Median PFS was 8.6 months (95% CI: 7.2, 9.3) for patients treated with talazoparib and 5.6 months (95% CI: 4.2, 6.7) for those treated with chemotherapy [HR: 0.54 (95% CI: 0.41, 0.71), $p < 0.0001$]. In addition, objective response rate in the talazoparib group was more than twice that of the control arm (62.6% for talazoparib *vs* 27.2% for chemotherapy [OR: 4.99 (95% CI: 2.9–8.8), $p < 0.0001$]). Neoadjuvant treatment with talazoparib in operable breast cancer patients with a gBRCAmt was reported recently in the 2018 Annual meeting of American Society of Clinical Oncology. Twenty patients with $\geq$1 cm tumor and gBRCAmt (16 patients with *BRCA1*, 4 with *BRCA2*) received 6 months of once daily oral talazoparib 1 mg, followed by definitive surgery. Among 19 patients who completed the treatment, 10 patients (53%) achieved pathologic complete response or a score of RCB 0. This high pCR rate seems promising and warrants further investigation [52].

gBRCAmt and other HRD markers determine the response to olaparib and that PARP inhibitors could be applied to patients with other HRD markers as well. Our in vitro data also confirm that olaparib has antitumor effects in BC and gastric cancer cell lines with wild-type gBRCA, based on which we suggested that RAD51C deficiency caused by promoter methylation can serve as a sensitive marker for olaparib responsiveness [53]. Furthermore, ATM is a key sensor of the DNA damage response pathway and ATM expression deficiency is frequently observed in gastric cancer [54]. A Phase II study (Study 39, NCT01063517) showed that the oral PARP inhibitor olaparib combined with paclitaxel provided a statistically significant improvement in overall survival (OS) versus paclitaxel alone as second-line therapy in Asian patients with advanced gastric cancer. A greater OS benefit was seen in patients whose tumor was ATM protein negative by immunochemistry (ATM) [55]. In a global phase III GOLD trial, advanced gastric cancer patients who failed first line treatment randomly assigned 1:1 to receive 80 mg/m^2 IV paclitaxel (days 1, 8, 15 per 28-day cycle) with placebo ($n = 262$; ATM negative, $n = 46$) or with 100 mg of olaparib twice daily ($n = 263$, ATM negative, $n = 47$), median OS was 8.8 months among patients assigned olaparib and 6.9 months among patients assigned placebo (HR 0.79, p-0.0262). Although the addition of olaparib to paclitaxel demonstrated a trend toward an OS benefit independent of ATM protein status, p-value did not meet the study's predefined criteria for significance of $p < 0.025$ [56]. Olaparib tended to demonstrate a benefit in terms of PFS, ORR (37.5% *vs* 16.1%, $p = 0.0309$), and time to deterioration of health-related quality of life among ATM patients. The pitfall in this trial was only 18% (94/525) ATM, which was much lower than phase II study 39 (50% ATM) [55, 56]. The study generated informative efficacy and safety data regarding the use of olaparib in combination with a chemotherapeutic agent and provides a foundation for future studies on patients with non-g*BRCA* tumors who might get benefit from adding PARP inhibitor to chemotherapy [56]. A TOPARP-1 trial conducted on metastatic castrate-resistant prostate cancer with *BRCA1/2* or *ATM* mutation proved that olaparib is effective on *ATM* mutation in addition to *BRCA* [57].

In addition to efforts to discover HRD markers other than gBRCAmt, there are active efforts underway to develop combinatorial treatment strategies using PARP inhibitors (Table 8.1).

A combination study for iniparib with platinum and gemcitabine in metastatic TNBC has been conducted to develop a combination strategy with platinum agents [58, 59]. For gastric cancer, olaparib is used with paclitaxel [55, 56]. Since PARP inhibitors or platinum-based regimens were proven to be effective in patients with HRD, combination strategies with HRD induction therapy have been proposed as an effort to expand responders to PARP inhibitors, DDR inhibitors, and DNA damaging agents. First, based on in vitro data suggesting that inhibition of the PI3K/AKT/mTOR pathway suppresses DDR, it has been reported that everolimus, an mTOR inhibitor, increases the effects of talazoparib, a PARP inhibitor, by lowering HRR capacity in *BRCA* proficient BC cells [60]. The findings of this study demonstrated that mTOR inhibition sensitizes cells to PARP inhibitors despite the fact that mTOR inhibition does not suppress the protein expression of multiple HR genes, including *BRCA1* and *RAD51*. A phase I study on the combination of olaparib with PI3K inhibitors BKM120 or BYL719 for recurrent TNBC patients, a phase Ib trial on

Table 8.1 Ongoing clinical trials of PARP inhibitors in breast cancer

Drug	Tumor type	Strategy	Phase	Trial
Olaparib	Recurrent TNBC	With PI3K inhibitors (BKM120 and BYL719)	I	NCT01623349
	TNBC	mTORC1/2 inhibitor (AZD2014) or AKT inhibitor (AZD5363)	Ib	NCT02208375
	Metastatic TNBC	With carboplatin and/or paclitaxel	II	NCT00516724
	TNBC with g*BRCA* mutation	With antiangiogenic agent (cediranib)	Ib	NCT01116648
	Breast cancer, ovarian, SCLC, and gastric cancer	With PDL-1 inhibitor (MEDI4736)	I/II	NCT02734004
Niraparib	HER2 and g*BRCA* mutation	Niraparib versus chemotherapeutics	III	NCT01905592
Rucaparib	TNBC with g*BRCA1/2* mutation	With cisplatin	II	NCT01074970
Veliparib	HER2-metastatic or locally advanced unresectable g*BRCA* associated BC	With carboplatin and paclitaxel	III	NCT02163694
	Metastatic and g*BRCA1/2* mutation	With temozolomide	II	NCT01009788
	Locally advanced or metastatic BC	With cyclophosphamide	I	NCT01351909
	Stage III-IV BC and g*BRCA1/2* mutation	With/without carboplatin	II	NCT01149083
	Stage III TNBC with g*BRCA* mutation	With carboplatin	I	NCT01251874
	Metastatic BC with g*BRCA* mutation	With temozolomide or carboplatin plus paclitaxel	II	NCT01506609
Talazoparib	Advanced cancer with somatic or germline *BRCA 1/2* mutation, PTEN loss, or HRD	Monotherapy	II	NCT02286687

olaparib and mTORC1/2 or AKT inhibitors AZD2014 or AZD5363, and a phase II trial on advanced solid tumors, including BC, is underway [61]. We have studied the possibilities of PARP inhibitors in various combinations and reported that suberoylanilide hydroxamic acid (SAHA), a histone deacetylase inhibitor, increases the antitumor effects of olaparib by suppressing DDR-related protein expression and RAD51 foci formation in a TNBC cell line [62]. We also reported that androgen receptor inhibition suppresses HR capacity and increases the efficacy of olaparib by inactivating ATM in an androgen receptor (AR)-expressing BC cell line. Using HRD induction as a strategy is meaningful in that it not only increases the utility of PARP inhibitors but also uncovers novel biological functions of signaling pathways on DDR pathways. Furthermore, we expect this could also broaden clinical application of multiple DDR inhibitors that are currently under development.

Table 8.2 Targeting DNA damage response beyond PARP inhibitors

Target	Agents	Company	Development stage
ATR	AZD6738	AstraZeneca	Phase I in refractory cancer with palclitaxel (NCT02630199) Phase II in NSCLC with durvalumab (NCT03334617)
	VX-970	Vertex	Phase I in refractory solid tumor with/without olaparib or cisplatin (NCT02723864)
	BAY1895344	Bayer	Phase I in advanced solid tumors and lymphomas (NCT03188965)
ATM	AZD0156	AstraZeneca	Phase I in advanced solid tumors (NCT02588105)
	AZD1390	AstraZeneca	Phase I in brain tumor with radiation (NCT03423628)
CHK1/2	Prexasertib (LY2606368)	Lilly	Phase II in TNBC, ovarian, and prostate cancer (NCT02203513)
CHK1	SRA737	Sierra oncology	Phase I in advanced solid tumors or Non-Hodgkin's lymphoma (NCT02797964)
CHK1	SCH900776	Merck	Phase II in acute myeloid leukemia (NCT01870596)
CHK1	AZD7762	AstraZeneca	Phase I termination in advanced solid tumor with irinotecan (NCT00473616)
DNA-PK	CC-115	Celgene	Phase I in prostate cancer with enzalutamide (NCT02833883)
DNA-PK	MSC2490484A	Merck	Phase I in advanced solid tumor (NCT02516813)
Wee 1	AZD1775	AstraZeneca	Phase II in breast cancer with cisplatin (NCT0301247)
PARP, ATR, and Wee1	Olaparib, AZD6738, and AZD1775	AstraZeneca	Phase II randomized study in metastatic triple-negative breast cancer stratified by alterations in homologous recombination repair (HRR)-related genes (including *BRCA1/2*) (VIOLETTE) (NCT03330847)

With PARP inhibitors successfully combining with DDR inhibitors, diverse DDR inhibitors that target various molecules and mechanisms have been developed based on the concept of synthetic lethality, and preclinical validation and clinical trials are underway (Table 8.2).

The ATR-CHK1 pathway plays an essential role in replication fork repair and stabilization. ATR inhibitors and CHK1 inhibitors have been developed as a strategy to aggravate DNA damage due to replication, and preclinical as well as clinical phase I and II trials have been conducted [21]. Our team also confirmed the antitumor effects of ATR inhibitors in gastric cancer and breast cancer; particularly, we confirmed that sensitivity to ATR inhibitors is altered in relation to CHK1 localization in HER2-positive BC and reported that ATR inhibitors sensitize cells to cisplatin and paclitaxel [63]. Importantly, we found that cells with ATM dysfunction were more sensitive to ATR inhibitor and inhibition of ATM in ATM proficient cells sensitizes to ATR inhibitor, which proved synthetic lethality between ATR inhibition and ATM deficiency [64]. Furthermore, Chris T. Williamson *et al.* suggested that ATR inhibitors are effective in a BC cell line with *ARID1A* mutation in their 2016 study published in Nature Communications [65]. An in vitro study found that ATR inhibition increases the antitumor effects of DNA damaging agents, topoisomerase inhibitors (SN38, etoposide, doxorubicin, and topotecan), platinum drugs such as cisplatin, and radiation. Currently, a phase I study is being conducted to investigate the effects of niraparib and an ATR inhibitor (VX-970) plus cisplatin regimen in refractory solid tumors [19]. According to recent study findings, IGF1R inhibition sensitizes BC cells to the effects of ATR inhibitors by increasing CHK1 phosphorylation and H2AX phosphorylation [66]. In addition, based on a report that replication origin firing is regulated by CDKs and Wee1 kinase activity, a strategy was developed in which DSBs are elevated by increasing replication firing and inducing nucleotide shortening by accelerating entry into an abnormal S phase by blocking Wee1, which inhibits CDK1/2 [67, 68]. A Wee1 inhibitor is currently being investigated in a phase II trial as a combination strategy with cisplatin in metastatic TNBC, and a phase I study investigating a combination of Wee1 inhibitor and olaparib on refractory solid tumors, including BC, is also underway [69, 70]. DDR inhibitors can be used alone or in combination with DNA damaging agents and radiation therapy or treatment with PARP inhibitors to induce synthetic lethality by blocking other DDR pathway mechanisms, and these strategies are being clinically tested.

Immune checkpoint inhibitors have emerged as promising therapeutic agents in oncology in recent years. Cytotoxic T lymphocyte antigen 4 (CTLA-4), programmed cell death-1 (PD-1), and programmed cell death ligand-1 (PD-L1) are clinically proven immune checkpoint inhibitors, and it has been suggested that severe genomic instability could be correlated with the effects of these drugs. Furthermore, multiple NGS studies have reported that HRD phenotype-related, 'mutational signature 3' tumors have elevated expression of CTLA-4, PD-L1, and Indoleamine 2,3-dioxygenase 1 (IDO-1) [39]. Currently, the argument that immune checkpoint inhibitors would be effective on patients with HRD is being accepted [39, 71, 72]. Specifically, those exhibiting *BRCA1* or *BRCA2* germline mutation had significantly higher expression of immunogenic and tumor- infiltrating lymphocytes (TILs) than those who did not have a *BRCA1* or *BRCA2* germline mutation [73]. Nolan *et al.* reported that *BRCA1*-associated TNBC cohorts showed higher TILs and mutation burden than those with wild-type *BRCA* TNBC [74]. Recently, immune checkpoint inhibitors are being actively investigated in breast cancer in combination with other agents with various mechanisms. PARP inhibitors have immunomodulatory effects in a *BRCA1*-deficient ovarian cancer mouse model, and talazoparib, a potent PARP inhibitor, has been found to increase cytotoxic CD8+ T cells. Furthermore, olaparib and talazoparib have been confirmed to increase PD-L1 expression, while combination therapy with PD-L1 blockade and PARP inhibitors has been confirmed to be effective in BC [75–77]. Based on these preclinical data, phase I/II trials on the combination of PD-L1 inhibitor durvalumab with olaparib and phase I/II trials on the combination of PD-L1 inhibitors pembrolizumab and niraparib are underway. In our institution, we start to recruit patients in a window of opportunity trial to investigate olaparib and durvalumab treatment prior to standard neoadjuvant chemotherapy in TNBC or low ER+ Stage II/III BC patients (NCT03594396). We expect that olaparib might increase the immune modulation efficacy of durvalumab by increasing genomic instability in BC patients. Owing to the development of diverse DDR inhibitors and the identification of new mechanisms, active research is ongoing to expand the utility of novel anticancer strategies and maximize antitumor effects.

8.4 Future Perspectives

DDR inhibitors have opened up possibilities of DNA damage pathway-driven treatment of intractable BC. Furthermore, DDR inhibitors offer great merits for cancer treatment in that they can overcome resistance and maximize antitumor effects in cases of resistance to the conventional targeted therapies or chemotherapeutics caused by elevated DDR activity. However, with the clinical application of DDR inhibitors, the problems of acquired resistance to DDR inhibitors are emerging. With regard to PARP inhibitors, the most well-known resistance mechanism involves the gain of HR function as a result of an indirect additional mutational event in a tumor [78–80]. More specifically, it has been discovered that acquired reversion mutations of *BRCA1* and *BRCA2* or loss of *BRCA1* promoter methylation lead to the recovery of HR function, which in turn results in a loss of response to PARP inhibitors and platinum drugs. Moreover, some *BRCA*-deficient cells have also been reported to be resistant to PARP inhibitors, as ATR controls RAD51 independent of BRCA. In such cases, combination therapy with ATR inhibitors and PARP inhibitors is expected to overcome the resistance. Yazinski *et al.* suggested that resistance in PARP inhibitor-resistant *BRCA*-deficient cancer cells can be overcome by inhibition of ATR inhibition owing to ATR's induction of HRR that bypasses *BRCA1/2* [81]. Similarly, it is expected that resistance to PARP inhibitors caused by the restoration of DDR activity can be overcome with a combination strategy with other DDR inhibitors. Because ATR inhibitors and PARP inhibitors have been reported to be effective in cancers with ATM loss, the response may be enhanced when combined with ATM inhibitors [17]. In particular, a combination of ATM and ATR inhibitors could also be considered to overcome resistance and maximize antitumor effects, as the resistance mechanisms of ATR inhibitors include crosstalk with ATM signals.

Overexpression/amplification of c-MET, which regulates PARP activity, has also been reported to suppress the response to PARP inhibitors in BC cells by increasing PARP1 enzymatic activity [82]. In fact, c-MET amplification is observed in BC, particularly after treatment. When cotreated with a c-MET inhibitor and PARP inhibitors, tumor growth was markedly inhibited in a TNBC xenograft model compared to treatment with either inhibitor alone, suggesting that c-MET overexpression may be another resistance mechanism for PARP inhibitors [82]. Another mechanism involves an increase of PARP inhibitor efflux through upregulation of the gene that encodes the P-glycoprotein (P-gp) efflux pump. In a *BRCA1*-deficient metastatic BC mouse model, continuous administration of olaparib induced resistance as a result of increased P-gp drug efflux transporter expression [83]. A novel PARP inhibitor called AZD2461 overcame this resistance with a low affinity for P-gp.

Although it is important to understand the mechanism of resistance, it is more important in clinical practice to define optimal treatment sequences after confirming resistance in patients using PARP inhibitors. In the recent TOPARP-A study on prostate cancer patients, a circulating cell-free DNA (cfDNA) analysis was performed to detect resistant clones, and the results showed that the aberration of cfDNA subclone was altered in tumor with germline *BRCA2* or somatic *BRCA2 and PALB2* mutation [84]. Based on these results, cfDNA analysis was proposed as a method of detecting real-time changes in resistance mechanisms without excessively straining patients. Furthermore, our team is currently conducting a genomic analysis of patients with PARP inhibitor resistance and attempting to discover effective therapies using patient-derived xenograft (PDX) models. We are investigating methods that offer a more durable response in cancer patients, such as identifying the resistance mechanism and discovering selective treatment regimens through genomic analysis in relation to the treatment process. In addition to overcoming resistance, we are seeking to identify methods to assess the efficacy of multiple novel DDR inhibitors including PARP inhibitors and maximize benefits by expanding the application of DDR inhibitors that target BC cells, which have high genomic instability and intracellular heterogeneity. Potential combination partners include other DDR inhibitors, immune checkpoint inhibitors, and signal pathway inhibitors of growth signals. Identification of the best candidates for these combination strategies remains to be investigated. The ultimate goal of these researches with DDR inhibitors would be the contribution to improve the quality of life and survival of patients who are suffering from breast cancer.

8.5 Summary

8.5.1 The Bench

Every cell undergoes more than tens of thousands of events everyday that damage DNA in various ways, including single-base mismatches, bulky adducts on DNA bases, intra- and interstrand DNA crosslinks, SSBs, and DSBs. Increased levels of DNA damage cause genomic instability, which is an underlying hallmark of cancer [1, 2]. DNA damage can be repaired by three different types of DNA repair pathways that are independently activated depending on the type of DNA damage. DSBs are repaired via the nonhomologous end joining (NHEJ) and homologous recombination (HR) repair pathways [3, 10]. Synthetic lethality is thought to be the explanation for the anticancer effects of DDR inhibitors and has become a promising new cancer treatment strategy [25–27]. Cell death increases as a result of an accumulation of unrepaired damage when the PARP-dependent pathway is inhibited by PARP inhibitors, which inhibit an enzyme that recognizes various types of DNA damage and is recruited to the damage site to induce recruitment of DDR molecules in other DDR pathway defective cells. PARP inhibitors including olaparib, rucaparib, and talazoparib showed dramatic antitumor effect in vitro and in vivo in gBRCAmt cell lines and cells with HRDs through defective DNA damage repair. Talazoparib showed the most potent PARP trapping activity. ATR inhibitors, ATM inhibitors, and DNA-PK inhibitors also showed antitumor efficacy as monotherapy and combination with PARP inhibitors and other immune checkpoint inhibitors. Mechanisms of acquired resistance against DDR inhibitors would be an important research topic.

8.5.2 *Translation*

Hereditary *BRCA1/2* mutation occurs in about 7% of all BC cases and in about 11–15% of triple-negative breast cancer (TNBC) subtypes. A tumor that lacks a *BRCA* mutation but results in HRD with similar responses to DNA damaging agents and clinicopathologic features is referred to as having “BRCAness”. The classic genetic alterations that induce BRCAness are mutations in *RAD51C, PALB2, BARD1, RAD51D,* and *CHEK2*, with recent reports suggesting that germline mutations such as *ATM, BAP1, CDK12*, and *FANCM* also cause HRD. Functional analysis that could assess HRD by observing the nuclear localization of RAD51, an essential component of HR response, was developed.

8.5.3 *The Bedside*

PARP inhibitors have demonstrated robust clinical benefit in patients with gBRCAmt. First-in-class PARP inhibitor, olaparib, and best-in-class talazoparib are approved for treating gBRCAmt breast cancer. Olaparib was also approved for maintenance treatment for platinum-sensitive serous ovarian cancer. The best molecular markers for determining HRD beyond *BRCA1/2* mutations, however, remain to be investigated. Active research is underway to develop various combination strategies to maximize the effect of DDR inhibitors. Moreover, combinations of DDR inhibitors and immune checkpoint inhibitors are being actively tested in clinical trials, based on the immune modulatory effect of DDR inhibitors. Acquired resistance mechanisms of DDR inhibitors, as well as defining best candidates and best combinations, would be future research topics for DDR inhibitors. It would also be crucial to establish a standardized method to detect HRD that is clinically relevant.

References

1. Broustas CG, Lieberman HB. DNA damage response genes and the development of cancer metastasis. Radiat Res. 2014;181(2):111–30.
2. Ciccia A, Elledge SJ. The DNA damage response: making it safe to play with knives. Mol Cell. 2010;40(2):179–204.
3. Ceccaldi R, Rondinelli B, D'Andrea AD. Repair pathway choices and consequences at the double-Strand break. Trends Cell Biol. 2016;26(1):52–64.
4. Hoeijmakers JH. Genome maintenance mechanisms for preventing cancer. Nature. 2001;411 (6835):366–74.
5. Caldecott KW. DNA single-strand break repair. Exp Cell Res. 2014;329(1):2–8.
6. Jiricny J. The multifaceted mismatch-repair system. Nat Rev Mol Cell Biol. 2006;7(5):335–46.
7. Prasad R, Dyrkheeva N, Williams J, Wilson SH. Mammalian Base excision repair: functional partnership between PARP-1 and APE1 in AP-site repair. PLoS One. 2015;10(5):e0124269.
8. van der Veen S, Tang CM. The BER necessities: the repair of DNA damage in human-adapted bacterial pathogens. Nat Rev Microbiol. 2015;13(2):83–94.
9. Scharer OD. Nucleotide excision repair in eukaryotes. Cold Spring Harb Perspect Biol. 2013;5 (10):a012609.
10. Branzei D, Foiani M. Regulation of DNA repair throughout the cell cycle. Nat Rev Mol Cell Biol. 2008;9(4):297–308.
11. Radhakrishnan SK, Jette N, Lees-Miller SP. Non-homologous end joining: emerging themes and unanswered questions. DNA Repair. 2014;17:2–8.
12. Michl J, Zimmer J, Tarsounas M. Interplay between Fanconi anemia and homologous recombination pathways in genome integrity. EMBO J. 2016;35(9):909–23.
13. Mateos-Gomez PA, Gong F, Nair N, Miller KM, Lazzerini-Denchi E, Sfeir A. Mammalian polymerase theta promotes alternative NHEJ and suppresses recombination. Nature. 2015;518 (7538):254–7.
14. Jasin M, Rothstein R. Repair of strand breaks by homologous recombination. Cold Spring Harb Perspect Biol. 2013;5(11):a012740.
15. Dudas A, Chovanec M. DNA double-strand break repair by homologous recombination. Mutat Res. 2004;566(2):131–67.
16. Bhargava R, Onyango DO, Stark JM. Regulation of single-Strand annealing and its role in genome maintenance. Trends Genet. 2016;32(9):566–75.
17. Cheng A, Zhao T, Tse KH, Chow HM, Cui Y, Jiang L, et al. ATM and ATR play complementary roles in the behavior of excitatory and inhibitory vesicle populations. Proc Natl Acad Sci U S A. 2018;115(2):E292–301.
18. Smith TR. DNA damage and breast cancer risk. Carcinogenesis. 2003;24(5):883–9.
19. Carrassa L, Damia G. DNA damage response inhibitors: mechanisms and potential applications in cancer therapy. Cancer Treat Rev. 2017;60:139–51.
20. Gavande NS, VanderVere-Carozza PS, Hinshaw HD, Jalal SI, Sears CR, Pawelczak KS, et al. DNA repair targeted therapy: the past or future of cancer treatment? Pharmacol Ther. 2016;160:65–83.
21. O'Connor MJ. Targeting the DNA damage response in Cancer. Mol Cell. 2015;60(4):547–60.
22. O'Neil NJ, Bailey ML, Hieter P. Synthetic lethality and cancer. Nat Rev Genet. 2017;18 (10):613–23.
23. Shaheen M, Allen C, Nickoloff JA, Hromas R. Synthetic lethality: exploiting the addiction of cancer to DNA repair. Blood. 2011;117(23):6074–82.
24. Beijersbergen RL, Wessels LFA, Bernards R. Synthetic lethality in Cancer therapeutics. Annual Review of Cancer Biology. 2017;1(1):141–61.
25. Ashworth A. A synthetic lethal therapeutic approach: poly(ADP) ribose polymerase inhibitors for the treatment of cancers deficient in DNA double-strand break repair. J Clin Oncol. 2008;26 (22):3785–90.

26. Rouleau M, Patel A, Hendzel MJ, Kaufmann SH, Poirier GG. PARP inhibition: PARP1 and beyond. Nat Rev Cancer. 2010;10(4):293–301.
27. Bryant HE, Schultz N, Thomas HD, Parker KM, Flower D, Lopez E, et al. Specific killing of BRCA2-deficient tumours with inhibitors of poly(ADP-ribose) polymerase. Nature. 2005;434 (7035):913–7.
28. Bartsch R, Bergen E. ASCO 2017: highlights in breast cancer. Memo. 2017;10(4):228–32.
29. Tappenden P, Harnan S, Ren S, Thokala P, Wong R, Mukuria C, et al. Olaparib for maintenance treatment of BRCA 1 or 2 mutated, relapsed, platinum-sensitive ovarian, fallopian tube and peritoneal Cancer in people whose relapsed disease has responded to platinum-based chemotherapy: an evidence review group perspective of a NICE single technology appraisal. PharmacoEconomics. 2017;35(1):97–109.
30. Robson M, Im SA, Senkus E, Xu B, Domchek SM, Masuda N, et al. Olaparib for metastatic breast Cancer in patients with a Germline BRCA mutation. N Engl J Med. 2017;377(6):523–33.
31. Pujade-Lauraine E, Ledermann JA, Selle F, Gebski V, Penson RT, Oza AM, et al. Olaparib tablets as maintenance therapy in patients with platinum-sensitive, relapsed ovarian cancer and a BRCA1/2 mutation (SOLO2/ENGOT-Ov21): a double-blind, randomised, placebo-controlled, phase 3 trial. Lancet Oncol. 2017;18(9):1274–84.
32. Polak P, Kim J, Braunstein LZ, Karlic R, Haradhavala NJ, Tiao G, et al. A mutational signature reveals alterations underlying deficient homologous recombination repair in breast cancer. Nat Genet. 2017;49(10):1476–86.
33. O'Kane GM, Connor AA, Gallinger S. Characterization, detection, and treatment approaches for homologous recombination deficiency in Cancer. Trends Mol Med. 2017;23(12):1121–37.
34. Riaz N, Blecua P, Lim RS, Shen R, Higginson DS, Weinhold N, et al. Pan-cancer analysis of bi-allelic alterations in homologous recombination DNA repair genes. Nat Commun. 2017;8 (1):857.
35. Mutter RW, Riaz N, Ng CK, Delsite R, Piscuoglio S, Edelweiss M, et al. Bi-allelic alterations in DNA repair genes underpin homologous recombination DNA repair defects in breast cancer. J Pathol. 2017;242(2):165–77.
36. Alexandrov LB, Nik-Zainal S, Wedge DC, Aparicio SA, Behjati S, Biankin AV, et al. Signatures of mutational processes in human cancer. Nature. 2013;500(7463):415–21.
37. Nik-Zainal S, Davies H, Staaf J, Ramakrishna M, Glodzik D, Zou X, et al. Landscape of somatic mutations in 560 breast cancer whole-genome sequences. Nature. 2016;534(7605):47–54.
38. Davies H, Glodzik D, Morganella S, Yates LR, Staaf J, Zou X, et al. HRDetect is a predictor of BRCA1 and BRCA2 deficiency based on mutational signatures. Nat Med. 2017;23(4):517–25.
39. Connor AA, Denroche RE, Jang GH, Timms L, Kalimuthu SN, Selander I, et al. Association of Distinct Mutational Signatures with Correlates of increased immune activity in pancreatic ductal adenocarcinoma. JAMA Oncol. 2017;3(6):774–83.
40. Mirza MR, Monk BJ, Herrstedt J, Oza AM, Mahner S, Redondo A, et al. Niraparib maintenance therapy in platinum-sensitive, recurrent ovarian Cancer. N Engl J Med. 2016;375(22):2154–64.
41. Naipal KA, Verkaik NS, Ameziane N, van Deurzen CH, Ter Brugge P, Meijers M, et al. Functional ex vivo assay to select homologous recombination-deficient breast tumors for PARP inhibitor treatment. Clin Cancer Res. 2014;20(18):4816–26.
42. Graeser M, McCarthy A, Lord CJ, Savage K, Hills M, Salter J, et al. A marker of homologous recombination predicts pathologic complete response to neoadjuvant chemotherapy in primary breast cancer. Clin Cancer Res. 2010;16(24):6159–68.
43. Gyawali B. The OlympiAD trial: who won the gold? Ecancermedicalscience. 2017;11:ed75.
44. Gelmon KA, Tischkowitz M, Mackay H, Swenerton K, Robidoux A, Tonkin K, et al. Olaparib in patients with recurrent high-grade serous or poorly differentiated ovarian carcinoma or triple-negative breast cancer: a phase 2, multicentre, open-label, non-randomised study. Lancet Oncol. 2011;12(9):852–61.
45. Ledermann J, Harter P, Gourley C, Friedlander M, Vergote I, Rustin G, et al. Olaparib maintenance therapy in patients with platinum-sensitive relapsed serous ovarian cancer: a

preplanned retrospective analysis of outcomes by BRCA status in a randomised phase 2 trial. Lancet Oncol. 2014;15(8):852–61.
46. Ang YLE, Tan DSP. Development of PARP inhibitors in gynecological malignancies. Curr Probl Cancer. 2017;41(4):273–86.
47. Kaufman B, Shapira-Frommer R, Schmutzler RK, Audeh MW, Friedlander M, Balmana J, et al. Olaparib monotherapy in patients with advanced cancer and a germline BRCA1/2 mutation. J Clin Oncol. 2015;33(3):244–50.
48. Ledermann J, Harter P, Gourley C, Friedlander M, Vergote I, Rustin G, et al. Olaparib maintenance therapy in platinum-sensitive relapsed ovarian cancer. N Engl J Med. 2012;366 (15):1382–92.
49. Swisher EM, Lin KK, Oza AM, Scott CL, Giordano H, Sun J, et al. Rucaparib in relapsed, platinum-sensitive high-grade ovarian carcinoma (ARIEL2 part 1): an international, multicentre, open-label, phase 2 trial. Lancet Oncol. 2017;18(1):75–87.
50. Coleman RL, Oza AM, Lorusso D, Aghajanian C, Oaknin A, Dean A, et al. Rucaparib maintenance treatment for recurrent ovarian carcinoma after response to platinum therapy (ARIEL3): a randomised, double-blind, placebo-controlled, phase 3 trial. Lancet. 2017;390 (10106):1949–61.
51. Litton JK, Rugo HS, Ettl J, Hurvitz SA, Gonçalves A, Lee K-H, et al. Talazoparib in patients with advanced breast cancer and a germline BRCA mutation. N Engl J Med. 2018;379:753–63. https://doi.org/10.1056/NEJMoa1802905.
52. Litton JK, Scoggins M, Hess KR, Adrada B, Barcenas CH, Murthy RK, et al. Neoadjuvant talazoparib (TALA) for operable breast cancer patients with a BRCA mutation (BRCA+). J Clin Oncol. 2018;36((15_suppl)):508.
53. Min A, Im SA, Yoon YK, Song SH, Nam HJ, Hur HS, et al. RAD51C-deficient cancer cells are highly sensitive to the PARP inhibitor olaparib. Mol Cancer Ther. 2013;12(6):865–77.
54. Kim JW, Im SA, Kim MA, Cho HJ, Lee DW, Lee KH, et al. Ataxia-telangiectasia-mutated protein expression with microsatellite instability in gastric cancer as prognostic marker. Int J Cancer. 2014;134(1):72–80.
55. Bang YJ, Im SA, Lee KW, Cho JY, Song EK, Lee KH, et al. Randomized, double-blind phase II trial with prospective classification by ATM protein level to evaluate the efficacy and tolerability of Olaparib plus paclitaxel in patients with recurrent or metastatic gastric Cancer. J Clin Oncol. 2015;33(33):3858–65.
56. Bang YJ, Xu RH, Chin K, Lee KW, Park SH, Rha SY, et al. Olaparib in combination with paclitaxel in patients with advanced gastric cancer who have progressed following first-line therapy (GOLD): a double-blind, randomised, placebo-controlled, phase 3 trial. Lancet Oncol. 2017;18(12):1637–51.
57. Mateo J, Carreira S, Sandhu S, Miranda S, Mossop H, Perez-Lopez R, et al. DNA-repair defects and Olaparib in metastatic prostate Cancer. N Engl J Med. 2015;373(18):1697–708.
58. Oza AM, Cibula D, Benzaquen AO, Poole C, Mathijssen RH, Sonke GS, et al. Olaparib combined with chemotherapy for recurrent platinum-sensitive ovarian cancer: a randomised phase 2 trial. Lancet Oncol. 2015;16(1):87–97.
59. Schouten PC, Dackus GM, Marchetti S, van Tinteren H, Sonke GS, Schellens JH, et al. A phase I followed by a randomized phase II trial of two cycles carboplatin-olaparib followed by olaparib monotherapy versus capecitabine in BRCA1- or BRCA2-mutated HER2-negative advanced breast cancer as first line treatment (REVIVAL): study protocol for a randomized controlled trial. Trials. 2016;17(1):293.
60. Mo W, Liu Q, Lin CC, Dai H, Peng Y, Liang Y, et al. mTOR inhibitors suppress homologous recombination repair and synergize with PARP inhibitors via regulating SUV39H1 in BRCA-proficient triple-negative breast Cancer. Clin Cancer Res. 2016;22(7):1699–712.
61. Matulonis UA, Wulf GM, Barry WT, Birrer M, Westin SN, Farooq S, et al. Phase I dose escalation study of the PI3kinase pathway inhibitor BKM120 and the oral poly (ADP ribose) polymerase (PARP) inhibitor olaparib for the treatment of high-grade serous ovarian and breast cancer. Ann Oncol. 2017;28(3):512–8.

62. Min A, Im SA, Kim DK, Song SH, Kim HJ, Lee KH, et al. Histone deacetylase inhibitor, suberoylanilide hydroxamic acid (SAHA), enhances anti-tumor effects of the poly (ADP-ribose) polymerase (PARP) inhibitor olaparib in triple-negative breast cancer cells. Breast Cancer Res. 2015;17:33.
63. Kim HJ, Min A, Im SA, Jang H, Lee KH, Lau A, et al. Anti-tumor activity of the ATR inhibitor AZD6738 in HER2 positive breast cancer cells. Int J Cancer. 2017;140(1):109–19.
64. Min A, Im SA, Jang H, Kim S, Lee M, Kim DK, et al. AZD6738, a novel Oral inhibitor of ATR, induces synthetic lethality with ATM deficiency in gastric Cancer cells. Mol Cancer Ther. 2017;16(4):566–77.
65. Williamson CT, Miller R, Pemberton HN, Jones SE, Campbell J, Konde A, et al. ATR inhibitors as a synthetic lethal therapy for tumours deficient in ARID1A. Nat Commun. 2016;7:13837.
66. O'Flanagan CH, O'Shea S, Lyons A, Fogarty FM, McCabe N, Kennedy RD, et al. IGF-1R inhibition sensitizes breast cancer cells to ATM-related kinase (ATR) inhibitor and cisplatin. Oncotarget. 2016;7(35):56826–41.
67. Otto T, Sicinski P. Cell cycle proteins as promising targets in cancer therapy. Nat Rev Cancer. 2017;17(2):93–115.
68. Caiola E, Frapolli R, Tomanelli M, Valerio R, Iezzi A, Garassino MC, et al. Wee1 inhibitor MK1775 sensitizes KRAS mutated NSCLC cells to sorafenib. Sci Rep. 2018;8(1):948.
69. Leijen S, van Geel RM, Sonke GS, de Jong D, Rosenberg EH, Marchetti S, et al. Phase II study of WEE1 inhibitor AZD1775 plus carboplatin in patients with TP53-mutated ovarian Cancer refractory or resistant to first-line therapy within 3 months. J Clin Oncol. 2016;34(36):4354–61.
70. Leijen S, van Geel RM, Pavlick AC, Tibes R, Rosen L, Razak AR, et al. Phase I study evaluating WEE1 inhibitor AZD1775 as Monotherapy and in combination with gemcitabine, Cisplatin, or carboplatin in patients with advanced solid tumors. J Clin Oncol. 2016;34 (36):4371–80.
71. Mao Y, Qu Q, Chen X, Huang O, Wu J, Shen K. The prognostic value of tumor-infiltrating lymphocytes in breast Cancer: a systematic review and meta-analysis. PLoS One. 2016;11(4): e0152500.
72. McAlpine JN, Porter H, Kobel M, Nelson BH, Prentice LM, Kalloger SE, et al. BRCA1 and BRCA2 mutations correlate with TP53 abnormalities and presence of immune cell infiltrates in ovarian high-grade serous carcinoma. Mod Pathol. 2012;25(5):740–50.
73. Bertucci F, Goncalves A. Immunotherapy in breast Cancer: the emerging role of PD-1 and PD-L1. Curr Oncol Rep. 2017;19(10):64.
74. Nolan E, Savas P, Policheni AN, Darcy PK, Vaillant F, Mintoff CP, et al. Combined immune checkpoint blockade as a therapeutic strategy for BRCA1-mutated breast cancer. Sci Transl Med. 2017;9(393):eaal4922.
75. Huang J, Wang L, Cong Z, Amoozgar Z, Kiner E, Xing D, et al. The PARP1 inhibitor BMN 673 exhibits immunoregulatory effects in a Brca1(−/−) murine model of ovarian cancer. Biochem Biophys Res Commun. 2015;463(4):551–6.
76. Higuchi T, Flies DB, Marjon NA, Mantia-Smaldone G, Ronner L, Gimotty PA, et al. CTLA-4 blockade synergizes therapeutically with PARP inhibition in BRCA1-deficient ovarian Cancer. Cancer Immunol Res. 2015;3(11):1257–68.
77. Jiao S, Xia W, Yamaguchi H, Wei Y, Chen MK, Hsu JM, et al. PARP inhibitor Upregulates PD-L1 expression and enhances Cancer-associated immunosuppression. Clin Cancer Res. 2017;23(14):3711–20.
78. Lim JSJ, Tan DSP. Understanding resistance mechanisms and expanding the therapeutic utility of PARP inhibitors. Cancers. 2017;9(8):109.
79. Montoni A, Robu M, Pouliot E, Shah GM. Resistance to PARP-inhibitors in Cancer therapy. Front Pharmacol. 2013;4:18.
80. Bitler BG, Watson ZL, Wheeler LJ, Behbakht K. PARP inhibitors: clinical utility and possibilities of overcoming resistance. Gynecol Oncol. 2017;147(3):695–704.

81. Yazinski SA, Comaills V, Buisson R, Genois MM, Nguyen HD, Ho CK, et al. ATR inhibition disrupts rewired homologous recombination and fork protection pathways in PARP inhibitor-resistant BRCA-deficient cancer cells. Genes Dev. 2017;31(3):318–32.
82. Du Y, Yamaguchi H, Wei Y, Hsu JL, Wang HL, Hsu YH, et al. Blocking c-met-mediated PARP1 phosphorylation enhances anti-tumor effects of PARP inhibitors. Nat Med. 2016;22 (2):194–201.
83. Henneman L, van Miltenburg MH, Michalak EM, Braumuller TM, Jaspers JE, Drenth AP, et al. Selective resistance to the PARP inhibitor olaparib in a mouse model for BRCA1-deficient metaplastic breast cancer. Proc Natl Acad Sci U S A. 2015;112(27):8409–14.
84. Goodall J, Mateo J, Yuan W, Mossop H, Porta N, Miranda S, et al. Circulating cell-free DNA to guide prostate Cancer treatment with PARP inhibition. Cancer Discov. 2017;7(9):1006–17.

Part III
Cancer Stem Cell and Tumor Heterogeneity in Breast Cancer

Chapter 9
Breast Cancer Metastasis

Mi Young Kim

Abstract Owing to increased awareness of the importance of mammogram and advances in surgical technology, survival rate of patients with primary breast cancer has dramatically increased. Despite all these advances in breast cancer treatment, there are no currently available treatments for this disease once it metastasizes to distant organs including bones, lungs, brain, and liver. This is mainly attributed to the complexity of metastatic process. Recent advances in technology enabled cancer biologists to dissect each step of the metastatic process, and this led to discovery of major players and molecules in this process. In this section, we will discuss recent discovery and advances in the field of breast cancer metastasis research.

Keywords Breast cancer metastasis · Metastasis model · Metastasis mechanisms · Pre-metastatic niche · Immune cells

9.1 Introduction

Breast cancer metastasis to distant organs is a deadly process and accounts for a majority of breast cancer-related deaths. This is mainly because (1) it is hard to perform a surgery once it is metastasized and (2) there are no effective drugs that can be used for the treatment of metastatic breast cancer. Thus, it is essential to identify prognostic markers that can accurately predict potential risks of metastasis and therapeutic targets that can be used to treat patients with metastatic breast cancer. A prerequisite achieving these goals is to gain a comprehensive understanding of the process of breast cancer metastasis.

Like in other cancers, breast cancer metastasis starts from invasion of cancer cells into the surrounding tissue, followed by dissemination, survival in circulation, arrest

M. Y. Kim (✉)
Department of Biological Sciences, Korea Advanced Institute of Science and Technology (KAIST), Daejeon, South Korea
e-mail: miyoungkim@kaist.ac.kr

D.-Y. Noh et al. (eds.), *Translational Research in Breast Cancer*, Advances in Experimental Medicine and Biology 1187,
https://doi.org/10.1007/978-981-32-9620-6_9

at the distant site, extravasation, and formation of micro- and macro-metastasis. Each of these steps is a rate-limiting process for the successful formation of metastasis and requires functions of various genes. Breast cancer metastasizes to bones, lungs, brain, and liver [1–3], and accumulating evidence indicates that metastatic breast cancer cells possess different molecular and cellular characteristics compared to the primary breast cancer cells. Furthermore, many studies have reported that different sets of genes are used for organ-specific metastasis [4–7] and this is because metastatic cancer cells, once they land on a secondary organ, must adapt to different environments presented by each organ. The expression of these sets of genes in primary tumor could be used as possible prognostic markers for predicting risks for metastasis [4, 5, 8]. Also, pharmacological inhibition of these genes has potential to be used in clinic alone or in combination with traditional chemotherapy [4, 5, 8, 9].

Recently, technological development such as single cell sequencing allowed us to investigate the heterogeneity of the metastatic cancer cells. In addition, improvement of live imaging technology enabled us to monitor metastatic processes in animal models.

Our understanding of the breast cancer metastasis has dramatically improved in the past 10 years, and some potentially promising targets have been identified. In the below sections, we will discuss recent studies that have provided insights into the process of metastasis and potential therapeutic targets.

9.2 Review of Past Studies

9.2.1 Mouse Models of Breast Cancer Metastasis

The use of various mouse models has significantly advanced our understanding of breast cancer metastasis. Each model presents advantages and disadvantages. Thus, it is recommended to choose appropriate models for a study depending on the questions to be addressed. In the below section, we will discuss some of the mouse models used in the field of breast cancer metastasis research.

9.2.1.1 Tumor Implantation Models

Tumor implantation models include xenograft and syngeneic mouse model. Both these models involve transplantation of cancer cells into mice except that human cancer cells were injected into immuno-deficient mice in xenograft, whereas mouse cancer cells are introduced into immuno-competent mice (xenograft) in syngeneic mouse model [10, 11]. While syngeneic model allows investigation of cancer cell-microenvironment interaction including immune cells, this does not accurately recapitulate human cancer. On the other hand, xenograft overcomes the shortcome of syngeneic model, but interaction between cancer cells and immune cells cannot be studied in this model [10, 11]. The major advance in field of breast cancer metastasis was achieved by the in vivo selection in xenograft model use of xenograft in in vivo selection. This method allows isolation of more homogeneous population of cancer cells with enriched organ-tropic metastatic ability. The use of in vivo selection enabled us to investigate genetic and biological differences of breast cancers with different organ-tropic metastatic activity [4, 5, 7].

Recent efforts to overcome the shortcome of a xenograft model include development of humanized mice. In addition, direct implantation of human tumor biopsies, which is referred to as patient-derived xenograft (PDX), has been attempted in order to minimize potential issues such as changes in characteristics of cancer cells, caused by the use of in vitro cultured cancer cell lines [12, 13]. However, the rate of metastasis in PDX is variable, and thus, it requires a large number of cohorts. At current stage, PDX is mainly used in studying primary breast cancer such as investigation of cancer cell heterogeneity [14].

9.2.1.2 Genetically Engineered Mouse Model (GEMM)

Several GEMM models have been used to study breast cancer metastasis including oncogene-derived (MMTV-neu, myc, wnt, and pyMT) [15] or in combination deletion of tumor suppressor (BRCA1/2, p53) [16]. A major limitation of conventional GEMM is that the expression of oncogene or tumor suppressor genes cannot be controlled. To resolve this issue, next generation of GEMM has been developed, which enables temporal and/or spatial regulation of oncogenes or TSG, therefore allowing study of metastatic process in more controlled manner [17, 18]. In addition, CRIPR/Cas9 technology is broadly used for rapid generation of GEMM [19].

9.2.2 Mechanisms Involved in Breast Cancer Metastasis

9.2.2.1 Local Invasion

Invasion of surrounding tissue by breast cancer cells is the first step of metastatic process, which involves changes in a variety of migration and cell adhesion molecules. One of the most extensively studied mechanisms that lead to local invasion is a phenomenon called "epithelial to mesenchymal transition" or EMT. The EMT process comprises loss of cell-cell adhesion between epithelial cells and acquisition of mesenchymal characteristics [20–22]. Early studies of EMT have revealed that EMT plays a critical role in various steps of developmental process such as gastrulation, neural crest cell formation, and etc. [20–22]. In addition, EMT is known to be associated with inflammation-induced fibrosis [20–22]. Furthermore, several studies suggest that EMT contributes to local invasion [23, 24]. EMT can be initiated by activation of several pathways including TGF-b, wnt, Notch, etc., and several studies have reported that stromal cells (e.g., cancer associated-fibroblasts or myeloid-derived suppressor cells), comprising tumor microenvironment contribute to activation of these pathways [25]. Subsequently, activation of aforementioned pathways induces EMT regulators such as TWIST1, ZEB1/2, and SNAIL, which leads to downregulation of epithelial markers (e.g, E-cadherin and ZO-1) as well as overexpression of mesenchymal markers (e.g., vimentin, fibronectin, and N-cadherin) [20–22]. As a consequence, cancer cells acquire invasiveness. However, it should be noted that previous notion that EMT is required for the metastatic process has been challenged. For example, a recent study by Fischer et al., by using elegant mouse models, have suggested that EMT process is not required for breast cancer metastasis to the lung, but leads to chemoresistance [26].

Interaction between stromal cells and breast cancer cells can also promote local invasion by secreting several proteases, which degrade cell adhesion molecules and extracellular matrix (ECM) and activate cyto/chemokine [27, 28]. One of the well-studied stromal cells that play such functions is macrophage [29]. In addition, mesenchymal stem cell (MSC) has been reported to contribute to the local invasion. Furthermore, recent studies have indicated that myeloid-derived suppressive cells (MDSCs) also promote cancer cell invasion through secretion of MMPs [30].

While prometastatic roles of macrophages are well-established, the underlying molecular mechanisms are still unclear. Some recent studies have shed light on this process. Cyclooxygenase 2 (COX2) has been shown to inhibit expression of prometastatic factors such as VEGFa and MMPs from macrophages [31]. In addition, GM-CSF also promotes production of M2-like macrophages [32].

In summary, constant communication between stromal cells and breast cancer cells can lead to activation of EMT program or other mechanisms, which eventually allows breast cancer cells to invade surrounding tissue.

9.2.2.2 Intravasation and Survival in Circulation

Cancer cell dissemination has been considered a very late event in cancer progression [33]. However, studies with transgenic mouse models and patient samples have revealed that dissemination can take place at very early stage of cancer progression [34, 35]. Breast cancer cells can be disseminated by lymphatic and/or hematogenous route. Lymphatic vessels, unlike the blood vessels, lack tight interendothelial junctions and have discontinuous basement membrane, making it easier for cancer cells to enter the lymphatic circulation. Indeed, the lymph node is often the first site of metastasis and the lymph node metastasis is an important marker for staging of breast cancer and increases risks for the distant metastasis [36, 37]. On the other hand, intravasation into blood vessel requires help of several non-cancer cells including perivascular macrophages [29]. These cells first secrete EGF and promote cancer cell migration as well as secretion of colony stimulating factor 1(CSF-1) by cancer cells [38]. Subsequently, cancer cell-derived CSF-1 recruits and stimulates the growth macrophages [38]. These macrophages then secrete proteases and degrade vascular base membrane, enabling cancer cells to enter the blood circulation

[38]. Other examples include pericytes that secrete CXCL12 to direct cancer to the blood vessel [39].

Once cancer cells intravasate into circulation, referred to as circulating tumor cells (CTCs), they now confront three major obstacles: (1) anoikis (detachment-induced apoptosis), (2) immune attack, and (3) physical damage by shear force. To survive under this hostile condition in the blood circulation, breast cancer cells employ several mechanisms. First, in order to overcome anoikis, breast cancer cells activate several signaling pathways including TrKB, EMT, PI3K, etc. [40]. In addition, platelet forms aggregates with cancer cells to protect them, and this is mediated by the interaction between coagulation factors VIIa and X in platelet and their receptor expressed in cancer cells [41, 42]. In addition, platelets protect cancer cells by bringing cancer cells and macrophages together and form microclot [41, 42]. The close association between high platelet counts and decreased survival in breast cancer patients further supports the importance of platelet in the metastasis process [41, 42].

As close association between number of CTCs and the risks in distant metastasis is well-accepted phenomenon, detecting the accurate numbers of CTCs in the patient blood has been a focus of recent technical development. Detection of CTCs is based on the physical and molecular characteristics of CTCs [43–45]. The first generation of CTC detection method uses antibodies against epithelial cell markers including EpCAM (epithelial cell adhesion molecule) and cytoketatin that are absent in blood and immune cells. Cell Search by Veridex (Raritan, NJ) is the only CTC detection kit that is currently used in clinic [46]. Briefly, this method uses 7.5 mL of patient blood sample, which is subject to negative selection with CD45 (leukocyte marker) and positive selection with EpCAM and cytoketatin [46]. More than 5 CTCs in 7.5 mL of blood are considered as a high-risk group for distant metastasis [46].

In addition to its use as a diagnostic/prognostic marker, CTCs can also be used to evaluate the efficacy of treatment in a given patient, allowing personalized medicine.

9.2.2.3 Arrest and Extravasation

Once CTCs are arrested at the distant organ, each organ presents different barriers. One of these barriers is the different structure of vasculature. For example, lung capillary is very tight compared to the leaky nature of primary tumors. Therefore, breast cancer cells must actively disrupt tight junction between endothelial cells and this is mediated by the function of several proteins. For example, angiopoietin-like 4 (ANGPTL4) has been shown to contribute to extravasation of breast cancer cells into lung parenchyma by disrupting endothelial layers [47]. In addition, COX2/MMP1,2/Epiregulin in combination also helps extravasation into the lung [9]. On the other hand, blood brain barrier (BBB) is the major barrier for the brain metastasis and it can be overcome by several genes including ST6GalNac5, COX2, HBEGF, MMP2, and cathepsin S [4, 48]. In contrast to these two organs, the existence of sinusoid in bones provides more permissive environment for cancer cells to extravasate into the bones, and thus, it is considered that extravasation is not a rate-limiting step in bone metastasis.

The role of macrophages in cancer extravasation has also been demonstrated in breast cancer. The association between macrophages and extravasating breast cancer cells has been observed, and depletion of macrophage significantly reduces number of extravasating breast cancer cells [49]. Studies have suggested VEGFa as one of the major macrophage-derived factors, which promotes cancer cell extravasation [50].

9.2.2.4 Formation of Micro- and Macrometastasis

Once breast cancer cells extravasate into the parenchyma of the secondary organ, they need to reinitiate the colonies against several obstacles presented by each organ. It includes (1) secretion of anti-metastatic signals from the stromal cells, (2) attack by immune cells, and (3) different microenvironment from the primary site. To overcome this, breast cancer cells must be able to survive against the anti-metastatic signals and to modify the microenvironment to hospitable for their growth. Several studies have revealed various genes that contribute to organ-specific metastasis of breast cancer, which is summarized below.

Lung Metastasis

Several genes have been identified to contribute to the formation of micro- and macrometastasis in the lung. These genes include Coco, ID1/3, Tenascin C, CXCL1, VCAM, miR-200, periostin, etc. [51–57].

A recent study has shown that BMP is one of the major anti-metastatic signals in the lung. This study also revealed that Coco, the inhibitor of BMP pathway, is overexpressed in lung metastatic breast cancer cells and allows breast cancer cells to overcome the inhibitory effect of BMP in self-renewal, therefore promoting reinitiation of new colonies in the lung environment [57].

On the other hand, some molecules confer BCCs with stem cell-like properties through exploiting the microenvironment such as ECM and stromal cells. Evidence suggests that the interaction between ECM of the lung parenchyma and the incoming breast cancer cells is essential in initiation of new colonies in the lung. In this regard, a recent study showed that breast cancer cells with lung metastasis-initiating ability secrete TGFb to promote the production of periostin, an ECM protein, from lung fibroblast. This then activates WNT signaling in the breast cancer cells that eventually promotes lung metastasis initiation [54].

In addition, glycoprotein Tenascin C increases stem cell-like properties of breast cancer cells by activating NOTCH pathway and also plays a role in interaction between cancer cells and lung fibroblast to support the initial growth of breast cancer cells [55]. On the other hand, VCAM1 promotes the interaction between breast cancer cells and macrophages, which subsequently protects breast cancer cells from apoptosis [52].

The last class of genes contributes to lung colonization by promoting MET (mesenchymal-epithelial transition), a reverse process of EMT. Recently, MET has been proposed to be an important step for the formation of full-grown lung metastases and several genes (e.g., inhibitor of differentiation1 (ID1)) have been shown to contribute to this process [51].

Brain Metastasis

As described in the previous section, brain presents a specialized environment including BBB and the presence of specialized cells such as astrocytes, microglia, etc. It has been observed that breast cancer cells escape from astrocyte-induced apoptosis by expressing molecules that neutralize the apoptotic molecules. For example, astrocyte secretes plasminogen activator (PA) that releases apoptotic FAS ligand from the membrane, which promotes apoptosis of incoming breast cancer cells [58]. To overcome this, breast cancer cells with brain metastatic activity secrete Serpin to inhibit the function of PA, sparing breast cancer cells from apoptosis [58]. Once breast cancer cells survive the astrocyte-induced death, they modify brain microenvironment to be more favorable for the growth of new colonies, in which astrocytes and microglia play essential roles.

The brain metastasis-promoting role of astrocytes and the underlying molecular mechanisms have been uncovered by several studies. First, a recent study showed that astrocytes play a role in self-renewal of breast cancer cells within the brain. In this study, the authors showed that brain-metastatic breast cancer cells secrete IL-1b, which upregulates JAG-1 expression in the astrocytes. Subsequently, this protein binds to its receptor NOTCH on the surface of brain-metastatic breast cancer cells and activates the downstream pathway, promoting the self-renewal of breast cancer cells [59].

In another study, it was demonstrated that astrocytes produce exosomes containing PTEN-targeting miRNAs. These exosome are then taken into the extravasated breast cancer cells and lead to the reduction of PTEN. Subsequently, PTEN loss increases the production of CCL2, which recruits myeloid cells to the metastatic sites. Finally, these myeloid cells promote the outgrowth of metastatic colonies [60]. In another study, it was reported that brain metastatic breast cancer cells express connexin 43 and protocadherin 7 (PCDH7), which promotes the formation of gap junction with astrocytes. This interaction triggers production of several inflammatory cytokines, which in turn activate STAT1 and NF-KB pathways in breast cancer cells. Ultimately, this not only enhances metastatic growth of breast cancer cells within the brain but also increases chemoresistance of the breast cancer cells [61]. While most studies have been focused on the role for astrocytes in brain metastasis, the contributions of other types of brain-specific stromal cells in this process still remain to be investigated.

Bone Metastasis

It has been shown that bone-resident cells secrete chemokine CXCL12 and this molecule functions to attract breast cancer cells expressing CXCR4, the receptor of CXCL12, promoting recruitment of breast cancer cells. Supporting this, CXCR4 is highly expressed in bone metastatic breast cancer cells in experimental models and associated with a higher risk for the bone metastasis in breast cancer patients [7].

Once breast cancer cells extravasate into the bone marrow, they also encounter several apoptotic signals including TRAIL (tumor necrosis factor (TNF)-related apoptosis inducing ligand). To escape the TRAIL-induced apoptosis, bone metastatic cancer cells activate SRC signaling, which turns on the survival pathways to promote their survival [8, 62].

Bone microenvironment is composed of several types of cells including osteoblasts and osteoclasts [63]. Under normal physiological conditions, osteoblasts and osteoclasts mediate a remodeling process, during which bone matrix is dissolved by osteoclast-derived acids and collagenases, while osteoblasts deposit organic matrix as well as minerals, completing a remodeling cycle [64].

Osteoclasts and osteoblasts also play critical roles in bone metastasis of breast cancer. These cells are known to secrete several factors that can promote the formation of bone metastases, and this is modulated by communication with bone metastatic breast cancer cells.

Studies support that bone metastatic breast cancer cells secrete several factors including PTHrP, IL11, IL6, and TNFa, which promote the release of RANKL from the osteoblasts that in turn binds to its receptor RANK [1, 65]. Activation of RANK pathway in osteoclasts stimulates bone resorption, which leads to the secretion of several growth factors such as TGFb and IGFs that promotes the growth of bone metastases. These factors stimulate cancer growth and further release of osteolytic factors, creating a vicious cycle [66].

Some of the newly identified players in breast cancer metastasis to the bones include JAG1, VCAM-1 [67, 68], as well as a set of miRNAs including miR-16, 141, 219, and 378 [69]. JAG1, a ligand of NOTCH1, has been shown to be overexpressed breast cancer cells with high bone metastatic activity and clinically associated with increased risk for bone metastasis. Mechanistically, JAG1 presented by breast cancer cells activates NOTCH pathway in osteoblast, which induces production of IL6 from osteoblast and subsequent differentiation of osteoclast. This series of events ultimately promotes bone metastasis [67]. As described above, VCAM-1 has been shown to play a role in lung metastasis of breast cancer. In addition, this molecule also promotes bone metastasis by recruiting osteoblast progenitors and thus activating osteoclast, indicating multifaceted roles of VCAM-1 in breast cancer [68].

Cancer-derived soluble ICAM1 has been shown to cause global miRNA expression changes, some of which promote osteoblast differentiation. Among these miRNAs, miR-141 and 219 were demonstrated to promote bone metastasis in experimental metastasis [7].

9.3 Current Evidence and Concept

9.3.1 Pre-metastatic Niche

Pre-metastatic niche refers to a tissue environment of the destination organ that has undergone changes to provide a supportive environment for the metastatic growth even prior to the cancer cell arrival [70–72]. The primitive concept of pre-metastatic niche was first formulated by Paget who suggested "Seed and soil" hypothesis in which tumor cells and the destination organs were referred to as "seeds' and "soil," respectively [33, 73]. This theory has been further expanded and supported by recent experimental evidence, which we will summarize below.

9.3.1.1 Process of Pre-metastatic Niche Formation

The formation of pre-metastatic niche is initiated by tumor-derived secreted factors as well as extracellular vesicles (e.g., exosomes and microvesicles). Hypoxia and inflammation within the primary breast cancer have been suggested as major causes for production of these factors [74, 75]. These factors then cause vascular leakiness and alter properties of ECM and the resident cells (e.g., fibroblasts) in the secondary organs. In addition, tumor-derived factors mobilize bone marrow-derived cells (BMDCs) to the destination organ [70, 71]. Pre-metastatic niche formed by the aforementioned events contributes to attraction and extravasation of CTCs to the destination organs and provides hospitable environment for the growth of incoming cancer cells.

9.3.1.2 Major Players in Formation of the Pre-metastatic Niche

As described above, tumor-derived factors, recruited BMDCs as well as immune cells, and changes in properties of local stromal cells play important roles in the formation of pre-metastatic niches [70, 71]. Recent studies have identified tumor-derived factors that contribute to the recruitment of BMDC to the secondary organs [72, 76, 77]. First, Osteopontin (OPN) has been shown to promote recruitment of several types of BMDCs [78], while P2Y2R contributes to recruitment of $CD11b^+$ BMDCs to the pre-metastatic lung [79]. Secretion of lysyl oxidase (LOX) by breast cancer cells also promotes accumulation of $CD11b^+$ cells [80]. In addition, tumor-derived factors induce stromal changes in the secondary organ to produce soluble factors, which in turn promotes infiltration of BMDCs and CTCs to the destination organ. For example, lung epithelial cells have been shown to produce chemokines upon the activation by tumor-derived RNAs and this leads to recruitment of BMDCs and breast cancer cell adhesion to the lung [81].

Mobilized BMDCs and immune cells are the second major players of pre-metastatic niche formation. Several types of BDMCs and immune cells contribute to the alteration of stromal components to prepare for the arrival of CTCs. These cells include VEGFR1-expressing hematopoietic progenitor cells, $CD11b^{+}$-myeloid cells, $CD11b^{+}Ly6C^{+}$ monocytes, and $CD11b^{+}Ly6C^{+}Ly6G^{+}$granulocytes [50, 82, 83]. In addition, several regulatory and immune suppressive cells such as macrophages, Treg, and neutrophils have been suggested to contribute to CTC extravasation and/or growth of incoming CTCs [84–86].

The final players in the formation of pre-metastatic niches are resident stromal cells in the destination organ. One of the most studied stromal cells are fibroblasts, which have been shown to be educated by tumor-derived factors and subsequently produce several inflammatory cytokines, chemokines, and ECM remodeling enzymes to shape a pre-metastatic niche [87]. Some studies have also shown that endothelial cells and osteoclasts are also involved in the formation of pre-metastatic niche [69, 85, 87].

9.3.1.3 Hallmarks of Pre-metastatic Niche

As the ultimate goal of pre-metastatic niches is to prepare the “soil” for the incoming “seeds”, pre-metastatic niche exhibits common characteristic regardless of the destination organs. First, pre-metastatic niche creates an immune-suppressive environment so that incoming CTCs can escape attack by immune cells [70, 71, 88]. Second, pre-metastatic niches provide inflammatory environment, which can foster the growth of disseminated cancer cells [70, 71, 88]. Third, increased angio and/or lymphangiogenesis is another characteristic of pre-metastatic niches, and these changes have been linked to the increased extravasation of CTCs as well as BMDCs [70, 71, 88]. For example, it has been shown that accumulation of $CD11b^{+}$ BMDCs has been indicated in inhibition of NK cells’ cytotoxic function in pre-metastatic lung [89].

9.3.2 Metastatic Cancer Stem Cells

Cancer stem cells have received tremendous attention because they exhibit drug resistance [90–92]. In primary breast cancer, the CD44 high/CD24 low cells have been first shown to possess stem cell properties: (1) self-renewal abilities, (2) expression of specific cell surface markers, and (3) high tumorigenic abilities [93]. In addition to CD44 and CD24, ALDH has also been identified as breast CSC markers, indicating heterogeneity of breast CSC population [94].

Similar to CSC, metastatic cancer stem cell (MCSC) was originally defined as a subpopulation of CSCs with metastatic ability. However, more broad definition has been used, that is, “cancer cells with an ability to reinitiate metastatic colonies in a secondary organ”. This is often referred to as “metastatic stem cells (MetSCs)”

[95, 96]. Compared to the CSCs in primary breast cancer, the information on MCSC is very limited. Thus, in this section, we will use more broad definition of MetSC.

There are several studies that support the role of MetSC in the initiation of metastasis. First, it has been shown that CD44 high/CD24 low cells are enriched in the population of disseminated cancer cells (DTCs) [35]. In addition, $CD44^+$ cells isolated from breast tumors were shown to be highly metastatic [97, 98]. Additional molecules suggested as MetSC markers include TAZ1 and ANTXR1 [92, 99]. Recently, analysis of single cells from breast cancer PDX model reported that early stage metastatic cells exhibit stem cell-like signature including increased expression of LGR5, NOTCH4, BMI1, and JAG1 and downregulation of CD24, MUC1, and EMP1 [14].

Currently, two models regarding the origin of MetSCs exist. The first one is CSCs in primary breast tumors pre-possess metastatic abilities. The second model involves acquiring metastasis-initiating abilities by several mechanisms. Experimental data supporting this model include the observation of transition from non-stem to stem cell population in breast cancer and TGF and WNT pathways have been shown to contribue to this process (For example, [95, 96, 100, 101]). However, the mechanisms by which MetSCs contribute to the initiation of metastasis still warrant further investigation.

9.3.3 Noncoding RNAs

Noncoding RNAs such as microRNAs and long noncoding RNAs (LncRNAs) have been shown to contribute to numerous cellular processes, and deregulation of noncoding RNAs is associated with several diseases such as cancers. In breast cancer, microRNAs and lncRNAs contribute to the general and/or organ-specific metastasis. Especially, the role of lncRNAs in breast cancer metastasis has been one of the recent focuses in the field.

LncRNAs function to regulate gene expression both in *cis* and *trans* via various mechanisms. The first class of lncRNAs transcriptionally controls their target genes by recruiting epigenetic modifiers. For example, HOTAIR, one of the lncRNAs transcribed from HOXC locus, has been shown to recruit polycomb repressive complex 2 (PRC2) to their target genes and change their expression. As a consequence, breast cancer cells acquire invasive ability, one of the first steps in the metastatic process. The metastasis-promoting role of HOTAIR was supported by the increased metastatic ability of HOTAIR-overexpressing breast cancer cells to the lung [102].

Action of the second class of lncRNAs also involves chromatin modification. However, instead of recruiting histone modifiers, they modulate the activities of histone modifiers and lncRNA BCAR4 is one of the well-studied examples. BCAR4 has been shown to bind to SNIP1, which originally functions as the inhibitor of histone acetyltransferase p300. Binding of BCAR to SNIP1 suppresses the inhibitory effects of SNIP1 on p300, thus leading to the histone acetylation. At the same time, BCAR also interacts with PNUT1, which eventually results in the dephosphorylation of RNA polymerase II at ser5. These two events lead to the transcriptional activation of GLI 2 target genes, which then promotes cancer cell migration. Interestingly, this study also demonstrated that interaction between BACR and its binding partners is induced by chemokine CCL21 [103].

In addition to modulating the transcription, some lncRNAs have been shown to regulate metastasis via affecting translation of target genes. One of the first lncRNAs identified to be involved in translational control and contribute to metastasis is treRNA (translational regulatory lncRNAs). TreRNA is implicated in suppression of E-cadherin translation, an epithelial marker, thus promoting EMT process. Consistent with this, TreRNA-overexpressing breast cancer cells possess increased migratory/invasive and metastatic abilities to the lung in vivo. Furthermore, clinical sample analysis revealed that TreRNA is overexpressed in lymph-node metastases compared to the matched primary breast cancer.

The final class of lncRNAs regulates expression of target genes by modulating protein-protein interaction. A recent study has elegantly demonstrated that NKILA (NF-kB interacting long noncoding RNA) interacts with NF-KB/IkB complex and interferes with IkB phosphorylation, which leads to the suppression of NF-kB pathway. As activation of NF-kB pathway plays an important role in breast cancer metastasis, inhibition of the pathway by NKILA results in the decreased breast cancer metastasis. Supporting the metastasis-suppressive role NKILA in breast cancer, decreased NKILA is correlated with poor outcome in breast cancer patients.

Adding more complex NKILA is regulated by microRNA 103/107. Thus, reduced expression of NKILA in aggressive breast cancer is attributed to the overexpression of miRNA 103/107 [104]. This strongly supports the interplay between microRNAs and lncRNAs in the process of breast cancer metastasis. Another example includes MAYA, which functions as a scaffold between MST1 and NSUN6. The formation of ternary complex leads to the methylation of MST1 and subsequent inactivation of the protein. This then activates the YAP target genes including CTGF and CYT61, which are known to contribute to the breast cancer metastasis to the lung [105].

While most of the studies on lncRNA and breast cancer metastasis have focused on the properties of cancer cell themselves such as their migratory ability and proliferation, recent studies have started to uncover the role of lncRNAs in the interaction between cancer cells and microenvironment of the secondary organ. A very recent study by Wang et al has identified lncRNA called LNC-BM, which is associated with brain metastasis of breast cancer. The authors have revealed that LNC-BM plays a role in vascular co-option and macrophage recruitment in brain. LNC-BM executes this by associating with JAK2, which then activates STAT3 pathway. Subsequently, transcription of CCL2 and ICAM1, STAT3 target genes, induces the infiltration of macrophages and vascular co-option, respectively [106].

Taken together, the studies on lncRNAs have provided a broader spectrum of players in the breast cancer metastasis.

9.3.4 *Immune Cells in Breast Cancer Metastasis*

9.3.4.1 Role of Immune-Suppressive Cells in Breast Cancer Metastasis

In the above section, we have described a few examples of contributions that immune cells make to promote breast cancer metastasis. In this section, we will review the role of specific types of cells in creation of immune-suppressive environment.

As discussed above, one of the prerequisites for the successful formation of metastasis is evading immune attack. Several types of immune-suppressive cells including myeloid, T_{Reg}, and other adaptive immune cells contribute to this process. Myeloid cells includng macrophages and neutrophils are a type of cells with very well-established immune suppressive function. Specifically, macrophages interfere with $CD8^{+}T$ cell functions by producing inhibitor ligands or by recruiting T_{Reg} cells [107]. Tumor-associated NK cells are also suggested to function in a similar way, while the molecular mechanisms warrant further investigation [108]. In addition to these fully differentiated myeloid cells, immature population of myeloid cells also plays a role in inhibition of T cell cytotoxicity [109].

T_{Reg} cells like in other types of cancers have shown to play an important role in immune suppression and thus promote metastasis of breast cancer. Metastasis-promoting roles of T_{Reg} cell have been supported by many studies. For example, positive correlation between number of T_{Reg} and lung metastatic burden was observed. In addition, increased T_{Reg} causes T cell death and is associated with increased bone metastasis [110, 111]. One of the molecules identified to play a role in increased number of T_{Reg} in breast cancer is galectin 1, which promotes expansion of T_{Reg} cells [112].

In addition to myeloid and T_{Reg} cells, TH_{17} and B_{Reg} cells have also been shown to be involved in breast cancer metastasis by promoting MDSC recruitment and conversion of T_{Reg} cells, respectively [113, 114]. Depletion or coinjection of these cells with breast cancer cells has been shown to reduce and promote lung metastasis in breast cancer, respectively [113, 114].

9.3.4.2 Immunotherapy in Breast Cancer

Immunotherapy is being intensively studied and successful in treatment of metastatic cancers such as metastatic melanoma, non-small cell lung carcinoma (NSCLC), and renal cell carcinoma [115–117]. Nivolumab and pembrolizumab are two FDA approved antiPD1 antibodies used in treatment of the aforementioned cancers [115–117]. The use of immunotherapy in treating breast cancer has not been actively pursued until recently because breast cancer is generally not considered as immunogenic. However, several recent studies indicated that PD-1 inhibitors may benefit patients with aggressive breast cancer and several PD-1 inhibitors are currently under clinical trial phases I and II [118].

9.3.5 Glycosylation

Glycosylation is one of the most ubiquitous protein modifications in the cells. However, the role of protein glycosylation in breast cancer metastasis has been very limited.

A recent study has shown that GALNT14 (polypeptide N-acetylgalactosaminyltransferase 14), a member of O-linked glycosylation-initiating enzymes, contributes to the lung metastasis by modulating communication between breast cancer cells and lung microenvironment [119]. This study demonstrated that GALNT14 promotes lung metastasis at the later stage of lung metastasis, which includes (1) overcoming inhibitory effects of BMPs, an anti-metastatic signal from the lung, (2) recruitment of macrophages by inducing production of cancer cell-derived chemokines, and (3) exploiting macrophage-secreted growth factors (e.g., FGFs) by breast cancer cells. During these processes, BMP receptor1A (BMPR1A) and FGF receptor 1 (FGFR1) are the O-glycosylated by GALNT14, which inhibits and promotes the activation of BMP and FGF pathway, respectively [119]. (Fig. 9.1).

Another recent study has shown that targeting glycosylation of PD-L1 could be used to eliminate TNBCs. This study has demonstrated that EGFR pathway promotes N-linked glycosylation by inducing expression of β-1,3-N-acetylglucosaminyltransferase (B3GNT3). Subsequently, this stimulates interaction between interaction between PD-L1 and PD1, which leads to immune suppression. Interestingly, administration of antibody against glycosylated PD-L1 not only inhibits immune suppression by promoting PD-L1 internalization but also leads to cancer cell death lacking PD-L1 receptor as a bystander effect [120]. This indicates that targeting glycosylated-protein may be used as a potential therapeutic strategy for breast cancer treatment.

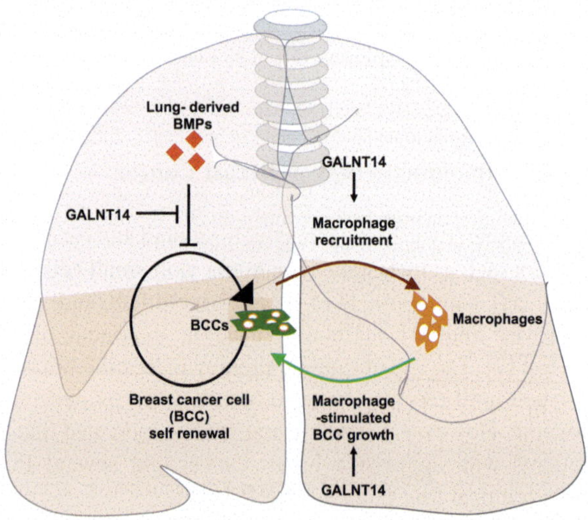

Fig. 9.1 Proposed model of GALNT14-mediated lung metastasis in breast cancer (modified from 119)

9.4 Future Research Direction

Accurate prediction and effective treatment of metastasis are the two ultimate goals of the metastasis research. The issue with currently reported prognostic markers is that their use is often very limited to the specific cohort of patients used in the study. Thus, systematic approach to identify prognostic markers is warranted.

In addition to analysis of primary breast cancer aimed for discovery of prognostic markers, early detection of CTCs will benefit breast cancer patients. While significant advances have been made in the detection of CTCs, plasticity and heterogeneity of CTCs make CTC detection very complicated. In order to improve the sensitivity and the specificity in CTC detection, further investigation of biological properties of CTCs should be proceeded.

Despite the decade of active metastasis research, we have no effective treatment for the metastatic breast cancer. This is mainly attributed to the fact that metastatic breast cancer cells possess different biological characteristics compared to the major population of the cancer cells comprising the primary cancer. Thus, drugs that are based on the properties of primary cancer cells are destined to fail. In addition, cancer cells are very heterogeneous and develop drug resistance. One solution for this issue could be targeting the stromal cells with pro-metastatic functions. As accumulating evidence supports that the close communication between stromal cells and breast cancer cells is required for the successful metastasis, drugs that can intervene this communication have potential to be used in treatment of breast cancer metastasis. Major advantages of targeting stromal cells are these cells (1) are more homogenous than cancer cells and (2) have lower mutation rate. Experimental results in a limited number of preclinical studies support the possibility of controlling metastasis by targeting stromal-cancer interaction [121]. However, our understanding of the molecular mechanisms governing the crosstalk between stromal cells and breast cancer cells is still very limited. Therefore, further investigations to identify mediators of cancer-stromal interaction are warranted.

9.5 Summary

- Breast cancer metastasis is very complicated process, and metastatic breast cancer cell-stroma interaction is required in each step of the metastatic process.
- Intervention of metastatic breast cancer cell-stromal interaction could provide new therapeutic drugs for effective treatment of patients with metastatic breast cancer.
- Identification and systematic use of prognostic markers as well as early detection will provide opportunity for the personalized therapy.
- Drugs based on cancer cell-stromal interaction may lead to significant advance in treatment of breast cancer metastasis.

References

1. Hofbauer LC, Rachner T, Singh SK. Fatal attraction: why breast cancer cells home to bone. Breast Cancer Res. 2008;10(1):101.
2. Eichler AF, Chung E, Kodack DP, Loeffler JS, Fukumura D, Jain RK. The biology of brain metastases-translation to new therapies. Nat Rev Clin Oncol. 2011;8(6):344–56.
3. Disibio G, French SW. Metastatic patterns of cancers: results from a large autopsy study. Arch Pathol Lab Med. 2008;132(6):931–9.
4. Bos PD, Zhang XH, Nadal C, Shu W, Gomis RR, Nguyen DX, et al. Genes that mediate breast cancer metastasis to the brain. Nature. 2009;459(7249):1005–9.
5. Minn AJ, Gupta GP, Siegel PM, Bos PD, Shu W, Giri DD, et al. Genes that mediate breast cancer metastasis to lung. Nature. 2005;436(7050):518–24.
6. Kang Y, He W, Tulley S, Gupta GP, Serganova I, Chen CR, et al. Breast cancer bone metastasis mediated by the Smad tumor suppressor pathway. Proc Natl Acad Sci U S A. 2005;102(39):13909–14.
7. Kang Y, Siegel PM, Shu W, Drobnjak M, Kakonen SM, Cordon-Cardo C, et al. A multigenic program mediating breast cancer metastasis to bone. Cancer Cell. 2003;3(6):537–49.
8. Zhang XH, Wang Q, Gerald W, Hudis CA, Norton L, Smid M, et al. Latent bone metastasis in breast cancer tied to Src-dependent survival signals. Cancer Cell. 2009;16(1):67–78.
9. Gupta GP, Nguyen DX, Chiang AC, Bos PD, Kim JY, Nadal C, et al. Mediators of vascular remodelling co-opted for sequential steps in lung metastasis. Nature. 2007;446(7137):765–70.
10. Bos PD, Nguyen DX, Massague J. Modeling metastasis in the mouse. Curr Opin Pharmacol. 2010;10(5):571–7.
11. Lee JW, Komar CA, Bengsch F, Graham K, Beatty GL. Genetically engineered mouse models of pancreatic cancer: the KPC model (LSL-Kras(G12D/+); LSL-Trp53(R172H/+); Pdx-1-Cre), its variants, and their application in immuno-oncology drug discovery. Curr Protoc Pharmacol. 2016;73:14.39.1–14.39.20.
12. Landis MD, Lehmann BD, Pietenpol JA, Chang JC. Patient-derived breast tumor xenografts facilitating personalized cancer therapy. Breast Cancer Res. 2013;15(1):201.
13. Marangoni E, Vincent-Salomon A, Auger N, Degeorges A, Assayag F, de Cremoux P, et al. A new model of patient tumor-derived breast cancer xenografts for preclinical assays. Clin Cancer Res. 2007;13(13):3989–98.
14. Lawson DA, Bhakta NR, Kessenbrock K, Prummel KD, Yu Y, Takai K, et al. Single-cell analysis reveals a stem-cell program in human metastatic breast cancer cells. Nature. 2015;526 (7571):131–5.
15. Sinn E, Muller W, Pattengale P, Tepler I, Wallace R, Leder P. Coexpression of MMTV/v-Ha-ras and MMTV/c-myc genes in transgenic mice: synergistic action of oncogenes in vivo. Cell. 1987;49(4):465–75.
16. Henneman L, van Miltenburg MH, Michalak EM, Braumuller TM, Jaspers JE, Drenth AP, et al. Selective resistance to the PARP inhibitor olaparib in a mouse model for BRCA1-deficient metaplastic breast cancer. Proc Natl Acad Sci U S A. 2015;112(27):8409–14.
17. Dickins RA, McJunkin K, Hernando E, Premsrirut PK, Krizhanovsky V, Burgess DJ, et al. Tissue-specific and reversible RNA interference in transgenic mice. Nat Genet. 2007;39 (7):914–21.
18. Premsrirut PK, Dow LE, Kim SY, Camiolo M, Malone CD, Miething C, et al. A rapid and scalable system for studying gene function in mice using conditional RNA interference. Cell. 2011;145(1):145–58.
19. Sanchez-Rivera FJ, Jacks T. Applications of the CRISPR-Cas9 system in cancer biology. Nat Rev Cancer. 2015;15(7):387–95.
20. Nieto MA. Epithelial plasticity: a common theme in embryonic and cancer cells. Science. 2013;342(6159):1234850.
21. Thiery JP, Acloque H, Huang RY, Nieto MA. Epithelial-mesenchymal transitions in development and disease. Cell. 2009;139(5):871–90.

22. Kalluri R, Weinberg RA. The basics of epithelial-mesenchymal transition. J Clin Invest. 2009;119(6):1420–8.
23. Zheng H, Shen M, Zha YL, Li W, Wei Y, Blanco MA, et al. PKD1 phosphorylation-dependent degradation of SNAIL by SCF-FBXO11 regulates epithelial-mesenchymal transition and metastasis. Cancer Cell. 2014;26(3):358–73.
24. Labelle M, Begum S, Hynes RO. Direct signaling between platelets and cancer cells induces an epithelial-mesenchymal-like transition and promotes metastasis. Cancer Cell. 2011;20 (5):576–90.
25. Bill R, Christofori G. The relevance of EMT in breast cancer metastasis: correlation or causality? FEBS Lett. 2015;589(14):1577–87.
26. Gao D, Joshi N, Choi H, Ryu S, Hahn M, Catena R, et al. Myeloid progenitor cells in the premetastatic lung promote metastases by inducing mesenchymal to epithelial transition. Cancer Res. 2012;72(6):1384–94.
27. Clark AG, Vignjevic DM. Modes of cancer cell invasion and the role of the microenvironment. Curr Opin Cell Biol. 2015;36:13–22.
28. Lopez-Novoa JM, Nieto MA. Inflammation and EMT: an alliance towards organ fibrosis and cancer progression. EMBO Mol Med. 2009;1(6–7):303–14.
29. Condeelis J, Pollard JW. Macrophages: obligate partners for tumor cell migration, invasion, and metastasis. Cell. 2006;124(2):263–6.
30. Yang L, Huang J, Ren X, Gorska AE, Chytil A, Aakre M, et al. Abrogation of TGF beta signaling in mammary carcinomas recruits Gr-1+CD11b+ myeloid cells that promote metastasis. Cancer Cell. 2008;13(1):23–35.
31. Na YR, Yoon YN, Son DI, Seok SH. Cyclooxygenase-2 inhibition blocks M2 macrophage differentiation and suppresses metastasis in murine breast cancer model. PLoS One. 2013;8(5): e63451.
32. Su S, Liu Q, Chen J, Chen J, Chen F, He C, et al. A positive feedback loop between mesenchymal-like cancer cells and macrophages is essential to breast cancer metastasis. Cancer Cell. 2014;25(5):605–20.
33. Fidler IJ. The pathogenesis of cancer metastasis: the 'seed and soil' hypothesis revisited. Nat Rev Cancer. 2003;3(6):453–8.
34. Weng D, Penzner JH, Song B, Koido S, Calderwood SK, Gong J. Metastasis is an early event in mouse mammary carcinomas and is associated with cells bearing stem cell markers. Breast Cancer Res. 2012;14(1):R18.
35. Balic M, Lin H, Young L, Hawes D, Giuliano A, McNamara G, et al. Most early disseminated cancer cells detected in bone marrow of breast cancer patients have a putative breast cancer stem cell phenotype. Clin Cancer Res. 2006;12(19):5615–21.
36. Karaman S, Detmar M. Mechanisms of lymphatic metastasis. J Clin Invest. 2014;124 (3):922–8.
37. de Boer M, van Dijck JA, Bult P, Borm GF, Tjan-Heijnen VC. Breast cancer prognosis and occult lymph node metastases, isolated tumor cells, and micrometastases. J Natl Cancer Inst. 2010;102(6):410–25.
38. Roussos ET, Condeelis JS, Patsialou A. Chemotaxis in cancer. Nat Rev Cancer. 2011;11 (8):573–87.
39. Keskin D, Kim J, Cooke VG, Wu CC, Sugimoto H, Gu C, et al. Targeting vascular pericytes in hypoxic tumors increases lung metastasis via angiopoietin-2. Cell Rep. 2015;10(7):1066–81.
40. Douma S, Van Laar T, Zevenhoven J, Meuwissen R, Van Garderen E, Peeper DS. Suppression of anoikis and induction of metastasis by the neurotrophic receptor TrkB. Nature. 2004;430 (7003):1034–9.
41. Kopp HG, Placke T, Salih HR. Platelet-derived transforming growth factor-beta down-regulates NKG2D thereby inhibiting natural killer cell antitumor reactivity. Cancer Res. 2009;69 (19):7775–83.
42. Gay LJ, Felding-Habermann B. Contribution of platelets to tumour metastasis. Nat Rev Cancer. 2011;11(2):123–34.

43. Ilie M, Hofman V, Long E, Bordone O, Selva E, Washetine K, et al. Current challenges for detection of circulating tumor cells and cell-free circulating nucleic acids, and their characterization in non-small cell lung carcinoma patients. What is the best blood substrate for personalized medicine? Ann Transl Med. 2014;2(11):107.
44. Racila E, Euhus D, Weiss AJ, Rao C, McConnell J, Terstappen LW, et al. Detection and characterization of carcinoma cells in the blood. Proc Natl Acad Sci U S A. 1998;95 (8):4589–94.
45. Takao M, Takeda K. Enumeration, characterization, and collection of intact circulating tumor cells by cross contamination-free flow cytometry. Cytometry A. 2011;79(2):107–17.
46. Allard WJ, Matera J, Miller MC, Repollet M, Connelly MC, Rao C, et al. Tumor cells circulate in the peripheral blood of all major carcinomas but not in healthy subjects or patients with nonmalignant diseases. Clin Cancer Res. 2004;10(20):6897–904.
47. Padua D, Zhang XH, Wang Q, Nadal C, Gerald WL, Gomis RR, et al. TGFbeta primes breast tumors for lung metastasis seeding through angiopoietin-like 4. Cell. 2008;133(1):66–77.
48. Sevenich L, Bowman RL, Mason SD, Quail DF, Rapaport F, Elie BT, et al. Analysis of tumour- and stroma-supplied proteolytic networks reveals a brain-metastasis-promoting role for cathepsin S. Nat Cell Biol. 2014;16(9):876–88.
49. Qian B, Deng Y, Im JH, Muschel RJ, Zou Y, Li J, et al. A distinct macrophage population mediates metastatic breast cancer cell extravasation, establishment and growth. PLoS One. 2009;4(8):e6562.
50. Qian BZ, Li J, Zhang H, Kitamura T, Zhang J, Campion LR, et al. CCL2 recruits inflammatory monocytes to facilitate breast-tumour metastasis. Nature. 2011;475(7355):222–5.
51. Gupta GP, Perk J, Acharyya S, de Candia P, Mittal V, Todorova-Manova K, et al. ID genes mediate tumor reinitiation during breast cancer lung metastasis. Proc Natl Acad Sci U S A. 2007;104(49):19506–11.
52. Chen Q, Zhang XH, Massague J. Macrophage binding to receptor VCAM-1 transmits survival signals in breast cancer cells that invade the lungs. Cancer Cell. 2011;20(4):538–49.
53. Korpal M, Ell BJ, Buffa FM, Ibrahim T, Blanco MA, Celia-Terrassa T, et al. Direct targeting of Sec23a by miR-200s influences cancer cell secretome and promotes metastatic colonization. Nat Med. 2011;17(9):1101–8.
54. Malanchi I, Santamaria-Martinez A, Susanto E, Peng H, Lehr HA, Delaloye JF, et al. Interactions between cancer stem cells and their niche govern metastatic colonization. Nature. 2011;481(7379):85–9.
55. Oskarsson T, Acharyya S, Zhang XH, Vanharanta S, Tavazoie SF, Morris PG, et al. Breast cancer cells produce tenascin C as a metastatic niche component to colonize the lungs. Nat Med. 2011;17(7):867–74.
56. Acharyya S, Oskarsson T, Vanharanta S, Malladi S, Kim J, Morris PG, et al. A CXCL1 paracrine network links cancer chemoresistance and metastasis. Cell. 2012;150(1):165–78.
57. Gao H, Chakraborty G, Lee-Lim AP, Mo Q, Decker M, Vonica A, et al. The BMP inhibitor Coco reactivates breast cancer cells at lung metastatic sites. Cell. 2012;150(4):764–79.
58. Valiente M, Obenauf AC, Jin X, Chen Q, Zhang XH, Lee DJ, et al. Serpins promote cancer cell survival and vascular co-option in brain metastasis. Cell. 2014;156(5):1002–16.
59. Xing F, Kobayashi A, Okuda H, Watabe M, Pai SK, Pandey PR, et al. Reactive astrocytes promote the metastatic growth of breast cancer stem-like cells by activating Notch signalling in brain. EMBO Mol Med. 2013;5(3):384–96.
60. Zhang L, Zhang S, Yao J, Lowery FJ, Zhang Q, Huang WC, et al. Microenvironment-induced PTEN loss by exosomal microRNA primes brain metastasis outgrowth. Nature. 2015;527 (7576):100–4.
61. Chen Q, Boire A, Jin X, Valiente M, Er EE, Lopez-Soto A, et al. Carcinoma-astrocyte gap junctions promote brain metastasis by cGAMP transfer. Nature. 2016;533(7604):493–8.
62. Xu J, Xu Z, Zhou JY, Zhuang Z, Wang E, Boerner J, et al. Regulation of the Src-PP2A interaction in tumor necrosis factor (TNF)-related apoptosis-inducing ligand (TRAIL)-induced apoptosis. J Biol Chem. 2013;288(46):33263–71.

63. Guise TA, Mohammad KS, Clines G, Stebbins EG, Wong DH, Higgins LS, et al. Basic mechanisms responsible for osteolytic and osteoblastic bone metastases. Clin Cancer Res. 2006;12(20 Pt 2):6213s–6s.
64. Raggatt LJ, Partridge NC. Cellular and molecular mechanisms of bone remodeling. J Biol Chem. 2010;285(33):25103–8.
65. Jones DH, Nakashima T, Sanchez OH, Kozieradzki I, Komarova SV, Sarosi I, et al. Regulation of cancer cell migration and bone metastasis by RANKL. Nature. 2006;440(7084):692–6.
66. Obenauf AC, Massague J. Surviving at a distance: organ-specific metastasis. Trends Cancer. 2015;1(1):76–91.
67. Sethi N, Dai X, Winter CG, Kang Y. Tumor-derived JAGGED1 promotes osteolytic bone metastasis of breast cancer by engaging notch signaling in bone cells. Cancer Cell. 2011;19(2):192–205.
68. Lu X, Mu E, Wei Y, Riethdorf S, Yang Q, Yuan M, et al. VCAM-1 promotes osteolytic expansion of indolent bone micrometastasis of breast cancer by engaging alpha4beta1-positive osteoclast progenitors. Cancer Cell. 2011;20(6):701–14.
69. Ell B, Mercatali L, Ibrahim T, Campbell N, Schwarzenbach H, Pantel K, et al. Tumor-induced osteoclast miRNA changes as regulators and biomarkers of osteolytic bone metastasis. Cancer Cell. 2013;24(4):542–56.
70. Liu Y, Cao X. Characteristics and significance of the pre-metastatic niche. Cancer Cell. 2016;30(5):668–81.
71. Peinado H, Zhang H, Matei IR, Costa-Silva B, Hoshino A, Rodrigues G, et al. Pre-metastatic niches: organ-specific homes for metastases. Nat Rev Cancer. 2017;17(5):302–17.
72. Kaplan RN, Riba RD, Zacharoulis S, Bramley AH, Vincent L, Costa C, et al. VEGFR1-positive haematopoietic bone marrow progenitors initiate the pre-metastatic niche. Nature. 2005;438(7069):820–7.
73. Paget S. The distribution of secondary growths in cancer of the breast. 1889. Cancer Metastasis Rev. 1989;8(2):98–101.
74. Deng J, Liu Y, Lee H, Herrmann A, Zhang W, Zhang C, et al. S1PR1-STAT3 signaling is crucial for myeloid cell colonization at future metastatic sites. Cancer Cell. 2012;21(5):642–54.
75. Chafe SC, Lou Y, Sceneay J, Vallejo M, Hamilton MJ, McDonald PC, et al. Carbonic anhydrase IX promotes myeloid-derived suppressor cell mobilization and establishment of a metastatic niche by stimulating G-CSF production. Cancer Res. 2015;75(6):996–1008.
76. Peinado H, Lavotshkin S, Lyden D. The secreted factors responsible for pre-metastatic niche formation: old sayings and new thoughts. Semin Cancer Biol. 2011;21(2):139–46.
77. Hiratsuka S, Watanabe A, Sakurai Y, Akashi-Takamura S, Ishibashi S, Miyake K, et al. The S100A8-serum amyloid A3-TLR4 paracrine cascade establishes a pre-metastatic phase. Nat Cell Biol. 2008;10(11):1349–55.
78. Fremder E, Munster M, Aharon A, Miller V, Gingis-Velitski S, Voloshin T, et al. Tumor-derived microparticles induce bone marrow-derived cell mobilization and tumor homing: a process regulated by osteopontin. Int J Cancer. 2014;135(2):270–81.
79. Joo YN, Jin H, Eun SY, Park SW, Chang KC, Kim HJ. P2Y2R activation by nucleotides released from the highly metastatic breast cancer cell MDA-MB-231 contributes to pre-metastatic niche formation by mediating lysyl oxidase secretion, collagen crosslinking, and monocyte recruitment. Oncotarget. 2014;5(19):9322–34.
80. Erler JT, Bennewith KL, Cox TR, Lang G, Bird D, Koong A, et al. Hypoxia-induced lysyl oxidase is a critical mediator of bone marrow cell recruitment to form the premetastatic niche. Cancer Cell. 2009;15(1):35–44.
81. Liu Y, Gu Y, Han Y, Zhang Q, Jiang Z, Zhang X, et al. Tumor exosomal RNAs promote lung pre-metastatic niche formation by activating alveolar epithelial TLR3 to recruit neutrophils. Cancer Cell. 2016;30(2):243–56.

82. Gil-Bernabe AM, Ferjancic S, Tlalka M, Zhao L, Allen PD, Im JH, et al. Recruitment of monocytes/macrophages by tissue factor-mediated coagulation is essential for metastatic cell survival and premetastatic niche establishment in mice. Blood. 2012;119(13):3164–75.
83. Kowanetz M, Wu X, Lee J, Tan M, Hagenbeek T, Qu X, et al. Granulocyte-colony stimulating factor promotes lung metastasis through mobilization of Ly6G+Ly6C+ granulocytes. Proc Natl Acad Sci U S A. 2010;107(50):21248–55.
84. Wu CF, Andzinski L, Kasnitz N, Kroger A, Klawonn F, Lienenklaus S, et al. The lack of type I interferon induces neutrophil-mediated pre-metastatic niche formation in the mouse lung. Int J Cancer. 2015;137(4):837–47.
85. Zhao E, Wang L, Dai J, Kryczek I, Wei S, Vatan L, et al. Regulatory T cells in the bone marrow microenvironment in patients with prostate cancer. Onco Targets Ther. 2012;1 (2):152–61.
86. Giles AJ, Reid CM, Evans JD, Murgai M, Vicioso Y, Highfill SL, et al. Activation of hematopoietic stem/progenitor cells promotes immunosuppression within the pre-metastatic niche. Cancer Res. 2016;76(6):1335–47.
87. Yamamura Y, Asai N, Enomoto A, Kato T, Mii S, Kondo Y, et al. Akt-Girdin signaling in cancer-associated fibroblasts contributes to tumor progression. Cancer Res. 2015;75 (5):813–23.
88. Chin AR, Wang SE. Cancer tills the premetastatic field: mechanistic basis and clinical implications. Clin Cancer Res. 2016;22(15):3725–33.
89. Sceneay J, Chow MT, Chen A, Halse HM, Wong CS, Andrews DM, et al. Primary tumor hypoxia recruits CD11b+/Ly6Cmed/Ly6G+ immune suppressor cells and compromises NK cell cytotoxicity in the premetastatic niche. Cancer Res. 2012;72(16):3906–11.
90. Baumann M, Krause M, Hill R. Exploring the role of cancer stem cells in radioresistance. Nat Rev Cancer. 2008;8(7):545–54.
91. Prieto-Vila M, Takahashi RU, Usuba W, Kohama I, Ochiya T. Drug resistance driven by cancer stem cells and their niche. Int J Mol Sci. 2017;18(12):2574.
92. Chen D, Bhat-Nakshatri P, Goswami C, Badve S, Nakshatri H. ANTXR1, a stem cell-enriched functional biomarker, connects collagen signaling to cancer stem-like cells and metastasis in breast cancer. Cancer Res. 2013;73(18):5821–33.
93. Al-Hajj M, Wicha MS, Benito-Hernandez A, Morrison SJ, Clarke MF. Prospective identification of tumorigenic breast cancer cells. Proc Natl Acad Sci U S A. 2003;100(7):3983–8.
94. Ginestier C, Hur MH, Charafe-Jauffret E, Monville F, Dutcher J, Brown M, et al. ALDH1 is a marker of normal and malignant human mammary stem cells and a predictor of poor clinical outcome. Cell Stem Cell. 2007;1(5):555–67.
95. Oskarsson T, Batlle E, Massague J. Metastatic stem cells: sources, niches, and vital pathways. Cell Stem Cell. 2014;14(3):306–21.
96. Liao WT, Ye YP, Deng YJ, Bian XW, Ding YQ. Metastatic cancer stem cells: from the concept to therapeutics. Am J Stem Cells. 2014;3(2):46–62.
97. Liu H, Patel MR, Prescher JA, Patsialou A, Qian D, Lin J, et al. Cancer stem cells from human breast tumors are involved in spontaneous metastases in orthotopic mouse models. Proc Natl Acad Sci U S A. 2010;107(42):18115–20.
98. Baccelli I, Schneeweiss A, Riethdorf S, Stenzinger A, Schillert A, Vogel V, et al. Identification of a population of blood circulating tumor cells from breast cancer patients that initiates metastasis in a xenograft assay. Nat Biotechnol. 2013;31(6):539–44.
99. Bartucci M, Dattilo R, Moriconi C, Pagliuca A, Mottolese M, Federici G, et al. TAZ is required for metastatic activity and chemoresistance of breast cancer stem cells. Oncogene. 2015;34(6):681–90.
100. Scheel C, Eaton EN, Li SH, Chaffer CL, Reinhardt F, Kah KJ, et al. Paracrine and autocrine signals induce and maintain mesenchymal and stem cell states in the breast. Cell. 2011;145 (6):926–40.

101. Oft M, Peli J, Rudaz C, Schwarz H, Beug H, Reichmann E. TGF-beta1 and Ha-Ras collaborate in modulating the phenotypic plasticity and invasiveness of epithelial tumor cells. Genes Dev. 1996;10(19):2462–77.
102. Gupta RA, Shah N, Wang KC, Kim J, Horlings HM, Wong DJ, et al. Long non-coding RNA HOTAIR reprograms chromatin state to promote cancer metastasis. Nature. 2010;464 (7291):1071–6.
103. Xing Z, Lin A, Li C, Liang K, Wang S, Liu Y, et al. lncRNA directs cooperative epigenetic regulation downstream of chemokine signals. Cell. 2014;159(5):1110–25.
104. Liu B, Sun L, Liu Q, Gong C, Yao Y, Lv X, et al. A cytoplasmic NF-kappaB interacting long noncoding RNA blocks IkappaB phosphorylation and suppresses breast cancer metastasis. Cancer Cell. 2015;27(3):370–81.
105. Li C, Wang S, Xing Z, Lin A, Liang K, Song J, et al. A ROR1-HER3-lncRNA signalling axis modulates the Hippo-YAP pathway to regulate bone metastasis. Nat Cell Biol. 2017;19 (2):106–19.
106. Wang S, Liang K, Hu Q, Li P, Song J, Yang Y, et al. JAK2-binding long noncoding RNA promotes breast cancer brain metastasis. J Clin Invest. 2017;127(12):4498–515.
107. Kuang DM, Zhao Q, Peng C, Xu J, Zhang JP, Wu C, et al. Activated monocytes in peritumoral stroma of hepatocellular carcinoma foster immune privilege and disease progression through PD-L1. J Exp Med. 2009;206(6):1327–37.
108. Fridlender ZG, Sun J, Kim S, Kapoor V, Cheng G, Ling L, et al. Polarization of tumor-associated neutrophil phenotype by TGF-beta: "N1" versus "N2" TAN. Cancer Cell. 2009;16 (3):183–94.
109. Sawant A, Hensel JA, Chanda D, Harris BA, Siegal GP, Maheshwari A, et al. Depletion of plasmacytoid dendritic cells inhibits tumor growth and prevents bone metastasis of breast cancer cells. J Immunol. 2012;189(9):4258–65.
110. Yang P, Li QJ, Feng Y, Zhang Y, Markowitz GJ, Ning S, et al. TGF-beta-miR-34a-CCL22 signaling-induced Treg cell recruitment promotes venous metastases of HBV-positive hepatocellular carcinoma. Cancer Cell. 2012;22(3):291–303.
111. Karavitis J, Hix LM, Shi YH, Schultz RF, Khazaie K, Zhang M. Regulation of COX2 expression in mouse mammary tumor cells controls bone metastasis and PGE2-induction of regulatory T cell migration. PLoS One. 2012;7(9):e46342.
112. Dalotto-Moreno T, Croci DO, Cerliani JP, Martinez-Allo VC, Dergan-Dylon S, Mendez-Huergo SP, et al. Targeting galectin-1 overcomes breast cancer-associated immunosuppression and prevents metastatic disease. Cancer Res. 2013;73(3):1107–17.
113. Novitskiy SV, Pickup MW, Gorska AE, Owens P, Chytil A, Aakre M, et al. TGF-beta receptor II loss promotes mammary carcinoma progression by Th17 dependent mechanisms. Cancer Discov. 2011;1(5):430–41.
114. Olkhanud PB, Damdinsuren B, Bodogai M, Gress RE, Sen R, Wejksza K, et al. Tumor-evoked regulatory B cells promote breast cancer metastasis by converting resting CD4(+) T cells to T-regulatory cells. Cancer Res. 2011;71(10):3505–15.
115. Hodi FS, O'Day SJ, McDermott DF, Weber RW, Sosman JA, Haanen JB, et al. Improved survival with ipilimumab in patients with metastatic melanoma. N Engl J Med. 2010;363 (8):711–23.
116. Borghaei H, Paz-Ares L, Horn L, Spigel DR, Steins M, Ready NE, et al. Nivolumab versus Docetaxel in advanced nonsquamous non-small-cell lung cancer. N Engl J Med. 2015;373 (17):1627–39.
117. Valsecchi ME. Combined nivolumab and ipilimumab or monotherapy in untreated melanoma. N Engl J Med. 2015;373(13):1270.
118. Katz H, Alsharedi M. Immunotherapy in triple-negative breast cancer. Med Oncol. 2017;35 (1):13.
119. Song KH, Park MS, Nandu TS, Gadad S, Kim SC, Kim MY. GALNT14 promotes lung-specific breast cancer metastasis by modulating self-renewal and interaction with the lung microenvironment. Nat Commun. 2016;7:13796.

120. Li CW, Lim SO, Chung EM, Kim YS, Park AH, Yao J, et al. Eradication of triple-negative breast cancer cells by targeting glycosylated PD-L1. Cancer Cell. 2018;33(2):187–201.e10.
121. Swierczak A, Cook AD, Lenzo JC, Restall CM, Doherty JP, Anderson RL, et al. The promotion of breast cancer metastasis caused by inhibition of CSF-1R/CSF-1 signaling is blocked by targeting the G-CSF receptor. Cancer Immunol Res. 2014;2(8):765–76.

Chapter 10
Single Cell Genomics for Tumor Heterogeneity

Hae-Ock Lee and Woong-Yang Park

Abstract Single cell genomics became a universal and powerful tool to study cellular diversity at genomic levels in normal and disease conditions. Cancer is a disease of genomic instability which instigates clonal evolution and intra-tumoral heterogeneity. Cancer progression also accompanies gross alterations in the microenvironment, and the stromal or immune cell types comprising the tumor microenvironment can be explored by single cell genomics. So far, breast cancer has been analyzed by single cell genomic tools for the clonal evolution, inter- and intra-tumoral heterogeneity in molecular signatures, and tumor microenvironment. We will briefly go over those studies and discuss the potential application of single cell genomics for the diagnostics and management of cancer.

Keywords Single cell genomics · Tumor heterogeneity · Breast cancer · Tumor evolution · Treatment resistance

10.1 Introduction

Cancer is a disease of genomic instability and heterogeneity. Tumor heterogeneity and its importance in tumor progression have been recognized for a long time and extensively studied at morphological and molecular level [1]. Artlessly, single cell genomics is the most comprehensive tool, currently available, to study the identity and function of heterogeneous subpopulations in cancer. Both DNA and RNA materials are targets of genomic analysis at single cell level. For DNA, genetic aberrations have qualitative characteristics, its diversity can be analyzed with bulk

H.-O. Lee (✉)
Department of Microbiology, College of Medicine, The Catholic University of Korea, Seoul, Republic of Korea
e-mail: haeocklee@catholic.ac.kr

W.-Y. Park
Samsung Medical Center, Samsung Genome Institute, Seoul, South Korea

D.-Y. Noh et al. (eds.), *Translational Research in Breast Cancer*, Advances in Experimental Medicine and Biology 1187,
https://doi.org/10.1007/978-981-32-9620-6_10

deep sequencing, and single cell DNA analysis can provide complementary information. On the other hand, transcriptome analysis in RNA measures quantitative characteristics. Therefore, bulk transcriptome analysis averages transcriptomes of diverse subpopulations within sample, and the heterogeneity within cannot be assessed. This quantitative nature of transcriptome data makes single cell analysis an essential and powerful tool for gene expression analysis on heterogeneous subpopulations in both normal and disease conditions.

Heterogeneity in cancer may be found between patients, which is defined as intertumoral heterogeneity and forms the basis for current practice of personalized cancer medicine. In recent years, precision medicine targeting genetic mutations, fusions, or copy number aberrations has expanded treatment choices and improved patient outcomes [2]. The cancer genome changes over time, and intratumoral heterogeneity may arise during cancer evolution. The intratumoral heterogeneity in advanced cancer and metastasis may evoke treatment resistance [3]. Through single cell DNA analysis, diverse tumor clones can be identified and clonal evolution of cancer genome is reconstructed. In addition, detection of genetic aberrations with small number of tumor cells or tumor DNAs can be used for screening and monitoring purposes. Gene expression pattern also has important prognostic or predictive values for the tumor progression and drug sensitivity. Single cell RNA sequencing can be adopted to resolve the cellular gene expression heterogeneity. Further, single cell analysis would sort out contaminating nontumor cells, allowing more accurate characterization of tumor cells, and even provide transcriptome landscape for tumor microenvironment. Breast cancer is one of the prototype cancers that single cell genomics has been applied for, to address genetic and gene expression heterogeneity in the hope of monitoring, finding better treatment targets, and overcoming the treatment resistance.

10.2 Review of Past Studies

In the past, intratumoral heterogeneity in cancer has been studied by low throughput methods such as histology, immunohistochemistry (IHC), fluorescence in situ hybridization (FISH), and flow cytometry. In many cancers, studies of intratumoral heterogeneity have focused on the potential mechanisms of treatment resistance. Estrogen receptor (ER) positive tumor is the most prevalent subtype in breast cancer, and adjuvant endocrine therapy is recommended for patients with as low as 1–2% ER positivity [4]. This criterion introduces broad range of ER expression within a tumor, and the presence or outgrowth of ER negative tumor cells may cause treatment resistance to the endocrine therapy. HER2 (human epidermal growth factor receptor 2) subtype comprises 15–20% breast cancer and shows aggressive clinical behavior [5]. HER2 amplification is also tested by IHC, and complementary FISH is performed for those with borderline staining results. Similar to ER, HER2 staining or FISH signals differ between tumor cells, and the presence or outgrowth of HER2 negative tumor cells may confer treatment resistance to HER2-targeted therapy. Despite continuous expression of ER or HER2, treatment resistance developed for the targeted therapies [6, 7] and search for the underlying mechanisms required systematic tools, genomics.

Large-scale sequencing analysis enabled comprehensive understanding of cancer genome [8] and revealed diverse mechanisms for treatment resistance. Mutations in ER coding gene (ESR1) were found to confer acquired endocrine resistance in metastatic breast cancer [9, 10]. Mutations in PIK3CA gene or pathway were associated with treatment resistance in HER2-targeted therapies [11, 12]. Moreover, computational methods were developed to infer intratumoral genetic heterogeneity from bulk sequencing data. Clonal heterogeneity in cancer cells could be inferred by frequencies of mutations and copy number aberrations (CNA) at DNA level [13–17]. Cellular composition could be inferred by deconvolution of gene expression data from tissues [18, 19]. Formerly, direct evidence for the genetic intratumoral heterogeneity in a large scale came from multiregional genome array and sequencing analysis [20, 21]. In breast cancer, macrodissection and array-based copy number analysis revealed different regional pattern of crude copy number aberrations [21]. Based on the heterogeneous multiregional CNA, phylogenetic tree could be reconstructed and clonal evolution inferred. Application of sequencing further extended the scope of regional heterogeneity. In renal cell carcinoma sampled from different primary cancer sectors, whole exome sequencing demonstrated intratumoral heterogeneity in mutation profiles and linked them with heterogeneity in gene expression and ploidy levels [20]. Finally, single cell DNA sequencing elaborated the heterogeneity to the cellular resolution [22].

While tumor DNA analysis is utilized to find genetic alterations and to reconstruct the paths of tumor evolution, gene expression analysis gives information more directly related to the tumor phenotype. In breast cancer, expression of ER, PR, and HER2 is the only decision criteria for specific treatment choices [23]. Use of gene expression profiling to determine ER/PR or HER2 positive breast cancer subtypes or to provide prognostic information has gained positive feedbacks, yet has not reached to a consensus of making absolute clinical decisions [24]. The concordance of breast cancer subtype analysis between using IHC and transcript expression is >90% [25]. Multigene expression profiling such as Oncotype DX, Mammaprint, and Prosigna can be used to tailor adjuvant endocrine and chemotherapy [26]. When the breast cancer subtype was analyzed by single cell RNA sequencing, mixed subtype cells were present with variable ER/PR/HER2 gene expression and downstream signaling pathway activation [27]. Intratumoral heterogeneity was also found in many cancer-related pathway gene expressions such as for proliferation, stemness, and metastasis.

Tumor tissues inherently contain stromal and immune cells, and these nontumor cells in the tumor microenvironment play critical roles in tumor progression. Stromal cells such as cancer-associated fibroblasts (CAF) may promote tumor growth and metastasis by stimulating growth factor signaling and tissue remodeling [28]. Tumor-infiltrating immune cells can control tumor progression in opposite direction by activating or suppressing the antitumor immunity [29]. Tumor-associated macrophages are known to possess immune suppressive characteristics, whereas cytotoxic T cells may target and kill tumor cells. Immune cell types, their numbers, and functional status have been studied by histology and inference from bulk data and linked with patient survival [30, 31]. In breast cancer, a high number of tumor infiltrating lymphocytes (TILs) were associated with good prognosis in TNBC subtype [32] and with good treatment response in HER2 subtype [33]. However, some cell types such as FOXP3-positive lymphocytes were associated with poor survival. In ER subtype, numbers of TILs were small and showed negative correlation with overall survival [34]. These reports demonstrated the necessity of determining specific immune cell types and status to properly define the immune status of cancer. Through single cell RNA sequencing, genome-wide characterization of individual TILs could be accomplished [27].

10.3 Current Evidence and Concepts

Detection of genetic aberrations in individual cells has important practical implications, as real-time screening or monitoring for cancer genome can be made using circulating tumor cells (CTCs) from liquid biopsies in noninvasive manner [35]. Monitoring of CTCs has relied on the immunomagnetic antibody staining of the epithelial cell adhesion molecule (EpCAM), and the number of CTCs gave predictive values for patient survival in multiple cancer including breast [36–38]. Single cell genomics even enabled genome-wide characterization of CTCs for their mutational, CNA, and gene expression profiles. CTCs recapitulated the genetic aberrations found in the primary tumor tissues, acting as surrogate biomarkers for tumor heterogeneity [39–41]. Single CTC RNA sequencing also revealed prognostic gene expression signatures [42]. These results suggested that genome profiling of CTCs may reveal genetic and gene expression heterogeneity associated with drug sensitivity or resistance. However, CTCs can be detected in relatively small proportion of cancer patients, and the low sensitivity limits their use for disease monitoring purposes. This limitation may be overcome by the complementary use of circulating tumor DNAs (ctDNA) [35]. Research progress on ctDNAs has paralleled CTCs as technical challenges in the detection of small amount of genomic materials are similar in both targets.

The technical development in single cell RNA sequencing is allowing genome wide characterization of tumor phenotype in association with tumor microenvironment. In breast cancer, single cell dissociation and RNA sequencing allowed isolation and characterization of tumor infiltrating immune cells [27]. In colon cancer, similar method allowed characterization of cancer-associated fibroblasts [43]. Both immune cells and fibroblasts play critical roles in tumor progression. Use of high-throughput single cell capture platform is allowing more thorough characterization of tumor microenvironment [44]. Characterization of tumor microenvironment is necessarily related to the paired assessment of normal cellular compartment. Use of single cell genomics to define cell types and status improves our understanding of normal human body, which is fundamental to detail damaged cellular phenotype in many disease conditions including cancer.

Large-scale RNA sequencing allows identification of subpopulations with gene expression features important in tumor progression, metastasis, and drug resistance

[44–47]. For most single cell genomic studies, freshly obtained tissues were enzymatically digested to get single cell suspension. The requirement of freshly prepared tissues is limiting the use of single cell genomics in archived tumor tissues. Analyzing archived tissues can facilitate longitudinal studies, which are crucial for the understanding of tumor evolution for extended periods. In DNA analysis, nuclei isolation technique has enabled the use of frozen or formalin-fixed paraffin-embedded tissues for single cell genomics [22]. In a similar manner, using nuclear RNAs for gene expression profiling would facilitate longitudinal analysis, which may demonstrate the changes of gene expression profiles along with tumor progression. The technique has been broadly adopted for the neuronal single cell analysis [48, 49]. In a recent publication, scientists at MD Anderson applied nanogrid nuclear RNA sequencing to demonstrate phenotypic diversity in archived frozen breast cancer [50]. Results of nuclear RNA sequencing revealed gene expression profiles comparable to total RNA sequencing, suggesting that the technique can be used for the frozen-archived tumor tissues.

Single cell or nuclei isolation and sequencing inevitably destroy the tissue architecture, and the spatial characteristics of tumor become lost. Low throughput methods such as immunohistochemistry or FISH preserve the spatial information yet have limitations by the number of molecules that can be detected. Therefore, combining the spatial information and high-throughput detection methods is being explored, on genetic aberrations, gene expression profiles, and protein expression. In situ RNA sequencing explores the genome wide gene expression analysis directly on preserved tissue sections [51, 52]. Targeted sequencing allows detection of genetic aberrations as well. In breast cancer tissue sections, targeted in situ RNA sequencing allowed gene expression profiling for as many as 31 transcripts including 21 transcripts used in a breast cancer prognostic expression panel [52]. At protein level, both multiplexed ion beam imaging (MIBI) and a CYTOF instrument adopt mass cytometry utilize antibodies labeled with rare lanthanide metals with a unique mass [53, 54]. With these techniques, up to a 100 of protein expression can be detected with spatial information in a similar way to the IHC. With MIBI, Garry Nolan's group at Stanford has demonstrated intratumoral heterogeneity using ten different antibodies in formalin fixed primary breast cancer tissues. Introduction of high-throughput genome/proteome detection methods in the spatial context is expected to bring up new findings in cancer research.

Simultaneous analysis of DNA and RNA enables tracking of clonal evolution together with gene expression pattern, which may provide causal relationship between genotype and gene expression phenotype [55–59]. Overall, heterogeneity in CNAs affected gene expression profiles in various cell lines and hepatocellular carcinoma. In a Trio-seq study where single cell genome, methylome, and transcriptome were simultaneously analyzed [58], CNAs had direct impact on gene expression but no impact on the methylation pattern. In the study, tumor cell heterogeneity was conferred at genetic, epigenetic, and transcriptomic levels. Combining antibody staining together with gene expression profiling allows better characterization of tumor phenotype as proteins are the ultimate functional unit of cells. Recently developed methods such as CITE-seq (Cellular indexing of transcriptomes and epitopes by sequencing) and REAP-seq (RNA expression and protein sequencing) allow more accurate characterization of cellular phenotypes [60, 61]. These methods have been used in the characterization of immune cells, due to antibody availability for surface molecules on immune cells and predefined immune cell phenotypes with protein markers. Thus, these methods will be extensively used for the characterization of tumor-associated immune microenvironment.

10.4 Future Research Directions

In recent years, new methods and platforms have been developed to realize single cell genomics, and their application in cancer expanded our knowledge on tumor heterogeneity in genome, transcriptome, and proteome level. Through these developments, we are equipped with single cell genomic tools to make new discoveries and to assess useful information that can directly improve patient outcome in cancer. However, most single cell genomics data production remains at the proof-of-concept level and the new methods and platforms need improvements for the clinical implementation. In the next step, we are expecting ample production of single cell genomic data from diverse clinical settings, in normal and disease conditions, as well as improvements or fine tuning of single cell genomics tools. The fulfillment will lead us to direct application of single cell genomics to cancer management.

Massive production of single cell genomics data has already begun. The human cell atlas [62], an international collaborative effort of building a human cellular reference map, is at the center of it, as normal human cell data would be a cornerstone to understand any disease conditions. The largest number of data production is expected to be made by commercial easy-to-use platforms like 10X genomics gemcode system [63] and to be supplemented by other multidimensional methods. Development of new methods is ongoing; yet, researchers in this field have reached a consensus that generation and standardization of human cell reference is an impending subject that can be accomplished with currently available technologies. Based on these, parallel data production in cancer will be directed toward tumor populations as well as stromal and immune cells in the tumor microenvironment. Surgical specimens from adjacent normal and tumor sites, small biopsies, and liquid biopsies from early to advanced stages of cancer will be analyzed. Experimental designs will encompass tumors of the primary or metastatic sites, of good or bad prognosis, and of responders or nonresponders to particular drugs including chemotherapeutic and immunotherapeutic agents. Based on the findings, our efforts will be directed to find therapeutic targets and ways to improve current practice of cancer medicine.

There are much to be done to improve current technologies or invent new ones to implement single cell genomics to clinical diagnosis and management of cancer. Fields closely awaiting for the direct use of single cell genomics would be related to the blood or body fluids and diagnosis and monitoring of diseases exploiting blood/fluid cells or related materials. Detection of malignant cells in the blood or body fluids has been diagnostic criteria for many hematologic cancers. For the diagnostic purposes, cell smears and suspensions from the blood, bone marrow aspirates, and body fluids are examined for their morphology and antibody staining of disease markers. These processes can be replaced by single cell genomics as gene expression profiling has potential to identify cell types and functional status more accurately and thoroughly compared to the conventional diagnostics that utilize small number of molecular parameters. To reach a goal of replacing current diagnostic methods, cost, turnaround time, and throughput need to be improved. With the conventional diagnostic methods using microslides or flow cytometry tubes, millions of cells can be examined for the presence of malignant cells. Current single cell genomics platform easily detects thousands of cells, but for more cell detection, linear increase in number of tests and cost is required. Even after those issues resolved, well-designed clinical trials would be required for each specific cancer cell type, validating single cell genomic profiling as a superior method compared to the conventional diagnostics. For solid tissue malignancies like breast cancer, routine diagnosis would rely on the examination of tissue biopsies as current single cell dissociation methods may not faithfully capture cell populations of diagnostic interest. Detection of circulating tumor cells or tumor DNAs may be utilized instead, if detection sensitivity and specificity are guaranteed. Capture and identification of one CTC in over millions of white blood cells or ctDNAs over a pool of normal cell-free DNAs still remain a challenge. Resolving this limitation will open up a new era of cancer management in screening, monitoring disease progression and recurrence, and matching best drug combinations, with the aid of single cell genomics.

References

1. Welch DR. Tumor heterogeneity--a 'contemporary concept' founded on historical insights and predictions. Cancer Res. 2016;76(1):4–6.
2. Schwartzberg L, Kim ES, Liu D, Schrag D. Precision oncology: who, how, what, when, and when not? Am Soc Clin Oncol Educ Book. 2017;37:160–9.
3. McGranahan N, Swanton C. Clonal heterogeneity and tumor evolution: past, present, and the future. Cell. 2017;168(4):613–28.
4. Goldhirsch A, Ingle JN, Gelber RD, Coates AS, Thurlimann B, Senn HJ, et al. Thresholds for therapies: highlights of the St Gallen international expert consensus on the primary therapy of early breast cancer 2009. Ann Oncol. 2009;20(8):1319–29.
5. Yersal O, Barutca S. Biological subtypes of breast cancer: prognostic and therapeutic implications. World J Clin Oncol. 2014;5(3):412–24.
6. Johnston SR, Dowsett M, Smith IE. Towards a molecular basis for tamoxifen resistance in breast cancer. Annals of oncology: official journal of the European society for. Med Oncol. 1992;3(7):503–11.
7. Mohd Sharial MS, Crown J, Hennessy BT. Overcoming resistance and restoring sensitivity to HER2-targeted therapies in breast cancer. Ann Oncol. 2012;23(12):3007–16.
8. Kandoth C, McLellan MD, Vandin F, Ye K, Niu B, Lu C, et al. Mutational landscape and significance across 12 major cancer types. Nature. 2013;502(7471):333–9.
9. Robinson DR, Wu YM, Vats P, Su F, Lonigro RJ, Cao X, et al. Activating ESR1 mutations in hormone-resistant metastatic breast cancer. Nat Genet. 2013;45(12):1446–51.

10. Toy W, Shen Y, Won H, Green B, Sakr RA, Will M, et al. ESR1 ligand-binding domain mutations in hormone-resistant breast cancer. Nat Genet. 2013;45(12):1439–45.
11. Shi W, Jiang T, Nuciforo P, Hatzis C, Holmes E, Harbeck N, et al. Pathway level alterations rather than mutations in single genes predict response to HER2-targeted therapies in the neo-ALTTO trial. Ann Oncol. 2017;28(1):128–35.
12. Loibl S, von Minckwitz G, Schneeweiss A, Paepke S, Lehmann A, Rezai M, et al. PIK3CA mutations are associated with lower rates of pathologic complete response to anti-human epidermal growth factor receptor 2 (her2) therapy in primary HER2-overexpressing breast cancer. J Clin Oncol. 2014;32(29):3212–20.
13. Roth A, Khattra J, Yap D, Wan A, Laks E, Biele J, et al. PyClone: statistical inference of clonal population structure in cancer. Nat Methods. 2014;11(4):396–8.
14. Li B, Li JZ. A general framework for analyzing tumor subclonality using SNP array and DNA sequencing data. Genome Biol. 2014;15(9):473.
15. Ha G, Roth A, Khattra J, Ho J, Yap D, Prentice LM, et al. TITAN: inference of copy number architectures in clonal cell populations from tumor whole-genome sequence data. Genome Res. 2014;24(11):1881–93.
16. Oesper L, Mahmoody A, Raphael BJ. THetA: inferring intra-tumor heterogeneity from high-throughput DNA sequencing data. Genome Biol. 2013;14(7):R80.
17. Miller CA, White BS, Dees ND, Griffith M, Welch JS, Griffith OL, et al. SciClone: inferring clonal architecture and tracking the spatial and temporal patterns of tumor evolution. PLoS Comput Biol. 2014;10(8):e1003665.
18. Newman AM, Liu CL, Green MR, Gentles AJ, Feng W, Xu Y, et al. Robust enumeration of cell subsets from tissue expression profiles. Nat Methods. 2015;12(5):453–7.
19. Yoshihara K, Shahmoradgoli M, Martinez E, Vegesna R, Kim H, Torres-Garcia W, et al. Inferring tumour purity and stromal and immune cell admixture from expression data. Nat Commun. 2013;4:2612.
20. Gerlinger M, Rowan AJ, Horswell S, Math M, Larkin J, Endesfelder D, et al. Intratumor heterogeneity and branched evolution revealed by multiregion sequencing. N Engl J Med. 2012;366(10):883–92.
21. Navin N, Krasnitz A, Rodgers L, Cook K, Meth J, Kendall J, et al. Inferring tumor progression from genomic heterogeneity. Genome Res. 2010;20(1):68–80.
22. Navin N, Kendall J, Troge J, Andrews P, Rodgers L, McIndoo J, et al. Tumour evolution inferred by single-cell sequencing. Nature. 2011;472(7341):90–4.
23. Krop I, Ismaila N, Andre F, Bast RC, Barlow W, Collyar DE, et al. Use of biomarkers to guide decisions on adjuvant systemic therapy for women with early-stage invasive breast cancer: American Society of Clinical Oncology clinical practice guideline focused update. J Clin Oncol. 2017;35(24):2838–47.
24. Henry NL, Bedard PL, DeMichele A. Standard and genomic tools for decision support in breast cancer treatment. Am Soc Clin Oncol Educ Book. 2017;37:106–15.
25. Mer AS, Klevebring D, Gronberg H, Rantalainen M. Study design requirements for RNA sequencing-based breast cancer diagnostics. Sci Rep. 2016;6:20200.
26. Myers MB. Targeted therapies with companion diagnostics in the management of breast cancer: current perspectives. Pharmacogenom Person Med. 2016;9:7–16.
27. Chung W, Eum HH, Lee HO, Lee KM, Lee HB, Kim KT, et al. Single-cell RNA-seq enables comprehensive tumour and immune cell profiling in primary breast cancer. Nat Commun. 2017;8:15081.
28. Erdogan B, Webb DJ. Cancer-associated fibroblasts modulate growth factor signaling and extracellular matrix remodeling to regulate tumor metastasis. Biochem Soc Trans. 2017;45 (1):229–36.
29. Gajewski TF, Schreiber H, Fu YX. Innate and adaptive immune cells in the tumor microenvironment. Nat Immunol. 2013;14(10):1014–22.

30. Salgado R, Denkert C, Demaria S, Sirtaine N, Klauschen F, Pruneri G, et al. The evaluation of tumor-infiltrating lymphocytes (TILs) in breast cancer: recommendations by an international TILs Working Group 2014. Ann Oncol. 2015;26(2):259–71.
31. Galon J, Costes A, Sanchez-Cabo F, Kirilovsky A, Mlecnik B, Lagorce-Pages C, et al. Type, density, and location of immune cells within human colorectal tumors predict clinical outcome. Science. 2006;313(5795):1960–4.
32. Mao Y, Qu Q, Chen X, Huang O, Wu J, Shen K. The prognostic value of tumor-infiltrating lymphocytes in breast cancer: a systematic review and meta-analysis. PLoS One. 2016;11(4): e0152500.
33. Solinas C, Ceppi M, Lambertini M, Scartozzi M, Buisseret L, Garaud S, et al. Tumor-infiltrating lymphocytes in patients with HER2-positive breast cancer treated with neoadjuvant chemotherapy plus trastuzumab, lapatinib or their combination: a meta-analysis of randomized controlled trials. Cancer Treat Rev. 2017;57:8–15.
34. Krishnamurti U, Wetherilt CS, Yang J, Peng L, Li X. Tumor-infiltrating lymphocytes are significantly associated with better overall survival and disease-free survival in triple-negative but not estrogen receptor-positive breast cancers. Hum Pathol. 2017;64:7–12.
35. Alix-Panabieres C, Pantel K. Clinical applications of circulating tumor cells and circulating tumor DNA as liquid biopsy. Cancer Discov. 2016;6(5):479–91.
36. Allard WJ, Matera J, Miller MC, Repollet M, Connelly MC, Rao C, et al. Tumor cells circulate in the peripheral blood of all major carcinomas but not in healthy subjects or patients with nonmalignant diseases. Clin Cancer Res. 2004;10(20):6897–904.
37. Cristofanilli M, Budd GT, Ellis MJ, Stopeck A, Matera J, Miller MC, et al. Circulating tumor cells, disease progression, and survival in metastatic breast cancer. N Engl J Med. 2004;351 (8):781–91.
38. Cristofanilli M, Hayes DF, Budd GT, Ellis MJ, Stopeck A, Reuben JM, et al. Circulating tumor cells: a novel prognostic factor for newly diagnosed metastatic breast cancer. J Clin Oncol. 2005;23(7):1420–30.
39. Pestrin M, Salvianti F, Galardi F, De Luca F, Turner N, Malorni L, et al. Heterogeneity of PIK3CA mutational status at the single cell level in circulating tumor cells from metastatic breast cancer patients. Mol Oncol. 2015;9(4):749–57.
40. Jiang R, Lu YT, Ho H, Li B, Chen JF, Lin M, et al. A comparison of isolated circulating tumor cells and tissue biopsies using whole-genome sequencing in prostate cancer. Oncotarget. 2015;6 (42):44781–93.
41. Bingham C, Fernandez SV, Fittipaldi P, Dempsey PW, Ruth KJ, Cristofanilli M, et al. Mutational studies on single circulating tumor cells isolated from the blood of inflammatory breast cancer patients. Breast Cancer Res Treat. 2017;163(2):219–30.
42. Lohr JG, Kim S, Gould J, Knoechel B, Drier Y, Cotton MJ, et al. Genetic interrogation of circulating multiple myeloma cells at single-cell resolution. Sci Transl Med. 2016;8 (363):363ra147.
43. Li H, Courtois ET, Sengupta D, Tan Y, Chen KH, Goh JJL, et al. Reference component analysis of single-cell transcriptomes elucidates cellular heterogeneity in human colorectal tumors. Nat Genet. 2017;49(5):708–18.
44. Tirosh I, Izar B, Prakadan SM, Wadsworth MH 2nd, Treacy D, Trombetta JJ, et al. Dissecting the multicellular ecosystem of metastatic melanoma by single-cell RNA-seq. Science. 2016;352 (6282):189–96.
45. Patel AP, Tirosh I, Trombetta JJ, Shalek AK, Gillespie SM, Wakimoto H, et al. Single-cell RNA-seq highlights intratumoral heterogeneity in primary glioblastoma. Science. 2014;344 (6190):1396–401.
46. Puram SV, Tirosh I, Parikh AS, Patel AP, Yizhak K, Gillespie S, et al. Single-cell transcriptomic analysis of primary and metastatic tumor ecosystems in head and neck cancer. Cell. 2017;171(7):1611–24.e24.

47. Suva ML, Rheinbay E, Gillespie SM, Patel AP, Wakimoto H, Rabkin SD, et al. Reconstructing and reprogramming the tumor-propagating potential of glioblastoma stem-like cells. Cell. 2014;157(3):580–94.
48. Krishnaswami SR, Grindberg RV, Novotny M, Venepally P, Lacar B, Bhutani K, et al. Using single nuclei for RNA-seq to capture the transcriptome of postmortem neurons. Nat Protoc. 2016;11(3):499–524.
49. Ofengeim D, Giagtzoglou N, Huh D, Zou C, Yuan J. Single-cell RNA sequencing: unraveling the brain one cell at a time. Trends Mol Med. 2017;23(6):563–76.
50. Gao R, Kim C, Sei E, Foukakis T, Crosetto N, Chan LK, et al. Nanogrid single-nucleus RNA sequencing reveals phenotypic diversity in breast cancer. Nat Commun. 2017;8(1):228.
51. Lee JH, Daugharthy ER, Scheiman J, Kalhor R, Ferrante TC, Terry R, et al. Fluorescent in situ sequencing (FISSEQ) of RNA for gene expression profiling in intact cells and tissues. Nat Protoc. 2015;10(3):442–58.
52. Ke R, Mignardi M, Pacureanu A, Svedlund J, Botling J, Wahlby C, et al. In situ sequencing for RNA analysis in preserved tissue and cells. Nat Methods. 2013;10(9):857–60.
53. Angelo M, Bendall SC, Finck R, Hale MB, Hitzman C, Borowsky AD, et al. Multiplexed ion beam imaging of human breast tumors. Nat Med. 2014;20(4):436–42.
54. Giesen C, Wang HA, Schapiro D, Zivanovic N, Jacobs A, Hattendorf B, et al. Highly multiplexed imaging of tumor tissues with subcellular resolution by mass cytometry. Nat Methods. 2014;11(4):417–22.
55. Dey SS, Kester L, Spanjaard B, Bienko M, van Oudenaarden A. Integrated genome and transcriptome sequencing of the same cell. Nat Biotechnol. 2015;33(3):285–9.
56. Han KY, Kim KT, Joung JG, Son DS, Kim YJ, Jo A, et al. SIDR: simultaneous isolation and parallel sequencing of genomic DNA and total RNA from single cells. Genome Res. 2018;28 (1):75–87.
57. Han L, Zi X, Garmire LX, Wu Y, Weissman SM, Pan X, et al. Co-detection and sequencing of genes and transcripts from the same single cells facilitated by a microfluidics platform. Sci Rep. 2014;4:6485.
58. Hou Y, Guo H, Cao C, Li X, Hu B, Zhu P, et al. Single-cell triple omics sequencing reveals genetic, epigenetic, and transcriptomic heterogeneity in hepatocellular carcinomas. Cell Res. 2016;26(3):304–19.
59. Macaulay IC, Haerty W, Kumar P, Li YI, Hu TX, Teng MJ, et al. G&T-seq: parallel sequencing of single-cell genomes and transcriptomes. Nat Methods. 2015;12(6):519–22.
60. Peterson VM, Zhang KX, Kumar N, Wong J, Li L, Wilson DC, et al. Multiplexed quantification of proteins and transcripts in single cells. Nat Biotechnol. 2017;35(10):936–9.
61. Stoeckius M, Hafemeister C, Stephenson W, Houck-Loomis B, Chattopadhyay PK, Swerdlow H, et al. Simultaneous epitope and transcriptome measurement in single cells. Nat Methods. 2017;14(9):865–8.
62. Rozenblatt-Rosen O, Stubbington MJT, Regev A, Teichmann SA. The human cell atlas: from vision to reality. Nature. 2017;550(7677):451–3.
63. Zheng GX, Terry JM, Belgrader P, Ryvkin P, Bent ZW, Wilson R, et al. Massively parallel digital transcriptional profiling of single cells. Nat Commun. 2017;8:14049.

Chapter 11
Advances in Tumor Sampling and Sequencing in Breast Cancer and their Application in Precision Diagnostics and Therapeutics

Amos Chungwon Lee, Han-Byoel Lee, Huiran Yeom, Seo Woo Song, Su Deok Kim, Ahyoun Choi, Sumin Lee, Yongju Lee, Wonshik Han, and Sunghoon Kwon

Abstract Intra- and Inter-tumoral heterogeneity is one of the main hurdles in diagnosing and treating breast cancer. Selecting, sampling, and sequencing the

---

Amos Chungwon Lee and Han-Byoel Lee contributed equally with all other contributors.

A. C. Lee
Interdisciplinary Program in Bioengineering, Seoul National University, Seoul, South Korea

Bio-MAX Institute, Seoul National University, Seoul, South Korea

H.-B. Lee · W. Han (✉)
Department of Surgery, Seoul National University College of Medicine, Seoul, South Korea

Biomedical Research Institute, Seoul National University Hospital, Seoul, South Korea

Cancer Research Institute, Seoul National University, Seoul, South Korea
e-mail: hanw@snu.ac.kr

H. Yeom · S. D. Kim · S. Lee · Y. Lee
Department of Electrical and Computer Engineering, Seoul National University, Seoul, South Korea

S. W. Song
Bio-MAX Institute, Seoul National University, Seoul, South Korea

A. Choi
Interdisciplinary Program in Bioengineering, Seoul National University, Seoul, South Korea

S. Kwon (✉)
Interdisciplinary Program in Bioengineering, Seoul National University, Seoul, South Korea

Biomedical Research Institute, Seoul National University Hospital, Seoul, South Korea

Department of Electrical and Computer Engineering, Seoul National University, Seoul, South Korea

Bio-MAX Institute, Seoul National University, Seoul, South Korea
e-mail: skwon@snu.ac.kr

D.-Y. Noh et al. (eds.), *Translational Research in Breast Cancer*, Advances in Experimental Medicine and Biology 1187,
https://doi.org/10.1007/978-981-32-9620-6_11

samples appropriately provide unique opportunities in realizing precision medicine. This chapter reviews some of the past landmarks, state-of-the-art technologies, and future directions of translational research in terms of tumor sampling technologies and sequencing in breast cancer. In the state-of-the-art technologies section, the technologies are categorized in terms of scientific, precision diagnostic, and precision therapeutic tools. Finally, limitations and future directions regarding various translational research for clinical applications using these technologies will be discussed.

Keywords Tumor heterogeneity · Single-cell sequencing · Liquid biopsy · Spatially resolved sequencing · Laser-induced cell sorting · Circulating tumor cells · Circulating tumor DNA · Drug screening

11.1 Introduction

Advances in next-generation sequencing (NGS) technologies have revolutionized oncology, especially in terms of understanding genetic composition of cancer. Extensive research in cancer began with The Cancer Genome Atlas (TCGA), a project that began in 2005 to categorize different genomic alterations of different cancers in a comprehensive atlas of cancer genomes [1–3]. TCGA has now produced over 2.5 petabytes of cancer genomes of 11,000 patients typing 33 different cancers. It provided insights into inter-tumoral genetic heterogeneity, indicating the need for precision medicine. The analysis of patient-specific genetic alterations harbored in the tumor has gained interests for their potential to be used as precision diagnostics for effective treatment of cancer. However, the complexity in precision medicine due to intra-tumoral genetic heterogeneity impeded translating these researches directly into clinical practice. The intra-tumoral genetic heterogeneity in breast cancer was first reported by Navin et al. where they sequenced single cells [4]. This study by Navin et al. first revealed tumor evolution of different subclones with different genetic alterations in a single tumor, raising a technological need for single-cell analysis and rare mutation detection. In other words, simply sequencing the bulk tumor will produce averaged out genetic information, in which the rare but clinically important mutations could be buried, hindering the realization of precision medicine (Fig. 11.1a). To disentangle and extract out the clinically important mutations from the complex nature of cancer, several strategies were reported to address the issue of tumor sampling (Fig. 11.1b). In this chapter, we categorized various state-of-the-art technologies according to three different sampling sources in breast cancer: tumor, peripheral blood, and primary cells. Technologies that utilize the tumor have potential to reveal tumorigenesis and tumor development. Those that utilize the blood show promise in liquid biopsy for precision diagnosis of breast cancer. Furthermore, those that use primary cells can screen the right drug precisely to the breast cancer patients. Altogether, these translational researches will bring breast cancer research from bench to bedside.

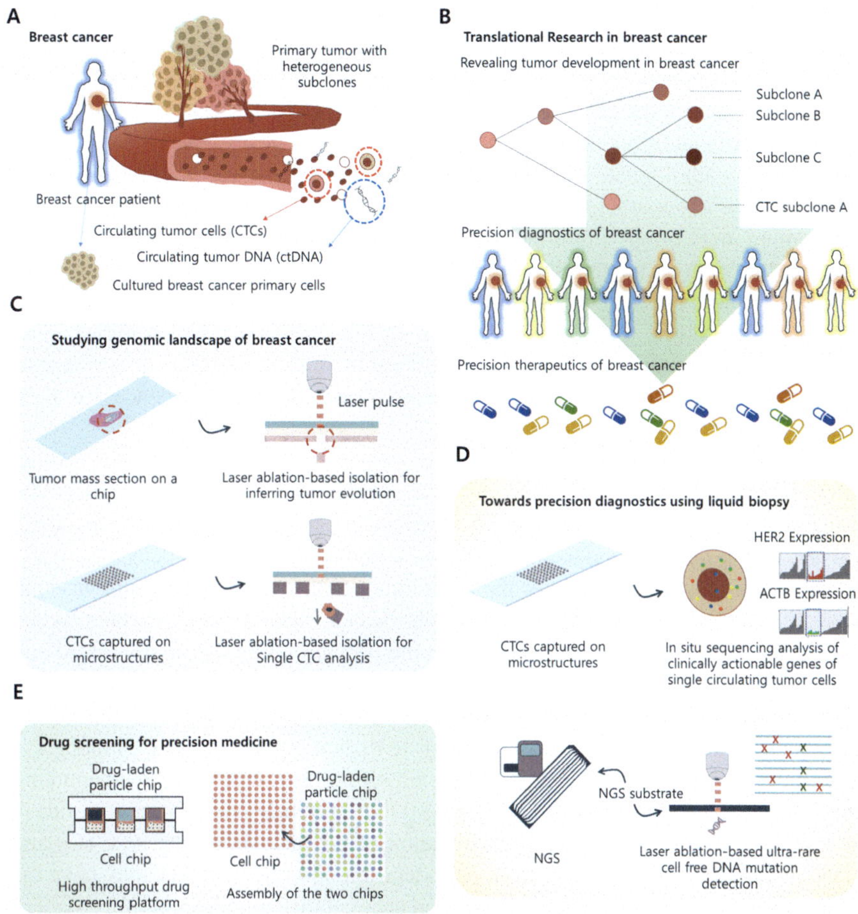

Fig. 11.1 Advances in tumor sampling and sequencing in breast cancer and their application in precision diagnostics and therapeutics. (**a**) Acquirable samples from breast cancer patients. (**b**) Translational research strategies in breast cancer. (**c**) Genomic research in breast cancer. (**d**) Precision diagnostics using liquid biopsy. (**e**) Drug screening for precision medicine

In contrast to traditional approaches that explored and analyzed the overall genomic landscape of a heterogeneous mass [5], emerging technologies that can specifically select samples for precise analysis of cancer were developed to unravel the heterogeneity of tumors. The most conventional approaches are technologies that utilize needle and surgical biopsy, invasive methods that remove parts of biological mass. Using these methods, a solid tumor can be analyzed both in bulk and at single-cell level. Genetic alterations detection from a bulk tumor is sufficient for quantitative analysis of non-rare variations [6]. On the other hand, single-cell sequencing methods provide a useful tool to discover rare tumor activating mutations that can be clinically actionable and have been extensively used for studying tumor evolution in breast cancer [4, 7–9]. Recent studies showed its potential to be used practically in the clinic for diagnosis, prognosis, and therapeutics [10]. Furthermore, studies exploring the transcriptome have revealed functional and immune landscape of breast cancer, and others have shown relationships between these single-cell RNA sequencing data and drug sensitivity [11–14].

However, pathological analysis is the basis of modern cancer medicine, and connecting the histopathological information to the molecular profile of the tumor is becoming increasingly important for practical use of molecular profiling technologies. Later in this chapter, some technologies that integrate morphological and spatial information of a single tumor cell or a cluster of cells are introduced [15, 16] (Fig. 11.1c). Likewise with further advancements in multi-omics technologies, more studies involving tissue sampling are necessary to fully understand tumorigenesis and the evolution of tumor, and eventually provide enough evidence for their translation to the clinic.

In addition to the conventional tissue biopsy methods mentioned above, other sampling modalities to detect and analyze various sources of breast cancer are available. Because cancer leaves its traces inside and throughout the patient's body, it is important to understand different sampling strategies to detect clinically significant genetic alterations. For the solid tumor to grow, it must acquire vasculature for the delivery of nutrition to the neoplastic cells that the tumor harbors. When the tumor outgrows, some of the cells from the primary tumor are disseminated and circulate throughout the body [17] (Fig. 11.1a). When these circulating tumor cells (CTCs) go through epithelial-to-mesenchymal transition (EMT), they may acquire the potential to become a seed for metastasis to distant organs [18, 19]. Tumors also shed out circulating tumor DNA (ctDNA) which can also represent the originating primary tumor [20–23]. Hence, CTCs and ctDNAs provide unique opportunities in the diagnosis, monitoring, and prognostication of cancer. Also, because CTCs and ctDNAs can be simply obtained from peripheral blood of the patients, they have the advantage of less invasiveness and increased accessibility to molecular information. The term liquid biopsy describes the method that extracts peripheral blood from the cancer patients, as an alternative to the invasive tissue biopsy methods. However, one limitation that impedes the translation of liquid biopsy is that CTCs are very rare (approximately 5 in 1 ml of peripheral blood) and clinically important genetic aberrations can be buried in ctDNAs, below frequency of 1%. In the next section, we discuss some strategies in translational medicine that can be used for liquid biopsy (Fig. 11.1d).

Primary tumor cells of breast cancer patients are another source of sampling that can be used in translational research. Although discovering genetic heterogeneity and tumor evolution in a solid tumor will reveal several important target genetic markers in applying the findings to precision diagnostics using liquid biopsy, tools that can screen the appropriate drug for the patient need to be developed for full realization of translational medicine in breast cancer.

When these different sources of sampling breast cancer meet appropriate technologies, various types of translational researches can be performed. In this chapter, we discuss translational researches in breast cancer from spatially resolved sequencing technologies to sequential drug screening methods that were applied using different sampling methods.

11.2 Review of Past Studies

11.2.1 Sampling Solid Tumor: Single-Cell Sequencing to Spatially Resolved Sequencing in Breast Cancer

Navin et al. reported intra-tumoral heterogeneity in breast cancer by sequencing single-cell genomes and revealed complex evolution in breast cancer [4]. They used flow cytometry to sort out single nuclei of cells in a tumor and analyzed their genomes using NGS. After the tumor was macro-dissected into individual portions of the mass, each went through fluorescence-activated cell sorting (FACS) technique. FACS uses laser beams to sort out differently marked fluorescence tags according to their emission spectrum [24]. It is now one of the most widely used technologies to sort out single cells from a mass, allowing differentiation of four to tens of different cells according to its characteristics. In case of the study by Navin et al., DAPI staining was used to select out nuclei in a mixture of lysed cells. The genomic DNA (gDNA) inside the nuclei is then fragmented and amplified using polymerase chain reaction (PCR)-based whole genome amplification (WGA) methods. Among several types of WGA methods, the degenerate oligonucleotide-primed PCR (DOP-PCR) used in this particular study was shown to be efficient in analyzing the copy number alterations (CNA) of the genomes, which are inferred from the NGS read counts of the gene fragments. DOP-PCR uses oligonucleotide primers which have partial degenerate sequences to effectively amplify the genome [25]. By analyzing the CNAs of the single cells in breast cancer, cell types can be determined and categorized into different subclones. By measuring the genetic distance between the subclones, the evolution of the tumor can be inferred, providing clues to understanding tumor development. Navin et al. claimed that subclones evolved in punctuated evolution and that the same applied to metastasis by comparing the genetic distances between the subclones of the primary breast tumor and the metastatic liver tumor. This work not only showed that tumors in breast cancer patients evolve with punctuated evolution, but also produced a basis for understanding the molecular biology of breast cancer. Similar work was done in mouse xenografts of human breast cancer. Eirew et al. analyzed the dynamics of genomic clones in breast cancer patient xenografts at single-cell resolution by applying targeted-amplicon deep sequencing [9].

The science behind tumor evolution in breast cancer using single-cell analysis is further elaborated by Gao et al. in their study of punctuated evolution in triple-negative breast cancer (TNBC) [26]. Using the same FACS and DOP-PCR platform, they successfully isolated single nuclei inside TNBC tumor samples and analyzed their CNAs to explore the tumor development within. TNBC is a subtype of breast cancer that is characterized by the lack of estrogen receptor (ER), progesterone receptor (PR), and human epidermal growth factor receptor 2 (HER2) amplification [27]. TNBC is also notorious for poor survival rates of the patients [28]. Gao et al. analyzed the CNAs to categorize subclones and observed clues of punctuated evolution in TNBC. Similar efforts to molecularly differentiate different subtypes of breast cancer have shown the possibility of applying tumor sampling in the diagnosis and treatment of patients [9, 28, 29]. For example, the relationship between the pathological subtypes of ductal carcinoma in situ (DCIS) and invasive ductal carcinoma (IDC) has long been an issue of interest [31, 32]. Especially, there has been substantial debate on whether DCIS precedes IDC or not. There are patients who develop both in the same mass, and sampling the tumor mass in these cases provides opportunity to differentiate the two subclones independently. However, because the subtyping system of DCIS and IDC is based on their histopathological information, simply sequencing single-cell genomes cannot explicitly explore the genomic relationships between the two. Instead, it requires a special technique that can connect the histopathological information and the genomic information in these subclones. Recently, Casasent et al. reported that genomic evolution occurred prior to invasion in DCIS-IDC patients [31]. To do so, they developed spatially resolved single-cell genome sequencing by combining laser catapulting technique and DOP-PCR, and analyzing CNAs and single nucleotide variations (SNVs) of the single cells. Laser catapulting is a similar technique to laser capture microdissection (LCM) techniques, which use laser to micro-dissect parts of interest and catapult the portion to the conventional PCR tubes. Casasent et al. used the laser catapulting system to dissect out single cells that are not interconnected to other parts of the tissue and analyzed their genomes. They used both CNAs and SNVs and connected to the pathological information and discovered how subclones evolved during invasion in ten breast cancer patients.

To unveil molecular footprints in the development of breast cancer, solid tumor has been sampled by FACS, LCM, and other sampling techniques. Although we are just beginning to understand the relationship between different subtypes of breast cancer, multimodal analyses of breast cancer in relation to the histopathological information will advance our knowledge. An example of translational research was done by Yates et al., in which 303 samples from tumors in 50 patients went through multiregion sequencing [30]. They investigated the landmarks of disease progression, such as resistance to chemotherapy and the acquisition of invasive or metastatic potential, through multiregion sequencing of breast cancer and connecting them to histopathological information.

11.2.2 Sampling Blood: CTC Enumeration to Single CTC Characterization in Breast Cancer

Circulating tumor cells reflect the characteristics of the primary tumor from which they originated. Accordingly, efforts to capture these rare cells have propagated the development of various techniques. The most famous platform to enrich CTCs from the peripheral blood is the CellSearch system, which utilizes magnetic beads coated with anti-epithelial cell adhesion molecule (EpCAM) antibodies. For epithelial cancers like breast cancer, it was thought that the CTCs, which are disseminated from the primary tumor, will retain its epithelial-like characteristics. EpCAM is one of the most common surface proteins that epithelial cells possess while blood cells do not. CellSearch is currently the only platform that has been approved by the Food and Drug Administration (FDA). An example of translational research in breast cancer using the CellSearch system is a study by Baccelli et al. [33]. Using the CellSearch system, they isolated EpCAM-positive CTCs and found that metastasis-initiating cells containing CTC populations expressed EpCAM, CD44, CD47, and MET. They show that the number of CTCs that express these four molecules were highly correlated with lower survival rates in breast cancer patients. However, it is reported that the false positive rates (i.e., capture rate of white blood cells, etc) are too high, hindering the purity of CTC during enrichment [34]. Enumerating CTCs was originally believed to be related to the patient survival of breast cancer. However, the study by Cristofanilli et al. proved this theory to be wrong by observing the relationship between the number of CTCs detected and the survival rate of breast cancer patients [35]. Although this study has debunked the hype in enumeration of CTCs, a new interest in CTC characterization in terms of their genomic and transcriptomic landscape grew.

The CTC chip developed by Nagrath et al. was proposed to overcome the purity issue of CellSearch by integrating microfluidics technology [36]. Nagrath et al. designed and built a microfluidic device, namely CTC chip, comprised of hundreds of micropillars (100 μm in diameter and height) that are coated with anti-EpCAM antibodies. Taking advantages of fluid mechanics in microscale, they aimed to increase the capture rate and the true positive rates of captured epithelial cells from whole blood samples. This effort was further shown in a study by Stott et al. from the same group, where they designed a herringbone structured micro biochip in which the micro-grooves were coated with anti-EpCAM antibodies [37]. Similar to the micropillars, the herringbone grooves generate microvortex, causing CTCs to interact more with the antibodies. The chip showed better efficiency in capturing epithelial CTCs than the CTC chip developed by Nagrath et al. One example of translating this technology to medicine is a study by Aceto et al. [38]. Using the herringbone CTC chip, they captured single and clustered CTCs, and observed whether they have metastatic potential in mouse models. Also, they investigated that the abundance of CTC clusters in patients denoted adverse outcome for the patients.

However, because these anti-EpCAM antibody-based CTC capturing methods cannot capture non-epithelial CTCs, which seem to have higher potential in metastasizing (especially when they go through EMT), researchers began to seek other CTC capturing methods [18, 39]. Some researchers have isolated EpCAM-negative CTCs using FACS technology by targeting CD45-negative cells (i.e., white blood cells). One example is a study by Zhang et al. in which they identified and characterized breast cancer CTCs that are competent for brain metastasis [40]. They isolated and enriched EpCAM-negative CTCs overexpressing the "brain metastasis selected markers (BMSMs)," cultured them in long-term, and found the BMSM protein signature that is suggestive of CTC metastatic competency to the brain. As mentioned earlier, FACS can be very useful in isolating single cells from a large pool of cells and isolating the specific single cells of interest by fluorescently labeling them. However, because CTCs are already rare and have various surface markers, FACS is an inefficient and a non-universal way of isolating CTCs. Accordingly, more efficient and universal methods for isolating CTCs were designed and investigated.

One method uses the physical properties of CTCs to enrich them. Sollier et al. developed a microfluidic device that utilizes inertial flow, taking advantage of the meniscus in laminar flow [41]. Because CTCs are usually larger and heavier than any other types of blood cells, they tend to slide to the sides of the channels and are captured in the micro-chambers located in the perimeter. This technology was commercialized by Vortex Biosciences and currently has specifications of 60–70% recovery of CTCs that are unlabeled, intact, and viable [42–44]. This technology was translated in a study by Ramani et al. [45], where they developed patient-derived orthotopic xenograft models of TNBC that have potential to be used in drug screening, etc.

Parsortix is another platform developed by ANGLE Inc. (Surrey, United Kingdom) that utilizes the physical properties of CTCs. The system is comprised of micro-filters that can filter out larger cells (i.e., CTCs) while other smaller blood cells pass through. A notable work from Gkountela et al. used the Parsortix system to isolate CTCs and CTC clusters [46]. They showed that CTC clustering shapes DNA methylation, which enables metastasis seeding in breast cancer. This hypomethylation profile of the CTC clusters is a promising target and the study also tested the potential of FDA-approved Na^+/K^+-ATPase inhibitors for their ability to dissociate CTC clusters. Another work by Vetter et al. showed that denosumab treatment is associated the absence of CTCs in breast cancer [47]. Through analyzing the blood counts of single CTCs and CTC clusters that are enriched by the Parsortix system, they found that patients treated with denosumab lacked CTCs, possibly indicating that it may prevent CTC generation.

Although CTC enrichment methods that utilize physical properties of CTCs have strength in capturing EpCAM-negative CTCs, it also has its own disadvantages of low specificity and low capture rate for small CTCs. Consequently, various types of CTC separation methods are being developed and translated to realize precision medicine through CTC liquid biopsy. They could be categorized into (1) immune-affinity selection, (2) size selection, (3) deformability selection, (4) dielectrophoresis selection, (5) hydrodynamics selection, and (6) selection through nanostructured surface [36, 41, 48–51]. However, all CTC separation platforms categorized above are usually suitable for separation or enumeration, not for extensive multi-omics analysis after they are collected. Additionally, platforms to retrieve the CTCs and also analyze their genomes have been developed, such as the reverse flow and the stimulus responsive polymers [51–54]. However, using these technologies, the captured CTCs must be pooled into a solution, hindering single-cell analysis in multi-omics. In addition to the efforts to enrich CTCs and analyze them in single-cell level, it is necessary to develop multi-omics approach in single CTC analysis.

11.2.3 Sampling Blood: ctDNA Fragment Enumeration to Ultrarare Variant Detection in Breast Cancer

In addition to CTCs, ctDNAs also provide an important source for liquid biopsy, especially when monitoring the status of a cancer patient in a less-invasive manner [21, 55]. ctDNAs can constitute as low as 0.01% of cell-free DNAs (cfDNAs) in a cancer patient [56]. In contrast to CTCs that have unique properties compared to normal blood cells, ctDNAs are DNA fragments with clinically valuable sequences that have properties very similar to other cfDNAs. Therefore, strategies to extract ctDNAs usually are associated with molecular technologies such as PCR, digital PCR, SNP array, and NGS, and technologies that can complement them [20, 56]. One landmark study by Dawson et al. is a proof-of-concept analysis of ctDNA in metastatic breast cancer, showing that the ctDNA levels were in greater correlation with tumor burden than the CTCs in 30 patients [21]. They used tagged-amplicon deep sequencing for *PIK3CA* and *TP53* to quantify ctDNA fragments. Deep sequencing generates more reads to the DNA clusters of cfDNA, providing higher chances of generating reads for ctDNAs. However, to sequence with higher depths, the number of samples or the sites of the genomes to be analyzed must be traded-off. Droplet digital PCR (ddPCR) is another tool that can accurately quantify ctDNA levels. ddPCR utilizes droplets, which is an individual picoliter chamber for PCR reactions. Due to the ultra-low volume of each partition, the sensitivity in PCR increases with less PCR bias. The ctDNA fragments can be quantified by assessing the fluorescent signals in the droplets. After performing whole genome sequencing of breast cancers to identify tumor-specific chromosomal rearrangements, or molecular "fingerprints" of each tumor, Olsson et al. used ddPCR to identify ctDNA and monitor breast cancer patients [23]. The study demonstrated the potential of ctDNA identified by ddPCR for detecting asymptomatic metastasis in breast cancer patients. In contrast to deep sequencing methods, ddPCR allows analysis of structural variation of the genome, but many of the clinically important genetic aberrations for breast cancer have been reported to be single nucleotide variations [6].

Instead of simply identifying and enumerating the abundance of ctDNA fragments, digging out rare mutations from the mixture of DNA fragments provides more insight into the status of cancer patients. Cohen et al. developed CancerSEEK, a blood test comprised of multiplex PCR primers that were optimally designed to detect rare mutations in the cfDNA, and therefore identify the presence of cancers and localize them [22]. This is a very useful tool that can inform us on different types of cancer present in a patient, whom may have asymptomatic early-stage tumor or even metastasis. However, variants are often insufficient to be able to identify and localize the cancer. Kinde et al. developed a technique using Safe-Sequencing System (Safe-SeqS) to analyze rare variants using unique identifiers (UIDs) and solid phase capture. After UIDs are assigned to the DNA fragments, adapters for universal PCR are ligated to the fragments with UIDs. Then fragments of interests are captured via a solid phase containing complementary DNA of interest. Using NGS, these captured fragments are amplified to analyze variants of interest in the fragments. Using Safe-SeqS, Bettegowda et al. showed the potential of ctDNA liquid biopsy for early detection of localized cancers by sequencing clinically important mutation in metastatic breast cancer [57]. They claimed that ctDNA is a broadly applicable biomarker that has clinical potential in various types of cancers. Similarly, McDonald et al. developed targeted digital sequencing (TARDIS) for multiplexed analysis of ctDNA in breast cancer [58]. TARDIS uses barcoding methods similar to Safe-SeqS, but instead uses hairpin adapters with UMIs and target-specific primers to increase specificity in ctDNA analysis. The authors claim that they have achieved 100-fold better sensitivity than the current limit of detection of ctDNAs. They showed that TARDIS-detected rare variant burden was associated with residual disease after neoadjuvant therapy in breast cancer. However, the DNA barcode-based methods have limitations that when an NGS error occurs in approximately 1%, additional methods for distinguishing the true variant from false ones must be complemented.

11.2.4 Sampling Primary Cells: Drug Screening Technologies in Breast Cancer

Advances in sequencing technology have contributed in detecting somatic mutations in tumors for sophisticated target identification and discovering effective targeted therapies. However, only a small percentage of cancer patients are treated according to the identification of specific genetic mutations [59]. Furthermore, responses to targeted therapies among genetically defined patients are inconsistent. Since the causality and correlation between tumor genetics and drug responses is yet to be understood in detail, there are limitations in matching appropriate treatment with genetic mutations. Functional screening of primary cancer cells biopsied from the tumor of patients may have the potential to overcome current limitation of predicting drug response if it can be utilized together, not just depending on genetics-based strategies [60]. In leukemia and other hematological malignancies, for example, functional drug screening using primary cancer cells from patients offers a tractable clinical value for predicting response since it is relatively easy to obtain a large number of viable cancer cells. Several groups have reported high-throughput screening using primary cancer cells from leukemia patients for translational approaches and, in some cases, correlated them to patient responses [61].

In addition, combinatorial drug screening with patient-derived cells is considered as one of only few solutions for patients with highly progressive disease with acquired resistance [62]. Treating diseases with multiple drugs leads to more complex and elaborate cellular pathway regulation. For patients who no longer show therapeutic response to conventional single drug, it is important to find drug combinations showing therapeutic effect and it is mostly done by large-scale screening of the candidate library of anticancer drugs with patient-derived cells. However, it is currently not generally utilized in the clinic due to low accessibility and technical limitations of current screening technologies. Although personalized drug screening is considered as one of the primary objectives for next-generation cancer therapy, following reasons are hindering its widespread use.

Patients presenting with metastatic disease mostly undergo a diagnostic needle biopsy rather than surgical resection. However, the number of cells from biopsy samples, typically 10^6 cells or less, is insufficient to obtain clinically meaningful screening results, which would be a major hurdle to test drug response especially when using the conventional 96-well plate based platform [63]. With such small number of samples, the number of drug candidates that can be screened with 96-well plate is normally under ten. Accordingly, it is hard to draw meaningful results because there are numerous combinations to be tested. Furthermore, the 2–6 months' time that is required for the procedure of expanding cell number with established cell lines is not feasible, considering the disease condition of the patient and the possibility of additionally acquired mutations. It is important to screen as many drug candidates as possible using small amount of primary samples with low passage.

Many lab-on-a-chip-based platforms have been developed to find technical solution for the demands to screen with a small quantity of primary cancer cells. It has enabled the screening of many drug candidates with a limited number of cells, but the low accessibility of those platforms makes it difficult for them to be widely used by clinicians or researchers in a clinical laboratory [64]. Lab-on-a-chip-based screening platforms are mainly categorized into two types: microfluidic-based and microarray-based platforms. Microfluidic-based platforms require complex tubing, valves, and microfluidic controllers. These operating systems are usually unfamiliar to clinicians, and the system becomes tremendously complicated as the scale of screening becomes larger. Practically, this type of platform is rarely used for drug screening. In the case of microarray-based platforms, most recently developed technologies have employed a method combining a cell microarray and a drug microarray chip. In most cases, preparing such a microarray demands a number of liquid handling operation steps, and the tiny structures on the chip require highly accurate liquid handling equipment. Therefore, conventional microarray-based screening platforms all need elaborate, automated liquid handling machines, which are difficult to operate and expensive. For these reasons, the majority of worldwide hospitals and small-scale laboratories with limited resources are unable to implement large-scale screening, resulting in slow adoption of these miniaturized drug screening platform.

11.3 Current Evidence and Concepts

11.3.1 Science Behind Translational Research in Breast Cancer, Enabled by Image-Linked Genomics

Understanding the sampled solid tumor is perhaps the most important hurdle to overcome for full realization of translational research in breast cancer. NGS-based single-cell sequencing methods allowed the generation of enormous amount of molecular data in breast cancer, and the efforts to connect the molecular data to the histopathological information have produced many scientific findings, as discussed earlier in this chapter. Especially, because modern oncology lies its basis in histopathological studies, it is important to develop spatially resolved sequencing methodologies to connect the missing link between the histopathological knowledge and the newly generated molecular data. Because histopathological image is often an overview snapshot of a biological process, the molecular data can provide information on what exactly is going on at the genetic level. To link image information to the genomic information, Kim et al. developed a method that is very similar to laser capture microdissection (LCM) technologies [15]. (Fig. 11.2). Phenotype-based high-throughput laser-aided isolation and sequencing (PHLI-seq) utilizes the pulsed laser device to isolate target cells directly from the stained tissue for genomic analysis. The whole genomes within the isolated cells are amplified and analyzed through NGS. Although LCM technologies serve as a powerful tool in dissecting out cells and linking the genetic information to the histopathological information, extensive image-linked genomics with LCM technologies was hindered by two main technological issues. First, for LCM technologies that utilize lasers with low wavelength (i.e., near ultraviolet to ultraviolet (UV)), artifacts are generated in sequencing results. These LCM machines cut out the boundaries of the regions of interest by burning them and the region within is catapulted with the UV beam. The non-ionizing radiation with UV lasers has been reported to cause thymine dimers by forming covalent bonds between the thymine bases [65]. The thymine dimers result in "kinks" and fragmentations in the genome, by which the artifacts in sequencing are generated. Second, for LCM technologies that utilize lasers with high wavelength (i.e., near infrared to infrared (IR)), additional polymeric films are required to melt out regions of interests. Then, the regions of interest are stamped and transferred for analysis. This contact-based transferring method often causes cross-contaminations, hindering precise analysis of single cells or small number of cells. Overall, both types of LCMs require expertise in running the equipment and the selecting process is low throughput. PHLI-seq overcomes the two issues in

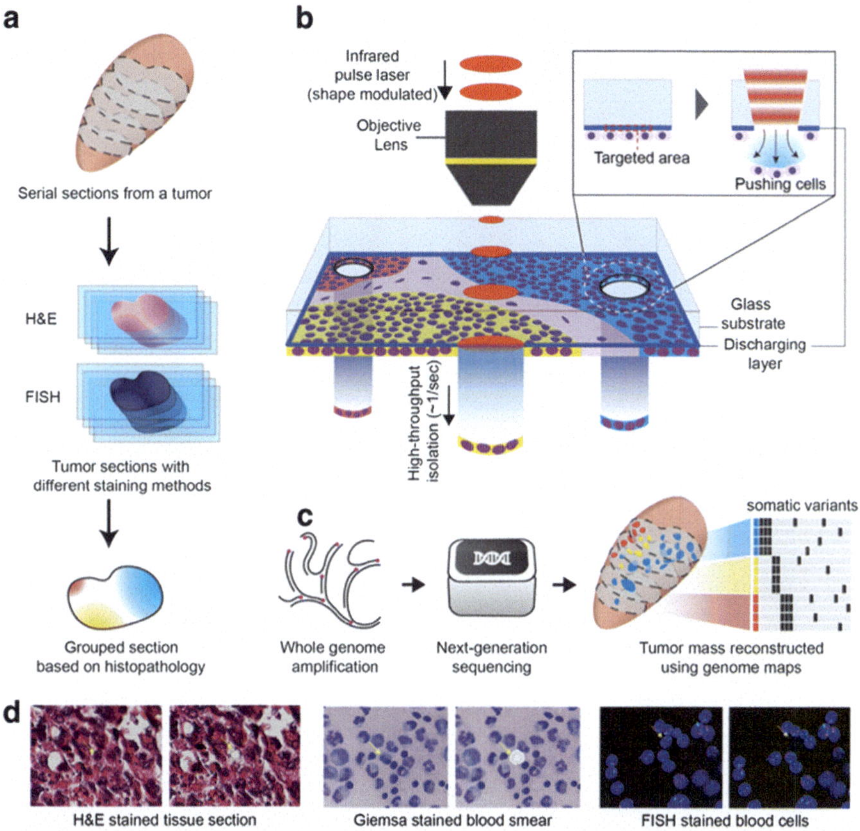

Fig. 11.2 Phenotype-based high-throughput laser-aided isolation and sequencing (PHLI-seq) method by Kim et al. (**a**) Overall workflow for preparation of PHLI-seq. (**b**) Main principle of PHLI-seq. (**c**) Post-processing workflow of PHLI-seq. (**d**) PHLI-seq applied to differently stained tissues. Figure adopted from Kim et al. [15]

conventional LCM methodologies by introducing pulsed laser with near-IR wavelength and indium tin oxide (ITO) sacrificial layer to robustly retrieve single cells in high-throughput (single target isolated in 1 s). The ITO layer serves as a protection layer against thermal damage and a vaporization source to generate light pressure onto the target region of interest. The authors used conventional cell lines to isolate single cells and performed low-depth whole genome sequencing (0.5x) to generate CNAs to validate the sequencing quality. When they compared the CNAs of the single cells isolated by PHLI-seq to those isolated by conventional LCM techniques, PHLI-seq outperformed the conventional LCM techniques. To demonstrate further, the authors applied PHLI-seq to a HR-positive/HER2-positive IDC. The tumor section was fixed with ethanol and stained via hematoxylin and eosin (H&E). With the help of pathologist and a trained pathology informatics algorithm, the tissue section was analyzed and categorized. Then the genomes from the target cells

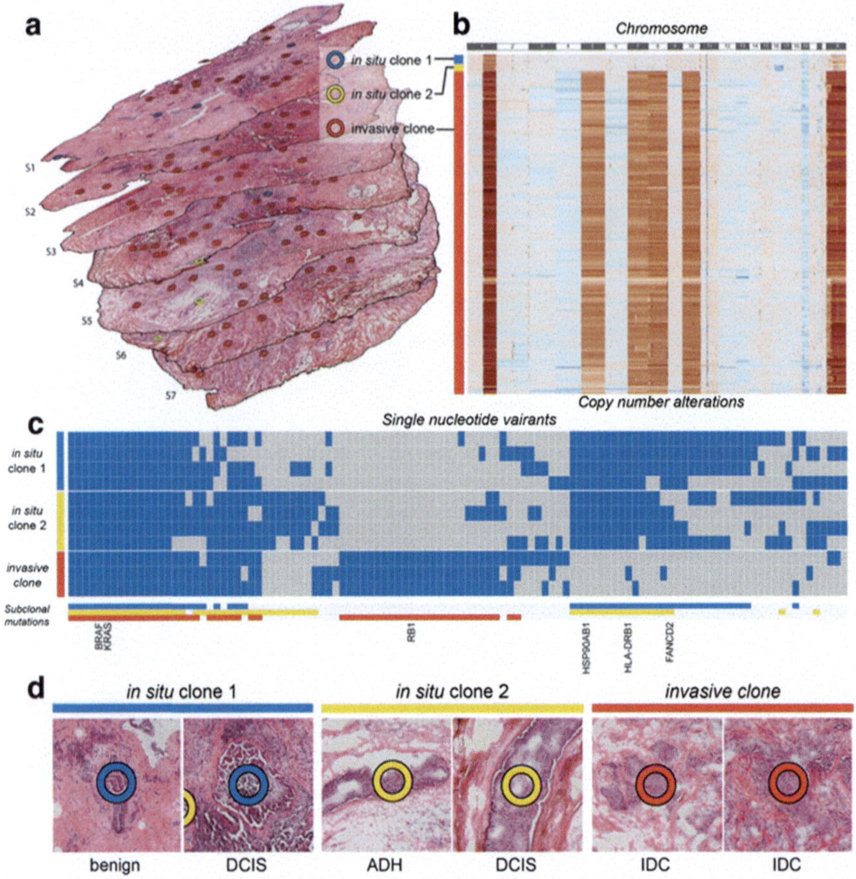

Fig. 11.3 PHLI-seq applied to depict a 3D map of a tumor from a breast cancer patient. (**a**) Serial sections from a tumor mass went through PHLI-seq. (**b**) Copy number alteration profiles of different regions of the tumor. (**c**) Information from single nucleotide variants revealed three intra-tumoral subclones. (**d**) Representative images of the three clones. Figure adopted from Kim et al. [15]

were amplified. The amplified genome samples were divided for three different sequencing purposes: low-depth whole genome sequencing, whole exome sequencing, and high-depth targeted sequencing. The low-depth whole genome sequencing was used to analyze the CNA landscape of the tumor, and whole exome sequencing and high-depth targeted sequencing were used to analyze the SNV landscape. Along with several driver and passenger mutations found from the samples, CNAs were used to discover three different subclones and their evolutionary relationships. Finally, the authors demonstrated application of PHLI-seq in serial tumor sections to display genetic hallmarks within histopathological images that were rendered in 3 dimensions. The H&E stained tissue sections showed evidences of mixed populations of IDC, DCIS, and atypical ductal hyperplasia (ADH). This further supported the theory that DCIS and IDC were developed in a separate divergent manner from a common subclonal ancestor (Fig. 11.3). PHLI-seq therefore effectively analyzes the genomes of small number of cells and links the genetic information to the image information. Serving as the bridge between the molecular biology to image analysis, PHLI-seq has potential to be developed in both ways, especially because novel molecular biology and image analysis methodologies that serve different purposes are explosively increasing.

Laser-induced isolation of micro-structure on optomechanically-transferrable-chip and sequencing (LIMO-seq) developed by the same group that developed PHLI-seq is a tool that analyzes single CTCs (Fig. 11.4) [16]. LIMO-seq also links the image information to the genomic information of the CTCs. Kim et al. fabricated microstructures on top of the ITO glass, building an array of thousands of 100 μm sized micropillars. Then, the micropillars are coated with anti-EpCAM antibodies, on which the CTCs from whole blood sample of a breast cancer patient were captured. The whole chip was imaged in three different fluorescence channels to analyze protein expression levels of cytokeratin (CK) and cluster of differentiation 45 (CD45) and adenine level with 4′,6-diamidino-2-phenylindole (DAPI). This linkage has several advantages in sorting out false positives and connecting protein expression levels to the genome of single CTCs. EpCAM-based enrichment of CTCs is notorious for the high false positive rates. Therefore, if CK and CD45 levels are analyzed, the captures can be distinguished between CTCs and leukocytes. CK levels are highly expressed in cancerous cells while CD45 is a marker for leukocytes. Kim et al. applied LIMO-seq to a whole blood sample from a treatment-naïve 53-year-old metastatic breast cancer patient who was diagnosed with invasive lobular carcinoma with negative ER, PR, and HER2 (Fig. 11.5). The patient had multiple bone metastases to the rib, scapulae, spine, and pelvic bones, as well as intraabdominal lymph nodes that were suggested on positron emission tomography-computed tomography (PET-CT) scan. 44 CTCs were enriched from 5 mL of whole blood and each and every single cells went through LIMO-seq. It produced low-depth whole genome sequencing results from which CNAs were inferred. Also, some of the CTCs went through targeted sequencing to infer SNV data. Although the authors demonstrated LIMO-seq with a simple micropillar array, the strength in this platform lies in the flexibility of the chip design. When the chip design is substituted with that of a different function, rare cells can be enriched via strategies different from immunoaffinity-based capture. Also, the potential for LIMO-seq when combined with different image analysis and molecular biology techniques is even larger. PHLI-seq and LIMO-seq are two examples of other image-linked genetic analyses technologies currently reported [66–68]. These are bimodal analysis techniques (image analysis plus genomic analysis), and when combined with other multi-omics strategy, the modality can be increased, providing larger insights into discovering science of breast cancer.

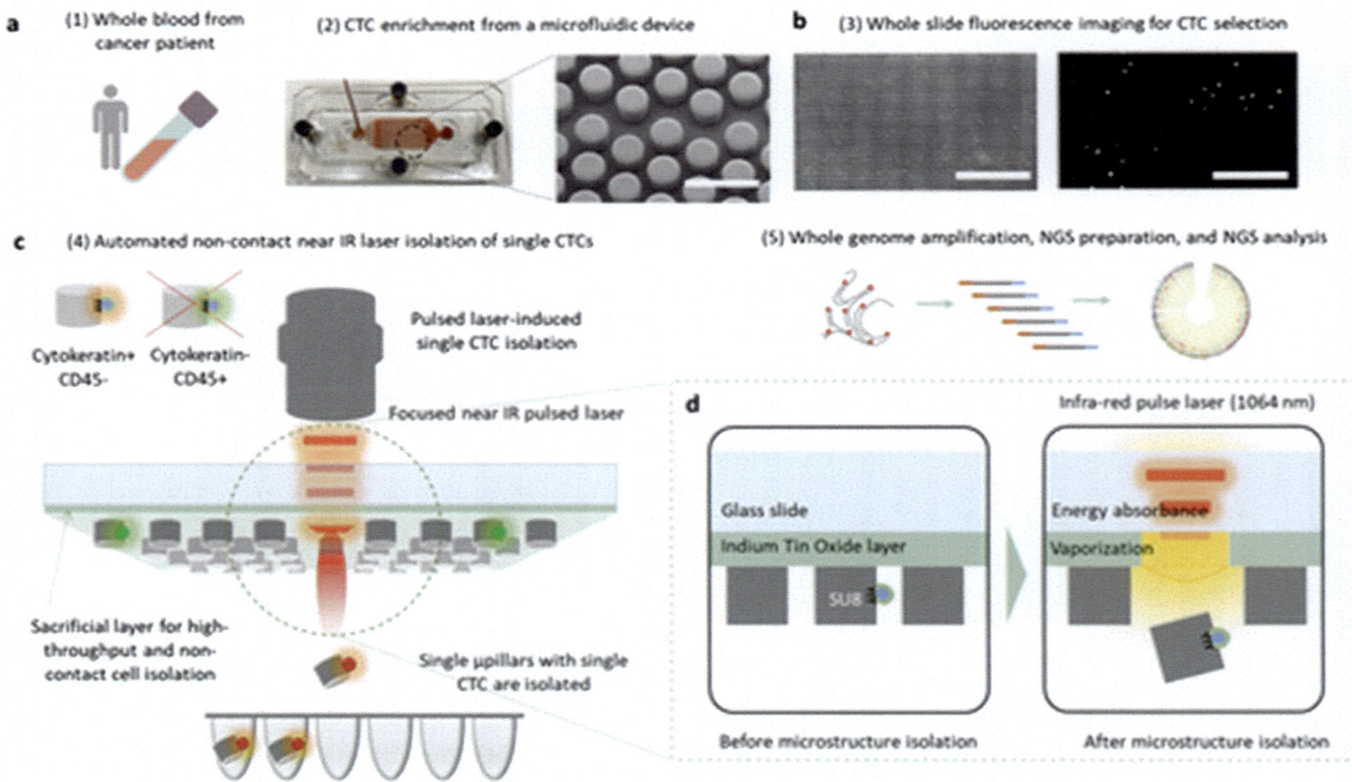

Fig. 11.4 Scheme of laser-induced isolation of microstructures on an optomechanically-transferrable-chip and sequencing (LIMO-seq). (**a**) Whole blood from cancer patient is run through a circulating-tumor-cell (CTC) capturing device. (**b**) Enriched CTCs are imaged with whole slide imaging. (**c**)–(**d**) principles of LIMO-seq. Figure adopted from Kim et al. [16]

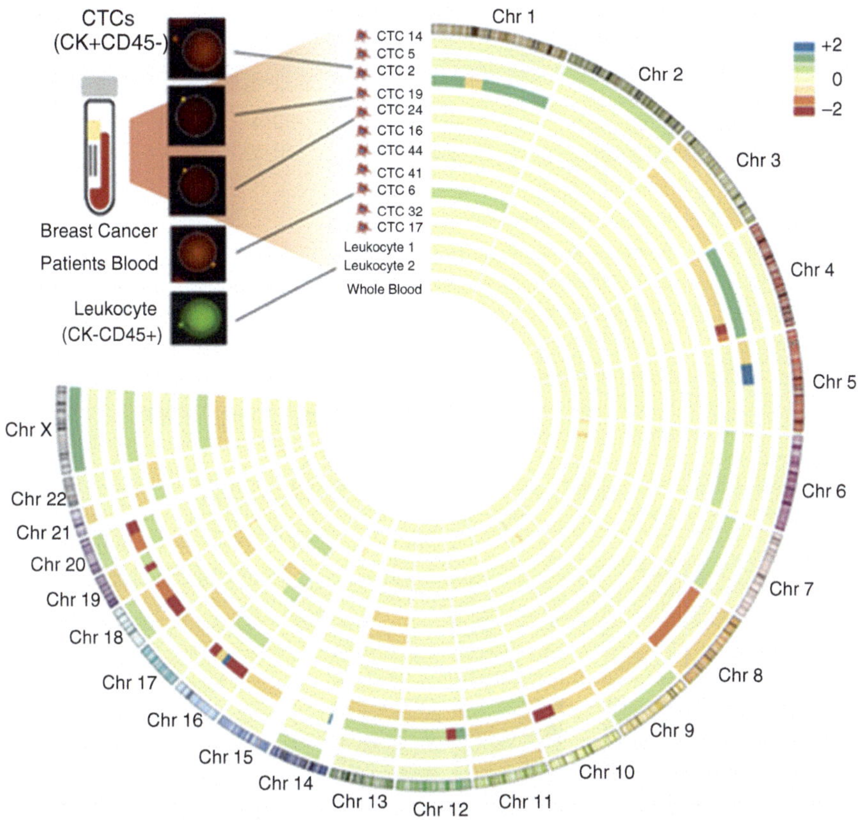

Fig. 11.5 Copy number alteration profiles of CTCs analyzed through LIMO-seq. Figure adopted from Kim et al. [16]

11.3.2 Precision Diagnostics Using Molecular Analysis of CTCs

By sampling peripheral blood, or in other words, by performing liquid biopsy, a less-invasive and therefore more frequent monitoring of cancer patients can be realized. Various strategies that can enrich and analyze CTCs and ctDNAs floating around the vasculature have been proposed by many research groups. One of them is a study by Lee et al., where the authors used immunoaffinity-based CTC capturing strategy and assessed clinically actionable genetic aberrations [69]. As we are beginning to understand some of the relationships between genetic aberrations and clinical information thanks to advances in sequencing technologies, some clinically actionable genetic aberrations are being tested in treating primary and metastatic tumors, and sometimes used in selecting drugs [6]. Therefore, Lee et al. adopted padlock probe-based rolling circle amplification (RCA) strategy to assess DNA mutations and RNA

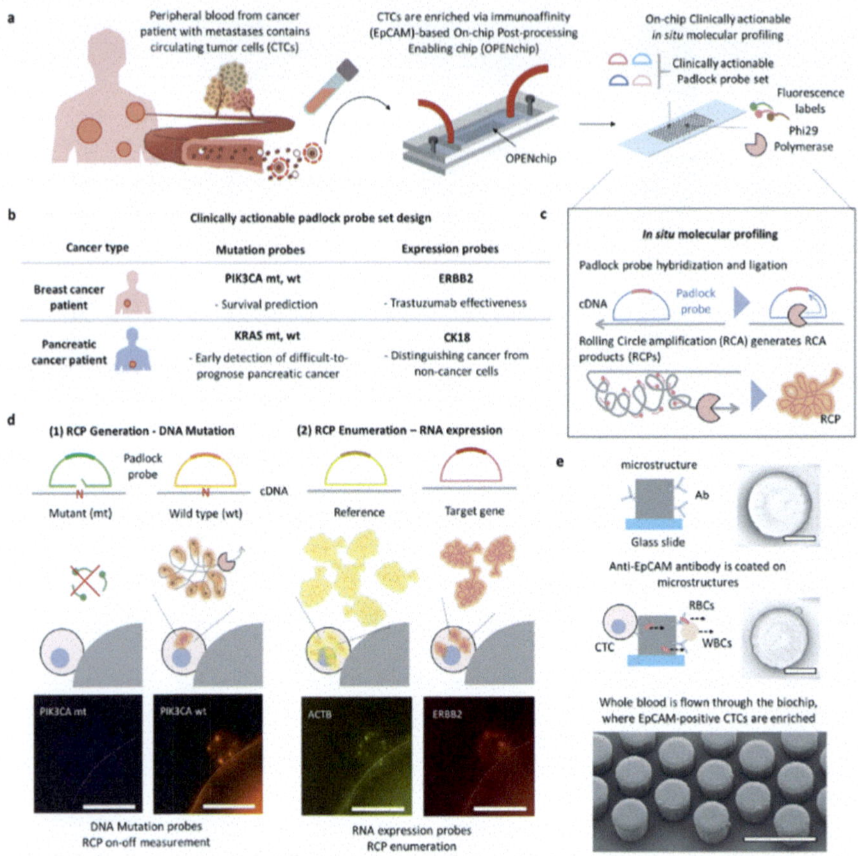

Fig. 11.6 Scheme of on-chip post-processing enabling chip (OPENchip). (**a**) Overall workflow of OPENchip. (**b**) Clinically actionable padlock probe set design for breast and pancreatic cancer patients. (**c**) In situ molecular profiling. (**d**) Rolling circle products (RCP) generated can indicate DNA mutation and RNA expression. (**e**) CTC capturing principle. Figure adopted from Lee et al. [69]

expressions simultaneously in situ (Fig. 11.6). After the CTCs are captured on the micropillars via immunoaffinity, the CTCs are fixed on chip for simultaneous in situ analysis of DNA variant and RNA expressions. Padlock probes, which are single stranded DNA fragments that can hybridize to a target of interest, are attached to mRNAs or genomic DNAs and if the padlock probes are connected, the phi29 polymerase repeatedly amplifies the target region via RCA. If there is a variant at a certain site and therefore bars the padlock probes to be linked, the RCA will not be performed. Therefore, one can test whether there is a DNA variant. Counting the rolling circle amplification product (RCP) will indicate RNA expression levels. To demonstrate, Lee et al. tested for PIK3CA variant and HER2 expression level in CTCs that were captured from whole blood from two breast cancer patients. They first designed the clinically actionable padlock probes and tested tin various cell lines. The results indicated that the epithelial CTCs can represent the primary tumor, from which the CTCs were disseminated. Using this monitoring system will provide a useful tool for precision diagnostics, especially when frequent monitoring can be important for patients with complicated metastasis status.

11.3.3 Precision Diagnostics Using Ultrarare Variant Detection in ctDNAs

The strategy for analyzing ctDNA by NGS is to filter out sequencing error and distinguish true variants (Fig. 11.7). Since NGS error rate is high (0.1–1%), rare variants at a frequency below 1% can be buried by the miscalled bases from NGS error. The source of the NGS is mostly from systematic errors such as de-phasing signal detection, signal cross-talk among DNA clusters, and overlap of emission frequency spectra [70]. It means that when the systematic error occurred during signal detection, the original DNA clusters on the NGS substrate remain unchanged. Therefore, one group approached to validate NGS error by isolating the DNA clusters from NGS substrate and amplifying to perform re-sequencing [71]. They used spike-in DNA libraries (variant frequency ranged from 0.002% to 90%) to verify the erroneous NGS reads, which have unintended variation compared to a reference sequence. Then they isolate the DNA clusters corresponding to the target reads through the laser retrieval system, which separates microscale objects through radiation pressure of a focused pulse laser. As a result, they verified that the true variant of frequency was as low as 0.003% by removing the systematic NGS error. Compared to conventional methods including molecular barcoding deep sequencing, this method could validate selectively only the reads of interest with low depth and reduce sequencing cost by excluding redundant consumption of non-interest NGS reads. In addition, conventional NGS error filtering methods depend on bioinformatics algorithm with the quality score (Q-score) generated by the NGS system itself. However, since the Q-score does not completely reflect NGS errors, a few important reads including critical variants of ctDNA can be removed during data quality control. In this manner, this method does not depend on Q-score because any DNA clusters corresponding to the erroneous reads before data trimming can be isolated and amplified before sequencing. Therefore, this method will be more effective in cases where there are few variant sites with ultrarare frequency such as in ctDNA analysis.

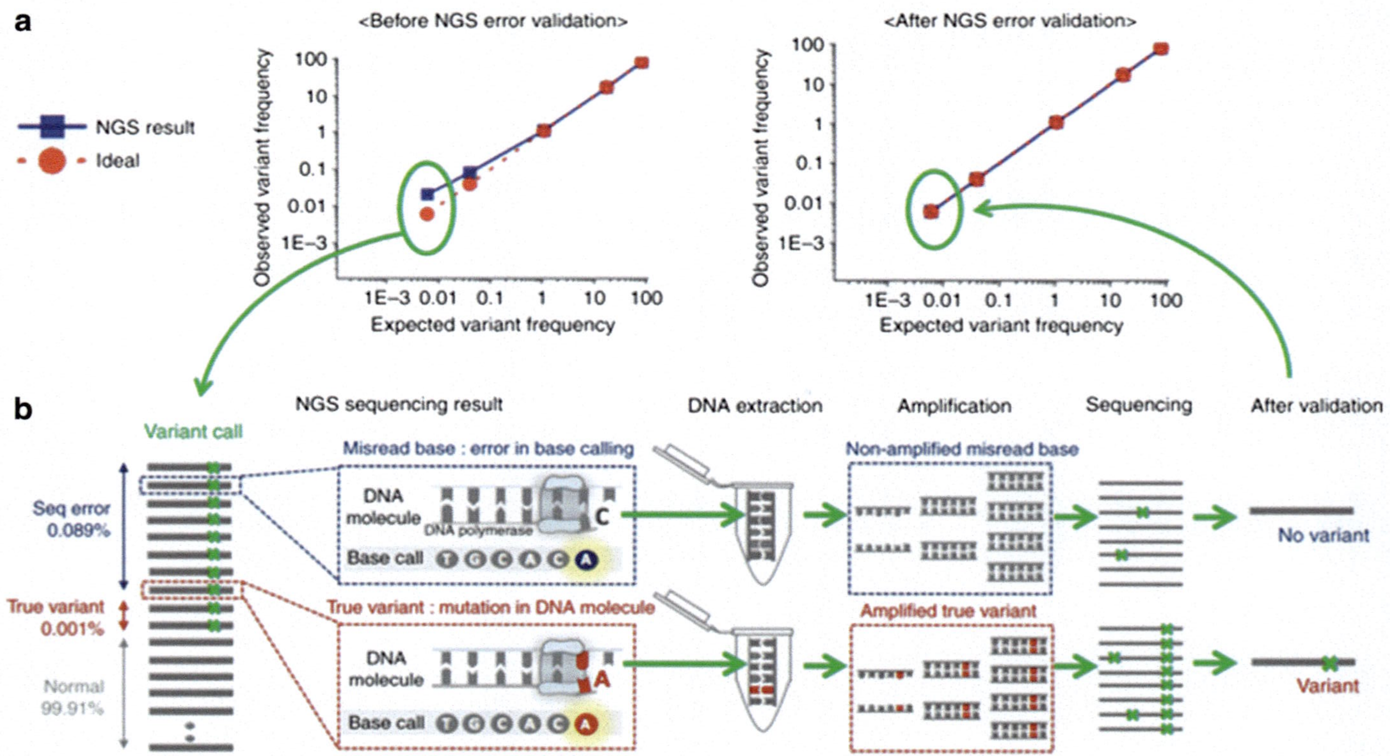

Fig. 11.7 Strategy to validate errors in sequencing results of circulating tumor DNA. (**a**) NGS error validation. (**b**) Strategy to validate the true variant. Figure adopted from Yeom et al. [71]

11.3.4 Precision Therapeutics Using Sequential Treatment Drug Screening

Great advancement on cancer therapy was achieved by genotype-based selection of targeted drugs for precision medicine. For example, tyrosine kinase inhibitors (TKIs) are now well-known and effective targeted drugs for cancers with mutations in *EGFR* (epidermal growth factor receptor) or *ALK* (anaplastic lymphoma kinase) translocations [72, 73]. Within few years, however, the tumor becomes non-responsive to the targeted therapy due to acquired resistance resulting from a variety of mechanisms [62]. For the patients with such a highly resistant cancer, combinatorial drugs enabling more complex and elaborate cellular pathway regulation can be one of the few solutions [74]. Therefore, screening drug combinations with primary cells or patient-derived tumor models from the biopsy samples and prescribing precision medicine based on the screening result has been of interest lately [75–79]. The major challenge here is that such screening generally requires unbiased large-scale screening, while the number of primary cells in the biopsy samples, typically under 10^6 cells, is not enough to test sufficient number of combinations [80]. Song et al. developed a lab-on-a-chip-based drug screening platform which only requires less than a hundred cells and 0.1 microliter of reagents per one reaction [81–83] (Fig. 11.8). They demonstrated a new method for drug treatment by utilizing self-assembly of drug-laden microparticles on the large-scale microarray, thereby removing thousands of pipetting steps and needs for the automated liquid handling machine [81, 84]. This can significantly lower the required cost for installing the high-throughput screening (HTS) platform. The authors demonstrated screening of sequential drug combinations against the highly resistant TNBC cells. Sequential administration of multiple drugs has received much attention recently, because concurrent application of combinatorial drugs increases dose exposure in patients and has potential for serious side effects [85]. Furthermore, recent findings that sequential application of drugs can dynamically modulate the intracellular pathways brighten the way for more powerful and elaborate treatment of resistant cancer with smaller incidence of side effects [74, 86]. Based on the knowledge that pre-treatment with EGFR inhibitors makes TNBC cells vulnerable to DNA-damage, the authors investigated the effect of 45 different combinations of DNA damaging drugs administered following EGFR inhibitor. From the screening results, the combination of erlotinib (ERL) followed by mitoxantrone (MTX) was revealed as the most synergistic sequential combination among the screened combinatorial library. With the technical advantages of the platform, 1600 independent assays on a single chip were possible with only two pipetting steps of drug-laden microparticles and a single step of the drug chip replacement, instead of numerous repeats of pipetting operations. The development of such low-cost and miniaturized HTS platform for primary cell drug screening will pave the way for the precision medicine based on the "personalized-optimal drug screening [87, 88]."

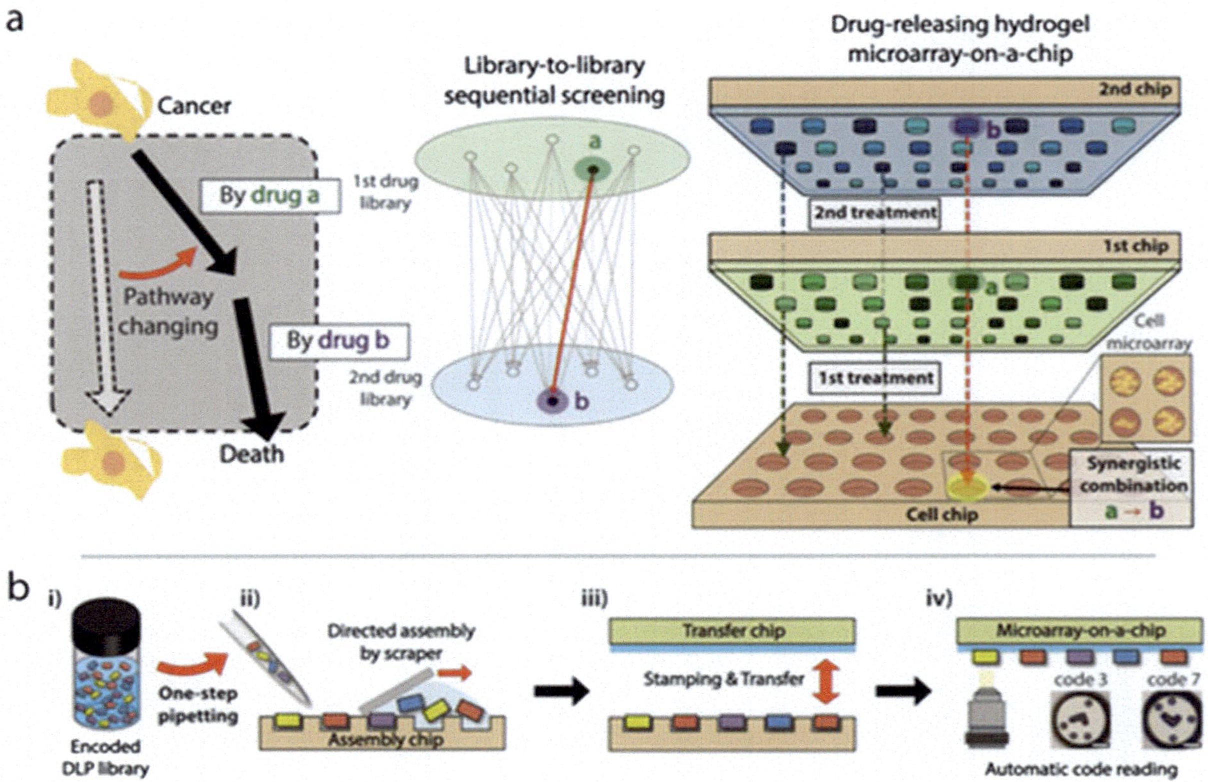

Fig. 11.8 Drug screening strategy using primary cancer cells for sequential treatment. (**a**) Strategy for sequential screening using drug-releasing hydrogel microarray-on-a-chip. (**b**) Overall workflow for construction drug-releasing hydrogel microarray-on-a-chip

11.4 Future Research Direction

Development in various molecular analysis strategies in genomics, transcriptomics, epigenomics, epitranscriptomics, proteomics, metabolomics, connectomics, and phenomics has exponentially increased since the development of NGS. We are beginning to understand breast cancer better as researchers are beginning to integrate two or three of these techniques. In the future, more integrated techniques with smart strategies should be developed in order to investigate and reveal the complexly entangled secrets in breast cancer. scTrio-seq is one example of a futuristic method for analyzing solid tumor in breast cancer [89]. Integrating single-cell whole genome bisulfite sequencing to transcriptome sequencing, Bian et al. reported CNAs, DNA methylation, and transcriptome information in multiregional sequencing of colorectal cancer. Also, Reyes et al. reported simultaneous profiling in gene expression and chromatin accessibility in single cells by integrating assay for transposase-accessible chromatin using sequencing (ATAC-seq) to single-cell RNA sequencing [90]. Alike these efforts, previous arts in integrating epigenomics to RNA expressions and genomic information have revealed intra-tumoral heterogeneity [91, 92]. If these efforts can further be integrated with spatially resolved technologies such as sequencing-based [66, 93] or in situ-based [67, 94, 95] techniques, our understanding in breast cancer in terms of its development, evolution, metastasis, diagnosis, and therapeutics will be augmented. As a specific example, assessing function and development of tumor-infiltrating lymphocytes [12, 96] that exist among different subclones in breast cancer will not only lead to development of tumor-targeting drugs (e.g., chimeric antigen receptor T cells), but also open up novel liquid biopsy target for breast cancer patients.

Along with the development in molecular technologies, liquid biopsy is emerging as a precise sampling method as an alternative to solid tumor biopsy. In the near future, thorough investigation in relationship between CTCs and their metastatic propensity will aid in targeting CTCs with metastatic potential. Few translational researches have begun to touch on EMT, mesenchymal-to-epithelial transition (MET), mechanical induction of stemness of CTCs, and CTC clustering [18, 19, 39, 97–99]. It seems that various cues work together to induce the metastatic potential of the disseminated CTCs, and when integrated with the solid tumor development studies, these investigations will provide powerful insights into how we can prevent metastasis. Also, capturing CTCs in a non-specific way will have to be developed [100]. A specific example of high potential is the use of VAR2CSA protein, originally expressed on the surface of malaria-causing *plasmodium*. These bacteria are known to have affinity against cancer cells, and few reports have investigated the use of VAR2CSA protein in capturing CTCs [101, 102]. For ctDNAs, more thorough clinical investigations must take place for interventional clinical trials [103]. Araujo et al. describe few examples of clinical trials concerning subjects without cancer but are at high risk, subjects with minimal residual disease post curative treatment, and subjects with advanced cancer. Although we mainly discussed CTC and ctDNA as possible candidates for translational medicine, miRNA, exosomes, tumor-educated platelets or immune cells also need to be investigated further for possibly better sources for clinical use [20, 99, 104, 105]. Taken together, a simple draw of blood will produce maximal insights into the subject status regarding breast cancer.

Making treatment decisions for cancer patients, or drug screening, by utilizing patient primary cells will also need to be integrated with the cutting-edge molecular analysis methods. As many strategies in combinatorial and sequential treatment on breast cancer are being developed, finding effective drugs in vitro by simply screening live or dead cells will be insufficient. Therefore, the next step toward drug screening methods lies in monitoring the changes in functional level by observing gene expression pattern changes. In situ sequencing methods enable observing the genetic effect of the small molecule drugs and therefore will provide insights into how the drugs work fundamentally, in terms of cellular mechanism. In situ profiling methods enable the genetic analysis of small molecule drugs in parallel. When combined with biochip, drug screening through high-throughput gene expression analysis on patient-derived cells would be possible and therefore provide insights into how drugs work fundamentally (i.e., mechanism of action (MOA)) in terms of cellular mechanism. This will guide better understanding of the biology of breast cancer.

11.5 Conclusion

Breast cancer can be devastating and is one of the most important issues in women's health. However, breast cancer is a very complex disease with many secrets not yet revealed. Advances in sequencing technologies and their strategic applications in scientific investigations, diagnostic tools, and therapeutic decision are actively being translated into the clinic and more are yet to come. In this chapter, we discussed different strategies for the translational medicine in breast cancer in terms of solid tumor, peripheral blood, and primary cell sampling methods. When these methods meet cutting-edge molecular analysis methods, experimental findings that were not discovered before the advancement of sequencing technologies can be realized on a daily basis. As discussed in future directions section of this chapter, a great variety of experimental methods and tools are available, enabling researchers to customize their studies according to their interests. Through development and integration of sequencing-based tools, we envision that the innovational translational researches in breast cancer will significantly contribute in promoting women's health and eventually human health.

References

1. The Cancer Genome Atlas Research Network. Comprehensive genomic characterization defines human glioblastoma genes and core pathways. Nature. 2008;455(7216):1061–8. http://www.nature.com/articles/nature07385
2. Kandoth C, McLellan MD, Vandin F, Ye K, Niu B, Lu C, et al. Mutational landscape and significance across 12 major cancer types. Nature. 2013;502(7471):333–9.
3. The Cancer Genome Atlas. Comprehensive molecular portraits of human breast tumours. Nature. 2012;490(7418):61–70.
4. Navin N, Kendall J, Troge J, Andrews P, Rodgers L, McIndoo J, et al. Tumour evolution inferred by single-cell sequencing. Nature. 2011;472(7341):90–4. https://doi.org/10.1038/nature09807.
5. Ciriello G, Gatza ML, Beck AH, Wilkerson MD, Rhie SK, Pastore A, et al. Comprehensive molecular portraits of invasive lobular breast Cancer. Cell. 2015;163(2):506–19.
6. El-Deiry WS, Goldberg RM, Lenz H, Shields AF, Gibney GT, Tan AR, et al. The current state of molecular testing in the treatment of patients with solid tumors. Cancer J Clin. 2019;69:305–43.
7. Casasent A, Edgerton M, Navin NE. Genome evolution in ductal carcinoma in situ: invasion of the clones. J Pathol. 2016;241(2):208–18.
8. Singh M, Al-Eryani G, Carswell S, Ferguson JM, Blackburn J, Barton K, et al. High-throughput targeted long-read single cell sequencing reveals the clonal and transcriptional landscape of lymphocytes. Nat Commun. 2019;10(1):3120.
9. Eirew P, Steif A, Khattra J, Ha G, Yap D, Farahani H, et al. Dynamics of genomic clones in breast cancer patient xenografts at single-cell resolution. Nature. 2014;518:422–6. https://doi.org/10.1038/nature13952.
10. Janiszewska M, Liu L, Almendro V, Kuang Y, Paweletz C, Sakr RA, et al. In situ single-cell analysis identifies heterogeneity for PIK3CA mutation and HER2 amplification in HER2-positive breast cancer. Nat Genet. 2015;47(10):1212–9. https://doi.org/10.1038/ng.3391.
11. Azizi E, Carr AJ, Plitas G, Cornish AE, Konopacki C, Prabhakaran S, et al. Single-cell map of diverse immune phenotypes in the breast tumor microenvironment. Cell. 174(5):1293–308.
12. Chung W, Eum HH, Lee H-O, Lee K-M, Lee H-B, Kim K-T, et al. Single-cell RNA-seq enables comprehensive tumour and immune cell profiling in primary breast cancer. Nat Commun. 2017;5(8):15081.
13. McGinnis CS, Patterson DM, Winkler J, Conrad DN, Hein MY, Srivastava V, et al. MULTI-seq: sample multiplexing for single-cell RNA sequencing using lipid-tagged indices. Nat Methods. 2019;17:1.
14. Kim K-T, Lee HW, Lee H-O, Kim SC, Seo YJ, Chung W, et al. Single-cell mRNA sequencing identifies subclonal heterogeneity in anti-cancer drug responses of lung adenocarcinoma cells. Genome Biol. 2015;16(1):127.
15. Kim S, Lee AC, Lee H-B, Kim J, Jung Y, Ryu HS, et al. PHLI-seq: constructing and visualizing cancer genomic maps in 3D by phenotype-based high-throughput laser-aided isolation and sequencing. Genome Biol. 2018;19(1):158.
16. Kim O, Lee D, Chungwon Lee A, Lee Y, Bae HJ, Lee H-B, et al. Whole genome sequencing of single circulating tumor cells isolated by applying a pulsed laser to cell-capturing micro-structures. Small. 2019;26:1902607.
17. Ashworth TR. A case of cancer in which cells similar to those in the tumours were seen in the blood after death. Aust Med J. 2017;14:146.
18. Gorges TM, Tinhofer I, Drosch M, Röse L, Zollner TM, Krahn T, et al. Circulating tumour cells escape from EpCAM-based detection due to epithelial-to-mesenchymal transition. BMC Cancer. 2012;12(1):178.
19. Maheswaran S, Haber DA. Cell fate: Transition loses its invasive edge. Nature. 2015;52:10–1.

20. Gorgannezhad L, Umer M, Islam MN, Nguyen N-T, MJA S. Circulating tumor DNA and liquid biopsy: opportunities, challenges, and recent advances in detection technologies. Lab Chip. 2018;18(8):1174–96.
21. Dawson S-J, Tsui DWY, Murtaza M, Biggs H, Rueda OM, Chin S-F, et al. Analysis of circulating Tumor DNA to monitor metastatic breast Cancer. N Engl J Med. 2013;368 (13):1199–209.
22. Cohen JD, Li L, Wang Y, Thoburn C, Afsari B, Danilova L, et al. Detection and localization of surgically resectable cancers with a multi-analyte blood test. Science. 2018;359 (6378):926–30.
23. Olsson E, Winter C, George A, Chen Y, Howlin J, Tang ME, et al. Serial monitoring of circulating tumor DNA in patients with primary breast cancer for detection of occult metastatic disease. EMBO Mol Med. 2015;7(8):1034–47.
24. Herzenberg LA, Sweet RG, Herzenberg LA. Fluorescence-activated cell sorting. In: Scientific American, vol. 234. New York: Scientific American, a division of Nature America; 1976. p. 108–18.
25. Telenius H, Carter NP, Bebb CE, Nordenskjold M, BAJ P, Tunnacliffe A. Degenerate oligonucleotide-primed PCR: General amplification of target DNA by a single degenerate primer. Genomics. 1992;13(3):718–25.
26. Gao R, Davis A, McDonald TO, Sei E, Shi X, Wang Y, et al. Punctuated copy number evolution and clonal stasis in triple-negative breast cancer. Nat Genet. 2016;48:1–15.
27. Rakha EA, Reis-Filho JS, Ellis IO. Basal-like breast cancer: a critical review. J Clin Oncol. 2008;26(15):2568–81.
28. Foulkes WD, Smith IE, Reis-Filho JS. Triple-negative breast cancer. N Engl J Med. 2010;363 (20):1938–48.
29. Hollestelle A, Elstrodt F, Nagel JH. a, Kallemeijn WW, Schutte M. Phosphatidylinositol-3-OH kinase or RAS pathway mutations in human breast cancer cell lines. Mol Cancer Res. 2007;5 (2):195–201.
30. Yates LR, Gerstung M, Knappskog S, Desmedt C, Gundem G, Van Loo P, et al. Subclonal diversification of primary breast cancer revealed by multiregion sequencing. Nat Med. 2015;21(7):751–9.
31. Casasent AK, Edgerton M, Navin NE. Genome evolution in ductal carcinoma in situ : invasion of the clones. J Pathol. 2017;241:208–18.
32. Casasent AK, Schalck A, Gao R, Sei E, Long A, Pangburn W, et al. Multiclonal invasion in breast tumors identified by topographic single cell sequencing. Cell. 2018;172(1–2):205–17.
33. Baccelli I, Schneeweiss A, Riethdorf S, Stenzinger A, Schillert A, Vogel V, et al. Identification of a population of blood circulating tumor cells from breast cancer patients that initiates metastasis in a xenograft assay. Nat Biotechnol. 2013;31(6):539–44. Available from: http://www.nature.com/articles/nbt.2576
34. Andree KC, van Dalum G, LWMM T. Challenges in circulating tumor cell detection by the cell search system. Mol Oncol. 2016;10(3):395–407.
35. Cristofanilli M, Budd GT, Ellis MJ, Stopeck A, Matera J, Miller MC, et al. Circulating tumor cells, disease progression, and survival in metastatic breast cancer. N Engl J Med. 2004;351 (8):781–91.
36. Nagrath S, Sequist LV, Maheswaran S, Bell DW, Irimia D, Ulkus L, et al. Isolation of rare circulating tumour cells in cancer patients by microchip technology. Nature. 2007;450 (7173):1235–9.
37. Stott SL, Hsu C-H, Tsukrov DI, Yu M, Miyamoto DT, Waltman BA, et al. isolation of circulating tumor cells using a microvortex-generating herringbone-chip. Proc Natl Acad Sci U S A. 2010;107(43):18392–7.
38. Aceto N, Bardia A, Miyamoto DT, Donaldson MC, Wittner BS, Spencer JA, et al. Circulating tumor cell clusters are oligoclonal precursors of breast cancer metastasis. Cell. 2014;158 (5):1110–22.

39. Lamouille S, Xu J, Derynck R. Molecular mechanisms of epithelial–mesenchymal transition. Nat Rev Mol Cell Biol. 2014;15(3):178–96.
40. Zhang L, Ridgway LD, Wetzel MD, Ngo J, Yin W, Kumar D, et al. The identification and characterization of breast cancer CTCs competent for brain metastasis. Sci Transl Med. 2013;5 (180):180ra48.
41. Sollier E, Go DE, Che J, Gossett DR, O'Byrne S, Weaver WM, et al. Size-selective collection of circulating tumor cells using vortex technology. Lab Chip. 2014;14(1):63–77.
42. Kidess-Sigal E, Liu HE, Triboulet MM, Che J, Ramani VC, Visser BC, et al. Enumeration and targeted analysis of KRAS, BRAF and PIK3CA mutations in CTCs captured by a label-free platform: Comparison to ctDNA and tissue in metastatic colorectal cancer. Oncotarget. 2016;7 (51):85349–64.
43. Che J, Yu V, Dhar M, Renier C, Matsumoto M, Heirich K, et al. Classification of large circulating tumor cells isolated with ultra-high throughput microfluidic Vortex technology. Oncotarget. 2016;7(11):12748–60.
44. Dhar M, Pao E, Renier C, Go DE, Che J, Montoya R, et al. Label-free enumeration, collection and downstream cytological and cytogenetic analysis of circulating tumor cells. Sci Rep. 2016;6(1):35474.
45. Ramani VC, Lemaire CA, Triboulet M, Casey KM, Heirich K, Renier C, et al. Investigating circulating tumor cells and distant metastases in patient-derived orthotopic xenograft models of triple-negative breast cancer. Breast Cancer Res. 2019;21(1):98.
46. Gkountela S, Castro-Giner F, Szczerba BM, Vetter M, Landin J, Scherrer R, et al. Circulating tumor cell clustering shapes DNA methylation to enable metastasis seeding. Cell. 2019;176 (1–2):98–112.
47. Vetter M, Landin J, Szczerba BM, Castro-Giner F, Gkountela S, Donato C, et al. Denosumab treatment is associated with the absence of circulating tumor cells in patients with breast cancer. Breast Cancer Res. 2018;20(1):141.
48. Shaw Bagnall J, Byun S, Begum S, Miyamoto DT, Hecht VC, Maheswaran S, et al. Deformability of tumor cells versus blood cells. Sci Rep. 2015;5:18542.
49. Faraghat SA, Hoettges KF, Steinbach MK, van der Veen DR, Brackenbury WJ, Henslee EA, et al. High-throughput, low-loss, low-cost, and label-free cell separation using electrophysiology-activated cell enrichment. Proc Natl Acad Sci U S A. 2017;114 (18):4591–6.
50. Cheng Y-H, Chen Y-C, Lin E, Brien R, Jung S, Chen Y-T, et al. Hydro-Seq enables contamination-free high-throughput single-cell RNA-sequencing for circulating tumor cells. Nat Commun. 2019;10(1):2163.
51. Zhao L, Lu YT, Li F, Wu K, Hou S, Yu J, et al. High-purity prostate circulating tumor cell isolation by a polymer nanofiber-embedded microchip for whole exome sequencing. Adv Mater. 2013;25(21):2897–902.
52. Ozkumur E, Shah AM, Ciciliano JC, Emmink BL, Miyamoto DT, Brachtel E, et al. Inertial focusing for tumor antigen-dependent and -independent sorting of rare circulating tumor cells. Sci Transl Med. 2013;5(179):179ra47.
53. Lin M, Chen J-F, Lu Y-T, Zhang Y, Song J, Hou S, et al. Nanostructure embedded microchips for detection, isolation, and characterization of circulating tumor cells. Acc Chem Res. 2014;47(10):2941–50.
54. Jiang R, Lu Y, Ho H, Li B, Chen J, Lin M, et al. (2015) A comparison of isolated circulating tumor cells and tissue biopsies using whole-genome sequencing in prostate cancer. Oncotarget
55. Alix-Panabieres C, Schwarzenbach H, Pantel K. Circulating tumor cells and circulating tumor DNA. Annu Rev Med. 2012;63:199–215.
56. Elazezy M, Joosse SA. Techniques of using circulating tumor DNA as a liquid biopsy component in cancer management. Comput Struct Biotechnol J. 2018;16:370.
57. Bettegowda C, Sausen M, Leary RJ, Kinde I, Wang Y, Agrawal N, et al. Detection of circulating tumor DNA in early- and late-stage human malignancies. Sci Transl Med. 2014;6(224):224ra24.

58. McDonald BR, Contente-Cuomo T, Sammut S-J, Odenheimer-Bergman A, Ernst B, Perdigones N, et al. Personalized circulating tumor DNA analysis to detect residual disease after neoadjuvant therapy in breast cancer. Sci Transl Med. 2019;11(504):eaax7392.
59. Dienstmann R, Jang IS, Bot B, Friend S, Guinney J. Database of genomic biomarkers for cancer drugs and clinical targetability in solid tumors. Cancer Discov. 2015;5(2):118–23.
60. Friedman AA, Letai A, Fisher DE, Flaherty KT. Precision medicine for cancer with next-generation functional diagnostics. Nat Rev Cancer. 2015;15:747–56.
61. Pemovska T, Kontro M, Yadav B, Edgren H, Eldfors S, Szwajda A, et al. Individualized systems medicine strategy to tailor treatments for patients with chemorefractory acute myeloid leukemia. Cancer Discov. 2013;3(12):1416–29.
62. Crystal AS, Shaw AT, Sequist LV, Friboulet L, Niederst MJ, Lockerman EL, et al. Patient-derived models of acquired resistance can identify effective drug combinations for cancer. Science. 2014;346(6216):1480–6.
63. Rajer M, Kmet M. Quantitative analysis of fine needle aspiration biopsy samples. Radiol Oncol. 2005;39(4):269–72.
64. Shirure VS, Bi Y, Curtis MB, Lezia A, Goedegebuure MM, Goedegebuure SP, et al. Tumor-on-a-chip platform to investigate progression and drug sensitivity in cell lines and patient-derived organoids. Lab Chip. 2018;18(23):3687–702.
65. Shibai A, Takahashi Y, Ishizawa Y, Motooka D, Nakamura S, Ying B-W, et al. Mutation accumulation under UV radiation in Escherichia coli. Sci Rep. 2017;7(1):14531.
66. Rodriques SG, Stickels RR, Goeva A, Martin CA, Murray E, Vanderburg CR, et al. Slide-seq: A scalable technology for measuring genome-wide expression at high spatial resolution. Science. 2019;363(6434):1463–7.
67. Ke R, Mignardi M, Pacureanu A, Svedlund J, Botling J, Wählby C, et al. In situ sequencing for RNA analysis in preserved tissue and cells. Nat Methods. 2013;10(9):857–60.
68. Nichterwitz S, Chen G, Aguila Benitez J, Yilmaz M, Storvall H, Cao M, et al. Laser capture microscopy coupled with Smart-seq2 for precise spatial transcriptomic profiling. Nat Commun. 2016;7(1):12139.
69. Lee AC, Svedlund J, Darai E, Lee Y, Lee D, Lee HB, et al. OPENchip: an on-chip: in situ molecular profiling platform for gene expression analysis and oncogenic mutation detection in single circulating tumour cells. Lab Chip. 2020;20(5):912–22.
70. Laehnemann D, Borkhardt A, McHardy AC. Denoising DNA deep sequencing data-high-throughput sequencing errors and their correction. Brief Bioinform. 2016;17(1):154–79.
71. Yeom H, Lee Y, Ryu T, Noh J, Lee AC, Lee H-B, et al. Barcode-free next-generation sequencing error validation for ultra-rare variant detection. Nat Commun. 2019;10(1):977.
72. Rosell R, Carcereny E, Gervais R, Vergnenegre A, Massuti B, Felip E, et al. Erlotinib versus standard chemotherapy as first-line treatment for European patients with advanced EGFR mutation-positive non-small-cell lung cancer (EURTAC): a multicentre, open-label, randomised phase 3 trial. Lancet Oncol. 2012 Mar;13(3):239–46.
73. Kwak EL, Bang YJ, Camidge DR, Shaw AT, Solomon B, Maki RG, et al. Anaplastic lymphoma kinase inhibition in non-small-cell lung cancer. N Engl J Med. 2010 Oct;363(18):1693–703.
74. Koplev S, Longden J, Ferkinghoff-Borg J, Bjerregård MB, Cox TR, Janine T. Erler, et al. Dynamic rearrangement of cell states detected by systematic screening of sequential anticancer treatments. Cell Rep. 2017 Sep;20(12):2784–91.
75. Hidalgo M, Amant F, Biankin AV, Budinská E, Byrne AT, Caldas C, et al. Patient-derived Xenograft models: an emerging platform for translational cancer research. Cancer Discov. 2014;4(9):998–1013.
76. Vlachogiannis G, Hedayat S, Vatsiou A, Jamin Y, Fernández-Mateos J, Khan K, et al. Patient-derived organoids model treatment response of metastatic gastrointestinal cancers. Science. 2018;359(6378):920–6.

77. Kim M, Mun H, Sung CO, Cho EJ, Jeon H-J, Chun S-M, et al. Patient-derived lung cancer organoids as in vitro cancer models for therapeutic screening. Nat Commun. 2019 Dec;10 (1):3991.
78. Wong AHH, Li H, Jia Y, Mak PI, Martins RPDS, Liu Y, et al. Drug screening of cancer cell lines and human primary tumors using droplet microfluidics. Sci Rep. 2017;7(1):1–15. https://doi.org/10.1038/s41598-017-08831-z.
79. Carstens MR, Fisher RC, Acharya AP, Butterworth EA, Scott E, Huang EH, et al. Drug-eluting microarrays to identify effective chemotherapeutic combinations targeting patient-derived cancer stem cells. Proc Natl Acad Sci U S A. 2015 Jul;112(28):8732–7.
80. Song SW. Introduction. In: One-step generation of a drug-releasing microarray for high-throughput small-volume bioassays. Singapore: Springer; 2019. p. 1–11.
81. Song SW, Kim SD, Oh DY, Lee Y, Lee AC, Jeong Y, et al. One-step generation of a drug-releasing hydrogel microarray-on-a-chip for large-scale sequential drug combination screening. Adv Sci. 2018;6(3):1801380. https://doi.org/10.1002/advs.201801380.
82. Song SW. One-step generation of a drug-releasing microarray for high-throughput small-volume bioassays. Singapore: Springer; 2019.
83. Song SW. System development. In: One-step generation of a drug-releasing microarray for high-throughput small-volume bioassays. Singapore: Springer; 2019. p. 13–40.
84. Song Y, Jeong Y, Kwon T, Lee D, Oh DY, Park T-J, et al. Liquid-capped encoded microcapsules for multiplex assays. Lab Chip. 2017;17(3):429–37.
85. Dear RF, McGeechan K, Jenkins MC, Barratt A, Tattersall MH, Wilcken N. Combination versus sequential single agent chemotherapy for metastatic breast cancer. Cochrane Database Syst Rev. 2013;3(5):3–8.
86. Lee MJ, Ye AS, Gardino AK, Heijink AM, Sorger PK, MacBeath G, et al. Sequential application of anticancer drugs enhances cell death by rewiring apoptotic signaling networks. Cell. 2012;149(4):780–94.
87. Yu M, Bardia A, Aceto N, Bersani F, Madden MW, Donaldson MC, et al. Ex vivo culture of circulating breast tumor cells for individualized testing of drug susceptibility. Science. 2014;345(6193):216–20.
88. Song SW. Conclusion and Discussion. In: One-step generation of a drug-releasing microarray for high-throughput small-volume bioassays. Singapore: Springer; 2019. p. 51–52.
89. Bian S, Hou Y, Zhou X, Li X, Yong J, Wang Y, et al. Single-cell multiomics sequencing and analyses of human colorectal cancer. Science. 2018;362(6418):1060–3.
90. Reyes M, Billman K, Hacohen N, Blainey PC. Simultaneous profiling of gene expression and chromatin accessibility in single cells. Adv Biosyst. 2019;3(11):1900065. Available from: https://onlinelibrary.wiley.com/doi/abs/10.1002/adbi.201900065
91. Viswanathan R, Cheruba E, Cheow LF. DNA Analysis by restriction enzyme (DARE) enables concurrent genomic and epigenomic characterization of single cells. Nucleic Acids Res. 2019;47(19):e122.
92. Cheow LF, Courtois ET, Tan Y, Viswanathan R, Xing Q, Tan RZ, et al. Single-cell multimodal profiling reveals cellular epigenetic heterogeneity. Nat Methods. 2016;13(10):833–6.
93. Vickovic S, Eraslan G, Salmén F, Klughammer J, Stenbeck L, Schapiro D, et al. High-definition spatial transcriptomics for in situ tissue profiling. Nat Methods. 2019;16 (10):987–90.
94. El-Heliebi A, Hille C, Laxman N, Svedlund J, Haudum C, Ercan E, et al. In situ detection and quantification of AR-V7, AR-FL, PSA, and KRAS point mutations in circulating tumor cells. Clin Chem. 2018;64(3):536–46.
95. Wu D, Yan J, Shen X, Sun Y, Thulin M, Cai Y, et al. Profiling surface proteins on individual exosomes using a proximity barcoding assay. Nat Commun. 2019;10(1):3854.
96. Li X, Warren S, Pelekanou V, Wali V, Cesano A, Liu M, et al. Immune profiling of pre- and post-treatment breast cancer tissues from the SWOG S0800 neoadjuvant trial. J Immunother Cancer. 2019;7(1):88.

97. Agnoletto C, Corrà F, Minotti L, Baldassari F, Crudele F, Cook W, et al. Heterogeneity in circulating tumor cells: the relevance of the stem-cell subset. Cancers. 2019;11(4):483.
98. Li Z, Wang Z, Tang Y, Lu X, Chen J, Dong Y, et al. Liquid biopsy-based single-cell metabolic phenotyping of lung cancer patients for informative diagnostics. Nat Commun. 2019;10 (1):3856.
99. Galanzha EI, Menyaev YA, Yadem AC, Sarimollaoglu M, Juratli MA, Nedosekin DA, et al. In vivo liquid biopsy using Cytophone platform for photoacoustic detection of circulating tumor cells in patients with melanoma. Sci Transl Med. 2019;11(496):eaat5857.
100. Raimondi C, Nicolazzo C, Gradilone A, Molecolare DM, Università S. Circulating tumor cells isolation: the "post-EpCAM era". Chin J Cancer Res. 2015;27(5):461–70.
101. Agerbæk MØ, Bang-Christensen SR, Yang M-H, Clausen TM, Pereira MA, Sharma S, et al. The VAR2CSA malaria protein efficiently retrieves circulating tumor cells in an EpCAM-independent manner. Nat Commun. 2018;9(1):3279.
102. Bang-Christensen SR, Pedersen RS, Pereira MA, Clausen TM, Løppke C, Sand NT, et al. Capture and detection of circulating glioma cells using the recombinant VAR2CSA malaria protein. Cells. 2019;8(9):998.
103. Araujo DV, Bratman SV, Siu LL. Designing circulating tumor DNA-based interventional clinical trials in oncology. Genome Med. 2019;11(1):22.
104. Int Veld SGJG, Wurdinger T. Tumor-educated platelets. Blood. 2019;133(22):2359–64.
105. Crowley E, Di Nicolantonio F, Loupakis F, Bardelli A. Liquid biopsy: monitoring cancer-genetics in the blood. Nat Rev Clin Oncol. 2013;10(8):472–84.

Chapter 12
Cancer Stem Cells in the Immune Microenvironment

Dong-Sup Lee and Keunhee Oh

Abstract Cancer stem cells are a subpopulation of cancer cells responsible for the most demanding and aggressive cancer cell phenotypes: therapy resistance, a self-protective feature of stem cells; distant metastasis, requiring anchorage independence for survival in the circulation; and recurrence, which is related to the dormant-active cycling of stem cells. Normal tissues are composed of parenchymal cells, supportive connective components, and cellular disposal systems for removing the products of physiological wear and tear. Cancer stem cells develop from normal counterparts and progressively interact with their microenvironments, modifying and conditioning the cancer microenvironment. Cancer-associated myeloid cells constitute a major element of the cancer microenvironment. During the process of carcinogenesis, cancer stem cells and their intimately associated myeloid cells mutually interact and evolve, such that the cancer cells potentiate the activity of the myeloid cells and, in return, the myeloid cells increase cancer stem cell characteristics. Normal myeloid cells function as key accessory cells to maintain homeostasis in normal tissues and organs; in cancers, these cells co-evolve with the malignant parenchymal cells and are involved in every aspect of cancer cell biology, including proliferation, invasion, distant metastasis, and the development of resistance to therapy. In this way, cancer-associated myeloid cells provide two of the key hallmarks of cancer: evasion of immune destruction and cancer-promoting inflammation.

Keywords Breast cancer · Cancer stem cell · Metastasis · STAT3 · MDSC · Cancer-promoting inflammation

---

D.-S. Lee (✉)
Seoul National University College of Medicine, Seoul, Republic of Korea
e-mail: dlee5522@snu.ac.kr

K. Oh
SillaJen, Inc., Seoul, Republic of Korea

D.-Y. Noh et al. (eds.), *Translational Research in Breast Cancer*, Advances in Experimental Medicine and Biology 1187,
https://doi.org/10.1007/978-981-32-9620-6_12

12.1 Introduction

Ever since the series of seminal papers by John Dick, which sequentially and systematically evaluated and proved the existence of leukemic stem cells in human acute myelogenous leukemia [1–3], the cancer stem cell hypothesis/theory has been tested in every solid cancer [4]. The cancer stem cell theory originally sought to explain cancer heterogeneity [5], and unlike the clonal evolution and stochastic models, which postulated the progressive development and existence of parallel heterogenic cancer cell subpopulations in cancers, the cancer stem cell theory stated that cancers are composed of a hierarchy of cells differentiated from rare cancer stem cells [6–8]. The two key features of stem cells are self-renewal, which maintains the cell entity (permanently), and differentiation, which produces serially differentiated progenitors and mature functioning cells. The criteria for proving the cancer stem cell theory in human cancer involve validating these two key characteristics of stem cells [9]. There are four essential criteria for cancer stem cells: (1) they involve a rare subpopulation among heterogeneous cancer cells; (2) they possess the capacity of in vivo tumorigenesis and correlated characteristics such as the capacity to form tumor spheres, side populations, and drug- and radiation-resistant cells, (3) they repopulate as original heterogeneous cancer cells when reconstituted in an in vivo (model); and (4) they possess the ability to be serially transferred, with a long-lasting (i.e., for generations) self-renewal capacity [9, 10]. Using these criteria, many groups have explored the existence of cancer stem cells in various human cancers. Leukemic stem cells, which completely reveal themselves, even have the long-term repopulating stem cells and short-term repopulating stem cells, as their internal hierarchy among leukemic stem cells [3]. Many studies have attempted to identity the cancer stem cells of solid cancers lacking at least one of the key criteria of cancer stem cells, typically the capacity for serial transfer, which could not be completely reconstituted in an in vivo model system [11–13].

Nevertheless, the cancer stem cell hypothesis/theory is still valid and has provided insight into in vivo cancer biology and led to the development of novel therapeutic interventions [14]. The characteristics of transformed cells, according to the well-known textbook of Weinberg, include loss of contact inhibition (the ability to grow over one another), the ability to grow without attachment to a solid substrate (anchorage independence), the ability to proliferate indefinitely (immortalization), a reduced requirement for mitogenic growth factors, a high saturation density (the ability to accumulate large numbers of cells in a culture dish), the inability to halt proliferation in response to the deprivation of growth factors, and finally and most importantly, the ability to form in vivo tumors [15]. These essential characteristics of cancer cells are reminiscent of the criteria for cancer stem cells, as follows: the most demanding and aggressive cancer cell phenotypes, such as those that are (1) therapy-resistant, which is the self-protective feature of stem cells, (2) distant metastasis, which requires anchorage independence for survival in the circulation, and (3) recurrence, which is related to the dormant-active cycling of stem cells [16–18]. Thus, we herein will consider cancer stem cells as a subpopulation of cancer cells, which show demanding and aggressive phenotypes that need to be treated using innovative interventions.

Because cancer is a malignant counterpart of an organ/tissue, it also consists of key tissue components involving the parenchyma and the connective tissue (i.e., the microenvironment) [19]. Among the essential components of the microenvironment of normal organs/tissues, fibroblasts are prototype connective tissue cells, and extensive interactions between parenchymal epithelial cells and fibroblasts are thus important for tissue organization. The basement membrane, which separates the epithelial and connective tissues and is an essential component of epithelial stem cell niche, is comprised of both components [20]. Cancer stem cells develop from normal counterparts that progressively interact with the microenvironment; this modifies and conditions them, resulting in a cancer microenvironment [21]. Thus, cancer-associated fibroblasts constitute the major element of the cancer microenvironment and have, thus far, been studied most intensively [22, 23].

For organ/tissue homeostasis, proper disposal of wear and tear products of tissue components is crucial [24]. Through the evolution of metazoan, progressive division of labor leads to the emergence of multiple specialized cell types. Further partitioning of primary and supportive functions of a given tissue leads to the appearance of accessory cell types [25]. Sertoli cells in the testis, Schwann cells in the peripheral nervous system, and tissue-resident macrophages, such as osteoclasts in the skeletal system and macrophages in various tissues, are typical examples [26]. Thus, like fibroblasts, tissue macrophages co-evolve with parenchymal epithelial cells, and these intimate interrelationships continue during the process of cancer formation. Thus, myeloid cells function as key accessory cells to maintain the homeostasis of normal organs/tissues [24–26]. In cancer tissues, these cells co-evolve with a malignant counterpart of parenchymal cells and intimately interact with each other during every cancer cell biology process, such as proliferation, invasion, distant metastasis, and the development of resistance to therapy [27, 28]. Inflammatory/immune cancer microenvironments are therefore mainly composed of myeloid cells and incoming adaptive components of the immune system.

12.2 Epithelial Cancer Stem Cells Actively Modulate Immune Microenvironments by Secreting Cytokines

12.2.1 Cytokine-Producing Parenchymal Epithelial Cells Initiate and Control Tissue Inflammatory/Immune Responses

Immune microenvironments are comprised of two key components involving soluble mediators, such as cytokines and chemokines, and inflammatory/immune cells. Interleukins (ILs), the prototypes of cytokines, were first shown to be expressed by white blood cells (leukocytes). Leukocytes were considered the main producers and effectors of cytokine networks; however, this paradigm has changed [29, 30]. Following parenchymal tissue damage by bleomycin, pulmonary epithelial cells initiate inflammatory responses by secreting the key inflammatory cytokine, IL-6, in a transglutaminase 2 (TG2)-NF-κB-dependent manner (Fig. 12.1a) [31]. This response represents a key step in the in situ differentiation of IL-17-producing T cells in the lung, with subsequent inflammatory amplification achieved by recruiting secondary neutrophilic infiltration into the lung, which leads to fibrosis (Fig. 12.1b). The critical role of epithelial cells, but not inflammatory cells, in initiating the inflammatory cascade through secreting cytokine IL-6 was confirmed in a bone marrow chimera study. Chimeras made in TG2-deficient recipients, i.e., lacking the TG2-NF-κB-IL-6 axis in epithelial components, showed reduced inflammation and fibrosis compared with those in wild-type mice, regardless of the bone marrow cell phenotype (Fig. 12.1c) [31].

12.2.2 Cytokine-Producing Malignant Epithelial Cells Show Cancer Stem Cell Characteristics

The critical role of cytokine mediators produced by epithelial cells also applies to the pathogenesis of malignant epithelial cells. Among the human breast cancer subtypes, TG2 expression was confined to some basal A, and all basal B, breast cancer cells tested. The most biologically aggressive types exhibited breast cancer stem cell phenotypes ($CD44^{+}CD24^{-}$), which were not present in ER^{+} or $ER^{+/-}Her\text{-}2^{+}$ luminal cell types or Her-2 overexpressing breast cancer cells (Fig. 12.2a) [32]. The TG2-NF-κB-IL-6 axis was also found in breast cancer stem cells. Breast cancer cells expressing a high level of TG2 secreted large amounts of IL-6 (Fig. 12.2a). IL-6 production was compared between control empty vector-transfected TG2 high-expressing basal B MDA-MB-231 breast cancer cells (MB231_Cont) and their TG2-knocked-down cells (MB231_shTG2); MB231_shTG2 cells showed reduced IL-6 production compared with MB231_Cont cells (Fig. 12.2b). Inhibition of TG2 activity using cysteamine reduced IL-6 production from TG2 high-expressing cells. IL-6 knockdown of basal B breast cancer cells (MB231_shIL-6) showed reduced IL-6 secretion, but TG2 expression levels were comparable to those of control cells, indicating TG2 activity was upstream of IL-6 production (Fig. 12.2c) [32]. These findings indicated that TG2-NF-κB-IL-6 signaling pathways were also critical in breast cancer stem cell cytokine production.

Cancer stem cell characteristics of TG2-IL-6 overexpressing breast cancer cells were evaluated. Cancer sphere formation decreased markedly both in TG2-knockdown and IL-6-knockdown breast cancer cells (MB231_shTG2 and MB231_shIL-6 cells) when compared with empty vector-transfected control cells (Fig. 12.3a) [32]. Both the numbers and sizes of spheres were reduced in TG2-knockdown and IL-6-knockdown cells. Control cancer cells (MB231_Cont)

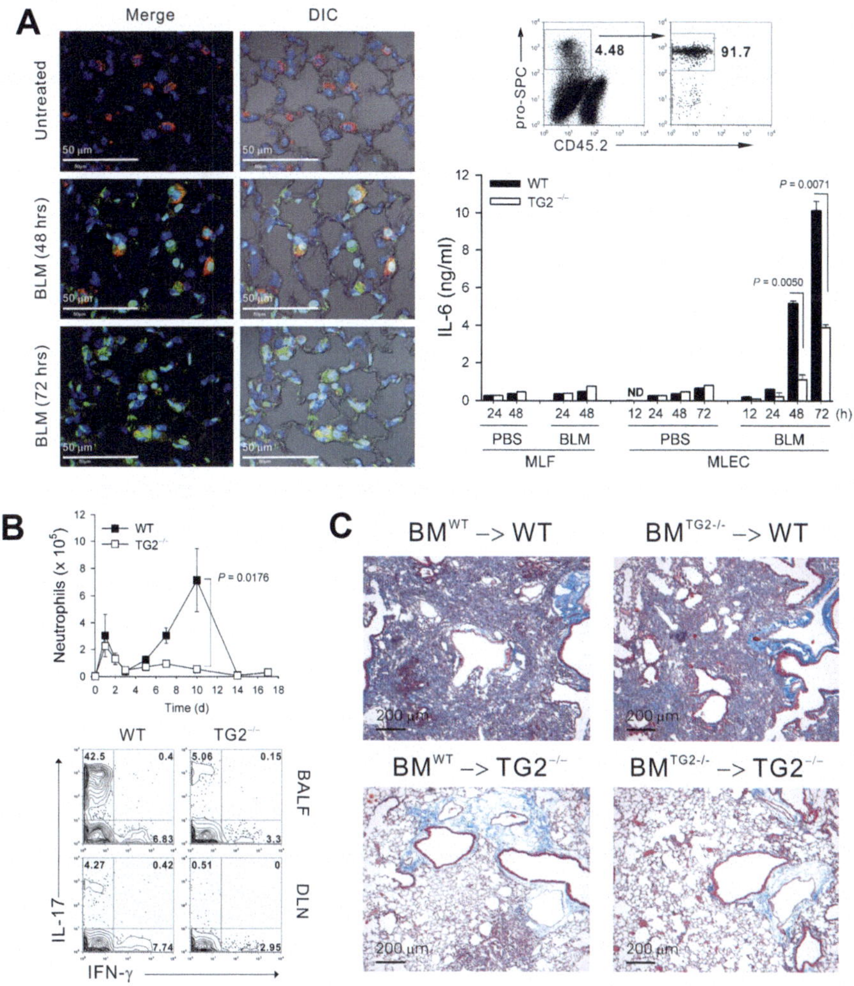

Fig. 12.1 Bleomycin-mediated pulmonary injury triggers a Th17 response. (**a**) Immunofluorescence staining of IL-6 production (green) from pro-SP-C (red)-expressing type II epithelial cells in the lungs of BLM-exposed wild-type B6 mice. Nuclei were counterstained with DAPI (blue) (left panel). Lung epithelial cells expressing pro-SP-C were sort-purified (upper panel). IL-6 levels in culture supernatants of sort-purified primary mouse lung epithelial cells (MLECs) and primary mouse lung fibroblasts (MLFs) from wild-type B6 mice as determined by ELISA. Cells (2×10^4) were treated with BLM (5 μg/mL) for the times indicated (right panel). (**b**) Neutrophils in BALF from wild-type B6 and TG2$^{-/-}$ mice were analyzed by flowcytometer on the indicated days following BLM treatment (upper panel). The percentages of CD4$^+$ cells producing IL-17 or IFN-γ in BALF and draining lymph nodes (DLN) of wild-type B6 and TG2$^{-/-}$ mice were determined 10 days after BLM exposure. Dot plots arc gated on CD4$^+$ T cells (lower panel). (**c**) Bone marrow chimeras were prepared by irradiation of wild-type B6 or TG2$^{/}$ mice, followed by T cell-depleted bone marrow cell reconstitution. Lung tissues were prepared 21 days after BLM instillation and stained with Masson's trichrome

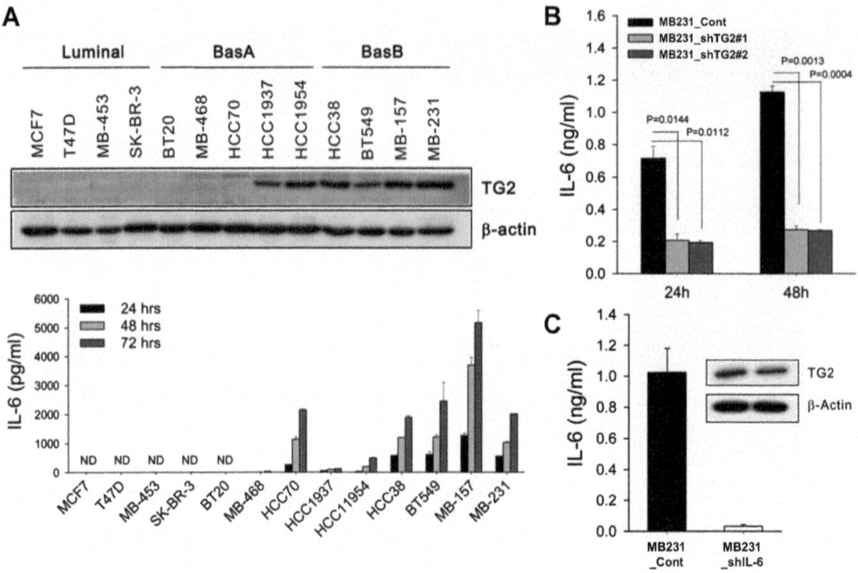

Fig. 12.2 TG2 expression levels in cancer cells correlated with IL-6 production. (**a**) TG2 expression in the 13 indicated human breast cancer cell lines was analyzed by Western blot (upper panel). IL-6 levels in culture supernatants of breast cancer cells were determined by ELISA (lower panel). Data represent mean ± SD. (**b**) IL-6 levels in the culture supernatants of control and TG2-knocked-down MDA-MB-231 cells were determined by ELISA. (**c**) IL-6 levels in the culture supernatants of control and IL-6-knocked-down MDA-MB-231 cells were determined by ELISA. TG2 expression was determined by RT-PCR analysis

cultured in sphere medium expressed more anti-apoptotic molecules, such as cIAP2 and Bcl-2, when compared with TG2-knockdown cells (MB231_shTG2) (Fig. 12.3b). Thus, TG2 supported cell survival via an anchorage-independent condition. Moreover, control cancer cells expressed more epithelial-to-mesenchymal transition (EMT)-related molecules such as N-cadherin and vimentin, compared with either TG2-knockdown (MB231_shTG2) or IL-6-knockdown cells (MB231_shIL-6) (Fig. 12.3c). When in vivo tumorigenic activity was measured using xenogeneic orthotopic transplantation in NOD-scid-IL2Rγ_c−/− (NSG) mice, breast cancer cells with high TG2 levels (MB231_Cont) showed rapid growth of primary tumor masses in the mammary fat pads when compared with TG2-knockdown cells (MB231_TG2) and IL-6-knockdown cells (MB231_shIL-6) (Fig. 12.3d). Notably, NSG mice inoculated with TG2 high-expressing MB231_Cont cells showed spontaneous distant hematogenous metastases, indicated by multiple visible metastatic nodules in the lung (Fig. 12.3e). In contrast, mice injected with TG2 knockdown cells (MB231_shTG2) showed reduced lung metastases. There was no metastasis in mice injected with IL-6-knockdown cells (MB231_shIL-6) (Fig. 12.3e) [32].

The clinical implications of the TG2-IL-6 axis in human breast cancer primary tumor tissues were assessed with a tissue microarray in 412 patients with operable

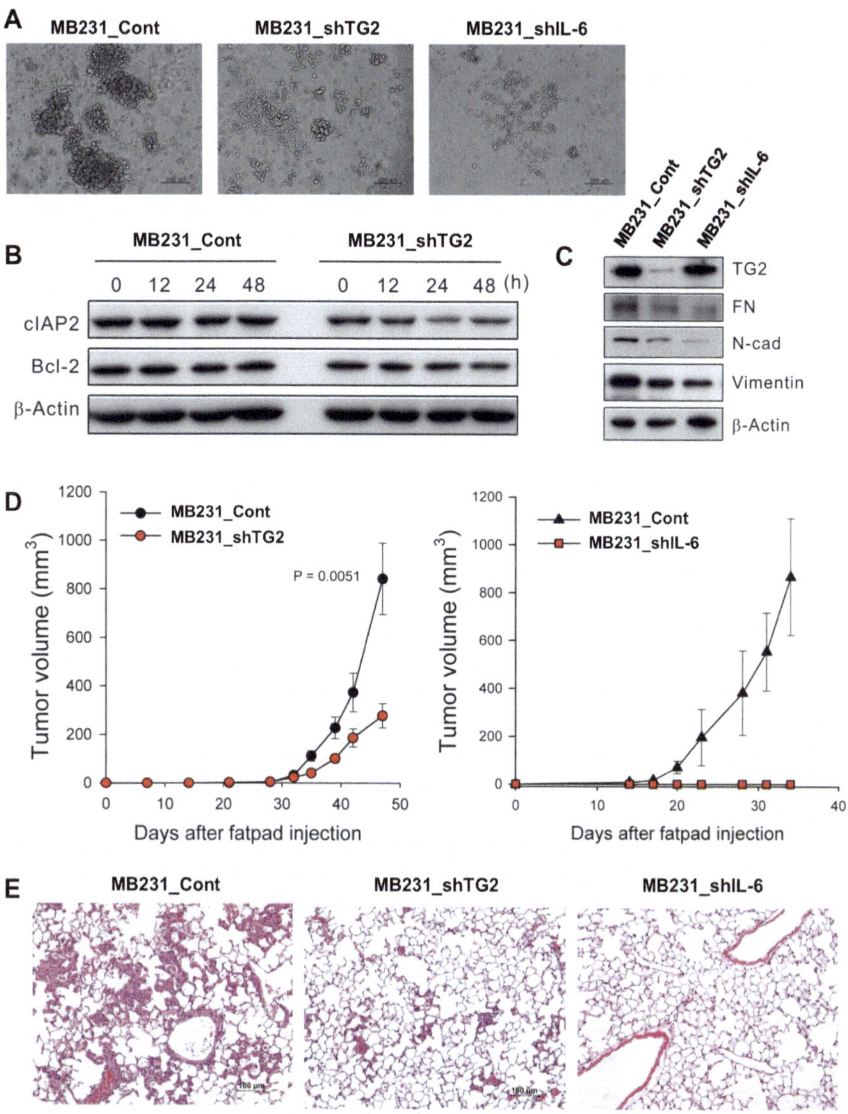

Fig. 12.3 TG2-mediated IL-6 allows anchorage-independent survival of cancer cells. (**a**) Control, TG2-knocked-down, and IL-6-knocked-down MDA-MB-231 cells were cultured in serum-free medium consisting of a 1:1 mixture of Ham's F-12 and DMEM, supplemented with growth factors. Visible spheres were counted under a microscope on day 8 post-plating. (**b**) cIAP2 and Bcl-2 expression was analyzed by Western blot after culture for indicated time in sphere medium. (**c**) TG2, fibronectin (FN), N-cadherin (N-Cad), and vimentin expression of control, TG2-knocked-down, and IL-6-knocked-down MDA-MB-231 cells analyzed by Western blot. (**d**) Control, TG2-knocked-down, and IL-6-knocked-down MDA-MB-231 cells (2×10^5 cells/each mouse) were injected in the fat pads of NSG mice. The growth of primary tumors was measured. Data are given as mean ± SD of 14 mice for each group. (**e**) Lung sections from mice xenografted with MDA-MB-231 cells at 45 days after the inoculation of cancer cells were analyzed

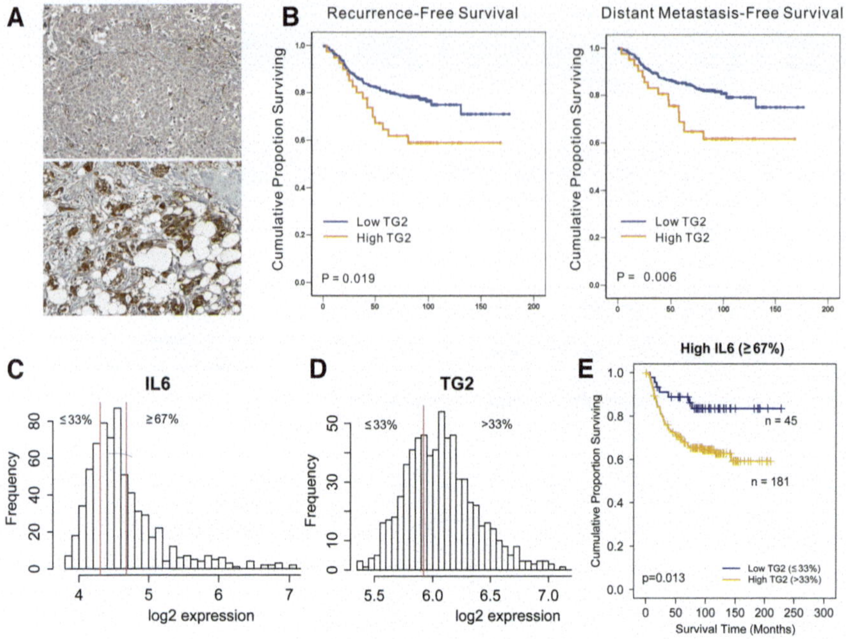

Fig. 12.4 Expression of TG2 and IL-6 in patients with breast cancer, and their relationship to distant metastasis-free survival. TG2 expression was analyzed by immunohistochemistry in a tissue microarray of primary tumors from patients with advanced breast cancer. (**a**) Immunohistochemical staining for TG2 in the primary tumors of patients with breast cancer showing negative (upper) and strong expression (lower) (×200). (**b**) Recurrence-free survival (left panel) and distant metastasis-free survival (right panel) according to TG2 expression adjusted for tumor size (≤2 cm vs. >2 cm), histological grade (1, 2 vs. 3), lymph node status (positive vs. negative), and hormone receptor status (positive vs. negative). The mean follow-up duration for patients after surgery was 83.6 ± 29.8 months. (**c–e**) In total, 684 human breast cancer gene expression profiles were obtained from three public datasets, and the association between the expression of TG2/IL-6 and distant metastasis-free survival (DMFS) was analyzed. The distributions of the log2 expression levels of IL-6 (C) and TG2 (**d**). (**e**) DMFS according to TG2 expression in the patients with high IL-6 expression

breast cancer treated at Seoul National University Hospital. The mean follow-up duration of these patients was 83.6 ± 29.8 months. Forty-two patients (10.2%) showed strong TG2 expression (Fig. 12.4a). Patients with high TG2-expressing tumors had significantly shorter recurrence-free survival and distant metastasis-free survival (DMFS) ($p = 0.019$ and $p = 0.006$, respectively; Fig. 12.4b). After adjusting for known prognostic factors using a Cox proportional hazard model, the expression level of TG2 remained an independent prognostic factor predicting recurrence and distant metastasis. These findings suggested that TG2 in human breast cancer primary tumors plays a critical role in metastasis and recurrence. To further validate the TG2-IL-6 signaling pathways in breast cancer progression, public datasets including a total of 684 breast cancer patients were collected, and the association between DMFS and TG2/IL-6 expression was investigated. The patients were classified into three groups based on the levels of IL-6 expression: high (patients with ≥67% IL-6 expression), medium (33~67%), and low IL-6 (≤33%) (Fig. 12.4c). The patients in each group were further stratified into two groups according to the expression level of TG2: the low TG2 group included patients with a ≤33% expression level of TG2, and the high TG2 group included all other patients (Fig. 12.4d). The results showed that among the high IL-6 group, most patients expressed high levels of TG2 ($n = 181$); only 20% of the patients ($n = 45$) expressed low levels of TG2 (Fig. 12.4e), suggesting that the TG2-IL-6 axis is also involved in human breast cancer primary tumors. In addition, high TG2 expression was associated with a significantly shorter DMFS compared with low TG2 in this group. The percentage of patients with low TG2 expression increased as the expression of IL-6 decreased (Fig. 12.4e), indicating that the expression levels of TG2 and IL-6 were also correlated in human breast cancer patients [32]. In conclusion, combined high expression of TG2 and IL-6, which conferred breast cancer stem cell characteristics, was related to a poor DMFS outcome in human breast cancer patients.

12.2.3 Microenvironmental Inflammatory Cytokines Supplement Cancer Stem Cell Characteristics

The signaling pathways involved in TG2-dependent IL-6 expression, which conferred breast cancer stem cell characteristics, were evaluated by overexpressing the whole sequence of human TG2 in otherwise TG2- and IL-6-negative luminal-type breast cancer cells (MCF7). The expression of E-cadherin was decreased and Snail2, an EMT inducer, as well as tissue inhibitors of metalloproteinases (TIMPs) 1, 2, and 3, was increased in MCF7_TG2 cells compared with control cells (Fig. 12.5a) [33]. MCF7_TG2 cells were $CD44^{+}CD24^{+}$, showing a partial gain of this breast cancer stem cell marker (Fig. 12.5b). In contrast to basal B breast cancer stem cells, which showed TG2-dependent IL-6 production, simple overexpression of TG2 in otherwise TG2- and IL-6-negative luminal-type breast cancer MCF7 cells (MCF7_TG2 cells) did not result in increased IL-6 expression (Fig. 12.5c). The behavior and gene expression of cancer cells were affected by the microenvironment surrounding the tumor, which included cytokines and growth factors released by stromal cells such as leukocytes and fibroblasts. To evaluate the effect of paracrine signals, MCF7 cells were treated with IL-1β, tumor necrosis factor (TNF)-α, transforming growth factor (TGF)-β, and epidermal growth factor (EGF). IL-1β treatment induced expression of IL-6 in breast cancer cells, and TG2-overexpressing cells expressed over 20 times more IL-6 than control cells after IL-1β treatment (Fig. 12.5c). Treating cells with TGF-β or EGF alone did not increase IL-6 expression, but TNF-α slightly increased IL-6 expression (Fig. 12.5c). Treatment with TGF-β, EGF, and TNF-α after IL-1β treatment further increased IL-6

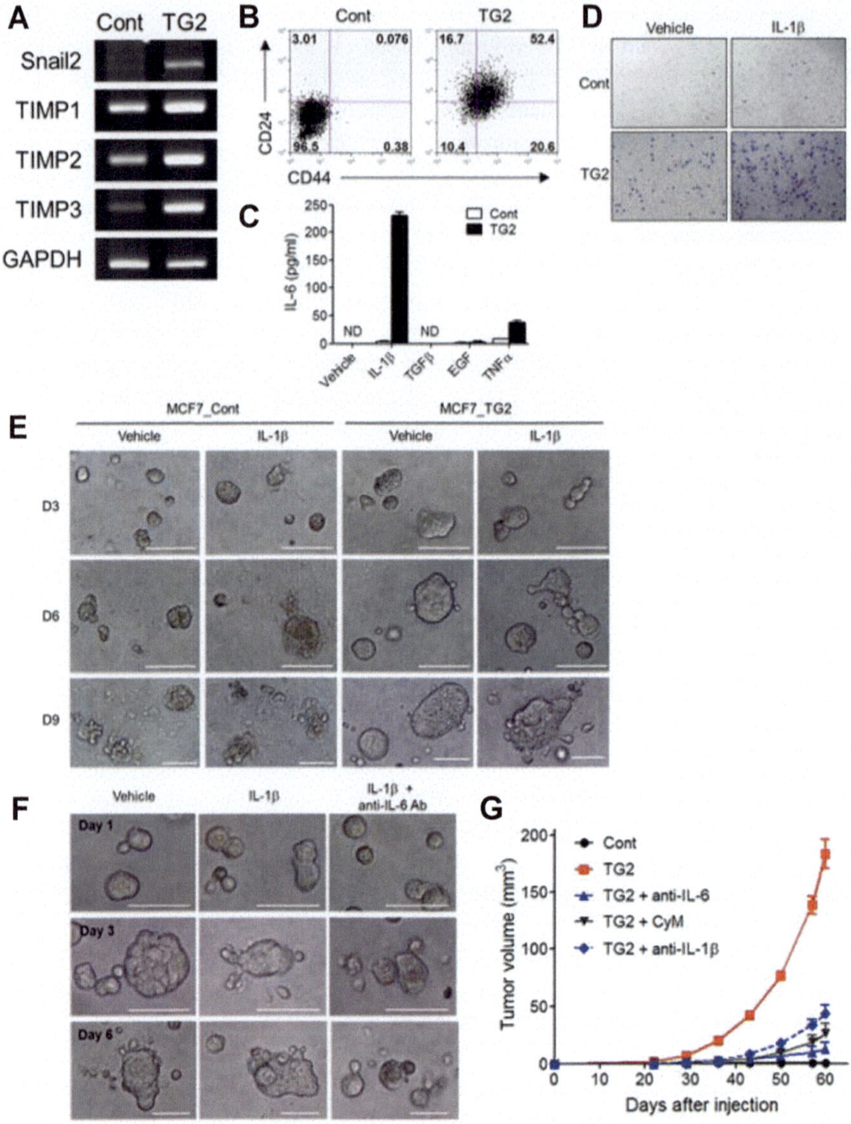

Fig. 12.5 IL-1β induced hormone-independent tumor growth of luminal-type breast cancer cells in a TG2-dependent manner. (**a**, **b**) MCF7 luminal-type breast cancer cells were stably transfected with TG2 (TG2) and control vector (Cont) and EMT and stem cell markers were compared using RT-PCR (**a**) and flow cytometry (**b**). (**c**) TG2-overexpressing MCF7 cells (TG2) and control vector-transfected MCF-7 cells (Cont) were treated with various cytokines (10 ng/mL) for 48 h, and IL-6 levels in culture supernatants were measured by ELISA. (**d**) MCF7_Cont and MCF7_TG2 cells were allowed to invade through Matrigel for 48 h in the presence or absence of IL-1β (10 ng/mL) (crystal violet). (**e**) MCF7_Cont and MCF7_TG2 cells were grown in 3D culture conditions in the presence or absence of IL-1β (10 ng/mL). (**f**) MCF7_TG2 cells were grown in 3D culture conditions in the presence or absence of IL-1β (10 ng/mL) and anti-IL-6 monoclonal antibody (10 μg/mL). (**g**) MCF7_Cont and MCF7_TG2 cells (1×10^6 cells/each mouse) were injected into the fat pads of NSG mice. Primary tumor growth was measured. Blocking anti-IL-6 antibody (100 μg/mouse) or

expression in MCF7_TG2 breast cancer cells. Other proinflammatory reagents, including lipopolysaccharide, Pam_3Cys, peptidoglycan, CpG, and bleomycin, did not induce IL-6 expression in either MCF7_Cont or MCF7_TG2 breast cancer cells [33].

Breast cancer cell behavior following TG2 overexpression and IL-1β stimulation was evaluated. MCF7_TG2 breast cancer cells showed increased invasiveness compared with MCF7_Cont cells, and IL-1β treatment further increased the invasiveness of MCF7_TG2 cells in a two-dimensional Matrigel® invasion assay (Fig. 12.5d) [33]. The synergistic effects of TG2 overexpression and IL-1β treatment on the invasion of MCF7 breast cancer cells were also revealed using a three-dimensional (3D) Matrigel® assay. MCF7_TG2 cells grew more rapidly and formed a larger spheroid in the 3D Matrigel® assay compared with MCF7_Cont cells, and IL-1β treatment further increased growth and conferred invasiveness in MCF7_TG2 cells (Fig. 12.5e). These cancer stem cell-like phenotypes were ameliorated by anti-IL-6 antibody treatment (Fig. 12.5f). Moreover, an in vivo tumorigenesis assay in NSG mice revealed that, unlike estrogen-dependent MCF7_Cont cells, MCF7_TG2 breast cancer cells obtained a tumorigenic capability in vivo without the addition of exogenous estrogen (Fig. 12.5g). This estrogen-independent growth was reduced in the presence of blocking anti-IL-6 or anti-IL-1β antibodies or the TG2 inhibitor, cysteamine (Fig. 12.5g) [33]. Together, the results showed that a microenvironment of IL-1β increased stem cell-like phenotypes, invasion, and estrogen-independent tumor growth of luminal-type breast cancer cells, thus completing the TG2-IL-6-STAT3 signaling axis of breast cancer stem cells.

12.3 Mutual Activation of Cancer Stem Cells and Microenvironmental Myeloid Cells Increase Cancer Stem Cell Characteristics and Distant Metastasis

12.3.1 Cytokine-Producing Cancer Stem Cells Showed Massive Myeloid-Derived Suppressor Cell (MDSC) Recruitment that Led to Distant Metastasis in Syngeneic Immunocompetent Hosts

High IL-6-secreting human breast cancer cells exhibit cancer stem cell phenotypes with enhanced distant metastasis and recruitment of more inflammatory cells when

Fig. 12.5 (continued) blocking anti-IL-1β antibody (100 μg/mouse) was injected intraperitoneally every third day, starting 1 day after tumor inoculation. The TG2 inhibitor cysteamine (CyM, 40 mg/kg/day) was injected intraperitoneally starting 1 day after tumor inoculation. Data are given as mean ± SEM of six mice for each group

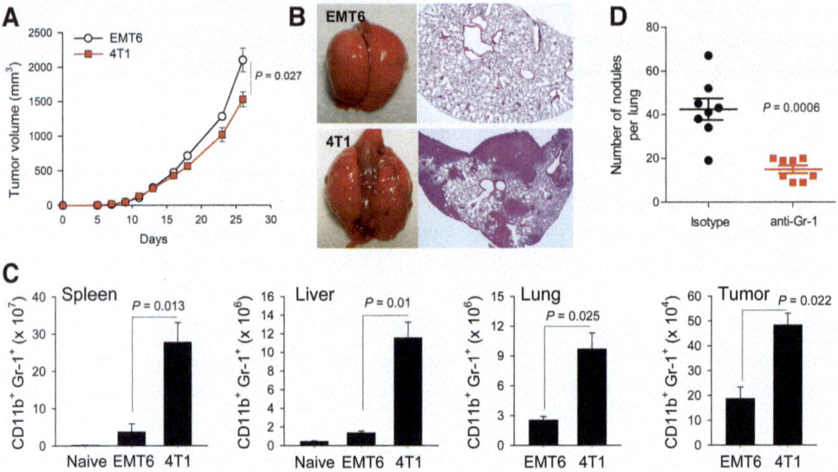

Fig. 12.6 Metastatic cancer cells facilitate recruitment of MDSCs. (**a**, **b**) EMT6 and 4T1 cells were injected into the mammary fat pads of BALB/c mice. (**a**) Primary tumor growth ($n = 8$). (**b**) Representative photographs of lungs 26 days after cell injection (H&E). (**c**) The absolute numbers of MDSCs ($CD11b^+Gr\text{-}1^+$) at 19 days (n = 4). (**d**) 4T1 cell-bearing mice were treated intraperitoneally with anti-Gr-1 antibodies. Numbers of tumor nodules in the lungs from 4T1 cell-bearing mice at 26 days ($n = 8$)

compared with low IL-6 expressing cells. Implementation and confirmation of these relationships in normal immunocompetent hosts was obtained by creating in vivo models using syngeneic murine breast cancer cells with differential IL-6 expression levels. IL-6 high-expressing 4T1 and low-expressing EMT6 cells were orthotopically grafted into the mammary fat pads of syngeneic BALB/c mice. Primary tumor growth was slightly greater for EMT6 cells when compared with 4T1 cells (Fig. 12.6a) [34]. At 26 days of grafting, 4T1 cancer cells showed extensive lung metastasis, while EMT6 cancer cells showed no distant metastasis in the lung, liver, or brain (Fig. 12.6b). IL-6 expressing 4T1 cell-bearing mice showed extensive recruitment of $CD11b^+Gr\text{-}1^+$ MDSCs in the lymphoid organ (spleen), metastasizing organs (lung and liver), and primary tumor masses. The number of MDSCs recruited was 2~8 times higher in 4T1 cell-bearing mice than in EMT6 cell-bearing mice (Fig. 12.6c). The critical role of MDSCs in distant metastasis was evaluated by depleting the MDSCs in 4T1 cell tumor-bearing mice, which resulted in reduced lung metastasis compared with the non-depleted controls (Fig. 12.6d) [34]. Together, these results showed that MDSCs expansion and recruitment in tumor-bearing mice were critically associated with the distant metastasis of IL-6-expressing breast cancer stem cells.

12.3.2 *Metastasizing, But Not Non-metastasizing Breast Cancer Cells, Activate MDSCs*

Whether IL-6-mediated MDSC recruitment promoted the metastasis of EMT6 cancer cells was evaluated using stably transfected EMT6 cells (EMT6_IL-6). EMT6_IL-6 cancer cell-bearing mice recruited more MDSCs to the spleen, lung, liver, and primary tumor masses when compared with the control EMT6_Con cell-bearing mice (Fig. 12.7a) [34]. The percentages and numbers of recruited MDSCs of EMT6_IL-6-bearing mice were comparable to 4T1 cell-bearing mice. However, distant lung metastasis was only slightly increased in EMT6_IL-6 cell-bearing mice when compared with EMT6_Con cell-bearing mice and was less than that seen in 4T1 cell-bearing mice (Fig. 12.7b). Thus, IL-6 secreted from breast cancer cells was important and sufficient for MDSC recruitment, but additional factors were required to fully induce the metastasis of cancer cells by recruited MDSCs. To reconstitute a local microenvironment that more closely resembled that of 4T1 cell-bearing mice, splenic MDSCs from 4T1 cell-bearing mice were adoptively transferred into EMT6 cell-bearing mice. The 4T1 splenic MDSC-transferred EMT6 cell-bearing mice showed only slightly increased lung metastases, compared with vehicle-treated control mice (Fig. 12.7c). Thus, neither repeated transfer of splenic MDSCs from metastatic 4T1-bearing mice nor IL-6 overexpression was sufficient to confer a metastasizing capacity on non-metastasizing EMT6 cancer cells comparable to that of 4T1 breast cancer cells [34]. Metastasizing cancer cells therefore produced additional components to potentiate the recruited MDSCs, thereby leading to distant metastasis.

To evaluate whether metastasizing, but not non-metastasizing, cancer cells further activated recruited MDSCs, splenic MDSCs from naïve and tumor-bearing mice were collected and co-cultured with 4T1 and EMT6 cells. Splenic MDSCs from naïve, EMT6 cell-bearing, or 4T1 cell-bearing mice co-cultured with 4T1 cells showed increased production of IL-6, irrespective of their source, when compared with those co-cultured with EMT6 cells (Fig. 12.7d) [34]. Splenic MDSCs became activated in co-cultures with 4T1 cells, either in the same chamber (lower) or a different chamber (upper) in a Transwell® culture assay (Fig. 12.7e), suggesting that contact-independent mediators were important for activation of these cells. The critical role of soluble factors was confirmed by incubating conditioned medium (CM) from breast cancer cells (4T1-CM and EMT6-CM) with splenic MDSCs. The 4T1-CM, but not the EMT6-CM, enhanced IL-6 production by splenic MDSCs (Fig. 12.7f). The 4T1-CM significantly increased IL-6 transcription in splenic MDSCs from both 4T1 cell- and EMT6 cell-bearing mice, while EMT6-CM and recombinant IL-6 only slightly induced IL-6 transcription. Splenic MDSCs treated with 4T1-CM showed activation of Stat3, NF-κB, JNK, ERK, and p38 signaling pathways. A signaling inhibitor study showed that the NF-κB, JNK, and p38 signaling pathways were important in IL-6 production by activated MDSCs (Fig. 12.7g). Importantly, 4T1 cell-bearing mice showed that MDSCs inside the primary tumor and lung strongly expressed IL-6, while those in the spleen from the

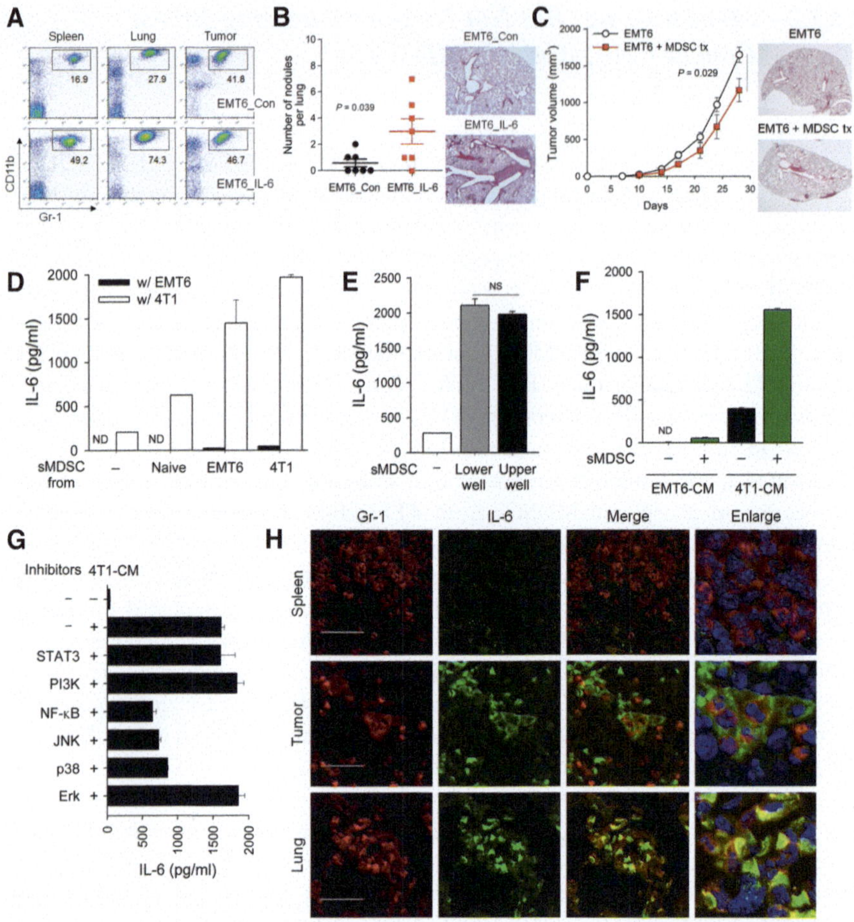

Fig. 12.7 Induction of recruitment and reconstitution of MDSCs in non-metastasizing EMT6 cell-bearing mice enhanced cancer cell metastasis. (**a**, **b**) EMT6_Con and EMT6_IL-6 cells were injected into the mammary fat pads of BALB/c mice. MDSCs were analyzed at 21 days. (**a**) Flowcytometric analysis of MDSCs at 21 days. (**b**) Numbers of metastatic nodules in the lungs at 26 days ($n = 7$) and lung sections at 26 days (H&E). (**c**) EMT6 cells were injected into the mammary fat pads. Three days later, mice were intravenously injected with splenic MDSCs (5×10^6/mouse) from 4T1 cell-bearing mice, a total of nine times. Primary tumor growth ($n = 5$) and representative photographs of lungs at 26 days. (**d**) Splenic MDSCs (4×10^5) were co-cultured with 4T1 cells (1×10^4) or EMT6 cells (1×10^4) for 48 h. IL-6 levels in the culture supernatants were measured by ELISA. (**e**, **f**) Splenic MDSCs from 4T1 cell-bearing mice were co-cultured with 4T1 cells in Transwell systems (**e**) or exposed to conditioned media (CM) for 24 h (**f**). (**g**) Splenic MDSCs were cultured with 4T1-CM in the presence of signaling inhibitors for 24 h. (**h**) Immunofluorescence staining of Gr-1 (red), IL-6 (green), and DAPI (blue) in the spleen, tumors, and lungs of 4T1 cell-bearing mice. Scale bar = 30 μm (original magnification, ×1000)

same mice expressed only small amounts of IL-6, and MDSCs in the primary tumor site of EMT6-bearing mice did not show increased IL-6 expression (Fig. 12.7g) [34]. Taken together, the results indicated that metastasizing, but not non-metastasizing, tumor-derived factors induced MDSCs to produce more IL-6, and full activation of recruited MDSCs occurred in the primary tumor site and metastatic organs in the vicinity of metastasizing cancer cells.

12.3.3 Activated MDSCs Increase Breast Cancer Stem Cell Characteristics and Stimulate Distant Metastasis Through IL-6 Trans-Signaling

Whether activated MDSCs in the metastasizing tumor microenvironment affect breast cancer cell behavior was evaluated by culturing 4T1 in CM from splenic MDSCs cultivated in the presence of 4T1-CM or EMT6-CM (4T1/MDSC-CM and EMT6/MDSC-CM, respectively) (Fig. 12.8a) [34]. The 4T1 cells cultured with 4T1/MDSC-CM, but not EMT6/MDSC-CM, showed significantly increased Stat3 phosphorylation within 10 min (Fig. 12.8b). Stat3 phosphorylation levels were increased for 48 h in 4T1 cells cultured with 4T1/MDSC-CM (Fig. 12.8c). Unlike 4T1/MDSC-CM, neither 4T1-CM nor recombinant IL-6 induced persistent activation of STAT3 (Fig. 12.8d) [34]. These results suggested that IL-6 is important for inducing Stat3 phosphorylation in 4T1 cells, but that soluble mediators other than IL-6 from tumor-infiltrating MDSCs are needed for persistent Stat3 phosphorylation of 4T1 cells.

Even though gp130, the common receptor chain for the IL-6 family of cytokines, was expressed ubiquitously, IL-6Rα was mainly expressed on hematopoietic cells [35]. To provide a strong signaling input leading to persistent STAT3 phosphorylation in 4T1 breast cancer cells, either IL-6Rα was expressed on these cells, which was not the case, or soluble IL-6Rα was provided *in trans*. To investigate which cells in the tumor microenvironment provided soluble IL-6Rα, the levels of soluble IL-6Rα secreted from ex vivo-cultured splenic MDSCs from naïve, EMT6 cell-bearing, and 4T1 cell-bearing mice were measured [34]. Splenic MDSCs from 4T1 cell-bearing mice produced more soluble IL-6Rα in ex vivo cultures compared with those from naïve and EMT6 cell-bearing mice (Fig. 12.8e). In contrast, the expression levels of the surface IL-6Rα chain on splenic MDSCs were similar between naïve, EMT6 cell-bearing, and 4T1 cell-bearing mice (Fig. 12.8f) [34].

Production of soluble IL-6Rα involves cell surface-associated proteases, such as the ADAM family proteases [36]. Among these proteases, Adam10 and Adam17 have been implicated in IL-6 trans-signaling [37, 38]. Non-stimulated splenic MDSCs from 4T1 cell-bearing mice expressed increased levels of both ADAM10 and ADAM17 when compared with splenic MDSCs from naïve and EMT6 cell-bearing mice (Fig. 12.8g) [34]. When splenic MDSCs from 4T1 cell-bearing mice were treated with broad spectrum protease inhibitors, the levels of soluble IL-6Rα

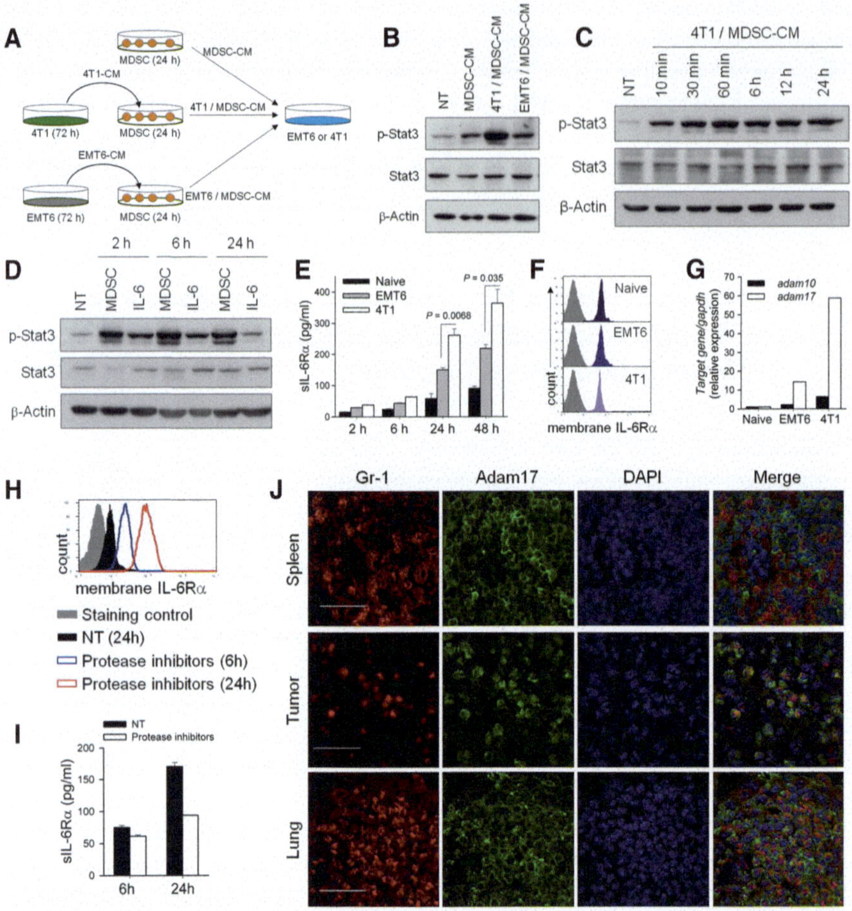

Fig. 12.8 Stimulation of MDSCs with metastasizing 4T1 cell-derived factors induced persistent Stat3 phosphorylation in cancer cells. (**a**) Splenic MDSCs from 4T1 cell-bearing mice were cultivated in the presence of 4T1-CM or EMT6-CM. The conditioned media (MDSC-CM, 4T1/MDSC-CM, EMT6/MDSC-CM) were harvested and applied to 4T1 and EMT6 cancer cells. (**b**, **c**) Phospho-Stat3 and Stat3 levels in 4T1 cells exposed to each CM for 10 min (**b**) and for the indicated periods of time (**c**). (**d**) 4T1 cells (1×10^4) were co-cultured with splenic MDSCs (4×10^5) from 4T1 cell-bearing mice or recombinant mouse IL-6 (1 ng/mL). Phospho-Stat3 and Stat3 levels in 4T1 cells were determined by Western blotting after the removal of MDSCs. (**e**) Soluble IL-6Rα levels in culture supernatants of splenic MDSCs were measured by ELISA and (**f**) surface IL-6Rα levels on splenic MDSCs were measured by FACS. (**g**) The mRNA expression of Adam10 and Adam17 in splenic MDSCs of naïve and tumor-bearing mice were determined by qRT-PCR. (**h**, **i**) Protease inhibitor cocktails were applied to cultures of splenic MDSCs from 4T1 cell-bearing mice for 6 or 24 h. (**h**) Membrane-bound IL-6Rα was detected by FACS and (**i**) soluble IL-6Rα levels were measured by ELISA. (**j**) Tissue sections were stained for Adam17 (green), Gr-1 (red), and DAPI (blue) to compare their localizations. Scale bar = 30 μm (original magnification, ×1000)

decreased and those of the membrane-bound form of IL-6Rα increased (Fig. 12.8h, i). To further evaluate the critical role of ADAM family proteases in IL-6Rα shedding, TAPI-2, a specific inhibitor of ADAM family proteases, was used. TAPI-2 treatment decreased shedding of surface IL-6Rα, as well as that of broad spectrum protease inhibitors. Confocal microscopy showed that MDSCs in the spleen, primary tumor mass, and lung metastatic lesions expressed increased levels of ADAM17 and IL-6Rα on their surfaces in 4T1 cell-bearing mice when compared with those in EMT6 cell-bearing mice (Fig. 12.8j) [34]. Thus, MDSCs that were recruited in the metastasizing 4T1-bearing mice were already capable of soluble IL-6Rα production, even in the spleen, a site remote from the metastasizing cancer cells. Because IL-6 levels of MDSCs were significantly increased only in the vicinity of metastasizing tumor cells, IL-6 trans-signaling occurred preferentially in primary tumor sites and the metastatic lung, but not in the spleen.

To evaluate whether IL-6 trans-signaling is important for activation of 4T1 breast cancer cells, 4T1 cells were cultivated in the presence of IL-6 and/or soluble IL-6Rα and were treated with an anti-IL-6R antibody (which blocks both conventional IL-6 signaling and IL-6 trans-signaling) or a gp130-Fc fusion protein (which blocks only IL-6 trans-signaling). IL-6, but not soluble IL-6Rα, increased Stat3 phosphorylation in 4T1 cells, and treatment with both IL-6 and soluble IL-6Rα further increased the phosphorylation of Stat3, suggesting that IL-6 trans-signaling functioned in 4T1 cell activation (Fig. 12.9a) [34]. Inhibition of IL-6 trans-signaling with gp130-Fc ameliorated Stat3 phosphorylation as efficiently as IL-6R blocking antibody (Fig. 12.9a). Treatment with gp130-Fc inhibited Stat3 phosphorylation in 4T1 cells cultured with 4T1/MDSC-CM, to an extent comparable to IL-6R antibody treatment (Fig. 12.9b). The significantly enhanced IL-6 trans-signaling of 4T1 cells resulted in increased invasiveness in a Matrigel® invasion assay, a response that was blocked by gp130-Fc treatment (Fig. 12.9c). The critical role of IL-6 trans-signaling in in vivo metastasis was confirmed by administration of gp130-Fc using osmotic pumps, which reduced primary tumor growth (Fig. 12.9d) and lung metastasis in a dose-dependent manner (Fig. 12.9e). Finally, whether the strong and persistent Stat3 phosphorylation in MDSC-potentiated cancer cells was crucial to spontaneous tumor metastasis was confirmed. Stat3 knockdown 4T1 (4T1_shStat3) cells showed similar levels of IL-6 production and MDSC recruitment, but markedly decreased invasiveness when compared with 4T1_Con cells (Fig. 12.9f). Primary tumor growth in the mammary fat pads was reduced in 4T1_shStat3 cell-bearing mice when compared with 4T1_Con cell-bearing mice (Fig. 12.7g), while the reduction in distant lung metastasis was greater in 4T1_shStat3 cell-bearing mice (Fig. 12.7h) [34]. Together, the results showed that cytokine-producing breast cancer stem cells and MDSCs formed a synergistic mutual feedback loop, and that the potentiated MDSCs directly increased cancer stem cell characteristics, leading to spontaneous metastasis.

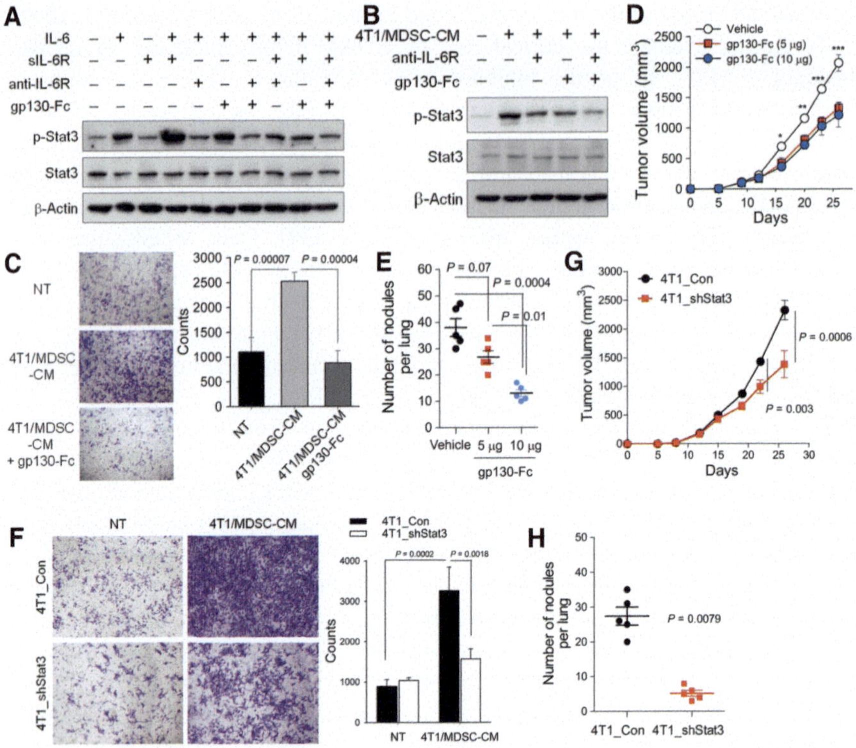

Fig. 12.9 Activated MDSCs contributed to tumor invasiveness through IL-6 trans-signaling. (**a**, **b**) 4T1 cells were treated with recombinant IL-6 plus soluble IL-6Rα (**a**) or 4T1/MDSC-CM (**b**) for 30 min in the presence of anti-IL-6R blocking antibody or gp130-Fc. (**c**) 4T1 cells were allowed to invade through Matrigel for 18 h in the presence or absence of 4T1/MDSC-CM and/or gp130-Fc (crystal violet). (**d**, **e**) 4T1 cells were injected into the mammary fat pads. Some mice underwent continuous administration using osmotic mini-pumps (5 or 10 μg for 14 days). (**d**) Primary tumor growth and (**e**) numbers of metastatic masses in the lungs at 26 days. (**f**) 4T1_Con and 4T1_shStat3 cells were allowed to invade through Matrigel for 18 h in the presence or absence of 4T1/MDSC-CM. (**f**) Invaded 4T1 cells (crystal violet) (left panel). Invaded cells were counted using ImageJ software (right panel). (**g**, **h**) 4T1_Con and 4T1_shStat3 cells were injected into the mammary fat pads. (**g**) Primary tumor growth. (**h**) Numbers of metastatic masses in the lungs at 26 days. Values are the means ± SEM of each group. $*P < 0.05$, $**P < 0.01$, $***P < 0.001$

12.4 The Immunogenicity of Cancer Stem Cells

During the progress of carcinogenesis, cancer stem cells and their intimately related myeloid cells mutually interact and evolve, so that cancer cells potentiate the myeloid cells, and in return, the myeloid cells increase their cancer stem cell characteristics [34, 39]. In addition to these direct contributions to cancer formation, invasion, distant metastasis, and therapy resistance, cancer stem cells possess the ability to manipulate host immunosurveillance [40]. For example, the abovementioned cytokine-producing breast cancer stem cells recruit MDSCs, and these cells are well-characterized suppressor cells of the adaptive immune responses involving several effector mechanisms, including induction of regulatory T (Treg) cell development or expansion of existing Treg cell populations, deprivation of T cells of amino acids that are essential for their growth and differentiation, and direct nitration and nitrosylation of components of the T cell receptor signaling complex and chemokines [27, 41, 42].

Recent advances in our knowledge of immunosuppressive cancer microenvironments have resulted in the identification of responsible effector cells and mediators [43]. Surrounded by the full repertoire of immunosuppressive mediators, cancer-specific T cells managing to reach tumor sites have difficulty in completely activating and thus performing all their effector cytotoxic functions, resulting in subsequent exhaustion [44, 45]. Negative immune regulators frequently expressed on exhausted T cells are PD-1, Tim-3, LAG3, and TIGIT [46]. The revival of exhausted cancer-specific T cells using specific blocking antibodies against these immune checkpoint molecules has been intensely studied [46, 47]. The leading antibodies, anti-CTLA-4 and anti-PD-1, provide dramatic improvements in long-term patient survival for several types of cancers, such as melanoma, non-small cell lung cancer, bladder cancer, and renal cell carcinoma [46–49]. However, the overall response rate for immune checkpoint blockade was rather low and varied by tumor type [50]. In terms of the reactivity of cancer-specific T cells, further mention should be made of the immunogenicity of cancer cells. The majority of cancer antigens are also expressed on their normal counterparts, and high-affinity T cells against these antigens are efficiently removed in the thymus through the mechanism of negative selection, thereby avoiding harmful autoimmune diseases [51]. Thus, the remaining tumor-specific T cells in the periphery are mostly of low-to-intermediate affinity and can easily be tolerized or exhausted [52]. The response rate to immune checkpoint inhibitors is higher in carcinogen-related tumors, such as sun exposure-associated melanoma and smoking-related lung and bladder carcinomas. These tumors are characterized by an increased burden of nonsynonymous DNA mutations, which are associated with the major molecular basis of anti-cancer T cell reactivity [52–54]. Somatic gene mutations resulting in single changes in amino acids can lead to the expression of mutated peptides on the major histocompatibility complex molecules, and these "neoepitopes" will attract high-affinity T cells that were never checked in the thymus during their development. Such T cell reactivity specific for either driver or passenger mutations can be characterized in cancer patients [52, 55]. Importantly, the mechanism of action of both anti-CTLA-4 and anti-PD-1 blocking antibodies has been linked to recurrence of neoepitope-specific high-affinity T cells in melanoma and lung cancer [56–58]. In this respect, characterization of the full antigenic repertoire of cancer stem cells is required, and novel therapeutic interventions, such as actively inducing neoepitopes on the cancer stem cells, are promising for successful and long-lasting precision cancer immunotherapy targeting cancer stem cells.

12.5 Summary

1. The bench
   Cytokine-producing breast cancer stem cells and their associated myeloid cells mutually interact and synergize through TG2/NF-κB/IL-6/STAT3 signaling pathways, leading to therapy resistance and distant metastasis.
2. Translation
   Combined high expression of TG2 and IL-6, which conferred stem cell characteristics, was associated with a poor DMFS outcome in human breast cancer patients.
3. The bedside
   Intervention in key cytokine pathways of breast cancer stem cells, such as IL-6 and downstream STAT signaling, using recently developed therapeutics, together with the depletion of tumor-promoting myeloid cells using novel therapeutics, will be critical to regulating both cancer stem cells and their microenvironments in patients with advanced, inoperable cancer.

References

1. Lapidot T, Sirard C, Vormoor J, Murdoch B, Hoang T, Caceres-Cortes J, et al. A cell initiating human acute myeloid leukaemia after transplantation into SCID mice. Nature. 1994;367 (6464):645–8.
2. Bonnet D, Dick JE. Human acute myeloid leukemia is organized as a hierarchy that originates from a primitive hematopoietic cell. Nat Med. 1997;3(7):730–7.
3. Hope KJ, Jin L, Dick JE. Acute myeloid leukemia originates from a hierarchy of leukemic stem cell classes that differ in self-renewal capacity. Nat Immunol. 2004;5(7):738–43.
4. O'Brien CA, Kreso A, Dick JE. Cancer stem cells in solid tumors: an overview. Semin Radiat Oncol. 2009;19(2):71–7.
5. Shackleton M, Quintana E, Fearon ER, Morrison SJ. Heterogeneity in cancer: cancer stem cells versus clonal evolution. Cell. 2009;138(5):822–9.
6. Huntly BJ, Gilliland DG. Leukaemia stem cells and the evolution of cancer-stem-cell research. Nat Rev Cancer. 2005;5(4):311–21.
7. Valent P, Bonnet D, De Maria R, Lapidot T, Copland M, Melo JV, et al. Cancer stem cell definitions and terminology: the devil is in the details. Nat Rev Cancer. 2012;12(11):767–75.
8. Kreso A, Dick JE. Evolution of the cancer stem cell model. Cell Stem Cell. 2014;14(3):275–91.
9. Clevers H. The cancer stem cell: premises, promises and challenges. Nat Med. 2011;17 (3):313–9.
10. Visvader JE, Lindeman GJ. Cancer stem cells: current status and evolving complexities. Cell Stem Cell. 2012;10(6):717–28. Review. https://doi.org/10.1016/j.stem.2012.05.007.
11. Al-Hajj M, Wicha MS, Benito-Hernandez A, Morrison SJ, Clarke MF. Prospective identification of tumorigenic breast cancer cells. Proc Natl Acad Sci U S A. 2003;100(7):3983–8.
12. Singh SK, Hawkins C, Clarke ID, Squire JA, Bayani J, Hide T, et al. Identification of human brain tumour initiating cells. Nature. 2004;432(7015):396–401.
13. Ricci-Vitiani L, Lombardi DG, Pilozzi E, Biffoni M, Todaro M, Peschle C, et al. Identification and expansion of human colon-cancer-initiating cells. Nature. 2007;445(7123):111–5.
14. Pützer BM, Solanki M, Herchenröder O. Advances in cancer stem cell targeting: how to strike the evil at its root. Adv Drug Deliv Rev. 2017;120:89–107.

15. Weinberg RA. The biology of cancer. 2nd ed. New York: Garland Science; 2014. p. 77–83.
16. Ablett MP, Singh JK, Clarke RB. Stem cells in breast tumours: are they ready for the clinic? Eur J Cancer. 2012;48(14):2104–16.
17. Yang F, Xu J, Tang L, Guan X. Breast cancer stem cell: the roles and therapeutic implications. Cell Mol Life Sci. 2017;74(6):951–66.
18. Batlle E, Clevers H. Cancer stem cells revisited. Nat Med. 2017;23(10):1124–34.
19. Rutkowski MR, Svoronos N, Perales-Puchalt A, Conejo-Garcia JR. The tumor macroenvironment: cancer-promoting networks beyond tumor beds. Adv Cancer Res. 2015;128:235–62.
20. Roberts KJ, Kershner AM, Beachy PA. The stromal niche for epithelial stem cells: a template for regeneration and a brake on malignancy. Cancer Cell. 2017;32(4):404–10.
21. Castaño Z, Fillmore CM, Kim CF, McAllister SS. The bed and the bugs: interactions between the tumor microenvironment and cancer stem cells. Semin Cancer Biol. 2012;22(5–6):462–70.
22. Bussard KM, Mutkus L, Stumpf K, Gomez-Manzano C, Marini FC. Tumor-associated stromal cells as key contributors to the tumor microenvironment. Breast Cancer Res. 2016;18(1):84.
23. Nair N, Calle AS, Zahra MH, Prieto-Vila M, Oo AKK, Hurley L, et al. A cancer stem cell model as the point of origin of cancer-associated fibroblasts in tumor microenvironment. Sci Rep. 2017;7(1):6838.
24. Kotas ME, Medzhitov R. Homeostasis, inflammation, and disease susceptibility. Cell. 2015;160 (5):816–27.
25. Okabe Y, Medzhitov R. Tissue biology perspective on macrophages. Nat Immunol. 2016;17 (1):9–17.
26. Perdiguero EG, Geissmann F. The development and maintenance of resident macrophages. Nat Immunol. 2016;17(1):2–8.
27. Gabrilovich DI, Ostrand-Rosenberg S, Bronte V. Coordinated regulation of myeloid cells by tumours. Nat Rev Immunol. 2012;12(4):253–68.
28. Ugel S, De Sanctis F, Mandruzzato S, Bronte V. Tumor-induced myeloid deviation: when myeloid-derived suppressor cells meet tumor-associated macrophages. J Clin Invest. 2015;125 (9):3365–76.
29. Korkaya H, Liu S, Wicha MS. Breast cancer stem cells, cytokine networks, and the tumor microenvironment. J Clin Invest. 2011;121(10):3804–9.
30. Chin AR, Wang SE. Cytokines driving breast cancer stemness. Mol Cell Endocrinol. 2014;382 (1):598–602. https://doi.org/10.1016/j.mce.2013.03.024.
31. Oh K, Park HB, Byoun OJ, Shin DM, Jeong EM, Kim YW, et al. Epithelial transglutaminase 2 is needed for T cell interleukin-17 production and subsequent pulmonary inflammation and fibrosis in bleomycin-treated mice. J Exp Med. 2011;208(8):1707–19.
32. Oh K, Ko E, Kim HS, Park AK, Moon HG, Noh DY, et al. Transglutaminase 2 facilitates the distant hematogenous metastasis of breast cancer by modulating interleukin-6 in cancer cells. Breast Cancer Res. 2011;13(5):R96.
33. Oh K, Lee OY, Park Y, Seo MW, Lee DS. IL-1β induces IL-6 production and increases invasiveness and estrogen-independent growth in a TG2-dependent manner in human breast cancer cells. BMC Cancer. 2016;16(1):724.
34. Oh K, Lee OY, Shon SY, Nam O, Ryu PM, Seo MW, et al. A mutual activation loop between breast cancer cells and myeloid-derived suppressor cells facilitates spontaneous metastasis through IL-6 trans-signaling in a murine model. Breast Cancer Res. 2013;15(5):R79.
35. Jones SA, Scheller J, Rose-John S. Therapeutic strategies for the clinical blockade of IL-6/ gp130 signaling. J Clin Invest. 2011;121(9):3375–83.
36. Scheller J, Chalaris A, Garbers C, Rose-John S. ADAM17: a molecular switch to control inflammation and tissue regeneration. Trends Immunol. 2011;32(8):380–7.
37. Pruessmeyer J, Ludwig A. The good, the bad and the ugly substrates for ADAM10 and ADAM17 in brain pathology, inflammation and cancer. Semin Cell Dev Biol. 2009;20 (2):164–74.

38. Chalaris A, Gewiese J, Paliga K, Fleig L, Schneede A, Krieger K, et al. ADAM17-mediated shedding of the IL6R induces cleavage of the membrane stub by gamma-secretase. Biochim Biophys Acta. 2010;1803(2):234–45.
39. Lu H, Clauser KR, Tam WL, Fröse J, Ye X, Eaton EN, et al. A breast cancer stem cell niche supported by juxtacrine signalling from monocytes and macrophages. Nat Cell Biol. 2014;16 (11):1105–17.
40. Bruttel VS, Wischhusen J. Cancer stem cell immunology: key to understanding tumorigenesis and tumor immune escape? Front Immunol. 2014;5:360.
41. Marvel D, Gabrilovich DI. Myeloid-derived suppressor cells in the tumor microenvironment: expect the unexpected. J Clin Invest. 2015;125(9):3356–64.
42. Kumar V, Patel S, Tcyganov E, Gabrilovich DI. The nature of myeloid-derived suppressor cells in the tumor microenvironment. Trends Immunol. 2016;37(3):208–20.
43. Chawla A, Alatrash G, Wu Y, Mittendorf EA. Immune aspects of the breast tumor microenvironment. Breast Cancer Manag. 2013;2(3):231–44.
44. Pauken KE, Wherry EJ. Overcoming T cell exhaustion in infection and cancer. Trends Immunol. 2015;36(4):265–76.
45. Speiser DE, Utzschneider DT, Oberle SG, Münz C, Romero P, Zehn D. T cell differentiation in chronic infection and cancer: functional adaptation or exhaustion? Nat Rev Immunol. 2014;14 (11):768–74. https://doi.org/10.1038/nri3740.
46. Sharma P, Allison JP. The future of immune checkpoint therapy. Science. 2015;348 (6230):56–61.
47. Sharma P, Allison JP. Immune checkpoint targeting in cancer therapy: toward combination strategies with curative potential. Cell. 2015;161(2):205–14.
48. Hamid O, Robert C, Daud A, Hodi FS, Hwu WJ, Kefford R, et al. Safety and tumor responses with lambrolizumab (anti-PD-1) in melanoma. N Engl J Med. 2013;369(2):134–44.
49. Collin M. Immune checkpoint inhibitors: the battle of giants. Pharm Pat Anal. 2017;6(4):135–7.
50. Xu-Monette ZY, Zhang M, Li J, Young KH. PD-1/PD-L1 blockade: have we found the key to unleash the antitumor immune response? Front Immunol. 2017;8:1597.
51. Klein L, Kyewski B, Allen PM, Hogquist KA. Positive and negative selection of the T cell repertoire: what thymocytes see (and don't see). Nat Rev Immunol. 2014;14(6):377–91.
52. Vonderheide RH, Domchek SM, Clark AS. Immunotherapy for breast cancer: what are we missing? Clin Cancer Res. 2017;23(11):2640–6.
53. Hirohashi Y, Torigoe T, Tsukahara T, Kanaseki T, Kochin V, Sato N. Immune responses to human cancer stem-like cells/cancer-initiating cells. Cancer Sci. 2016;107(1):12–7.
54. Fiori ME, Villanova L, De Maria R. Cancer stem cells: at the forefront of personalized medicine and immunotherapy. Curr Opin Pharmacol. 2017;35:1–11.
55. McGranahan N, Furness AJ, Rosenthal R, Ramskov S, Lyngaa R, Saini SK, et al. Clonal neoantigens elicit T cell immunoreactivity and sensitivity to immune checkpoint blockade. Science. 2016;351(6280):1463–9.
56. Kunz M, Hölzel M. The impact of melanoma genetics on treatment response and resistance in clinical and experimental studies. Cancer Metastasis Rev. 2017;36(1):53–75.
57. Nathanson T, Ahuja A, Rubinsteyn A, Aksoy BA, Hellmann MD, Miao D, et al. Somatic mutations and neoepitope homology in melanomas treated with CTLA-4 blockade. Cancer Immunol Res. 2017;5(1):84–91.
58. Cho JH. Immunotherapy for non-small-cell lung cancer: current status and future obstacles. Immune Netw. 2017;17(6):378–91.

Chapter 13
Theranostics for Breast Cancer Stem Cells

Woo Kyung Moon and Hoe Suk Kim

Abstract Effectively targeting and treating breast cancer stem cells (BCSCs), which have been linked to tumor development and metastasis, and recurrence still remains a challenging issue in preclinic and clinic. Screening and identifying characteristic BCSC biomarkers is important for distinguishing BCSCs from differentiated tumor cells within the tumor mass. Molecular imaging and nanotechnology are evolving as new fields that have a potentially high research and clinical impact. Developing the biocompatible contrast agents conjugated with high-affinity biomarker to selectively target BCSCs and is one of the key prerequisites for image-guided diagnosis and monitoring therapy of BCSCs. Very recently, we documented the extra domain-B fibronectin (EDB-FN), which is considered as a new putative biomarker for BCSCs (NDY-1 cell) derived from human breast carcinosarcoma. We here review BCSC-targeted theranostics in vitro and in vivo by delivering siRNA or drug using the nanoparticles conjugated with a small peptide specific to EDB-FN.

Keywords Breast cancer stem cell (BCSC) · Magnetic resonance imaging (MRI) · Thermally cross-linked superparamagnetic iron oxide nanoparticles (TCL-SPION) · extra domain-B fibronectin (EDB-FN) · Theranostics

13.1 Introduction

Advances in molecular imaging and nanotechnology allow us to explore the non-invasive diagnosis and monitoring therapy of cancers in living systems. Magnetic resonance imaging (MRI), because of its extremely high sensitivity in detecting cancer, can diagnose breast cancer without any radiation dose, and enhanced MRI can make earlier and differential diagnosis to evaluate equivocal mammographic

W. K. Moon (✉) · H. S. Kim
Department of Radiology, Seoul National University & Seoul National University Hospital, Seoul, Republic of Korea
e-mail: moonwk@snu.ac.kr

D.-Y. Noh et al. (eds.), *Translational Research in Breast Cancer*, Advances in Experimental Medicine and Biology 1187,
https://doi.org/10.1007/978-981-32-9620-6_13

findings [1]. Nanotechnological platform including clinically approved iron oxide nanoparticles has generated a great deal of attention for translational research, due to emerging applications for non-invasive imaging and therapy. Magnetic iron oxide nanoparticles, which are a well-known T2 contrast agents for MRI [2], can combine active drug compounds with selective targeting moieties and offer biomedical applications in clinic.

The science of cancer stem cells is still evolving and, despite the many unknowns, holds significant promise for the next phase of oncology therapeutics. Since cancer stem cells, a rare subpopulation of undifferentiated cells with embryonic stem cell characteristics within the tumor were first documented in patient samples with myeloid leukemia [3–5], such cells have been found in various types of human solid tumors [6, 7]. The self-renewal properties of cancer stem cells underlie the mechanisms of tumor initiation and recurrence and are implicated in the dissemination of the primary tumor to metastatic sites [6–8]. The cancer stem cell model accounts for important forms of the phenotypic and functional heterogeneity in cancer [9, 10]. Preclinical stem cell-based strategies show great promise for use in targeted anticancer therapy applications [2, 11, 12]. Since breast cancer stem cells (BCSCs), which displaying $CD44^{+}CD24^{-}$ phenotype, were first documented by Al-Hajj et al. [13]; several findings have reported that BCSCs exhibiting additional biomarkers such as $CD133^{+}$, integrins ($CD29^{+}$, $CD49^{+}$, and $CD61^{+}$), and ALDH activity are key contributors to the development and heterogeneity of the breast cancer [14–19].

Very recently, Dr. Noh's group reported the BCSC population (designated NDY-1) exhibiting $CD44^{+}CD24^{-}CD49^{+}ALDH^{+}$ phenotype marker in self-renewing sarcospheres derived from human breast carcinosarcoma [20]. More interestingly, in NDY-1 cells highly express the extra domain-B fibronectin (EDB-FN). We here review our recent studies regarding the extra domain-B fibronectin (EDB-FN), which considered as a putative additional BCSC marker and EDB-FN-targeted theranostics for BCSCs in cultured NDY-1 cells and xenograft tumor model.

13.2 Review of Past Studies

13.2.1 Heterogeneous Phenotype Markers for Breast Cancer Stem Cell (BCSC)

Like all stem cells, cancer stem cells, which are also called "tumor-initiating cells," represent a rare population of cells within a tumor and are defined by their ability for self-renewal; they are considered to be responsible for cancer progression, recurrence, and therapeutic resistance [21]. Cancer stem cells have been identified in a variety of human tumors, as assayed by their ability to initiate tumor growth in immunocompromised mice [3–9]. The attempts to identify, isolate, and characterize

Table 13.1 Aforementioned heterogeneous BCSC markers

BCSC markers	Reference
$CD44^{+}CD24^{-/low}$	[3, 13, 19, 27]
Sphere-forming	[17, 27, 28]
Hoechst 33342 Side population	[22, 29]
Aldehyde dehydrogenase (ALDH)	[14, 30]
$CD133^{+}$	[18, 23, 24]
$CD29^{+}CD49f^{+}CD61^{+}$	[25, 26]
$PROCR^{+}/ESA^{+}$	[31]

cancer stem cell populations in diverse types of tumors are mostly dependent on cell surface markers [7], sphere-forming abilities, aldehyde dehydrogenase (ALDH) activities [14], and Hoechst 33342 side population [22].

Breast cancer is a complex heterogeneous disease, and its management is tailored to the individual woman's cancer. Breast cancer stem cells (BCSCs) with $CD44^{+}CD24^{-/low}$ phenotype identified from metastatic pleural effusions of breast carcinoma patients are first reported by Al-Hajj et al. [13]. The combination of the BCSC markers CD44 and CD24 is by far the most extensively studied and undeniably the most contentious. However, different groups, together with the widespread expression of CD44, strongly suggest that the $CD44^{+}CD24^{-/low}$ phenotype maker is not sufficient to characterize BCSC [16, 17]. Aldehyde dehydrogenase (ALDH) which highly expressed in specific stem cells at several tissues is documented as another candidate marker of BCSCs [14, 15]. In addition to $CD44^{+}CD24^{-/low}$ and $ALDH^{+}$, CD133+ sorted cells harbor BCSC properties [18, 23, 24]. $CD24^{+}CD29^{+}$ cells in BRCA1 related mammary tumors retain their capacity for self-renewal and tumor formation [25, 26]. In aforementioned evidences (Table 13.1), BCSCs are a heterogeneous population similar to the heterogeneity seen in breast cancer; it is comprised of various histological subtypes, with variable clinical presentations and different underlying molecular signatures. Despite the many studies to demonstrate the presence of BCSCs based on cell surface marker profiles, there still remains a need for a universal marker or combination of markers able to identify and isolate BCSC from all breast cancers.

13.2.2 Translational Research for BCSC-Targeted Imaging and Therapy Using Magnetic Nanoparticle-Based MRI

Molecular imaging provides a powerful tool for patient-tailored therapy planning, therapy monitoring, and disease follow-up, as well as targeting non-invasive diagnostics and treatments, especially with the increasing use of theranostics in precision medicine. Advances of nanotechnology have led to the development of nanomaterials with both potential diagnostic and therapeutic applications. Commercially available magnetic iron oxide nanoparticles are most commonly used for

Table 13.2 Magnetic iron oxide nanoparticles currently approved or in clinical trial

Preclinical agent	Commercial name	MR target	Status
AMI-25	Ferumoxide, Feridex, Endoderm	Liver	Approved
OMP	Abdoscan	Bowel	Approved
AMI-121	Gastromark, Ferumoxsil, Lumirem	Bowel	Approved
SHU555A	Resovist	Liver	Approved (EU, Japan, Australia)
AMI-227	Combidex, Sinerem, Ferumoxtran	Lymph node metastases	Phase III
CODE 7228	Feraheme, Ferumoxytol	Vasculature	Phase II

biomedical application in clinic (Table 13.2) because of their excellent properties of biocompatibility and biodegradability [32, 33]. Active targeting, as opposed to passive targeting, should add value to selective and site-specific treatment. In order to be able to actively and specifically target BCSCs to a solid tumor, a pre-requisite is the presence of a target molecule, a tumor-specific epitope, expressed at the membrane surface of the tumor cells [12]. In most cases, the superparamagnetic iron oxide nanoparticles (SPIOs) are equipped with certain agents that recognize various BCSC surface proteins have received particular attention as nanotechnological platform to identify and treat image-guided BCSC within tumors.

13.3 Current Evidence and Concepts

13.3.1 A Novel Putative BSCS Marker, EDB-FN and BCSC-Targeted Therapy by Liposomal Delivery of EDB-FN siRNA

In breast cancer, several putative BCSC markers have already been reported, but the agreement on their phenotypic characterization is still absent. Lee et al. [20] first reported that CD49d$^{+/high}$ population (designated NDY-1 cells) derived from primary breast carcinosarcoma tissue of Korean patient displays long-term self-renewing spheres, high tumor-initiating ability in limiting dilution transplantation to NOD/SCID mice, low response rate to docetaxel treatment (Fig. 13.1). Sun Y et al. [34] demonstrated that NDY-1 cells express BCSC-related genes such as BCSC phenotype markers (CD44^{+}/CD24^{-}/ALDH^{+}) and self-renewal (KLF-4, c-Myc, Oct-4, and Nanog), and intriguingly, high level of EDB-FN (Fig. 13.2). EDB-FN is not found in normal adult tissues, but it is highly expressed in the blood vessels and extracellular matrices of aggressive solid tumors, which makes it a

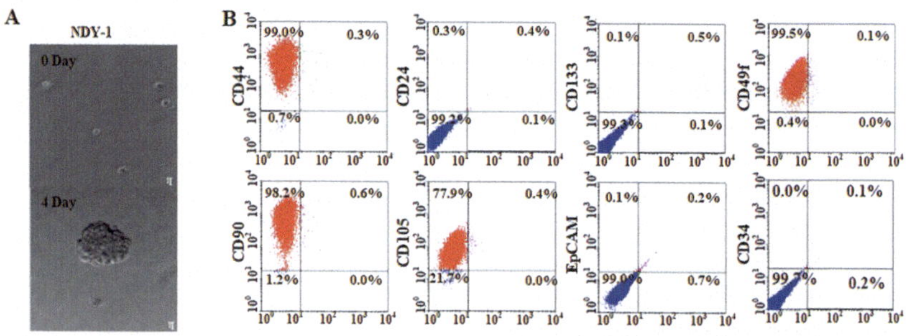

C

Injected cell No.	Tumorigenic Incidence (%)
1x10^6	3/3 (100%)
1x10^5	6/6 (100%)
1x10^4	4/4 (100%)
1x10^3	4/4 (100%)
2x10^2	1/4 (25%)

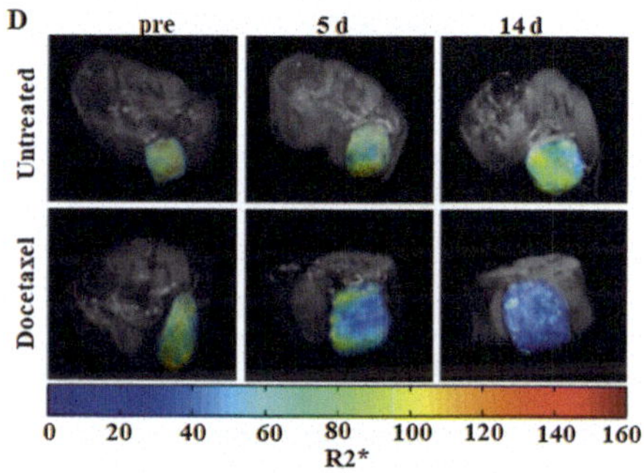

Fig. 13.1 In vitro and in vivo characterization of NDY-1 cells (**a**) Sphere-forming ability of NDY-1 cells in anchorage-independent conditions (**b**) Flow cytometric analysis for phenotypic markers. NDY-1 cells exhibit CD44high, CD24−, CD49fhigh, CD90high, EpCAM−, and CD34−. (**c**) Tumor formation in a non-obese diabetic-severe combined immunodeficiency (NOD/SCID) injected with NDY-1 cells in the mammary fat pads. NDY-1 cells populations induced tumor formation, even when as few as 200 cells were injected. (**d**) Comparative MRI and R2* value distribution analysis for therapeutic response to docetaxel treatment on NDY-1 xenograft tumors. NDY-1 xenograft tumors display low response rate to docetaxel treatment

promising tumor-associated biomarker [35–38]. In very recent study [39], siRNA-mediated EDB-FN knockdown NDY-1 cells display the significant reduction in the gene expression levels related with BCSC phenotype markers ($CD44^+/CD24^-/ALDH^+$), the self-renewal genes (KLF-4, c-Myc, Oct-4, and Nanog), drug resistance (ABCG-2), and mesenchymal marker (N-cadherin, Slug, Twist) and sphere-forming ability (Fig. 13.3). EDB-FN-specific peptides (APT_{EDB}) to preferentially target EDB-FN-positive BCSCs and EDB-FN targeting liposomes (APT_{EDB}-LS-$siRNA^{EDB}$) that encapsulate EDB-FN siRNA for the BCSC-targeted therapy were produced (Fig. 13.4a–d). The tumor volumes in the $siRNA^{EDB}$- and LS-siRNA-treated groups were slightly lower than those of saline-treated mice whereas those of the APT_{EDB}-LS-$siRNA^{EDB}$-treated group were much lower (Fig. 13.4e, f). Histological analysis further showed that treatment with APT_{EDB}-LS-$siRNA^{EDB}$ markedly reduced the expression of CD44 and KLF-4 and induced the translocation of integrin-α5 into the nucleus of the tumor (Fig. 13.4g). Collectively, our findings suggest that EDB-FN is an additional marker of BCSCs when combined with $CD44^+/CD24^-/ALDH^+$ for targeting and treating BCSCs, and a targeted delivery

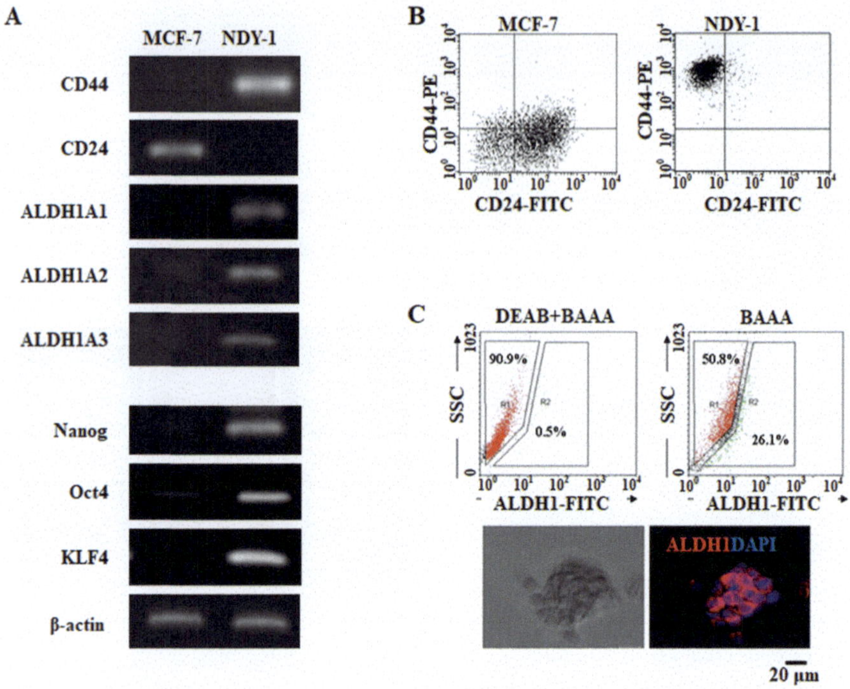

Fig. 13.2 Analysis of heterogeneous phenotype markers expressed in NDY-1. (**a**) RT-PCR analysis of the self-renewal- and phenotype marker-related genes in NDY-1 and MCF-7. Specific phenotype markers of BCSCs and self-renewal genes were highly expressed in NDY-1 cells but not in MCF-7 cells. (**b**) Flow cytometry analysis of the surface markers CD44 and CD24. NDY-1 exhibited a CD44+/CD24− BCSC phenotype. (**c**) ALDEFLUOR assay for ALDH1 activity and immunostaining analysis for ALDH1 expression. NDY-1 cells exhibited ALDH1 activity and NDY-1 spheroids strongly expressed the ALDH1 protein

of EDB-FN siRNA to BCSCs may be a conceivable option for treatment of the aggressive breast tumors.

13.3.2 MRI-Guided Diagnosis of BCSCs Using the EDB-FN Targeting SPIOs

The non-invasive targeted imaging of BCSCs is important for the diagnosis and therapy of breast cancers. Our collaborator developed the thermally cross-linked superparamagnetic iron oxide nanoparticles (TCL-SPION) achieving lower cytotoxicity and better tumor MR contrast than commercially available SPIONs, monocrystalline iron oxide nanoparticles (MION-47), and clinically approved SPIONs, Feridex, and Resovist [40], suggesting that TCL-SPION may be used as a new platform for tumor imaging and therapy monitoring. Recently, we prepared EDB-FN

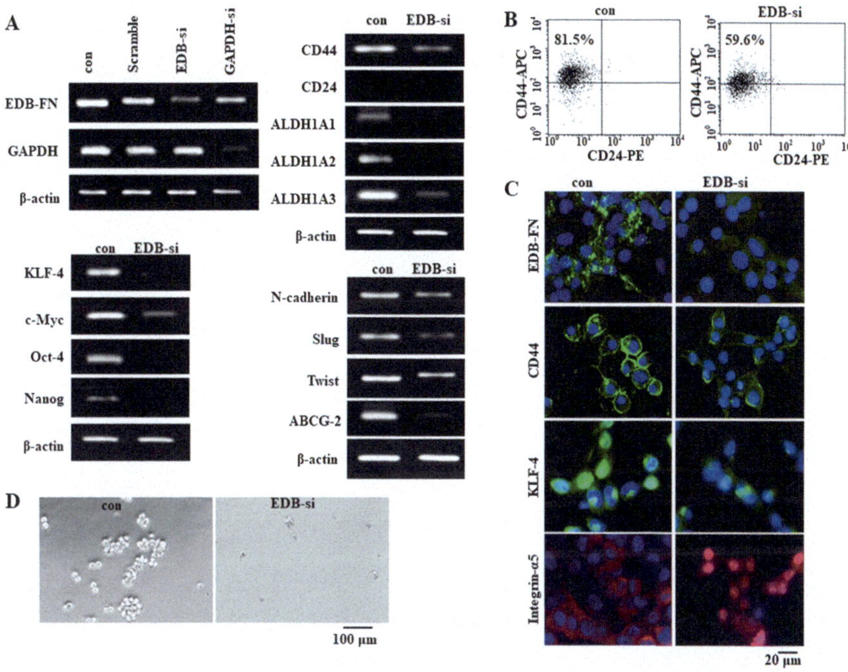

Fig. 13.3 Analysis of BCSC phenotype markers and sphere formation in EDB-FN knockdown NDY-1 cells (**a**) RT-PCR analysis of genes related with BCSC phenotype markers (CD44, CD24, and ALDH1A), self-renewal (KLF-4, c-Myc, Oct-4, and Nanog), mesenchymal marker (N-cadherin, Slug, and Twist), and drug resistance (ABCG-2) in EDB-FN knockdown NDY-1 cells. EDB-FN siRNA strongly silenced EDB-FN expression, as well as suppressing the expression of CD44, ALDH1A1-3, KLF-4, c-Myc, Oct-4, Nanog, N-cadherin, Slug, Twist, and ABCG-2 mRNAs. (**b**) Flow cytometry analysis of EDB-FN knockdown cells. EDB-FN knockdown resulted in decreasing CD44+/CD24 population. (**c**) Immunofluorescence images of EDB-FN, CD44, KLF-4, and integrin-α5 expression. EDB-FN knockdown downregulated expression of EDB-FN, CD44, and KLF-4 and caused integrin-α5 to localize to the nucleus. (**d**) Sphere formation of EDB-FN knockdown NDY-1 cells. The EDB-FN knockdown cells failed to form spheres efficiently in anchorage-independent conditions

targeting TCL-SPION (APT_{EDB}-TCL-SPIONs) conjugated with EDB-FN-specific peptides to evaluate whether could be applied for BSCS imaging in vitro and in vivo (Fig. 13.5a, b). In the in vitro MRI of cell phantoms, selective binding of APT_{EDB}-TCL-SPION to NDY-1 cells was evident (Fig. 13.5c). After the intravenous injection of APT_{EDB}-TCL-SPION into the NDY-1 mouse tumor xenograft model, a significant decrease in the signal within the tumor was observed in the T_2*-weighted images; however, there was only a marginal change in the signal of non-targeting SPIONs such as $APT_{scramble}$-TCL-SPION (Fig. 13.5d). EDB-FN proteins (dark brown) were abundantly detected in the NDY-1 tumor cells as well as the tumor vasculature and interstitium and prussian blue staining revealed that a large number

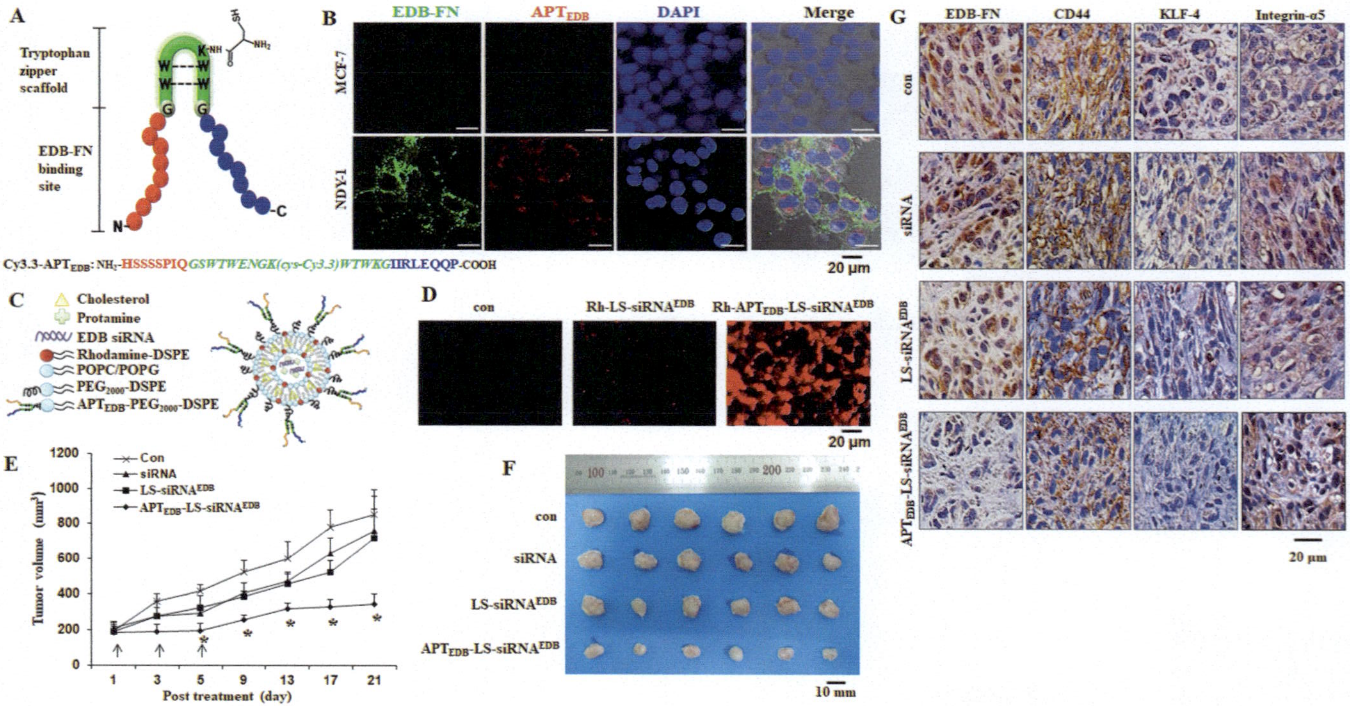

Fig. 13.4 EDB-FN-specific peptides (APT_{EDB}) to preferentially target EDB-FN-positive BCSCs and EDB-FN targeting liposomes (APT_{EDB}-LS-$siRNA^{EDB}$) that encapsulate EDB-FN siRNA for the BCSC-targeted therapy (**a**) A schematic depiction of EDB-FN-specific peptide structure. (**b**) EDB-FN targeting images of the Cy3.3-labeled APT_{EDB} (Cy3.3-APT_{EDB}, red fluorescence) and immunostained EDB-FN (green fluorescence) images in breast cancer cells. Cy3.3-APT_{EDB}-specific signals were observed in EDB-FN overexpressing NDY-1 cells but not in MCF-7 cells. (**c**) A schematic depiction of rhodamine-labeled APT_{EDB}-LS-$siRNA^{EDB}$ (Rh-APT_{EDB}-LS-$siRNA^{EDB}$). (**d**) Fluorescence images of the cellular uptake of Rh-LS-$siRNA^{EDB}$ or Rh-APT_{EDB}-LS-$siRNA^{EDB}$. Effective uptake of Rh-APT_{EDB}–LS-$siRNA^{EDB}$ by NDY-1 cells was observed at 4 h after treatment. (**e**) Volumes of subcutaneous xenograft tumors in NOG mice

after systemic treatment with $siRNA^{EDB}$, $LS\text{-}siRNA^{EDB}$, or $APT_{EDB}\text{-}LS\text{-}siRNA^{EDB}$. Three intravenous injections (arrows) of $APT_{EDB}\text{-}LS\text{-}siRNA^{EDB}$ (3 mg/kg) effectively suppressed tumor growth when compared with injection of EDB-FN siRNA, $LS\text{-}siRNA^{EDB}$, or saline. (**f**) Images of tumors isolated from NOG mice at 21 days after systemic treatment with $siRNA^{EDB}$, $LS\text{-}siRNA^{EDB}$, or $APT_{EDB}\text{-}LS\text{-}siRNA^{EDB}$. The tumors isolated from $APT_{EDB}\text{-}LS\text{-}siRNA^{EDB}$-treated mice were significantly smaller than those of the other groups. (**g**) Representative immunohistochemical staining of EDB-FN, integrin-α5, CD44, and KLF-4 in tumors treated with $siRNA^{EDB}$, $LS\text{-}siRNA^{EDB}$, or $APT_{EDB}\text{-}LS\text{-}siRNA^{EDB}$

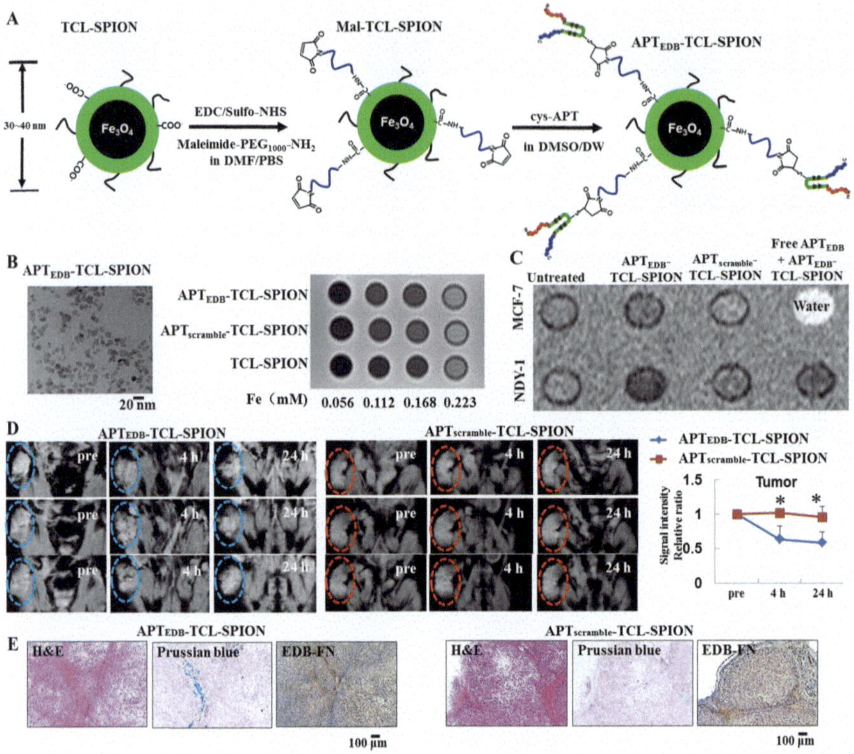

Fig. 13.5 Preparation of APT_{EDB}-TCL-SPION and in vitro and in vivo EDB-FN-targeted MRI (**a**) Schematic illustration of APT_{EDB}-TCL-SPIONs. (**b**) A TEM image of APT_{EDB}-TCL-SPION. (**c**) In vitro T2-weighted images of cell treated with APT_{EDB}-TCL-SPION and $APT_{scramble}$-TCL-SPION (11.2 μg Fe/mL) for 12 h at 37 °C after blocking with EDB-FN aptides (APT_{EDB}, 0.1 mg/mL) for 1 h. Hypointense signals were clearly detected in NDY-1 cells treated with APT_{EDB}-TCL-SPIONs but were reduced by pre-incubation with APT_{EDB}. (**d**) In vivo T2*-weighted multi-slice images and signal intensity of the NDY-1 tumor in the mouse obtained prior to injection and at 4 h and 24 h after the injection of APT_{EDB}-TCL-SPION or $APT_{scramble}$-TCL-SPION (20 mg Fe/kg). Multifocal hypointense spots and An apparent signal intensity decrease were observed in tumors obtained from mice injected with APT_{EDB}-TCL-SPION. (**e**) Hematoxylin and eosin (H&E) staining, Prussian blue staining, and EDB-FN immunostaining in tumor sections. EDB-FN proteins (dark brown) were abundantly detected in the NDY-1 tumors. Prussian blue staining showed that a larger number of accumulated SPIONs were detected as blue dots in the tumors obtained from mice injected with APT_{EDB}-TCL-SPION compared with $APT_{scramble}$-TCL-SPION

of blue dots were observed in the tumors obtained from mice injected with APT_{EDB}-TCL-SPION relative to $APT_{scramble}$-TCL-SPION (Fig. 13.5e). Taken together, we report for the first time that APT_{EDB}-TCL-SPION could be used as an MRI contrast agent for non-invasive BSCS imaging.

13.3.3 Delivery of Doxorubicin-Loaded Theranostics to BCSCs

Functionalized nanoparticles are ideal platform for successful BCSCs-specific therapies because they possess the properties of high drug loading capacity solubility enhancement effects, site-specific delivery mechanism that avoids drug deposition in normal tissues, and provides effective drug doses to the target site. Finally, we produced the doxorubicin (Dox)-loaded APT_{EDB}-TCL-SPIONs (Dox@APT_{EDB}-TCL-SPIONs) [41] (Fig. 13.6a), which can be employed for MRI-guided simultaneous diagnosis and therapy. The Dox@APT_{EDB}-TCL-SPIONs had a nine to ten fold higher area under the curve (AUC) and a lower clearance rate (CL) compared to free Dox (Fig. 13.6b). Dox@APT_{EDB}-TCL-SPIONs enabled more efficient delivery of Dox, thus exhibiting higher cytotoxic activity than non-targeted Dox@TCL-SPIONs (Fig. 13.6c). The therapeutic responses of individual BCSC tumors to doxorubicin (Dox) in 21 mice were evaluated by MRI finding and histological features. Because the mean SI ratio of the post-contrast to pre-contrast MR images of the tumor masses was 0.61 ± 0.94 after three injections of the Dox@APT_{EDB}-TCL-SPIONs, a cutoff value of 0.6 for the signal intensity (SI) ratio based on the predictive value for MRI-guided theranostic agents was selected. The decrease in tumor volume after 14 days (calculated as a ratio of the post-treatment volume compared to pre-treatment volume) was greater in the SI < 0.6 group compared to the SI > 0.6 group (Fig. 13.6d). The relative SI enhanced by Dox@APT_{EDB}-TCL-SPIONs on T_2*-weighted images of tumors was significantly correlated with the scores of EDB-FN and TUNEL staining at histology, thus demonstrating the ability of Dox@APT_{EDB}-TCL-SPIONs to identify the presence of a BCSC population within tumors and predict great therapeutic efficacy in tumors with high level of EDB-FN expression (Fig. 13.6e). Our data indicate Dox@APT_{EDB}-TCL-SPIONs can detect and treat BCSCs within tumors by targeting EDB-FN-expressing cells. These nanoparticles thus have MRI-guided theranostic potential in breast cancer.

13.4 Future Research Direction

Combination with molecular imaging and nanomedicines now represents an effective approach to accelerate the development of potential drugs against cancer. BCSCs markers are instable and substantially heterogeneous between patients. The recent advent of high-throughput sequencing platforms including single-cell RNA-sequencing opened a new window in identifying additional BCSC markers, understanding of BCSC heterogeneity, and the development of precision medicine for individual cancer patient. Before designing novel anti-BCSC strategies, most of all, available markers should be further tested in combination; additional markers, or specific gene signatures, are definitely needed to define, and possibly target, BCSC populations of the different breast cancer subtypes. Thus, taking a precision

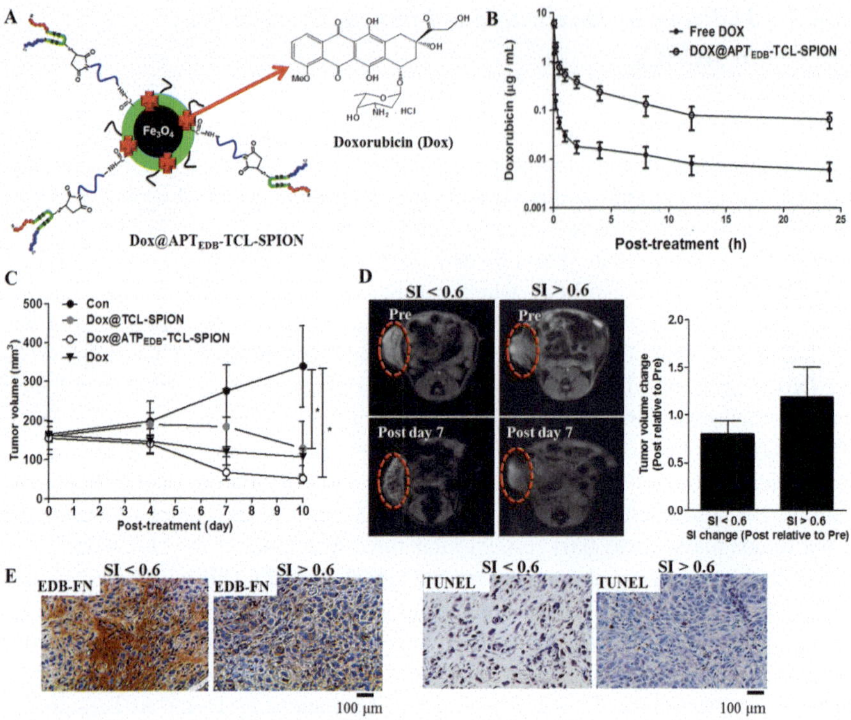

Fig. 13.6 Preparation of Dox@APT_{EDB}-TCL-SPION loaded with doxorubicin (Dox) and evaluation of the anti-tumor efficacy of the Dox@APT_{EDB}-TCL-SPIONs in vivo (**a**) Schematic illustration of Dox@APT_{EDB}-TCL-SPIONs. (**b**) In vivo pharmacokinetics of the Dox@APT_{EDB}-TCL-SPIONs. The total Dox concentration in blood samples of female BALB/c nude mice was quantified following administration of free Dox (2 mg/kg DOX) or Dox@APT_{EDB}-TCL-SPIONs (2 mg/kg Dox; 20 mg Fe/kg APT_{EDB}-TCL-SPIONs). The Dox@APT_{EDB}-TCL-SPIONs had a nine to tenfold higher area under the curve and a lower clearance rate compared to free Dox. (**c**) Evaluation of the anti-tumor efficacy of the Dox@APT_{EDB}-TCL-SPIONs in vivo. Dox@APT_{EDB}-TCL-SPIONs or Dox@TCL-SPIONs containing 2 mg Dox/kg and Dox were intravenously administered on days 0, 3, and 6. The greatest inhibition of tumor growth was observed after treatment with the Dox@APT_{EDB}-TCL-SPIONs. (**d**) Representative T2*-weighted MR images of tumors (red circle) with the indicated signal intensity (SI) ratios 7 days after treatment with Dox@APT_{EDB}-TCL-SPIONs according to a cut-off value of 0.6 for the SI ratio based on the predictive value for MRI-guided theranostic agents. The changes in tumor volume after 14 days (calculated as a ratio of the post-treatment volume compared to pre-treatment volume) was greater in the SI < 0.6 group compared to the SI > 0.6 group. (**e**) Correlation between the MRI SI ratio and the histological characteristics (EDB-FN and TUNEL staining) of tumors in mice treated with Dox@APT_{EDB}-TCL-SPIONs. As the SI ratio decreased, an increase in EDB-FN and TUNEL staining was observed

medicine approach to individual patients with different BCSCs markers, "personalized" nanoparticles conjugated with BCSCs marker-specific ligands/antibodies should be developed and approved in clinic. The distinct nano-scale material formulations to enhance co-delivery of chemotherapy drugs against conventional cancer cells and BCSC-targeting drugs and combine with thermal, radiation, and immunotherapeutic strategy may have great potential in facilitating BCSC therapy.

13.5 Summary

1. The bench
   NDY-1 cells derived from primary breast carcinosarcoma tissue exhibit BCSC characteristics including CD44+CD24−ALDH+ markers, long-term self-renewing spheres, and high tumor-initiating ability. Most importantly, EDB-FN highly expressed in NDY-1 cells is considered as a putative additional marker for BCSC derived from human breast carcinosarcoma.
2. Translation
   A liposomal system (APT_{EDB}-LS-$siRNA^{EDB}$) that enables simultaneous targeting and knockdown of EDB-FN shows potent therapeutic efficacy in the BCSC-derived tumors in vivo. The doxorubicin-loaded APT_{EDB}-TCL-SPIONs (Dox@APT_{EDB}-TCL-SPIONs) can detect and treat BCSCs within tumors by efficiently targeting EDB-FN and show MRI-guided theranostic potential to predict individual treatment responses.
3. The bedside
   Image-guided theranostics using these nanoparticles can offer clinicians a novel way to non-invasively analyze intra- or inter-different features of tumors and predict the therapeutic potency of anticancer medicines in a personalized manner. The emerging field of theranostics can improve precision medicine.

References

1. Cho N, Han W, Han BK, Bae MS, Ko ES, Nam SJ, Chae EY, Lee JW, Kim SH, Kang BJ, et al. Breast cancer screening with mammography plus ultrasonography or magnetic resonance imaging in women 50 years or younger at diagnosis and treated with breast conservation therapy. JAMA Oncol. 2017;3(11):1495–502.
2. Vinogradov S, Wei X. Cancer stem cells and drug resistance: the potential of nanomedicine. Nanomedicine (Lond). 2012;7:597–615.
3. Bonnet D, Dick JE. Human acute myeloid leukemia is organized as a hierarchy that originates from a primitive hematopoietic cell. Nat Med. 1997;3:730–7.
4. Wang JC, Lapidot T, Cashman JD, Doedens M, Addy L, Sutherland DR, Nayar R, Laraya P, Minden M, Keating A, et al. High level engraftment of NOD/SCID mice by primitive normal and leukemic hematopoietic cells from patients with chronic myeloid leukemia in chronic phase. Blood. 1998;91:2406–14.
5. Lapidot T, Sirard C, Vormoor J, Murdoch B, Hoang T, Caceres-Cortes J, Minden M, Paterson B, Caligiuri MA, Dick JE. A cell initiating human acute myeloid leukaemia after transplantation into SCID mice. Nature. 1994;367:645–8.
6. Clarke MF, Dick JE, Dirks PB, Eaves CJ, Jamieson CH, Jones DL, Visvader J, Weissman IL, Wahl GM. Cancer stem cells--perspectives on current status and future directions: AACR workshop on cancer stem cells. Cancer Res. 2006;66:9339–44.

7. Ailles LE, Weissman IL. Cancer stem cells in solid tumors. Curr Opin Biotechnol. 2007;18:460–6.
8. Fillmore CM, Kuperwasser C. Human breast cancer cell lines contain stem-like cells that self-renew, give rise to phenotypically diverse progeny and survive chemotherapy. Breast Cancer Res. 2008;10:R25.
9. Dick JE. Stem cell concepts renew cancer research. Blood. 2008;112:4793–807.
10. Meacham CE, Morrison SJ. Tumour heterogeneity and cancer cell plasticity. Nature. 2013;501:328–37.
11. He L, Gu J, Lim LY, Yuan ZX, Mo J. Nanomedicine-mediated therapies to target breast cancer stem cells. Front Pharmacol. 2016;7:313.
12. Shen S, Xia JX, Wang J. Nanomedicine-mediated cancer stem cell therapy. Biomaterials. 2016;74:1–18.
13. Al-Hajj M, Wicha MS, Benito-Hernandez A, Morrison SJ, Clarke MF. Prospective identification of tumorigenic breast cancer cells. Proc Natl Acad Sci U S A. 2003;100:3983–8.
14. Ginestier C, Hur MH, Charafe-Jauffret E, Monville F, Dutcher J, Brown M, Jacquemier J, Viens P, Kleer CG, Liu S, et al. ALDH1 is a marker of normal and malignant human mammary stem cells and a predictor of poor clinical outcome. Cell Stem Cell. 2007;1:555–67.
15. Charafe-Jauffret E, Ginestier C, Iovino F, Tarpin C, Diebel M, Esterni B, Houvenaeghel G, Extra JM, Bertucci F, Jacquemier J, et al. Aldehyde dehydrogenase 1-positive cancer stem cells mediate metastasis and poor clinical outcome in inflammatory breast cancer. Clin Cancer Res. 2010;16:45–55.
16. Abraham BK, Fritz P, McClellan M, Hauptvogel P, Athelogou M, Brauch H. Prevalence of CD44+/CD24−/low cells in breast cancer may not be associated with clinical outcome but may favor distant metastasis. Clin Cancer Res. 2005;11:1154–9.
17. Rappa G, Lorico A. Phenotypic characterization of mammosphere-forming cells from the human MA-11 breast carcinoma cell line. Exp Cell Res. 2010;316:1576–86.
18. Wright MH, Calcagno AM, Salcido CD, Carlson MD, Ambudkar SV, Varticovski L. Brca1 breast tumors contain distinct CD44+/CD24- and CD133+ cells with cancer stem cell characteristics. Breast Cancer Res. 2008;10:R10.
19. Honeth G, Bendahl PO, Ringner M, Saal LH, Gruvberger-Saal SK, Lovgren K, Grabau D, Ferno M, Borg A, Hegardt C. The CD44+/CD24- phenotype is enriched in basal-like breast tumors. Breast Cancer Res. 2008;10:R53.
20. Lee KM, Han W, Kim JB, Shin I, Ko E, Park IA, Lee DS, Oh K, Noh DY. The CD49d+/high subpopulation from isolated human breast sarcoma spheres possesses tumor-initiating ability. Int J Oncol. 2012;40:665–72.
21. Visvader JE. Cells of origin in cancer. Nature. 2011;469:314–22.
22. Hirschmann-Jax C, Foster AE, Wulf GG, Nuchtern JG, Jax TW, Gobel U, Goodell MA, Brenner MK. A distinct "side population" of cells with high drug efflux capacity in human tumor cells. Proc Natl Acad Sci U S A. 2004;101:14228–33.
23. Xiao Y, Ye Y, Yearsley K, Jones S, Barsky SH. The lymphovascular embolus of inflammatory breast cancer expresses a stem cell-like phenotype. Am J Pathol. 2008;173:561–74.
24. Storci G, Sansone P, Trere D, Tavolari S, Taffurelli M, Ceccarelli C, Guarnieri T, Paterini P, Pariali M, Montanaro L, et al. The basal-like breast carcinoma phenotype is regulated by SLUG gene expression. J Pathol. 2008;214:25–37.
25. Vassilopoulos A, Wang RH, Petrovas C, Ambrozak D, Koup R, Deng CX. Identification and characterization of cancer initiating cells from BRCA1 related mammary tumors using markers for normal mammary stem cells. Int J Biol Sci. 2008;4:133–42.
26. Vaillant F, Asselin-Labat ML, Shackleton M, Forrest NC, Lindeman GJ, Visvader JE. The mammary progenitor marker CD61/beta3 integrin identifies cancer stem cells in mouse models of mammary tumorigenesis. Cancer Res. 2008;68:7711–7.
27. Ponti D, Costa A, Zaffaroni N, Pratesi G, Petrangolini G, Coradini D, Pilotti S, Pierotti MA, Daidone MG. Isolation and in vitro propagation of tumorigenic breast cancer cells with stem/progenitor cell properties. Cancer Res. 2005;65:5506–11.

28. Fournier MV, Martin KJ. Transcriptome profiling in clinical breast cancer: from 3D culture models to prognostic signatures. J Cell Physiol. 2006;209:625–30.
29. Patrawala L, Calhoun T, Schneider-Broussard R, Zhou J, Claypool K, Tang DG. Side population is enriched in tumorigenic, stem-like cancer cells, whereas ABCG2+ and ABCG2- cancer cells are similarly tumorigenic. Cancer Res. 2005;65:6207–19.
30. Charafe-Jauffret E, Ginestier C, Iovino F, Wicinski J, Cervera N, Finetti P, Hur MH, Diebel ME, Monville F, Dutcher J, et al. Breast cancer cell lines contain functional cancer stem cells with metastatic capacity and a distinct molecular signature. Cancer Res. 2009;69:1302–13.
31. Hwang-Verslues WW, Kuo WH, Chang PH, Pan CC, Wang HH, Tsai ST, Jeng YM, Shew JY, Kung JT, Chen CH, et al. Multiple lineages of human breast cancer stem/progenitor cells identified by profiling with stem cell markers. PLoS One. 2009;4:e8377.
32. Weissleder R, Stark DD, Engelstad BL, Bacon BR, Compton CC, White DL, Jacobs P, Lewis J. Superparamagnetic iron oxide: pharmacokinetics and toxicity. AJR Am J Roentgenol. 1989;152:167–73.
33. Gupta AK, Naregalkar RR, Vaidya VD, Gupta M. Recent advances on surface engineering of magnetic iron oxide nanoparticles and their biomedical applications. Nanomedicine (Lond). 2007;2:23–39.
34. Sun Y, Kim HS, Park J, Li M, Tian L, Choi Y, Choi BI, Jon S, Moon WK. MRI of breast tumor initiating cells using the extra domain-B of fibronectin targeting nanoparticles. Theranostics. 2014;4:845–57.
35. Santimaria M, Moscatelli G, Viale GL, Giovannoni L, Neri G, Viti F, Leprini A, Borsi L, Castellani P, Zardi L, et al. Immunoscintigraphic detection of the ED-B domain of fibronectin, a marker of angiogenesis, in patients with cancer. Clin Cancer Res. 2003;9:571–9.
36. Mhawech P, Dulguerov P, Assaly M, Ares C, Allal AS. EB-D fibronectin expression in squamous cell carcinoma of the head and neck. Oral Oncol. 2005;41:82–8.
37. Kosmehl H, Berndt A, Strassburger S, Borsi L, Rousselle P, Mandel U, Hyckel P, Zardi L, Katenkamp D. Distribution of laminin and fibronectin isoforms in oral mucosa and oral squamous cell carcinoma. Br J Cancer. 1999;81:1071–9.
38. Ricci E, Cavalot AL, Sanvito F, Bussi M, Albera R, Staffieri A, Cortesina G, Marchisio PC. Differential expression and topography of adhesion molecules in laryngeal and oropharyngeal carcinomas. Acta Otolaryngol. 2002;122:234–40.
39. Sun Y, Kim HS, Saw PE, Jon S, Moon WK. Targeted therapy for breast cancer stem cells by liposomal delivery of siRNA against fibronectin EDB. Adv Healthc Mater. 2015;4:1675–80.
40. Li M, Kim HS, Tian L, Yu MK, Jon S, Moon WK. Comparison of two ultrasmall superparamagnetic iron oxides on cytotoxicity and MR imaging of tumors. Theranostics. 2012;2:76–85.
41. Yujin S, Hoe SK, Sukmo K, Yin JP, Sangyong J, Woo KM. Magnetic Resonance Imaging-Guided Drug Delivery to Breast Cancer Stem-Like Cells. Advanced Healthcare Materials. 2018;7(21):1800266.

Chapter 14
Patient-Derived Xenograft Models in Breast Cancer Research

Deukchae Na and Hyeong-Gon Moon

Abstract Patient-derived xenograft (PDX) model can be used as a platform to study the individual patient's sensitivity to targeted agents as well as its ability to guide our understanding in various aspects of tumor biology including the tumor's clonal evolution and interaction with microenvironment. In this chapter, we review the history of PDX models in various tumor types. Additionally, we highlight the key studies that suggested potential value of PDX models in cancer treatment. Specifically, we will briefly introduce several studies on the issue of PDX models for precision medicine. In latter part of this chapter, we focus on the studies that used PDX models to investigate the molecular biology of breast cancer that underlies the process of drug resistance and tumor metastasis. Also, we will address our own experience in developing PDX models using breast cancer tissues from Korean breast cancer patients.

Keywords Patient-derived xenograft model · Breast cancer · Genetics · Precision medicine · Drug resistance · Microenvironment

14.1 History of Establishing PDX Models Using Immunodeficient Mice

Patient-derived xenograft (PDX) models can be generated with the implantation of fresh pieces of the tumor in immunodeficient mice, subcutaneously or in a place that more closely resembles the original tumor location to expand and preserve individual tumors from cancer patients [1]. PDX models provide a powerful tool and have

D. Na
Institute of Convergence Medicine, Ewha Womans University Mokdong Hospital, Seoul, South Korea

H.-G. Moon (✉)
Department of Surgery, Seoul National University College of Medicine, Seoul, South Korea

D.-Y. Noh et al. (eds.), *Translational Research in Breast Cancer*, Advances in Experimental Medicine and Biology 1187,
https://doi.org/10.1007/978-981-32-9620-6_14

been widely used for studying cancer biology, assisting personalized cancer therapy and drug screening in a preclinical setting. As human cancer models for anticancer drug testing, PDX models receive attention compared with mouse tumors or human cancer cell lines transplanted into mice. Previous anticancer drug screening methods such as in vitro cell culture and organoid culture models are beneficial in genetic modification and high-throughput screening. However, these methods have limitations such as selective proliferation and adjustment to culture condition [2]. PDX models can preserve key characteristics of patient's tumors including histologic features, genomic signatures, and the heterogeneity of cancer cells [3]. Therefore, they highly recapitulate the original patient tumor and can serve as a predictive platform for therapeutic outcomes [4].

PDX models can be generated using a variety of immunodeficient mice: severely compromised immune deficient (SCID) mice, athymic nude mice, nonobese diabetic (NOD)–SCID mice, and recombination-activating gene 2 (Rag2)-knockout mice [5]. PDX models are generated by implantation of fresh human tumor tissues into immunodeficient mice. Tumors are generally dissected into fragments no larger than 10 mm^3 and are implanted 1–2 tumor tissues per mouse. For solid tumors the cells are grown to approximately 1000 mm^3 size and then can be cryopreserved or can be dissected again and reimplanted into new mice for next passaging (Fig. 14.1). The early success rate of PDX establishment is extremely low, which is largely due to the rejection of grafts by the host immune system. In 1968, Pantelouris reported a mutant mouse (BALB/c nu/nu) suitable for xenografting of human cancer tissue [6]. These nude mice have the *Foxn1* mutation, are athymic, and therefore lack the functional T cells. The take rate of immortalized cell lines in nude mice ranges from 50 to 100%, the take rate of tumor tissue implants is generally low and varies largely among tumors of different origins. Nude mice are still commonly used as hosts for xenotransplantation of human tumors. In 1983, Bosma et al. [7] reported the severe combined immunodeficiency (scid) mutant CB17 mice. The mice that were homozygous for the mutant $Prkdc^{scid}$ (protein kinase, DNA activated, catalytic polypeptide) were designated C.B-17 scid. Further crossing of SCID mice with the nonobese diabetic (NOD) strain led to the development of NOD-SCID mice, which lack both T- and B-lymphocytes [8]. Recently, NOD.Cg-$Prkdc^{scid}$ $Il2rg^{tm1Wjl/SzJ}$(NSG) mice have become the mouse strain of choice for such PDX studies because this mouse has no IL2 receptor gamma, which is an important component of the surface receptor of immune cells that transduce signals from six kinds of interleukins. Since the signaling pathway of IL2 receptor gamma is needed for the differentiation and function of many hematopoietic cells, absence of this receptor leads to dysfunction of innate immunity including natural killer (NK) cells. Therefore, it is considered to be a very effective model for the engraftment of primary tumor tissue or tumor cells (Table 14.1) [9, 10].

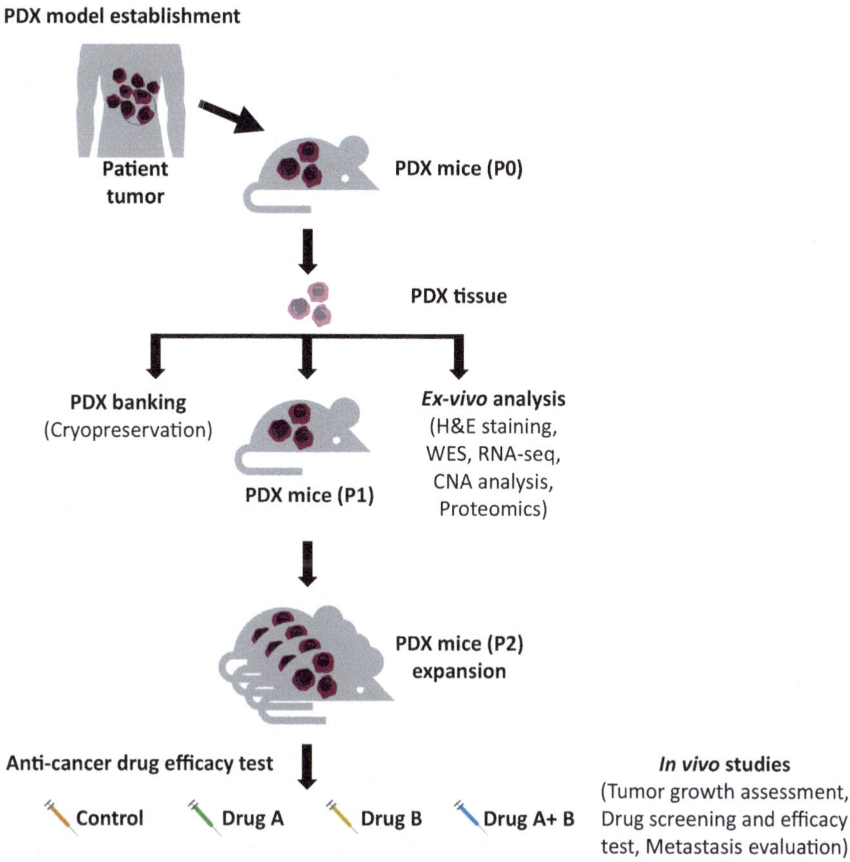

Fig. 14.1 Generation of the PDX models and anticancer drug efficacy testing. Tumor tissues from cancer patients are implanted into immunodeficient mice (P0) subcutaneously or orthotopically. After growth of tumor tissues in P0 mice, these tissues are used for genomic analysis such as whole exome sequencing (WES), RNA sequencing (RNA-seq) and copy number alteration analysis and then can be preserved or reimplanted into new mice for next passage. After more expanding tumor xenografts (P1 and more passages), diverse in vivo anticancer drug response will be tested in these models

14.2 Patient-Derived Xenografts as Cancer Models for the Drug Efficacy and Mechanism of Resistance

PDX models in breast, lung, colorectal, and renal cancers have been already widely used in diverse research projects and preclinical trials. Some studies have suggested that drug efficacy data obtained with PDX models correlates well with clinical data outcome [11]. For example, a study showed high correlation between PDX models and clinical trials for over 3300 drug response datasets [12]. In other study, PDX models of colorectal cancers treated with the epidermal growth factor receptor

Table 14.1 Comparison of immunodeficient mouse strains for PDX models

Mouse strain	Immune system deficiency	Advantage	Disadvantage
BALB/c nude	No mature T cells	Hairless phenotype	Functional B and NK cell
NOD/SCID	No mature T, B cells	Low leakiness with age Engrafts hematopoietic cancer cell lines	Relatively short life span (~36 weeks) Sensitive to irradiation and genome toxic drugs
NSG, NOG	No mature T, B cells, functional NK cells	Support engraftment of malignant hematopoietic cells, solid tumors	Sensitive to irradiation and genome toxic drugs

NOD nonobese diabetic, *SCID* severely compromised immune deficient, *NSG* NOD-SCID mice with $Il2rg^{tm1Wjl}$, *NOG* NOD-SCID mice with $Il2rg^{tm1Sug}$

Table 14.2 Representative commercial PDX models resources

Companies	Country	Homepage
Aveo Oncology	USA	http://www.aveooncology.com
Charles River Laboratories	USA	http://www.criver.com
The Jackson Laboratory	USA	https://www.jax.org
Champions Oncology	USA	https://championsoncology.com
Taconic	USA	http://www.taconic.com
Crownbio	USA	http://www.crownbio.com
WuXi AppTec	China	http://www.wuxiapptec.com
Oncodesign	France	http://www.oncodesign.com
Oncotest	Germany	http://www.oncotest.com

inhibitor, cetuximab, showed similar responses to that of the patients where tumor originated [13]. Similarly, responses to sirolimus and sunitinib and dovitinib, but not to erlotinib, were largely correlated between PDX models and corresponding clinical outcome results for renal cell cancer [14]. Moreover, rapamycin inhibitors showed a poor response in the PDX models of RAS-mutant colorectal carcinomas, which was identical to the results obtained in clinic [15].

Having good correlation between PDX models and clinical trials provides a chance to find novel biomarkers for drug reactivity. For example, in a melanoma PDX model introducing vemurafenib resistance, the resistant tumors showed dependency on BRAF signaling due to the elevated BRAF(V600E) expression [16]. These data suggest the possibility that elevated BRAF expression would be a biomarker for vemurafenib resistance. Another study found a molecular mechanism of gemcitabine resistance through the use of PDX models of pancreatic cancer [17]. Likewise, other prognostic biomarkers of drug reactivity could be identified by diverse drug sensitive and resistant PDX models. Systematic analysis of PDX models enables biobanking of genomically well-defined tumors. These biobanks are valuable resources for developing new predictive or prognostic biomarkers and individualized treatment strategies, thereby potentially guiding personalized medicine (Table 14.2) [18].

Co-clinical trials are preclinical research studies that can be in parallel with human patients in clinical trials. In this application, PDX models are generated from cancer tissues of patients in clinical trials and the PDXs are treated with the same and possibly additional therapies to follow clinical response [19]. Response to new agents, mechanisms underlying responses to the treatment, and exploring prognostic biomarkers can all be studied by using established PDXs from patients in clinical trials. Co-clinical trials have been designed, in which PDX models are treated with anticancer therapies in parallel with the same treatment of patients in clinical trials [20, 21]. The co-clinical trial concept allows integration of preclinical and clinical data, facilitating personalized treatment selection for patients, discovery of predictive biomarkers, and identification of resistance mechanisms. Whether responses to chemotherapy observed in PDX models resemble the response rates of patients in clinical trials still remain to be elucidated [22, 23]. Based on this, strategies for new combinations can also be suggested. For example, a phase II co-clinical trial of arsenic trioxide in relapsed small cell lung cancer revealed that PDX modeling reliably reproduced clinical outcome [24]. Another recent study revealed that the response to dovitinib in lung squamous cell carcinomas could be predicted by signatures of FGFR gene expression [25]. Such co-clinical trials give us a chance to evaluate drug efficacy in a cost-effective and efficient manner.

Although PDX models are excellent in vivo platforms for precision oncology medicine, there are several limitations that should be noted. The first disadvantage is the variable success rate of tumor engraftment [26]. Therefore, the variation observed in the cancer patient population may not be recapitulated faithfully in PDX models due to this selective engraftment rate [19]. Clinically aggressive tumors with many proliferative cancer cells have the highest engraftment rate [27, 28].

A second disadvantage is the long generation time of PDX models, which limits their use in personalized medicine. The time between implantation and progressive growth of the xenograft tumor can range from 2 to 9 months [29]. In general, those tumors that are further advanced tend to grow faster and are easier to establish. In addition, certain tumor types, such as prostate cancers, are difficult to establish as PDX models. In the case of metastasized disease, patients may not even survive the PDX generation time [30]. PDX models may have limited use in diagnostics due to their low-throughput character and relatively high costs. In addition to these practical problems for use of PDX models in personalized medicine, their use is also somewhat limited because of fundamental imperfections of the model. Although they retain intratumor heterogeneity, they fail to maintain the heterogeneity in the human tumor microenvironment, as the tumor stroma is slowly substituted by mouse stroma upon passaging. Therefore, the contribution of tumor–stroma interaction cannot be deduced faithfully from PDX models for drug screening.

Those tumors that have genetic heterogeneity cannot always be recapitulated in serial passages if the genetic heterogeneity is not all represented in the dissected tumor that is passaged. There is controversy in whether PDX mimics the clinical outcome in patients. Todd Golub et al. [31] have tracked 1110 PDX models covering 24 types of cancers, transferring tumor tissue from one mouse to the next and collecting the relevant genetic data. The results show that there is some variation in the data of mice compared to the genetic data of the tumor cells in the human body as the tumor tissue is delivered in mice. The researchers suppose that this change may be due to the different response of the PDX model to cancer drugs. On the contrary to this, David Sidransky et al. [32] have established PDX models of 92 patients with various solid cancers and conducted a dosing study, the results showed that the correlation is up to 87% between the response to drugs of patients and the associated PDX models.

PDX formation requires tumor implantation in severely immunocompromised host animals, complicating the evaluation of tumor immunology and drugs targeting the immune system [33]. This problem could be circumvented by using mice carrying a humanized immune system, although problems with graft-versus-host disease limit this approach severely [34]. Therefore, when studying immunotherapies or tumor–stromal interactions there is a need for alternative model systems that allow exploration of the tumor microenvironment.

Overall, PDX models have been exploited for drug screening, biomarker discovery, identification of resistance mechanisms, and preclinical evaluation of personalized treatment strategies. PDX models maintain several characteristics of the in vivo tumor, including histopathological features, gene expression profiles, copy number variation, and metastatic behavior. PDX models harbor more intratumor complexity because the tumor is not dissociated. Since the generation time of PDX models is rather long, this model is less suitable for drug screening and personalized medicine but is still important for drug validation, investigation of therapy resistance mechanisms and biomarker development.

14.3 Recent Development of PDX Models in Breast Cancer Research

During the last decades, there has been a wide scientific interest in developing PDX models from breast cancer tissues [1, 35–39]. Major studies reporting their experience of developing breast cancer PDX models are listed in the Table 14.1. Based on the advances in developing immunodeficient mouse models that can increase the engraftment rates of human cancer tissues, many studies have reported high numbers of stably maintained breast cancer PDX models more than 30 cases (Table 14.3).

There has been a shift of trends among the past PDX studies that more researchers now use highly immunodeficient mouse strains for developing PDX models, and many researchers focus on developing PDX models from primary tumor rather than metastatic tumors. Zhang et al. [40] have compared the effects of various transplant conditions including the types of mouse strains, the use of supplementary estradiol, and the use of co-injection of fibroblasts in developing successfully engrafted breast cancer PDX models. Using SCID mice, they have observed that while the initial engraftment rates do not vary (47.4% vs 40.0%), there was a significant increase in stable PDX model rates when the estradiol supplementation was used (2.6% vs

Table 14.3 Recent studies reporting the engraftment rate in breast cancer PDX models

	Cases	Strain	Xenograft method	Primary/ metastasis	Engraftment rate	Subtype	Metastasis
Outzen et al. [43]	1	Nude	Minced tissue	Not reported	Not reported	Not reported	Not reported
Sakakibara et al. [44]	37	SCID	Unknown	Unknown	76.1%	Not reported	8/12 (among 12 rapid growing tumors)
Al-Hajj et al. [45]	9	NOD/SCID	Minced tissues (cell suspension for pleural effusion samples), orthotopic	1 (11.1%)/ 8 (89.9%)	Not reported	Not reported	Not reported
Marangoni et al. [46]	22	Athymic nude	Subcutaneous	25 (75.8%)/ 8 (24.2%)	11.0%	5 ER+, 19 ER−	6/17 (lung metastasis)
Bergamaschi et al. [30]	2	SCID	Subcutaneous	All primary	20% (initial) and 6.7% (stable)	1 ER+/PR+, 1 ER−/PR−	Not reported
Liu et al. [47]	8	NOD/SCID	Minced tissues (cell suspension for pleural effusion samples), orthotopic	6 (75.0%)/2 (25.0%)	Not reported	2 HR+, 2 HER2+, 4 TNBC	+ in two TNBC models
Fleming et al. [48]	2	NOD/SCID	Cells from pleural effusion	0 (0%)/2 (100%)	100%	ER− PR−	Not reported
DeRose et al. [49]	12	NOD/SCID	Tissue fragments (cell suspension for pleural effusion and ascites samples), orthotopic	4 (33.3%)/ 8 (66.7%)	27%	2 ER+/PR+/HER2−, 1 ER+/PR+/HER2+, 2 ER−/PR−/HER2+, 5 ER−/PR−/HER2−	11/12 models
Ma et al. [50]	3	NOD/SCID	Tissue fragments	Not reported	Not reported	3 TNBC	Not reported
Kabos et al. [42]	10	NOD/SCID or NOD/SCID/ ILIIrg$^{-/-}$	Tissue fragments (cells in matrigel for pleural effusion and ascites samples), orthotopic	Not reported 4 (66.7%)/2 (33.3%) for	41.7%	8 ER+, 2 TNBC	Not reported

(continued)

Table 14.3 (continued)

	Cases	Strain	Xenograft method	Primary/ metastasis	Engraftment rate	Subtype	Metastasis
				6 models reported			
Valliant et al. [51], Oakes et al. [52]	37	NOD-SCID-IL2Rgc$^{-/-}$	Tissue fragments, orthotopic	Not reported	23.4%	13 HR+, 2 HR−, 5 HER2+	Not reported
Zhang et al. [53]	25	NOD/SCID or NSG	Tissue fragments (cell suspension for pleural effusion and ascites samples), orthotopic	Not reported 20 (80%)/5 (20%) for 25 models	31.3–47.4% according to the transplant condition	7 HER2+, 18 basal (PAM50 subtype)	12/25 models
Li et al. [54]	20	NOD/SCID	Dissociated cell suspension	60 from early, 132 from advanced tumors	14.5%	11 ER−/HER2−, 2 HER2+, 7 ER+/HER2−	Not reported
Du Manoir et al. [55]	20	Nude	Tissue fragments, interscapular fat pad	All primary	15.4%	2 ER+/PR+, 4 ER+/PR−, 14 ER−/PR−	Rare lung metastasis
Zhang et al. [56]	7	NOD/SCID	Tissue fragments, orthotopic	6 (85.7%)/1 (14.3%)	100%	All TNBC	Not reported
Eirew et al. [57]	30	NSG/ NRG	Tumor organoid injection, orthotopic	10 (66.7%)/5 (33.3%) for 16 models analyzed	54.5%	5 ER+, 4 HER2+, 6 TNBC	Not reported
Moon et al. [28]	19	NSG	Tissue fragment, orthotopic	78 (92.8%)/6 (7.2%)	22.6%	3 HR+/HER2−, 1 HR+/HER2+, 3 HR−/HER2+, 12 HR−/HER2−	Frequent lung and lymph node metastasis

21.4%). Interestingly, the concomitant use of immortalized human fibroblasts negated the pro-engraftment effect of estradiol suggesting potential tumor-suppressor effect of human fibroblasts in immunodeficient mice. However, the pro-engraftment effect of estradiol is still controversial since Zhang et al. used different tumors for different transplant conditions rather than randomizing same tumor tissues, and most of the successfully engrafted tumors were estrogen receptor negative tumors. Furthermore, other research groups show comparable success rates of PDX engraftment despite the use of concomitant use of the fibroblasts suggesting that the role of fibroblast requires further clarifications [41, 42].

14.4 Prognostic Implication of PDX Models in Breast Cancer

DeRose et al. [49] have reported the pivotal paper reporting their successful establishment of 12 breast cancer PDX models in 2013. Among the 24 patients with newly diagnosed breast cancer, only four resulted in viable xenograft tumors in NOD/SCID mouse. The patients whose tumors were successfully engrafted into mammary fat pads showed significant worse clinical outcome suggesting that the PDX engraftment can be used as a potential surrogate for tumor aggressiveness and poor clinical outcomes. However, since the authors did not stratify the patients according to the molecular subtypes, the poor clinical outcome in successful PDX engraftment tumors might be confounded by other features of tumor biology such as molecular subtypes. Du Manoir et al. [55] have reported their series of 20 breast cancer PDX models derived from diverse molecular subtypes of breast cancer with the engraftment rate of 15.4%. They have also observed that ER+ tumors showed significantly slower growth rate and successful engraftment rate. In their survival analysis, the PDX engraftment was significantly associated with the relapse-free survival in the breast cancer patients and this association was also observed after stratifying the patients according to the molecular subtypes.

Our initial experience with the PDX models of TNBC tumors included 84 breast cancer patients with different clinical characteristics [28]. When the transplanted cases were stratified according to the clinical and molecular parameters, we observed that the known clinical and molecular parameters, such as clinical presentation or molecular subtypes, which represent the biologic aggressiveness of breast cancer are significantly associated with the successful engraftment rates (Fig. 14.2a, b). The TNBC subtype, which is known to be the most aggressive breast cancer subtype [58], showed not only increased rate of engraftment but also more rapid in vivo tumor growth after transplantation (Fig. 14.2c).

After observing the association between the factors representing tumor aggressiveness and PDX engraftment rates, we sought to find a gene signature that is associated with successful PDX engraftment within the TNBC cases (Fig. 14.2d). Firstly, we observed that the PDX engraftment was associated with higher risk of

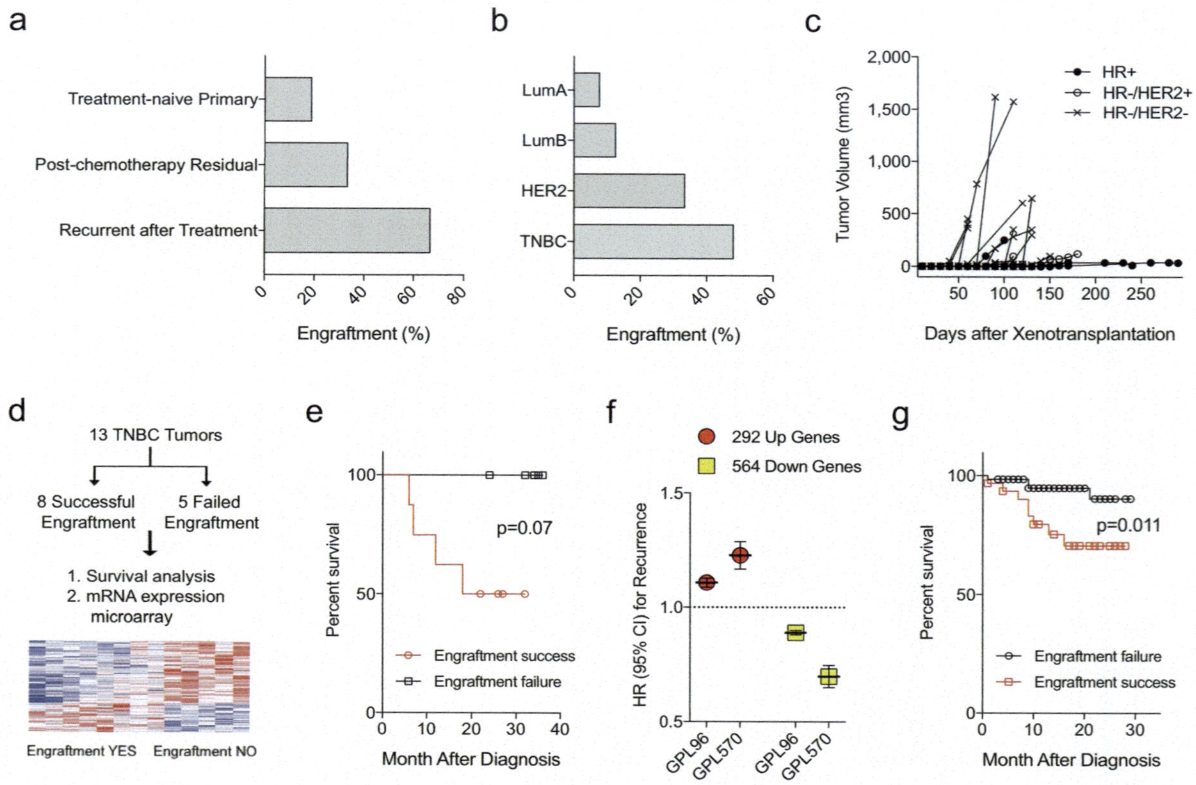

Fig. 14.2 PDX engraftment in breast cancer

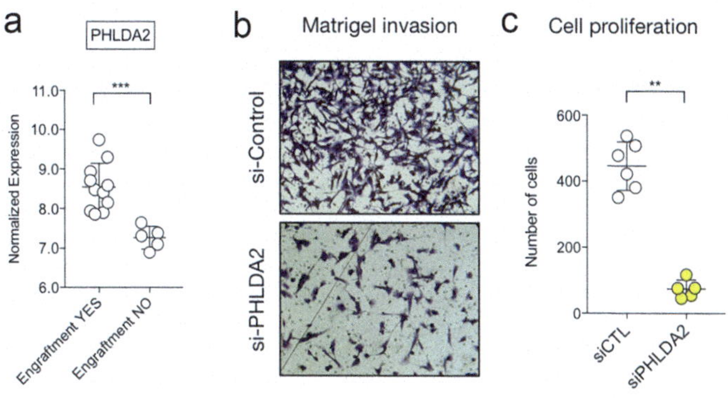

Fig. 14.3 Engraftment-related genes and breast cancer cell phenotype

tumor recurrence in TNBC patients (Fig. 14.2e). We were able to identify a gene signature that represents the TNBC tumor's likeliness to be successfully engrafted in the PDX models. The gene signature of PDX engraftment was significantly associated with patients' prognosis when it was examined in independent mRNA datasets of TNBC patients (Fig. 14.2f). After our initial report on the breast cancer PDX model [28], we have expanded our cases to more smaller and early-stage breast cancer patients, and our experience shows continuous findings that the successful PDX engraftment in TNBC tumors is significantly associated with worse clinical outcomes (Fig. 14.2g).

We then performed an in vitro screening to examine the effect of the PDX engraftment-related upregulated genes on the behaviors of the breast cancer cells. PHLDA2, which showed significant upregulation in TNBC tumors with successful engraftment (Fig. 14.3a), had significant impact on breast cancer cell's proliferation and invasion (Fig. 14.3b, c). Similar findings were shown for other PDX engraftment-related upregulated genes suggesting that the phenomenon of PDX engraftment can be used as an effective surrogate for tumor aggressiveness in TNBC tumors. The association between the successful PDX engraftment and the biologic aggressiveness of the primary tumor has also been reported in other tumor types such as pancreatic cancer or brain tumors [59, 60]. These observations suggest that the PDX engraftment process can be a useful translational platform for developing clinically relevant biomarkers and novel therapeutic targets.

14.5 Research on Breast Cancer Metastasis Using PDX Models

Distant metastatic lesions are the major causes of deaths in breast cancer patients. Although the survival of the stage IV breast cancer patients who carry distant metastasis has been improved due to the recent development in systemic therapies

[61], the efforts to understand the biologic mechanisms of metastasis remain to be a major research field in solid tumors [62]. Traditionally, researchers used archived tissue samples that correspond to primary tumor and metastasis from same patients to define the molecular changes occurring during the process of metastasis [63, 64]. Researchers have also used animal models of distant metastasis using established cancer cell lines. For example, Massagué and colleagues have shown a set of gene expression signatures associated with the lung or bone metastasis by enriching the cell population that drives the metastasis process [65]. In this approach, researchers usually repeat the process of in vivo metastasis to specific organs to detect the distinct molecular features of metastatic cells [66, 67]. While the above approaches resulted in improved insights into the process of metastasis in solid tumors, they also carried certain limitations such as the limited availability of primary and metastatic tumor tissues obtained from patients and the fact that the cell line models cannot fully represent the heterogeneity of human tumors.

PDX models can provide a unique opportunity to address the mechanisms of breast cancer metastasis since some of the models successfully develop distant metastasis in mouse. Sakakibara et al. [44] have shown that, among the twelve rapidly growing breast cancer PDX models, eight showed visible metastasis in distant organs. Marangoni et al. [46] have reported that six out of seventeen breast cancer PDX models showed metastatic lesions in the lung and DeRose et al. [49] have reported even higher rates of in vivo metastasis in their PDX models. Powell et al. [68] have also shown that in their model of a HER2-enriched case, the dissociated PDX tumor cells were able to develop metastasis to the lung, bone, liver, and brain.

Our experience with breast cancer PDX models has also demonstrated that the PDX models of triple negative breast cancers can successfully develop spontaneous metastasis to distant organs [28]. Many of our models showed the presence of metastatic lesions in distant organs such as the lung, liver, or lymph nodes (Fig. 14.4a). The cancer cells in the metastatic lesions showed similar histologic and cytologic features when compared to the cells in the primary transplanted tumors. Furthermore, when the primary tumors and the metastatic sites were profiled for their transcriptomic features, the lesions showed highly correlated profiles of gene expression patterns (Fig. 14.4b). However, some of the genes showed differential expression levels between the primary tumor and metastatic tumors suggesting these genes may play different roles according to the specific sites of tumor growth. These findings suggest that PDX models may provide novel molecular findings that can advance our insights on the process of metastasis.

Powell et al. [69] have used this approach to demonstrate the value of PDX model in identifying a novel CEACAM5 in breast cancer cell's metastasis to lungs. They have obtained lung metastasis cells using orthotopic PDX models and enriched the driver cells of lung metastasis by reimplanting the lung metastatic cells onto mammary fat pads. Genomic profiling of the lung metastatic tumor cells has suggested CEACAM5 as a potent regulator of breast cancer lung metastasis via mesenchymal–epithelial transition mechanisms. It is expected that the PDX model will continue to

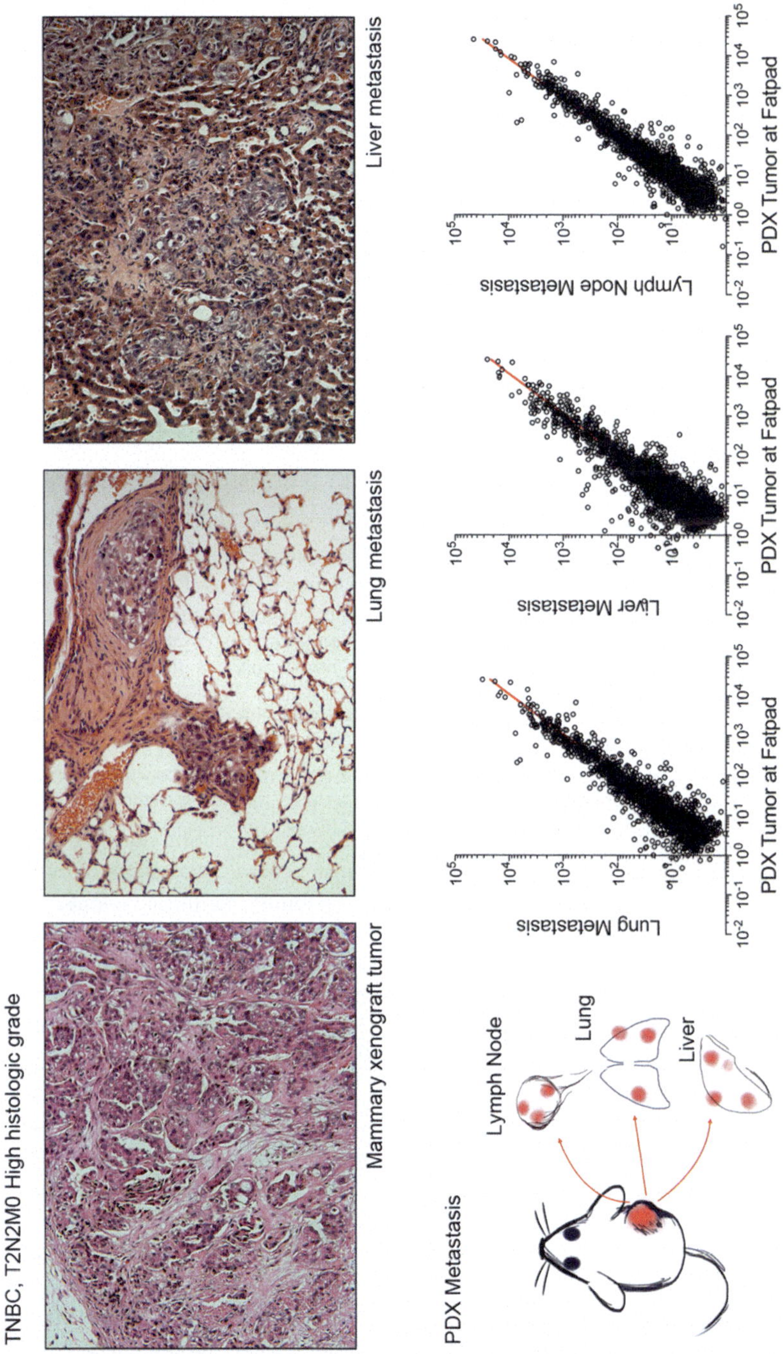

Fig. 14.4 Biological characteristics of PDX tumor and its metastases

serve as a valuable translational platform in exploring the underlying mechanism of breast cancer metastasis.

14.6 Limitations of the Breast Cancer PDX Models

Despite the potential advantages of PDX models for preclinical cancer research, the adoption of the PDX model is still limited. Obviously, the need for the fresh cancer tissues, the higher cost of the model, and the longer time required for initial model establishment are major factors behind the limited use of the PDX models [37]. Especially, in hormone receptor-positive breast cancers, the initial engraftment rate is quite low and the initial engraftment period can be longer than 12 months in some tumors [28]. Considering the high incidence of hormone receptor-positive breast cancers [70], further technical advances that improve the engraftment rate and growth rate are required.

Another important issue for PDX model is the possibility of ongoing genomic evolution of PDX tumors that are not seen in the primary tumor of the originating patients. Bergamaschi et al. [30] have reported the changes in the mutational profiles of PDX tumors including various cancer-driver genes such as TP53. Furthermore, the PDX tumors also showed higher prevalence of structural alterations and gene expression profiles. Our experience with PDX models has also suggested that while the gene expression profiles are generally maintained in PDX tumors, there are small subsets of mutational profiles and structural alterations that are specific to the PDX tumors (unpublished data).

Eirew et al. [71] have extensively analyzed the patterns of the genomic evolution occurring during the PDX engraftment and serial passages. Their findings suggest that breast cancer PDX models show either rapid clonal evolution during the early passages stages or moderate but sustained gain of genomic variations during the serial passages. Additionally, they suggest the possibility that these genomic alterations in PDX models are not stochastic events but rather biologically meaningful determinants of fitness since different PDX models originating from a same tumor show reproducible patterns of genomic evolution.

While the above findings suggest the need for more sophisticated methods for evaluating the authenticity of the PDX models as the PDX models may harbor different genetic characteristics compared to the primary tumors, the findings may also provide a unique window of opportunities to elucidate the process of tumor progression and metastasis in a group of heterogeneous human tumor cells. Indeed, Ding et al. [72] have shown that PDX tumors carry genomic alterations similar to those of metastatic sites that are not detected in the primary tumor.

Finally, the tumor-host interactions that are critical during the development of human solid tumors are not properly reproduced in PDX models due to the lack of adequate tumor-immune responses [73, 74]. This lack of physiologic tumor-immune interactions in the immunodeficient mice has become a more important challenge in the current era of solid tumor immunotherapies [75]. One effort to overcome this limitation is to develop a humanized PDX model by transplanting human hematopoietic stem cells which results in active human immune systems in mice. Wang et al. have showed that the humanized PDX models of triple negative breast cancer patients can be a valuable tool to test the in vivo efficacy of pembrolizumab and to understand the molecular mechanisms of resistance to the immunotherapy [76]. However, the humanized mouse models carry certain limitations according to the specific methods and cell types of transplantation [77]. Further research is needed to determine the optimal methods of humanized PDX models for tumor immunology studies.

References

1. Williams SA, Anderson WC, Santaguida MT, Dylla SJ. Patient-derived xenografts, the cancer stem cell paradigm, and cancer pathobiology in the 21st century. Lab Investig. 2013;93 (9):970–82.
2. Gao D, Chen Y. Organoid development in cancer genome discovery. Curr Opin Genet Dev. 2015;30:42–8.
3. Heid I, Steiger K, Trajkovic-Arsic M, Settles M, Esswein MR, Erkan M, Kleeff J, Jager C, Friess H, Haller B, et al. Co-clinical assessment of tumor cellularity in pancreatic cancer. Clin Cancer Res. 2017;23(6):1461–70.
4. Kopetz S, Lemos R, Powis G. The promise of patient-derived xenografts: the best laid plans of mice and men. Clin Cancer Res. 2012;18(19):5160–2.
5. Morton CL, Houghton PJ. Establishment of human tumor xenografts in immunodeficient mice. Nat Protoc. 2007;2(2):247–50.
6. Pantelouris EM. Absence of thymus in a mouse mutant. Nature. 1968;217(5126):370–1.
7. Bosma GC, Custer RP, Bosma MJ. A severe combined immunodeficiency mutation in the mouse. Nature. 1983;301(5900):527–30.
8. Shultz LD, Schweitzer PA, Christianson SW, Gott B, Schweitzer IB, Tennent B, McKenna S, Mobraaten L, Rajan TV, Greiner DL, et al. Multiple defects in innate and adaptive immunologic function in NOD/LtSz-scid mice. J Immunol. 1995;154(1):180–91.
9. Shultz LD, Lyons BL, Burzenski LM, Gott B, Chen X, Chaleff S, Kotb M, Gillies SD, King M, Mangada J, et al. Human lymphoid and myeloid cell development in NOD/LtSz-scid IL2R gamma null mice engrafted with mobilized human hemopoietic stem cells. J Immunol. 2005;174(10):6477–89.
10. Greiner DL, Hesselton RA, Shultz LD. SCID mouse models of human stem cell engraftment. Stem Cells. 1998;16(3):166–77.
11. Delyon J, Varna M, Feugeas JP, Sadoux A, Yahiaoui S, Podgorniak MP, Leclert G, Dorval SM, Dumaz N, Soulie J, et al. Validation of a preclinical model for assessment of drug efficacy in melanoma. Oncotarget. 2016;7(11):13069–81.
12. Gu Z, Jiang J, Yan Y, Tan T, Yu T, Liu Z, Du W, Yang X, Qiu L, Ye XK. Evaluation of the correlations between patient-derived xenograft (PDX) model-based mouse trials and cancer patient-based clinical trials. J Clin Oncol. 2017;35(15_suppl):e23140.
13. Bertotti A, Migliardi G, Galimi F, Sassi F, Torti D, Isella C, Cora D, Di Nicolantonio F, Buscarino M, Petti C, et al. A molecularly annotated platform of patient-derived xenografts ("xenopatients") identifies HER2 as an effective therapeutic target in cetuximab-resistant colorectal cancer. Cancer Discov. 2011;1(6):508–23.
14. Kerbel RS. Human tumor xenografts as predictive preclinical models for anticancer drug activity in humans: better than commonly perceived-but they can be improved. Cancer Biol Ther. 2003;2(4 Suppl 1):S134–9.

15. Migliardi G, Sassi F, Torti D, Galimi F, Zanella ER, Buscarino M, Ribero D, Muratore A, Massucco P, Pisacane A, et al. Inhibition of MEK and PI3K/mTOR suppresses tumor growth but does not cause tumor regression in patient-derived xenografts of RAS-mutant colorectal carcinomas. Clin Cancer Res. 2012;18(9):2515–25.
16. Das Thakur M, Salangsang F, Landman AS, Sellers WR, Pryer NK, Levesque MP, Dummer R, McMahon M, Stuart DD. Modelling vemurafenib resistance in melanoma reveals a strategy to forestall drug resistance. Nature. 2013;494(7436):251–5.
17. Sebastiani V, Ricci F, Rubio-Viqueira B, Kulesza P, Yeo CJ, Hidalgo M, Klein A, Laheru D, Iacobuzio-Donahue CA. Immunohistochemical and genetic evaluation of deoxycytidine kinase in pancreatic cancer: relationship to molecular mechanisms of gemcitabine resistance and survival. Clin Cancer Res. 2006;12(8):2492–7.
18. Dowst H, Pew B, Watkins C, McOwiti A, Barney J, Qu S, Becnel LB. Acquire: an open-source comprehensive cancer biobanking system. Bioinformatics. 2015;31(10):1655–62.
19. Hidalgo M, Amant F, Biankin AV, Budinska E, Byrne AT, Caldas C, Clarke RB, de Jong S, Jonkers J, Maelandsmo GM, et al. Patient-derived xenograft models: an emerging platform for translational cancer research. Cancer Discov. 2014;4(9):998–1013.
20. Nardella C, Lunardi A, Patnaik A, Cantley LC, Pandolfi PP. The APL paradigm and the "co-clinical trial" project. Cancer Discov. 2011;1(2):108–16.
21. Chen Z, Cheng K, Walton Z, Wang Y, Ebi H, Shimamura T, Liu Y, Tupper T, Ouyang J, Li J, et al. A murine lung cancer co-clinical trial identifies genetic modifiers of therapeutic response. Nature. 2012;483(7391):613–7.
22. Rubio-Viqueira B, Hidalgo M. Direct in vivo xenograft tumor model for predicting chemotherapeutic drug response in cancer patients. Clin Pharmacol Ther. 2009;85(2):217–21.
23. Pompili L, Porru M, Caruso C, Biroccio A, Leonetti C. Patient-derived xenografts: a relevant preclinical model for drug development. J Exp Clin Cancer Res. 2016;35(1):189.
24. Owonikoko TK, Zhang G, Kim HS, Stinson RM, Bechara R, Zhang C, Chen Z, Saba NF, Pakkala S, Pillai R, et al. Patient-derived xenografts faithfully replicated clinical outcome in a phase II co-clinical trial of arsenic trioxide in relapsed small cell lung cancer. J Transl Med. 2016;14(1):111.
25. Kim HR, Kang HN, Shim HS, Kim EY, Kim J, Kim DJ, Lee JG, Lee CY, Hong MH, Kim SM, et al. Co-clinical trials demonstrate predictive biomarkers for dovitinib, an FGFR inhibitor, in lung squamous cell carcinoma. Ann Oncol. 2017;28(6):1250–9.
26. Hidalgo M, Bruckheimer E, Rajeshkumar NV, Garrido-Laguna I, De Oliveira E, Rubio-Viqueira B, Strawn S, Wick MJ, Martell J, Sidransky D. A pilot clinical study of treatment guided by personalized tumorgrafts in patients with advanced cancer. Mol Cancer Ther. 2011;10(8):1311–6.
27. Lawrence MG, Pook DW, Wang H, Porter LH, Frydenberg M, Kourambas J, Appu S, Poole C, Beardsley EK, Ryan A, et al. Establishment of primary patient-derived xenografts of palliative TURP specimens to study castrate-resistant prostate cancer. Prostate. 2015;75(13):1475–83.
28. Moon HG, Oh K, Lee J, Lee M, Kim JY, Yoo TK, Seo MW, Park AK, Ryu HS, Jung EJ, et al. Prognostic and functional importance of the engraftment-associated genes in the patient-derived xenograft models of triple-negative breast cancers. Breast Cancer Res Treat. 2015;154 (1):13–22.
29. Dangles-Marie V, Pocard M, Richon S, Weiswald LB, Assayag F, Saulnier P, Judde JG, Janneau JL, Auger N, Validire P, et al. Establishment of human colon cancer cell lines from fresh tumors versus xenografts: comparison of success rate and cell line features. Cancer Res. 2007;67(1):398–407.
30. Bergamaschi A, Hjortland GO, Triulzi T, Sorlie T, Johnsen H, Ree AH, Russnes HG, Tronnes S, Maelandsmo GM, Fodstad O, et al. Molecular profiling and characterization of luminal-like and basal-like in vivo breast cancer xenograft models. Mol Oncol. 2009;3 (5–6):469–82.

31. Ben-David U, Ha G, Tseng YY, Greenwald NF, Oh C, Shih J, McFarland JM, Wong B, Boehm JS, Beroukhim R, et al. Patient-derived xenografts undergo mouse-specific tumor evolution. Nat Genet. 2017;49(11):1567–75.
32. Izumchenko E, Paz K, Ciznadija D, Sloma I, Katz A, Vasquez-Dunddel D, Ben-Zvi I, Stebbing J, McGuire W, Harris W, et al. Patient-derived xenografts effectively capture responses to oncology therapy in a heterogeneous cohort of patients with solid tumors. Ann Oncol. 2017;28(10):2595–605.
33. Cassidy JW, Caldas C, Bruna A. Maintaining tumor heterogeneity in patient-derived tumor Xenografts. Cancer Res. 2015;75(15):2963–8.
34. Shultz LD, Brehm MA, Garcia-Martinez JV, Greiner DL. Humanized mice for immune system investigation: progress, promise and challenges. Nat Rev Immunol. 2012;12(11):786–98.
35. Landis MD, Lehmann BD, Pietenpol JA, Chang JC. Patient-derived breast tumor xenografts facilitating personalized cancer therapy. Breast Cancer Res. 2013;15(1):201.
36. Whittle JR, Lewis MT, Lindeman GJ, Visvader JE. Patient-derived xenograft models of breast cancer and their predictive power. Breast Cancer Res. 2015;17(1):17.
37. Siolas D, Hannon GJ. Patient-derived tumor Xenografts: transforming clinical samples into mouse models. Cancer Res. 2013;73(17):5315.
38. DeRose YS, Gligorich Keith M, Wang G, Georgelas A, Bowman P, Courdy Samir J, Welm Alana L, Welm Bryan E. Patient-derived models of human breast cancer: protocols for in vitro and in vivo applications in tumor biology and translational medicine. Curr Protocols Pharmacol. 2013;60(1):14.23.11–43.
39. Kawaguchi T, Foster BA, Young J, Takabe K. Current update of patient-derived Xenograft model for translational breast cancer research. J Mammary Gland Biol Neoplasia. 2017;22 (2):131–9.
40. Zhang X, Claerhout S, Prat A, Dobrolecki LE, Petrovic I, Lai Q. A renewable tissue resource of phenotypically stable, biologically and ethnically diverse, patient-derived human breast cancer xenograft models. Cancer Res. 2013;73:4885.
41. Li S, Shen D, Shao J, Crowder R, Liu W, Prat A. Endocrine-therapy-resistant ESR1 variants revealed by genomic characterization of breast-cancer-derived xenografts. Cell Rep. 2013;4:1116.
42. Kabos P, Finlay-Schultz J, Li C, Kline E, Finlayson C, Wisell J, Manuel CA, Edgerton SM, Harrell JC, Elias A, et al. Patient-derived luminal breast cancer xenografts retain hormone receptor heterogeneity and help define unique estrogen-dependent gene signatures. Breast Cancer Res Treat. 2012;135(2):415–32.
43. Outzen HC, Custer RP. Growth of human normal and neoplastic mammary tissues in the cleared mammary fat pad of the nude mouse. J Natl Cancer Inst. 1975;55(6):1461–6.
44. Sakakibara T, Xu Y, Bumpers HL, Chen FA, Bankert RB, Arredondo MA, Edge SB, Repasky EA. Growth and metastasis of surgical specimens of human breast carcinomas in SCID mice. Cancer J Sci Am. 1996;2(5):291–300.
45. Al-Hajj M, Wicha MS, Benito-Hernandez A, Morrison SJ, Clarke MF. Prospective identification of tumorigenic breast cancer cells. Proc Natl Acad Sci U S A. 2003;100(7):3983–8.
46. Marangoni E, Vincent-Salomon A, Auger N, Degeorges A, Assayag F, de Cremoux P, de Plater L, Guyader C, De Pinieux G, Judde JG, et al. A new model of patient tumor-derived breast cancer xenografts for preclinical assays. Clin Cancer Res. 2007;13(13):3989–98.
47. Liu H, Patel MR, Prescher JA, Patsialou A, Qian D, Lin J, Wen S, Chang YF, Bachmann MH, Shimono Y, et al. Cancer stem cells from human breast tumors are involved in spontaneous metastases in orthotopic mouse models. Proc Natl Acad Sci U S A. 2010;107(42):18115–20.
48. Fleming JM, Miller TC, Meyer MJ, Ginsburg E, Vonderhaar BK. Local regulation of human breast xenograft models. J Cell Physiol. 2010;224(3):795–806.
49. DeRose YS, Wang G, Lin YC, Bernard PS, Buys SS, Ebbert MT, Factor R, Matsen C, Milash BA, Nelson E, et al. Tumor grafts derived from women with breast cancer authentically reflect tumor pathology, growth, metastasis and disease outcomes. Nat Med. 2011;17(11):1514–20.

50. Ma CX, Cai S, Li S, Ryan CE, Guo Z, Schaiff WT, Lin L, Hoog J, Goiffon RJ, Prat A, et al. Targeting Chk1 in p53-deficient triple-negative breast cancer is therapeutically beneficial in human-in-mouse tumor models. J Clin Invest. 2012;122(4):1541–52.
51. Vaillant F, Merino D, Lee L, Breslin K, Pal B, Ritchie ME, Smyth GK, Christie M, Phillipson LJ, Burns CJ, et al. Targeting BCL-2 with the BH3 mimetic ABT-199 in estrogen receptor-positive breast cancer. Cancer Cell. 2013;24(1):120–9.
52. Oakes SR, Vaillant F, Lim E, Lee L, Breslin K, Feleppa F, Deb S, Ritchie ME, Takano E, Ward T, et al. Sensitization of BCL-2-expressing breast tumors to chemotherapy by the BH3 mimetic ABT-737. Proc Natl Acad Sci U S A. 2012;109(8):2766–71.
53. Zhang X, Claerhout S, Prat A, Dobrolecki LE, Petrovic I, Lai Q, Landis MD, Wiechmann L, Schiff R, Giuliano M, et al. A renewable tissue resource of phenotypically stable, biologically and ethnically diverse, patient-derived human breast cancer xenograft models. Cancer Res. 2013;73(15):4885–97.
54. Li S, Shen D, Shao J, Crowder R, Liu W, Prat A, He X, Liu S, Hoog J, Lu C, et al. Endocrine-therapy-resistant ESR1 variants revealed by genomic characterization of breast-cancer-derived xenografts. Cell Rep. 2013;4(6):1116–30.
55. du Manoir S, Orsetti B, Bras-Goncalves R, Nguyen TT, Lasorsa L, Boissiere F, Massemin B, Colombo PE, Bibeau F, Jacot W, et al. Breast tumor PDXs are genetically plastic and correspond to a subset of aggressive cancers prone to relapse. Mol Oncol. 2014;8(2):431–43.
56. Zhang H, Cohen AL, Krishnakumar S, Wapnir IL, Veeriah S, Deng G, Coram MA, Piskun CM, Longacre TA, Herrler M, et al. Patient-derived xenografts of triple-negative breast cancer reproduce molecular features of patient tumors and respond to mTOR inhibition. Breast Cancer Res. 2014;16(2):R36.
57. Eirew P, Steif A, Khattra J, Ha G, Yap D, Farahani H, Gelmon K, Chia S, Mar C, Wan A, et al. Dynamics of genomic clones in breast cancer patient xenografts at single-cell resolution. Nature. 2015;518(7539):422–6.
58. Criscitiello C, Azim HA Jr, Schouten PC, Linn SC, Sotiriou C. Understanding the biology of triple-negative breast cancer. Ann Oncol. 2012;23(Suppl 6):vi13–8.
59. Garrido-Laguna I, Uson M, Rajeshkumar NV, Tan AC, de Oliveira E, Karikari C, Villaroel MC, Salomon A, Taylor G, Sharma R, et al. Tumor engraftment in nude mice and enrichment in Stroma- related gene pathways predict poor survival and resistance to gemcitabine in patients with pancreatic cancer. Clin Cancer Res. 2011;17(17):5793.
60. Zhao X, Liu Z, Yu L, Zhang Y, Baxter P, Voicu H, Gurusiddappa S, Luan J, Su JM, Leung H-cE, et al. Global gene expression profiling confirms the molecular fidelity of primary tumor-based orthotopic xenograft mouse models of medulloblastoma. Neuro-Oncology. 2012;14 (5):574–83.
61. Lee ES, Jung SY, Kim JY, Kim JJ, Yoo TK, Kim YG, Lee KS, Lee ES, Kim EK, Min JW, et al. Identifying the potential long-term survivors among breast cancer patients with distant metastasis. Ann Oncol. 2016;27(5):828–33.
62. Hanahan D, Weinberg RA. Hallmarks of cancer: the next generation. Cell. 2011;144 (5):646–74.
63. Ramaswamy S, Ross KN, Lander ES, Golub TR. A molecular signature of metastasis in primary solid tumors. Nat Genet. 2003;33(1):49–54.
64. Weigelt B, Glas AM, Wessels LF, Witteveen AT, Peterse JL, van't Veer LJ. Gene expression profiles of primary breast tumors maintained in distant metastases. Proc Natl Acad Sci U S A. 2003;100(26):15901–5.
65. Gupta GP, Minn AJ, Kang Y, Siegel PM, Serganova I, Cordon-Cardo C, Olshen AB, Gerald WL, Massague J. Identifying site-specific metastasis genes and functions. Cold Spring Harb Symp Quant Biol. 2005;70:149–58.
66. Minn AJ, Gupta GP, Siegel PM, Bos PD, Shu W, Giri DD, Viale A, Olshen AB, Gerald WL, Massague J. Genes that mediate breast cancer metastasis to lung. Nature. 2005;436 (7050):518–24.

67. Kang Y, Siegel PM, Shu W, Drobnjak M, Kakonen SM, Cordon-Cardo C, Guise TA, Massague J. A multigenic program mediating breast cancer metastasis to bone. Cancer Cell. 2003;3 (6):537–49.
68. Powell E, Shao J, Yuan Y, Chen HC, Cai S, Echeverria GV, Mistry N, Decker KF, Schlosberg C, Do KA, et al. p53 deficiency linked to B cell translocation gene 2 (BTG2) loss enhances metastatic potential by promoting tumor growth in primary and metastatic sites in patient-derived xenograft (PDX) models of triple-negative breast cancer. Breast Cancer Res. 2016;18(1):13.
69. Powell E, Shao J, Picon HM, Bristow C, Ge Z, Peoples M, Robinson F, Jeter-Jones SL, Schlosberg C, Grzeskowiak CL, et al. A functional genomic screen in vivo identifies CEACAM5 as a clinically relevant driver of breast cancer metastasis. NPJ Breast Cancer. 2018;4(1):9.
70. Howlader N, Altekruse SF, Li CI, Chen VW, Clarke CA, Ries LAG, Cronin KA. US incidence of breast cancer subtypes defined by joint hormone receptor and HER2 status. JNCI J Natl Cancer Inst. 2014;106(5):dju055.
71. Eirew P, Steif A, Khattra J, Ha G, Yap D, Farahani H. Dynamics of genomic clones in breast cancer patient xenografts at single-cell resolution. Nature. 2015;518:422.
72. Ding L, Ellis MJ, Li S, Larson DE, Chen K, Wallis JW, Harris CC, McLellan MD, Fulton RS, Fulton LL, et al. Genome remodelling in a basal-like breast cancer metastasis and xenograft. Nature. 2010;464:999.
73. Place AE, Jin Huh S, Polyak K. The microenvironment in breast cancer progression: biology and implications for treatment. Breast Cancer Res. 2011;13(6):227.
74. Hanahan D, Coussens Lisa M. Accessories to the crime: functions of cells recruited to the tumor microenvironment. Cancer Cell. 2012;21(3):309–22.
75. Binnewies M, Roberts EW, Kersten K, Chan V, Fearon DF, Merad M, Coussens LM, Gabrilovich DI, Ostrand-Rosenberg S, Hedrick CC, et al. Understanding the tumor immune microenvironment (TIME) for effective therapy. Nat Med. 2018;24:541.
76. Wang M, Yao L-C, Cheng M, Cai D, Martinek J, Pan C-X, Shi W, Ma A-H, De Vere White RW, Airhart S, et al. Humanized mice in studying efficacy and mechanisms of PD-1-targeted cancer immunotherapy. FASEB J. 2018;32(3):1537–49.
77. Walsh NC, Kenney LL, Jangalwe S, Aryee K-E, Greiner DL, Brehm MA, Shultz LD. Humanized mouse models of clinical disease. Ann Rev Pathol Mech Dis. 2017;12 (1):187–215.

Part IV
Biomarkers for Precision Medicine in Breast Cancer Patients

Chapter 15
Proteomic Interrogation in Cancer Biomarker

Un-Beom Kang

Abstract Biomarkers factor into the diagnosis and treatment of almost every patient with cancer. The innovation in proteomics follows improvement of mass spectrometry techniques and data processing strategy. Recently, proteomics and typical biological studies have been the answer for clinical applications. The clinical proteomics techniques are now actively adapted to protein identification in large patient cohort, biomarker development for more sensitive and specific screening based on quantitative data. And, it is important for clinical, translational researchers to be acutely aware of the issues surrounding appropriate biomarker development, in order to facilitate entry of clinically useful biomarkers into the clinic. Here, we discuss in detail include the case research for clinical proteomics. Furthermore, we give an overview on the current developments and novel findings in proteomics-based cancer biomarker research.

Keywords Cancer · Biomarker · Proteomics · Proteogenomics · Clinical application

15.1 Introduction

A biomarker refers to a factor that can be measured objectively as a response to an exposure or intervention in a pathology environment. It is recognized that discover appropriate cancer biomarker is essential to classify cancers for therapy, predict responses to treatments, and support treatment-related decision making [1]. The biomarker encompasses from small molecule such as blood glucose to polymer substance like proteins and nucleic acids. Blood glucose as a diagnosis method for diabetes is the most typical biomarker, and blood cholesterol or prostate-specific antigen is good example developed as biomarker. As the proteome is made through

U.-B. Kang (✉)
Core Protein Resources Center, Daegu Gyeongbuk Institute of Science and Technology, Daegu, South Korea
e-mail: unbeom.kang@bertis.com

D.-Y. Noh et al. (eds.), *Translational Research in Breast Cancer*, Advances in Experimental Medicine and Biology 1187,
https://doi.org/10.1007/978-981-32-9620-6_15

"central dogma" and functionally regulates cell behavior, proteomics is expected to expand our knowledge of the biology and disease mechanisms underlying carcinogenesis and cancer progression [2]. Moreover, the typical advantage of studying proteome including alternative splicing, post-translational modification, and flexible conversion through protein-protein interaction makes higher expectation for biomarker discovery.

Cancer biomarker, especially protein marker has become a vocation for the application of proteomic technologies [3, 4]. Protein discovery that should be related with canonical pathway for disease occurrence and progress, and adaptation as biomarker to classify the response to treatment and identify potential targets for development of drug and novel therapies has been actively thrusted in oncology by proteomic approaches. Indeed, proteomics tools are continuously enhanced to meet the needs for high-throughput and high sensitivity for convergence of a proteomics to cancer research. These methodological innovations and great improvement in mass spectrometry(MS) need particular attention to be paid to the study design and the data analysis, in order to minimize the chance of identifying associations that are subsequently determined to be false positives. Key aspects of biomarker development include careful study design to avoid bias, comprehensive testing and validation, and accurate reporting of the results.

Proteomics approaches were largely consisted with three different steps. The first step is the sample preparation represented as digestion and separation process using 2-dimensional electrophoresis gel or liquid chromatography. In the mass operation step, prepared samples were analyzed by various type of mass spectrometry as the purpose. Then, protein is identified through database searching with or without modifications. In this review, we will rather concentrate on the sample preparation step relevant to cancer biomarker which is the first and the most informants during the entire courses to guarantee a promising result. As well, for the purposes of this review, we would read future direction of proteomics in cancer biomarker by thinking current evidence and concepts.

15.2 Translate Proteomic Research into Cancer Biomarker

Biomarker development is one of the most efficient and valuable objective of proteomics studies. There was pioneer study of translational research in clinical proteomics. N.L. Anderson and N.G. Anderson reported in 2002 about an alternative and more comprehensive classification of the protein content in plasma [5]. They applied several categories to classify plasma proteome; (1) Proteins secreted by solid tissues that act in plasma, (2) Immunoglobulins, (3) "Long-distance" receptor ligands, (4) "Local" receptor ligands, (5) Temporary passengers, (6) Tissue leakage products, (7) Aberrant secretion, (8) Foreign proteins. Consequently, 289 plasma proteins were listed from public source in which concentrations of 70 proteins were estimated and plotted. The dynamic range across the high abundance end, serum albumin (35–10 mg/ml) protein and the low abundance end, interleukin 6 (0–5 pg/ml) protein covered a factor of 10^{10}. They mentioned that detection of disease marker in plasma, using mass spectrometry is probably challenging because of limitations associated with detection. The author suggested that further development of rational approach coupled with significantly collected clinical samples for developing disease biomarkers.

15.2.1 *Biomarker Discovery with Unbiased Proteomics*

Typically, a biomarker pipeline takes mainly two distinct steps from laboratory development to clinic: discovery as a first step and following confirmation step including qualification, verification, and validation phases (Fig. 15.1) [1]. In proteomics, biomarker development starts with comparative proteome profiling with small number of samples. As many different types of samples, such as tissue, body fluids, or even model cell line, are necessary to subtract a weighted output. On the contrary, hundreds to thousands of samples are evaluated for the clinical assessment of the biomarker candidate in the latest clinical validation stage. Putative biomarker candidates should be validated in specimens obtained by less invasive techniques are more desirable [1, 6].

In general, proteomic approach in biomarker discovery step takes two main tracks; unbiased low- throughput screening or high-throughput approach in the targeted analysis. The latter strategy is now being promoted as the preferred approach because of defining an intended use for the tumor marker at the early stages of the discovery process allows better control of the variables that may influence measured levels of the marker during the discovery process. However, it has to keep in mind that the candidates for targeted analysis should be from unbiased screening which is frequently used in proteomics.

15.2.1.1 Gel-Based Proteomics Approach

Different proteomics technologies have been developed to detect putative candidate for cancer biomarker. In the early days of proteomics, proteome was separated and identified in combination with two-dimensional polyacrylamide gel electrophoresis (2D-PAGE) and MALDI-TOF/TOF MS [7]. The nature of technology, it has been applied for direct compare of cancer cells proteins and is still preferred from many laboratories [8–10]. An example of application of this basic proteomics technique involving analysis on conditioned media of cultured breast cancer (BC) cell lines was obtained and validated on plasma from cancer patients [8]. Independently secreted proteins obtained from Hs578Bst (nontumor breast cell line) and Hs578T (malignant breast cell line) were resolved by 2D-PAGE and visualized with silver staining. A comparison of the 2D-PAGE images revealed that eight protein spots were changed in their expression levels more than two-fold. The eight proteins were identified by MALDI-TOF/TOF MS analysis and a database searching. One decreased protein spot was identified from the database search as perlecan, a huge

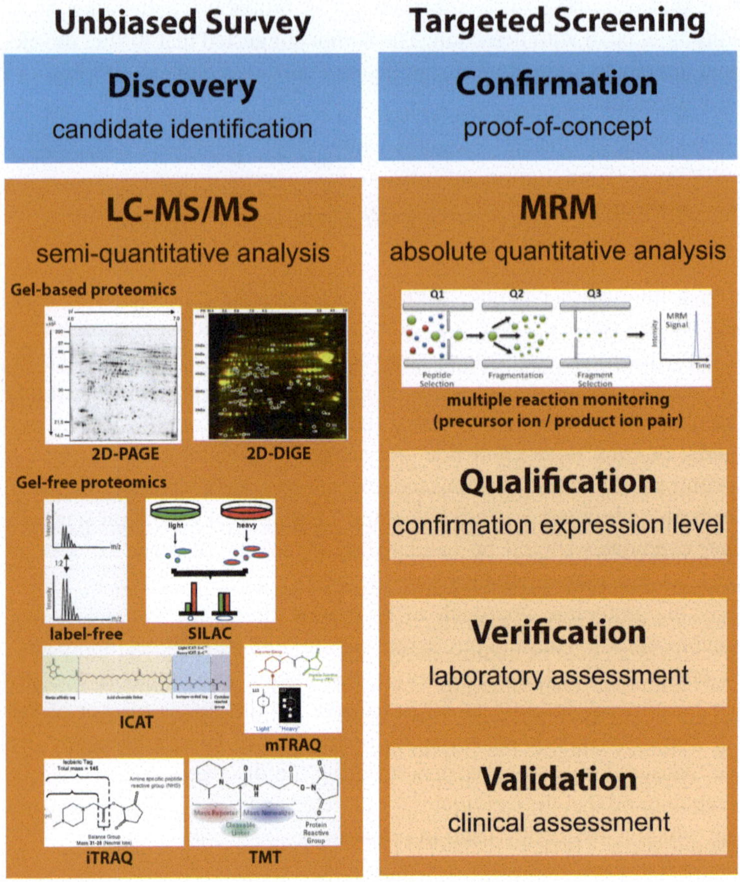

Fig. 15.1 Proteomic pipeline of biomarker discovery. A biomarker pipeline takes mainly two distinct steps which are discovery and confirmation. The first step takes unbiased survey scan based on semiquantification to identify disease specific proteins (left panel). The latter step is performing for proof of concept. In proteomics, MRM workflow is usually taken for selective and sensitive quantification in absolute protein level. Generally, large sample set is necessary to provide clinical assessment (right panel)

membrane protein of molecular weight 480 kDa. There was a gap between theoretical and real protein size, since the protein migrated to around 25 kDa on 2D-PAGE. The author made suspicion if the protein could be a specific proteolytic fragment or a nonspecific degradation product of perlecan. Targeted mass analysis to the n-terminus tryptic peptide of the 25 kDa protein revealed that it was the endorepellin LG3 fragment from large protein perlecan liberated by the action of BMP-1. The follow-up verification study based on western blot analysis demonstrated that plasma level of the endorepellin LG3 fragment was significantly lower in BC patients compared to healthy controls.

2D-PAGE provides direct visual confirmation of changes in protein or post-translational modifications (PTMs) abundance. These evidences make it easy to decide follow-up experimental steps because genomic analysis could not provide information about post or cotranslational modification. Despite this advantage there is inherent limitation as follows poorly reproducible and insufficient protein detection sensitivity. With the development of image technology, differential imaging gel electrophoresis (DIGE) technique has been introduced into proteomics. This method was designed in an attempt to figure out the limitation of 2D-PAGE using multiplexed fluorescent dyes. Proteins from different samples labeled with individual dye would be running on a single gel at once to address the issue of gel-to-gel variability. Moreover, it adds a quantitative component to conventional 2D-PAGE analyses [11]. Therefore, DIGE technology has been a good choice to biomarker discovery. For example, five proteins, Fatty acid-binding protein 1, Intelectin-1, Transitional endoplasmic reticulum ATPase, Transgelin, and Tropomyosin 2, were demonstrated as the proteins associated with high-risk recurrence of colorectal cancer (CRC) by using 2D-DIGE approach [12]. To investigate cancer prognostic marker, protein samples obtained from two different groups of stage IV CRC patients were separately labeled with cyanine fluorescent dyes. Good prognostic group (GPG) who had survived more than 5 years after palliative surgery and subsequent chemotherapy treatment was labeled with Cy3 fluorescent dye. The other poor prognostic group (PPG) who had died within 25 months was applied to Cy5 fluorescent dye. Each labeled protein samples were mixed together for running on a single gel. Around 1500 protein spots were detected in which differentially expressed 40 protein spots were picked for identification with mass analysis. Several proteins such as Actin, Desmin, and Transgelin were identified at multiple spots. The spots identified as same protein were migrated to similar molecular size but different isoelectric point. This pattern is usually shown when a protein has PTM. Take all together, the author emphasized that gel-based approach can be used to readily extract information on PTMs.

15.2.1.2 Gel-Free Comparative Proteome Profiling

Advancement in MS facilitated not only deep digging for plasma and other biofluids proteins that span more than six logs of protein abundance, but also systematically characterization of the proteome dynamics under quantity changing conditions. Quantitative proteome analysis accompanies the comparison of same sequences peptide across different samples. One can compare the intensities of respective peptide chromatographic peaks from one chromatogram to another, so-called label-free quantification. The others, peptides/proteins can be metabolically or chemically labeled prior to MS analysis then compare the intensities of each peptide against labeling moiety.

Shotgun proteomics and direct peak intensity comparison is a convenient approach for relative-quantitative profiling across large sample sets. The approach named as label-free is one of the widely applied for cancer biomarker research.

Accumulated experience of MS analysis demonstrated that protein abundancy is correlated with a larger number of MS2 spectra for peptides, thus relative quantitation of the identified proteins can be achieved. Untreated peptides are analyzed separately, and peak areas directly compared between runs for relative quantification. In order to quantify the proteins from complex biological mixture, sophisticated normalization methods are used to remove systematic artefacts in the peptide intensity values between MS measurements [13, 14]. By applying a label-free LC-MS/MS technique based on spectral counting to use urine as a source and identify the proteins for diagnosis and monitoring progression, Beretov et al. found altered expression of 59 urinary proteins in BC patients, in which significantly elevated expression of three proteins-Extracellular matrix protein 1 (*ECM1*), Microtubule-associated serine/threonine-protein kinase 4, and Filaggrin in a panel of human BC were subsequently validated in cell lines by western blotting [15]. Chen and coworkers implemented a label-free quantitative study to develop plasma protein biomarkers for distinguishing lymph node metastasis in breast cancer. They selected two representative proteins (RARB and FBLN5) out of 33 differentially expressed proteins and indicated that protein expression level resulting from label-free quantification is highly consistent with immunoblotting assay [16].

It is needless to say that the label-free is affordable proteomic technique for comparative profiling of clinical samples. However, MS has common problems something like the difficulty in predicting ionization efficiencies of peptides during electrospray makes reproducibility issues. Of course the reproducibility is a main caveat of label-free quantitative proteomic [17]. The pioneer researcher introduced stable isotope to a protein and compared two or more samples by MS. Because of the stable isotope-labeled peptides possess similar physical and chemical properties as their unlabeled counterparts that make equivalent movement during chromatographic separation. But the isotope introduced samples are recognized by mass spectrometry with a mass difference. Quantification is achieved by comparing their respective signal intensities [18, 19]. Labeling strategies can be subdivided into metabolic (stable isotope labeling in cell culture/SILAC) and chemical (isotope-coded affinity tag/ICAT, mass differential tags for relative and absolute quantification/mTRAQ, isobaric tags for relative and absolute quantitation/iTRAQ, and tandem mass tag/TMT) reactions.

The SILAC involves incorporation of isotopically stable amino acids into proteins during active cell proliferation. For the SILAC experiment, usually, two different culture conditions were taken with the medium containing light or heavy arginine/lysine. The latter is labeled with carbon-13 atoms (^{13}C) instead of the normal carbon-12 (^{12}C). When the cells are growing in this conditioned medium, they incorporate the heavy arginine/lysine into all of their proteins [20, 21]. SILAC has become an important method in secreted protein analysis especially for quantitative proteomics. It can be used to discriminate proteins secreted by cells from serum contaminants [22]. Originally, clinical samples and most animal-based samples would not be applicable for labeling based on metabolic reaction. Alternative SILAC technique, super-SILAC, was demonstrated to un-culturable sample.

Super-SILAC is a kind of internal standard which is a mixture of several cell lines cultured in heavy-SILAC condition and serves for normalization across different samples [23]. By performing quantitative profiling using the super-SILAC technique, Boersema et al. compared the N-glycosylated secretome of BC cell lines. To make super-SILAC mixture, BC cell lines-HCC1143, HCC1937, and HCC2218, were metabolic labeled by culturing in heavy isotope containing amino acid and culture media were collected together. Primary human mammary epithelial cells from two different sources were selected as control cell lines. MCF-10a and HMT-3522-S1 cells represent premalignant cells, HCC1143 and HCC1937 cells stage II tumors, HCC202, HCC2218, and HCC1599 cells stage III tumors, and finally, MFM223 and MDA-MB-453 are metastatic cells from pleural effusions. The secretome of these different cell lines was collected as conditioned medium. These conditioned medium of the control cell lines and the super-SILAC were then mixed. Proteins were digested with trypsin and N-glycosylated peptides were captured by two broad spectrum lectins—concanavalin A and wheat germ agglutinin on a 30 kDa filter. The N-glycosylated peptides were thereby separated from nonglycosylated peptides that were analyzed by highly sensitive LC-MS. In total, 1398 unique N-glycosylation sites were identified and quantified. They also applied this N-glyco secretome analysis strategy by super-SILAC to human plasma from female donor and demonstrated that the super-SILAC approach can distinguish classical plasma proteins from tissue leakage proteins by their SILAC ratios [24].

The stable isotope can be simply introduced by chemical reaction which would be affordable with mammalian samples in particular clinical purpose. Isotope-coded affinity tagging (ICAT) technique is the first commercial approach for engaging isotope containing label tag to quantitative analysis. The ICAT reagent consists of three elements: biotin affinity tag used to isolate ICAT-labeled peptides; a linker containing stable isotope signatures which can be differentiated by mass spectrometry; and a reactive group with specificity toward thiol groups [25]. This method has been developed to analyze relative amounts of cysteine containing peptides in tryptic digests of protein extracts. In-silico analysis indicates that cysteine is found in more than 90% of human proteins, in other words, most human proteins should be quantified by ICAT approach with reduced sample complexity [26]. For breast cancer biomarker discovery, the ICAT method was applied to screening of differentially expressed protein in plasma obtained from normal healthy controls and breast cancer patients. Plasma is the most popular clinical sample for biomarker discovery because it communicates cells, tissues, and organs in human body, however, the large dynamic range of this clinical relevant sample precludes a deep proteome coverage [5]. In the global proteomics, limited dynamic range of detection method is a prime issue. Indeed, just few hundreds of the most abundant plasma proteins can be analyzed in a single proteomic experiment [27]. To overcome this, mainly two strategies has been applied: the depletion of the highly abundant plasma proteins and the extensive sample fractionation. There are any single methods yet to remove high abundance proteins perfectly and to enrich low abundance proteins completely. But, antibody-based negative enrichment system has preferred to remove the specifically targeted proteins as well as both reproducibility and selectivity [28–30]. Depleted plasma was subjected to ICAT labeling and intensively fractionated with strong-cation exchange chromatography, then adapted tandem MS in search of new serological biomarkers for breast cancer. A total of 155 proteins were identified and quantified by ICAT method. Among them, 33 proteins showed abundance changes by more than 1.5-fold between the plasmas of breast cancer patients and healthy women. The two biomarker candidates, BTD and GPX3, were next tested with immunoblot assay in a blinded set of breast cancer and control to ascertain the markers ability to differentiate the two groups. Finally, BTD was a potential serological biomarker for the detection of breast cancer [31].

The ICAT technology basically provides quantitative information at MS1 spectra of each peptides. There is another approach for comparative profiling through full MS scans, mTRAQ method. The term has similar concept with super-SILAC, that is to serve as internal standard not for semiquantification but to measure absolute amount of protein in a sample [32]. There is a triplex mTRAQ set (Δ0, Δ4, Δ8) of nonisobaric (differing mass) reagents, three individual reagents are based on the same chemical structure but the mTRAQ Δ0 contains no isotopes and Δ8 has two ^{15}N and six ^{13}C isotope atoms, while Δ4 has one ^{15}N and three ^{13}C isotope atoms. Standard peptides for target proteins would be labeled with one or several mTRAQ reagents and the mixed labeled peptides added into sample, thus it can be distinguished by MS from endogenous peptide of sample. Interestingly, Kang et al. applied the method for a systematic study to evaluate the unconventional use of mTRAQ as an MS1-quantification tag in comparative profiling where chemical isotopic labeling is needed [33, 34]. Although ICAT method can detect low abundance proteins by reducing sample complexity, it would miss identification of proteins with few or no cysteine residues, and frequently lose information for post-translational modifications. These limitations have been somewhat solved by the mTRAQ method. They are labeled at lysine residue and N-terminal which should cover any peptides of a particular protein [35]. An example in cancer biomarker discovery using this reagent was when mTRAQ was used to measure changes in the proteome of plasma from breast cancer [36]. Peptides processed from depleted plasma of healthy control and breast cancer patients were labeled with mTRAQ Δ0 and Δ4, respectively. For the deep proteome coverage, the mTRAQ-labeled tryptic peptides were separated against isoelectric point of each peptide, OFFGEL fractionation technique, and analyzed by LC-MS/MS. The total numbers of unique peptides identified were 6984 mapping to 204 proteins. The data were compared with the previous report in which 155 proteins were identified by analyzing same plasma sample set in ICAT labeling [31]. There was intersection of only 86 proteins in both datasets. The author suggested that the low percentage of proteins shared was probably attributed to the difference of property in each labeling strategy, but it also strongly demonstrated that diverse technology can be adapted in complementary manner. Even though it was not detected through ICAT method, two proteins (THBS1 and BRWD3) showed significant increase in breast cancer plasma was evaluated by western-blot assay to confirm for their diagnostic value as serum markers.

The introduction of Isobaric tags such as TMT and iTRAQ enables more accurate quantification at MS2 spectra. These reagents are typically composed of a mass reporter, a mass normalizer and an amine reactive group. The mass reporter and mass normalizer moieties incorporate stable isotopes in multiple configurations such that each mass reporter's mass can be resolved in a MS2 spectrum. Resulting from substitution of ^{13}C and ^{15}N, TMT method has 16 individual channels and iTRAQ method is consisted with eight distinct channels to meet the demand for multiplexed experiment [37, 38]. The intact mass of each isobaric tag variant, however, is same. With this labeling technique, digested peptides from multiple samples are labeled in parallel, then mixed and simultaneously acquired fragment ions and reporter ions from tandem mass spectrum. Intensity of mass reporter ion is relevant amount of peptide quantity in corresponding sample [39]. The isobaric tags ensure same chemical property of labeled peptides derived from different sample will have the same chromatographic elution profile. This leads to improvement in the signal-to-noise ratio of MS2 spectrum and often makes enhanced identification. Labidi-Galy and her colleagues presented a desirable application of iTRAQ method to elucidate a mitogenic effect of Elafin protein in basal-like breast cancer (BLBC) [40]. They, recently, reported that Elafin is overexpressed by high-grade serous ovarian carcinoma (HGSOC) and it is associated with poor overall survival. Interestingly, HGSOC and BLBC share many features including TP53 mutations, genomic instability and poor prognosis. iTRAQ- based experiment was implemented to clarify differential phosphoproteome in BLBC cell line (BT549) stimulated with rElafin. Phosphopeptides were enriched by using affinity of metal ion to the phosphate group then analyzed with LC-MS/MS. In total, 7130 distinct phosphopeptides were quantified that mapped to 2742 unique gene IDs. There were observed changes in phosphorylation on 386 peptides, which mapped to 316 unique gene IDs. Elafin-mediated signaling appeared to target multiple pathways, including MAPK ($P < 0.001$, 12 genes).

15.2.2 Proteomic Approach for Clinical Validation in Biomarker Development

Once biomarker candidates were discovered, targeted analysis is always taken for verification and validation in necessarily large clinical sample cohorts (Fig. 15.1, right panel). In a targeted workflow, the MS is programmed to detect specific peptide ions which represent proteins of interest. Unlike the unbiased discovery-phase experiments, targeted analysis requires up-front investment to optimize assay condition against each target protein. In recent year, a kind of algorithm was introduced to support method optimization which accompanies triple quadrupole MS (QQQ) has been the most widespread instrument to measure concentrations of candidate biomarker proteins in plasma and cell lysates [41, 42]. Target peptide ions are selected to pass through the first quadrupole mass filter, which can be referred to as "precursor" ions for fragmentation in the second quadrupole. In the third mass filter, certain fragment ions referred to as "product" ions are selected and then guided to the detector for quantification. Finally, a signal intensity versus retention time is traced resulting in a selected (or single) reaction monitoring (SRM) workflow for each precursor ion/product ion pair represented as an ion transition. When multiple transitions are monitored, the overall process is termed multiple reaction monitoring (MRM). This workflow is a highly specific and sensitive MS technique that can selectively quantify compounds without interference from other components in the sample.

Lee and Kang et al. have adopted MRM workflow to develop a protein signature for breast cancer diagnosis, by screening hundreds of candidate proteins in human plasma [43]. Based on their previous works and literature review on breast cancer specific biomarkers [8, 31, 36, 44], 124 proteins were selected in verification phase of biomarker development. The optimization algorithm and synthetic peptide standard help to generate reliable MRM assay, resulting 56 proteins were implemented to investigate into plasma from 80 patients with breast cancer and 80 healthy women. Verification experiment revealed that binary regression analysis with three proteins (neural cell adhesion molecule L1-like protein, apolipoprotein C-1, and carbonic anhydrase-1) illustrated highest statistical significance, the sensitivity, specificity, and area under the curve (AUC) of the diagnostic model was 78.75%, 78.75%, and 0.831, respectively. The proteomic signature was then validated in plasma samples from 100 patients with breast cancer and 100 healthy women. The 3-protein model was capable of detecting breast cancer when tested in an independent large cohort, and its performance was higher in patients with stage I and stage II breast cancer, who may benefit from breast cancer screening by detecting tumors in the asymptomatic period.

Clinically available biomarker needs to build cut-off criteria to discriminate disease. The three proteins signature was optimized to a unique algorithm for blood-based test yield from absolute quantification. Weighted score against each protein is interpolated to reference value and guide to make a disease decision. The diagnostic algorithm, Mastocheck@, has meaning in terms of the first case of clinically approved blood test for breast cancer diagnosis with mass spectrometry by measuring absolute protein amount on disease condition.

Clinical validation in a relatively large cohort of cancer patients is an essential stage during cancer biomarker development. In the context of throughput, MRM workflow is commendable clinical proteomic choice. Kim and her colleagues have demonstrated that an MRM-based proteomic assay can be a useful tool for breast cancer screening and its accuracy is specific to breast cancer [45]. They measured amount of three proteins (neural cell adhesion molecule L1-like protein, apolipoprotein C-1, and carbonic anhydrase 1) present in human plasma by MRM workflow. An independent cohort of 1129 blood samples from 575 breast cancer patients, 454 healthy controls, and 100 patients with other malignancies were used to verify and optimize the assay. Each quantity data of three candidate proteins were applied to mass spectrometry-based breast cancer blood test algorithm and the output value clearly clarified breast cancer patients (Table 15.1).

Table 15.1 Biomarker effectiveness for breast cancer diagnosis

	Sensitivity (%)	Specificity (%)	PPV (%)	NPV (%)
Current protein marker (CA15-3)	23.2	95.3	83.3	55.4
Current protein marker (CEA)	17.4	83.7	51.7	50.3
Mass spectrometry-based breast cancer blood test	71.6	85.2	82.9	75.0

15.3 Translation in Clinical Application of Proteomics

Many proteomic researches in cancer biomarker presuppose through examination of proteome from whole individual. Tremendous improvement on the instrumental power makes it practical to identify hidden proteins beyond dynamic range with high confidence. It draws a hope that clinically promising biomarker will be identified someday. Anderson NL presented 109 unique protein targets in plasma or serum which have been cleared for clinical test from US Food and Drug Administration (FDA) since 1993. The rate of introduction of new protein-based tests approved by the FDA has fallen to an average of one per year [46]. Many laboratories make great effort and a lot of proteins were presented their promise as cancer biomarker. But, they have been hardly contributed to an improvement in clinical outcomes. Recently, a multiple MS search was used to produce the PTM-patterns for FDA-approved plasma proteins in glioblastoma multiforme (GBM) patients. Petushkova and coworker implemented LC-MS analysis in the context of proteomic profiling of PTM peptides of plasma proteins. They found one hundred unique PTM peptides proteotypic for FDA plasma markers in the control plasma samples including 33 phosphorylated, 38 acetylated, and 29 ubiquitinated peptides [47]. This evidence leads that quantitative monitoring PTM changes are useful biomarker to diagnose certain cancers and provide insight into therapeutic progress.

Post-translational modifications (PTMs) of proteins affect pathways linked to cellular lifespan and the affinity alteration cause serious health consequences including cancer. More than 100 different PTMs are reported in human [48], among the rest, several PTMs including phosphorylation, acetylation, methylation, glycosylation, and ubiquitination were routinely found in cancer [49]. It is well established that changes in gene expression levels may not fully reflect the true state of cancer progression or development [50, 51]. The clinical data have shown that the quantity of genomic and transcriptomic aberrations levels do not fully represent the structural variations such as PTM at the protein level. Further, recent studies in breast cancer suggested that PTM profiles can be used as alternative readout that reflect the function and activity of signaling pathways [52–54].

Being complexity and low stoichiometric nature of PTMs in whole proteome, PTM analysis is still an analytical challenge. Most PTMs are present at low levels in cells and tissues, and are therefore difficult to detect by MS. For this reason, characterization of cancer correlated PTMs typically involves enrichment step based on affinity isolation to separate and concentrate a specific type of PTM of interest from the rest in complex biological samples [55]. Moreover, enrichment methods can be combined with semiquantitative techniques with or without stable isotope labeling for determining changes of specific PTM on a proteome-wide [26].

Immobilized metal affinity chromatography (IMAC) using Fe(III) was initially used to isolate O-phosphopeptides for mapping phosphorylation sites [56]. This successful analytical strategy for enriching O-phosphopeptides takes a chemical feature of the phosphate group. Negative charge of phosphate group is ability to participate in covalent bonding with immobilized metal ions. A titanium dioxide (TiO2)-based solid matrix or combined use with IMAC has also applied to enrich phosphopeptides [57, 58].

A traditional biochemical experiments are widely used antibodies for the detection of PTMs in a protein. Immunoaffinity isolation of peptides of interest using an antibody are widely used for the detection of protein lysine acetylation [59], arginine methylation [60], ubiquitination [61], and tyrosine phosphorylation [62]. In addition, antibodies recognize specific PTM motifs sequence have been used to identify downstream target for kinase and trace the alteration of PTM-mediated signaling pathway [63].

Many proteomics studies of glycoproteins have been reported, however, only a few type can be routinely identified presumably by N-glycosylation. It is mainly affinity-based enrichment methods using lectin or chemical derivatization. Lectin-based affinity enrichment [64], in particular, combinations of different types of lectins provide comprehensive analysis of the N-glycosylated proteome [65]. Chemical derivatization involving oxidation of the carbohydrate side chain and coupling to hydrazide resin through hydrazone bond is another approach to enrich glycosylated peptides. In this case, N-glycopeptides are released by PNGase F and analyzed by MS [66].

The enriched PTM peptides are subjected to MS analysis and implemented to PTM peptide sequences, sites mapping, and even quantification. During the MS analysis, multidimensional MS techniques that further simplify PTM peptide mixtures can enhance the yield in modified peptide identification. Identification of PTMs commonly evaluated by preset with specific PTM moiety as variable modification during database searching [67]. But, specialized bioinformatics tools ensure the accuracy and statistical significance of the identification [68, 69].

15.4 Convergence of Proteomics for Cancer Genomics

The heterogeneity of cancer has tremendously concealed understanding of what is under pinnings of cancer signaling and its phenotypic manifestation. Although, genomic studies have allowed us evidence about the polygenetic nature of cancer, but its effect at the proteomic level is not fully understood. When the microarray is a primary technology in genomic research, an approach to understand the reciprocal action of genomic and proteomic alterations has been presented. However, microarray depends on hybridization between nucleic acid is not sufficient to cover the overall information of DNA or RNA. Consequently, a multidisciplinary convergence of genomic and proteomic observation was hindered beyond complementary strategy of each area with innate advantages and/or disadvantages.

Proteogenomics is the systematic and comprehensive integration of proteomics with genomics and so much as transcriptomics. Several studies have demonstrated the relevance of proteogenomics in cancer research. Proteogenomic approach in cancer research is starting from generation of whole exome sequencing (WES) and transcriptome RNA-seq data. The WES data are mapping to reference genome to find cancer-specific single nucleotide variant (SNV) and insertion deletion (Indel) by applying some variant calling pipeline. Once, exclude synonymous mutation unaffected to protein sequence, customized searching database for separate types of cancer sample can be generated [70]. The total variants are over tens of thousands, but, proteogenomics narrows it into hundreds to thousands results reducing driver gene candidates. In this context, proteogenomics has emerged as a useful tool in cancer research because it integrates genomic and transcriptomic data and tests with mass spectrometry.

A distinction of proteogenomic strategy in cancer research was successfully demonstrated when the proteomics data with exome sequences were integrated to identify genomic aberrations in triple-negative BC. Further, the combined approach successfully identified markers for drug sensitivity and understands the mechanisms of drug resistance [71]. Clearly, the proteogenomic approach will provide the basic molecular diagnostics toolbox for precision cancer medicine [72]. Using The Cancer Genome Atlas (TCGA) network data, Li et al. [73] integrated genomic, transcriptomic, and proteomic dataset to classify patients with nonsmall cell lung cancer by prognosis, and this approach has the ability to identify new cancer biomarkers. In another proteogenomic integration study, researchers found therapeutic targets from drug treatment experiment based on HER2 or the PI3K pathway in patient-derived xenograft (PDX) models [74]. This proteogenomic strategy in cancer research, also known as onco-proteogenomics, takes advantage of how the information as a whole can guide the understanding of physiologies and pathologies of cancer through identification of alterations in protein–protein interactions and protein kinases functional switches at the genomic-based proteome level, which are responsible for modifying cellular phenotypes. Furthermore, it provides a unified vision of proteome-wide understanding of cellular functions.

This convergence concept will increasingly exploit the unique possibilities of synergizing genomic, transcriptomic, proteomic, metabolomic, and lipidomic datasets. National Cancer Institute (NCI) has been progressed The Clinical Proteomic Tumor Analysis Consortium (CPTAC) for extensive survey in onco-proteogenomics. More recently, the NCI Office of Cancer Clinical Proteomics Research (OCCPR), part of the National Institutes of Health (NIH), and the FDA have signed a Memorandum of Understanding (MOU) in proteogenomic regulatory science. This will engage in scientific and programmatic collaborations in clinical proteomics and onco-proteogenomics. It may imply whenever another large coordinative groups or consortium will be undertaken for not only other widespread diseases but also rare diseases which precision personal medicine is desperately needed.

15.5 Summary

Biomarker paradigm has been unconverted in a generic frame, discovery cancer specific targets, and validates the clinical significance. The general thought is that MS and its proteomic applications will play a major role in cancer biomarker discovery. Indeed, a number of MS-based methods have been introduced for monitoring protein biomarkers and still in progress. Together with newer proteomic technologies could significantly contribute to the discovery and development of clinically efficient cancer biomarkers with diagnostic/prognostic values for monitoring the disease state and for drug discovery, but at the same time the limitation of single field is also clearly appeared. Nowadays, scientific research is also in convergence era, in other words, multilateral study underlying multiomics including DNA, RNA, proteins, epigenetics, and metabolites will be essential matters in cancer biomarker development.

References

1. Rifai N, Gillette MA, Carr SA. Protein biomarker discovery and validation: the long and uncertain path to clinical utility. Nat Biotechnol. 2006;24(8):971–83.
2. Gromov P, Moreira JM, Gromova I, Celis JE. Proteomic strategies in bladder cancer: from tissue to fluid and back. Proteomics Clin Appl. 2008;2(7–8):974–88.
3. Reymond MA, Schlegel W. Proteomics in cancer. Adv Clin Chem. 2007;44:103–42.
4. Cowan ML, Vera J. Proteomics: advances in biomarker discovery. Expert Rev Proteomics. 2008;5(1):21–3.
5. Anderson NL, Anderson NG. The human plasma proteome: history, character, and diagnostic prospects. Mol Cell Proteomics. 2002;1(11):845–67.
6. Hu S, Loo JA, Wong DT. Human body fluid proteome analysis. Proteomics. 2006;6 (23):6326–53.
7. Sallam RM. Proteomics in cancer biomarkers discovery: challenges and applications. Dis Markers. 2015;2015:321370.
8. Chang JW, Kang UB, Kim DH, Yi JK, Lee JW, Noh DY, et al. Identification of circulating endorepellin LG3 fragment: potential use as a serological biomarker for breast cancer. Proteomics Clin Appl. 2008;2(1):23–32.
9. Francis FL, Jankova L, Dent OF, Molloy MP, Kwun SY, Clarke C, et al. Identification of distinctive protein expression patterns in colorectal adenoma. Proteomics Clin Appl. 2010;4 (1):60–70.
10. Hamelin C, Cornut E, Poirier F, Pons S, Beaulieu C, Charrier JP, et al. Identification and verification of heat shock protein 60 as a potential serum marker for colorectal cancer. FEBS J. 2011;278(24):4845–59.
11. Magdeldin S, Enany S, Yoshida Y, Xu B, Zhang Y, Zureena Z, et al. Basics and recent advances of two-dimensional- polyacrylamide gel electrophoresis. Clin Proteomics. 2014;11(1):16.

12. Kim HJ, Kang UB, Lee H, Jung JH, Lee ST, Yu MH, et al. Profiling of differentially expressed proteins in stage IV colorectal cancers with good and poor outcomes. J Proteome. 2012;75 (10):2983–97.
13. Zhou W, Liotta LA, Petricoin EF. The spectra count label-free quantitation in cancer proteomics. Cancer Genomics Proteomics. 2012;9(3):135–42.
14. Zhu W, Smith JW, Huang CM. Mass spectrometry-based label-free quantitative proteomics. J Biomed Biotechnol. 2010;2010:840518.
15. Beretov J, Wasinger VC, Millar EK, Schwartz P, Graham PH, Li Y. Proteomic analysis of urine to identify breast cancer biomarker candidates using a label-free LC-MS/MS approach. PLoS One. 2015;10(11):e0141876.
16. Chen L, Zhao W, He J, Li L, Meng D, Cai D, et al. Label-free quantitative proteomic screening of candidate plasma biomarkers for the prognosis of breast cancer with different lymph node statuses. Proteomics Clin Appl. 2018;12(3):e1700117.
17. Rudnick PA, Wang X, Yan X, Sedransk N, Stein SE. Improved normalization of systematic biases affecting ion current measurements in label-free proteomics data. Mol Cell Proteomics. 2014;13(5):1341–51.
18. Nakamura T, Oda Y. Mass spectrometry-based quantitative proteomics. Biotechnol Genet Eng Rev. 2007;24:147–63.
19. Ciccimaro E, Blair IA. Stable isotope dilution LC-MS for quantitative biomarker analysis. Bioanalysis. 2010;2(2):311–41.
20. Ong SE, Blagoev B, Kratchmarova I, Kristensen DB, Steen H, Pandey A, et al. Stable isotope labeling by amino acids in cell culture, SILAC, as a simple and accurate approach to expression proteomics. Mol Cell Proteomics. 2002;1(5):376–86.
21. Blagoev B, Kratchmarova I, Ong SE, Nielsen M, Foster LJ, Mann M. A proteomics strategy to elucidate functional protein-protein interactions applied to EGF signaling. Nat Biotechnol. 2003;21(3):315–8.
22. Stastna M, van Eyk JE. Investigating the secretome: lessons about the cells that comprise the heart. Circ Cardiovasc Genet. 2012;5(1):o8–o18.
23. Geiger T, Cox J, Ostasiewicz P, Wisniewski JR, Mann M. Super-SILAC mix for quantitative proteomics of human tumor tissue. Nat Methods. 2010;7(5):383–5.
24. Boersema PJ, Geiger T, Wisniewski JR, Mann M. Quantification of the N-glycosylated secretome by super-SILAC during breast cancer progression and in human blood samples. Mol Cell Proteomics. 2013;12(1):158–71.
25. Gygi SP, Rist B, Gerber SA, Turecek F, Gelb MH, Aebersold R. Quantitative analysis of complex protein mixtures using isotope-coded affinity tags. Nat Biotechnol. 1999;17 (10):994–9.
26. Kang UB, Alexander WM, Marto JA. Interrogating the hidden phosphoproteome. Proteomics. 2017;17(6)
27. Schneider LV, Hall MP. Stable isotope methods for high-precision proteomics. Drug Discov Today. 2005;10(5):353–63.
28. Liu T, Qian WJ, Mottaz HM, Gritsenko MA, Norbeck AD, Moore RJ, et al. Evaluation of multiprotein immunoaffinity subtraction for plasma proteomics and candidate biomarker discovery using mass spectrometry. Mol Cell Proteomics. 2006;5(11):2167–74.
29. Yocum AK, Yu K, Oe T, Blair IA. Effect of immunoaffinity depletion of human serum during proteomic investigations. J Proteome Res. 2005;4(5):1722–31.
30. Brand J, Haslberger T, Zolg W, Pestlin G, Palme S. Depletion efficiency and recovery of trace markers from a multiparameter immunodepletion column. Proteomics. 2006;6(11):3236–42.
31. Kang UB, Ahn Y, Lee JW, Kim YH, Kim J, Yu MH, et al. Differential profiling of breast cancer plasma proteome by isotope-coded affinity tagging method reveals biotinidase as a breast cancer biomarker. BMC Cancer. 2010;10:114.
32. DeSouza LV, Taylor AM, Li W, Minkoff MS, Romaschin AD, Colgan TJ, et al. Multiple reaction monitoring of mTRAQ-labeled peptides enables absolute quantification of endogenous

levels of a potential cancer marker in cancerous and normal endometrial tissues. J Proteome Res. 2008;7(8):3525–34.
33. Kang UB, Yeom J, Kim H, Lee C. Quantitative analysis of mTRAQ-labeled proteome using full MS scans. J Proteome Res. 2010;9(7):3750–8.
34. Kang UB, Yeom J, Kim HJ, Kim H, Lee C. Expression profiling of more than 3500 proteins of MSS-type colorectal cancer by stable isotope labeling and mass spectrometry. J Proteome. 2012;75(10):3050–62.
35. Yoon JY, Lim KY, Lee S, Park K, Paek E, Kang UB, et al. Improved quantitative analysis of mass spectrometry using quadratic equations. J Proteome Res. 2010;9(5):2775–85.
36. Suh EJ, Kabir MH, Kang UB, Lee JW, Yu J, Noh DY, et al. Comparative profiling of plasma proteome from breast cancer patients reveals thrombospondin-1 and BRWD3 as serological biomarkers. Exp Mol Med. 2012;44(1):36–44.
37. Choe L, D'Ascenzo M, Relkin NR, Pappin D, Ross P, Williamson B, et al. 8-plex quantitation of changes in cerebrospinal fluid protein expression in subjects undergoing intravenous immunoglobulin treatment for Alzheimer's disease. Proteomics. 2007;7(20):3651–60.
38. Mertins P, Tang LC, Krug K, Clark DJ, Gritsenko MA, Chen L, et al. Reproducible workflow for multiplexed deep-scale proteome and phosphoproteome analysis of tumor tissues by liquid chromatography-mass spectrometry. Nat Protoc. 2018;13(7):1632–61.
39. Gingras AC, Gstaiger M, Raught B, Aebersold R. Analysis of protein complexes using mass spectrometry. Nat Rev Mol Cell Biol. 2007;8(8):645–54.
40. Labidi-Galy SI, Clauss A, Ng V, Duraisamy S, Elias KM, Piao HY, et al. Elafin drives poor outcome in high-grade serous ovarian cancers and basal-like breast tumors. Oncogene. 2015;34 (3):373–83.
41. Keshishian H, Addona T, Burgess M, Kuhn E, Carr SA. Quantitative, multiplexed assays for low abundance proteins in plasma by targeted mass spectrometry and stable isotope dilution. Mol Cell Proteomics. 2007;6(12):2212–29.
42. Kitteringham NR, Jenkins RE, Lane CS, Elliott VL, Park BK. Multiple reaction monitoring for quantitative biomarker analysis in proteomics and metabolomics. J Chromatogr B Analyt Technol Biomed Life Sci. 2009;877(13):1229–39.
43. Lee HB, Kang UB, Moon HG, Lee J, Lee KM, Yi M, et al. Development and validation of a novel plasma protein signature for breast cancer diagnosis by using multiple reaction monitoring-based mass spectrometry. Anticancer Res. 2015;35(11):6271–9.
44. Kim DH, Bae J, Lee JW, Kim SY, Kim YH, Bae JY, et al. Proteomic analysis of breast cancer tissue reveals upregulation of actin-remodeling proteins and its relevance to cancer invasiveness. Proteomics Clin Appl. 2009;3(1):30–40.
45. Kim Y, Kang UB, Kim S, Lee HB, Moon HG, Han W, et al. A validation study of a multiple reaction monitoring-based proteomic assay to diagnose breast cancer. J Breast Cancer. 2019;22 (4):579–86.
46. Anderson NL. The clinical plasma proteome: a survey of clinical assays for proteins in plasma and serum. Clin Chem. 2010;56(2):177–85.
47. Petushkova NA, Zgoda VG, Pyatnitskiy MA, Larina OV, Teryaeva NB, Potapov AA, et al. Post-translational modifications of FDA-approved plasma biomarkers in glioblastoma samples. PLoS One. 2017;12(5):e0177427.
48. Hornbeck PV, Kornhauser JM, Tkachev S, Zhang B, Skrzypek E, Murray B, et al. PhosphoSitePlus: a comprehensive resource for investigating the structure and function of experimentally determined post-translational modifications in man and mouse. Nucleic Acids Res. 2012;40(Database issue):D261–70.
49. Ryslava H, Doubnerova V, Kavan D, Vanek O. Effect of posttranslational modifications on enzyme function and assembly. J Proteome. 2013;92:80–109.
50. Chin L, Gray JW. Translating insights from the cancer genome into clinical practice. Nature. 2008;452(7187):553–63.
51. Sawyers CL. The cancer biomarker problem. Nature. 2008;452(7187):548–52.

52. Hanash SM, Pitteri SJ, Faca VM. Mining the plasma proteome for cancer biomarkers. Nature. 2008;452(7187):571–9.
53. Jensen ON. Interpreting the protein language using proteomics. Nat Rev Mol Cell Biol. 2006;7 (6):391–403.
54. Spickett CM, Pitt AR, Morrice N, Kolch W. Proteomic analysis of phosphorylation, oxidation and nitrosylation in signal transduction. Biochim Biophys Acta. 2006;1764(12):1823–41.
55. Pagel O, Loroch S, Sickmann A, Zahedi RP. Current strategies and findings in clinically relevant post-translational modification-specific proteomics. Expert Rev Proteomics. 2015;12 (3):235–53.
56. Ficarro SB, McCleland ML, Stukenberg PT, Burke DJ, Ross MM, Shabanowitz J, et al. Phosphoproteome analysis by mass spectrometry and its application to Saccharomyces cerevisiae. Nat Biotechnol. 2002;20(3):301–5.
57. Pinkse MW, Uitto PM, Hilhorst MJ, Ooms B, Heck AJ. Selective isolation at the femtomole level of phosphopeptides from proteolytic digests using 2D-NanoLC-ESI-MS/MS and titanium oxide precolumns. Anal Chem. 2004;76(14):3935–43.
58. Thingholm TE, Jensen ON, Robinson PJ, Larsen MR. SIMAC (sequential elution from IMAC), a phosphoproteomics strategy for the rapid separation of monophosphorylated from multiply phosphorylated peptides. Mol Cell Proteomics. 2008;7(4):661–71.
59. Zhang J, Sprung R, Pei J, Tan X, Kim S, Zhu H, et al. Lysine acetylation is a highly abundant and evolutionarily conserved modification in Escherichia coli. Mol Cell Proteomics. 2009;8 (2):215–25.
60. Zhan X, Desiderio DM. Nitroproteins from a human pituitary adenoma tissue discovered with a nitrotyrosine affinity column and tandem mass spectrometry. Anal Biochem. 2006;354 (2):279–89.
61. Udeshi ND, Mertins P, Svinkina T, Carr SA. Large-scale identification of ubiquitination sites by mass spectrometry. Nat Protoc. 2013;8(10):1950–60.
62. Pandey A, Podtelejnikov AV, Blagoev B, Bustelo XR, Mann M, Lodish HF. Analysis of receptor signaling pathways by mass spectrometry: identification of vav-2 as a substrate of the epidermal and platelet-derived growth factor receptors. Proc Natl Acad Sci U S A. 2000;97 (1):179–84.
63. Matsuoka S, Ballif BA, Smogorzewska A, McDonald ER 3rd, Hurov KE, Luo J, et al. ATM and ATR substrate analysis reveals extensive protein networks responsive to DNA damage. Science. 2007;316(5828):1160–6.
64. Kaji H, Saito H, Yamauchi Y, Shinkawa T, Taoka M, Hirabayashi J, et al. Lectin affinity capture, isotope-coded tagging and mass spectrometry to identify N-linked glycoproteins. Nat Biotechnol. 2003;21(6):667–72.
65. Yang Z, Harris LE, Palmer-Toy DE, Hancock WS. Multilectin affinity chromatography for characterization of multiple glycoprotein biomarker candidates in serum from breast cancer patients. Clin Chem. 2006;52(10):1897–905.
66. Ahn Y, Kang UB, Kim J, Lee C. Mining of serum glycoproteins by an indirect approach using cell line secretome. Mol Cells. 2010;29(2):123–30.
67. Chen Y, Kwon SW, Kim SC, Zhao Y. Integrated approach for manual evaluation of peptides identified by searching protein sequence databases with tandem mass spectra. J Proteome Res. 2005;4(3):998–1005.
68. Kim S, Na S, Sim JW, Park H, Jeong J, Kim H, et al. MODi: a powerful and convenient web server for identifying multiple post-translational peptide modifications from tandem mass spectra. Nucleic Acids Res. 2006;34(Web Server issue):W258–63.
69. Li Q, Shortreed MR, Wenger CD, Frey BL, Schaffer LV, Scalf M, et al. Global post-translational modification discovery. J Proteome Res. 2017;16(4):1383–90.
70. Yeom J, Kabir MH, Lim B, Ahn HS, Kim SY, Lee C. A proteogenomic approach for protein-level evidence of genomic variants in cancer cells. Sci Rep. 2016;6:35305.
71. Lawrence RT, Perez EM, Hernandez D, Miller CP, Haas KM, Irie HY, et al. The proteomic landscape of triple-negative breast cancer. Cell Rep. 2015;11(4):630–44.

72. Bertier G, Carrot-Zhang J, Ragoussis V, Joly Y. Integrating precision cancer medicine into healthcare-policy, practice, and research challenges. Genome Med. 2016;8(1):108.
73. Li L, Wei Y, To C, Zhu CQ, Tong J, Pham NA, et al. Integrated omic analysis of lung cancer reveals metabolism proteome signatures with prognostic impact. Nat Commun. 2014;5:5469.
74. Huang KL, Li S, Mertins P, Cao S, Gunawardena HP, Ruggles KV, et al. Proteogenomic integration reveals therapeutic targets in breast cancer xenografts. Nat Commun. 2017;8:14864.

Chapter 16
Next-Generation Sequencing-Based Biomarkers in Breast Cancer

Wonshik Han and Woosung Lim

Abstract For the realization of precision medicine in cancer treatment, discovery, and validation of clinically useful biomarker is the most important prerequisite. Biomarkers are needed and used for evaluation of cancer susceptibility, cancer screening (early detection), cancer subtyping, prediction of prognosis, decision of appropriate adjuvant therapy and duration of therapy, and for monitoring of recurrence. Biomarkers are also needed for decision of target therapy in metastatic cancer and monitoring of their response during follow-up. Now is the era of Next-Generation Sequencing (NGS). NGS technology can detect almost all kind of genomic changes that occur in cancer that is different from normal condition. The cost also is now reasonably low to use in routine clinical practice.

This chapter will review four kinds of NGS-based biomarkers that are already being used in clinical practice although the routine use is controversial, and that are promising and under active investigation focusing on studies done in Seoul National University Hospital (SNUH).

Keywords Breast neoplasms · Biomarkers, Tumor · Hereditary breast and ovarian cancer syndrome · Circulating tumor DNA · High-throughput nucleotide sequencing · Gene expression profiling · Molecular-targeted therapy · Precision medicine · Immunotherapy

---

W. Han (✉) · W. Lim
Department of Surgery, Seoul National University College of Medicine, Seoul, South Korea

Biomedical Research Institute, Seoul National University Hospital, Seoul, South Korea

Cancer Research Institute, Seoul National University, Seoul, South Korea
e-mail: hanw@snu.ac.kr

D.-Y. Noh et al. (eds.), *Translational Research in Breast Cancer*, Advances in Experimental Medicine and Biology 1187,
https://doi.org/10.1007/978-981-32-9620-6_16

16.1 Biomarkers for high-hereditary cancer risk

Cancers that run in families can be caused by an abnormal gene that is passed from generation to generation. Although this is often referred to as inherited cancer, what is inherited is the abnormal gene that can lead to cancer. Only about 5% to 10% of all cancers are thought to result directly from gene mutations inherited from a parent. Many hereditary cancer syndromes and the causative genes are already known such as, Cowden syndrome (*PTEN*), hereditary breast-ovarian cancer syndrome (*BRCA1* and *BRCA2*), and Li-Fraumeni syndrome (*TP53*). The most famous one of them is HBOC syndrome due to *BRCA1* or *BRCA2* mutations. The population incidence of this syndrome is about 1/500 to 1/1000 and the lifetime risk of breast cancer in affected women is about 50 to 85%. Usually *BRCA1* and *BRCA2* mutation tests using direct sequencing of the two genes have been done for women suspicious of hereditary cancer. Now due to the advancement in Next-Generation Sequencing (NGS) technology and decreasing cost of it, panel tests of multiple known hereditary cancer genes are available. The established breast cancer susceptibility genes are *ATM, BRCA1, BRCA2, CDH1, CHEK2, NBN, NF1, PALB2, PTEN, STK11*, and *TP53*. Genes with undefined risk of breast cancer but frequently included on multiplex sequencing panels are *BARD1, BLM, BRIP1, FAM175A, FANCC, MRE11A, RAD50, RAD51C, RAD51D*, and *XRCC2* [1]. The NCCN guideline is now recommending management strategies for breast and ovarian cancer based on genetic tests: Discussion of risk-reducing mastectomy with the patients who carry *CDH1, PALB2, PTEN, TP53, BRCA1*, and *BRCA2* mutation; Regular screening with breast magnetic resonance imaging (MRI) for women with *ATM, CHEK2*, and *STK11* mutation; Risk-reducing salphingo-oophorectomy for *BRIP1, RAD51C*, and *RAD51D* carriers.

Companies like Myriad, Invitae, and Ambry Genetics are providing their own hereditary cancer panel services. The number of genes included in the NGS panels are about 25 to 50 and most of the genes are overlapped between the services of each company. A hereditary cancer gene panel (64 genes) was also developed in SNUH and now is used in Hereditary Cancer Clinic of the hospital (Table 16.1).

The advantages of the panel test are (1) they provide broader picture of cancer risk, (2) it can find unexpected mutation associated with the familial cancer,

Table 16.1 Hereditary Cancer Gene Panel (64 genes) developed in Seoul National University Hospital

ALK	*APC*	*ATM*	*ATR*	*BAP1*	*BARD1*	*BLM*	*BMPR1A*
BRCA1	*BRCA2*	*BRIP1*	*CDH1*	*CDK4*	*CDKN2A*	*CHEK2*	*EPCAM*
FAM175A	*FANCA*	*FACB*	*FANCC*	*FANCD2*	*FANCE*	*FANCF*	*FANCG*
FANCI	*FANCL*	*FH*	*FLCN*	*GSTP1*	*HOXB13*	*KRAS*	*LIG4*
MEN1	*MET*	*MLH1*	*MRE11A*	*MSH2*	*MSH6*	*MUTYH*	*NAT*
NBN	*NF1*	*PALB2*	*PALLD*	*PMS2*	*PRKAR1A*	*PRSS1*	*PTEN*
RAD50	*RAD51*	*RAD51C*	*RAD51D*	*RB1*	*RET*	*SDHB*	*SDHC*
SDHD	*SLX4*	*SMAD4*	*SPINK1*	*STK11*	*TP53*	*VHL*	*XRCC2*

(3) convenience, time and cost saving compared to multiple single-syndrome tests, (4) it provide critical information when the family history is imperfect. Multigene panel test increases the yield of detection of deleterious mutation compared to targeted gene sequencing [2]. In a study of 10,000 patients referred for NGS panel testing (GeneDx), pathogenic or likely pathogenic variant prevalence was 9.0% in all patients [3]. The high frequency of positive results in a wide range of cancer genes shows genetic heterogeneity of hereditary cancer and the usefulness of multigene panels over genetic tests of one or two genes. The limitations of the NGS gene panel tests are 1) too many variants of unknown significance (VUS) are found and little information is available in many genes, 2) lack of clinical/screening guidelines for mutation carrier in many of the genes, 3) sometimes the result may increase anxiety for the patients. In a study Prospective Registry of Multiplex Testing (PROMPT), they collected data from commercial laboratories such as Ambry Genetics, Color Genomics, GeneDx, Invitae, Myriad Genetics, Pathway Genomics, and Quest Diagnostics, etc., and showed that 37% of the variants were VUS. Moreover, there were conflicting interpretations between the labs for up to 26% of the results [4].

In summary, recent advances in NGS technology have enabled far more rapid, less expensive sequencing of multiple genes than past. Multigene panel has about twice the yield of finding pathogenic mutation compared to conventional gene test. However, higher diagnostic yield comes with greater uncertainty. Expert counseling and tailoring to patient's preference is required. Adequate screening program and prophylactic treatment for the detected mutation carriers have to be established in the near future.

16.2 Biomarkers for Early Detection

Early detection of cancer in asymptomatic individuals with blood biomarker is the most challenging field in the cancer biomarker studies. As yet, there is no universal ctDNA signature for use in screening for any stage or type of cancer. This is due to the inability to detect low concentrations of ctDNA, and this limitation could be overcome with a more sensitive test. But increased sensitivity can lead to increased genetic noise, which in turn, can make it difficult to differentiate between tumor-associated DNA mutations and nontumor-associated DNA mutations, leading to an increased risk of false positives. Grail is an innovative company that is leading this technology using NGS-based circulating tumor DNA (ctDNA) detection. In the 2018 AACR meeting, they presented the initial findings of Circulating Cell-Free Genome Atlas (CCGA) study. They used blood samples from 878 participants with newly diagnosed treatment-naive cancer spanning 20 tumor types and across all clinical stages. Additionally, 580 participants with no clinical cancer diagnosis were enrolled and 169 technical assay controls were utilized. After isolating the cell-free DNA, samples were analyzed using three distinct sequencing methods: targeted sequencing, to measure nonsynonymous single nucleotide variants (SNVs) and indels in particular stretches of the genome; whole-genome sequencing, to measure

Table 16.2 Gene list of ctDNA NGS panel developed in SNUH

	Genes	No. of target region	Target size (bp)	Cumulative size (bp)
1	*ESR1*	9	1877	1877
2	*ERBB2*	28	3800	5677
3	*PIK3CA*	20	3207	8884
4	*TP53*	12	1263	10,147
5	*AKT1*	13	1443	11,590
6	*BRCA1*	23	5658	17,248
7	*BRCA2*	26	10,257	27,505
8	*FGFR1*	19	2635	30,140
9	*CCND1*	5	888	31,028
10	*PTEN*	9	1732	32,760
11	*MDM2*	11	1494	34,254
12	*IGF1R*	21	4104	38,358
13	*KIT*	21	2931	41,289
14	*EGFR*	30	3889	45,178
15	*NF1*	58	8581	53,759
16	*MYC*	3	1365	55,124
17	*GATA3*	5	1335	56,459
18	*MAP3K1*	20	4539	60,998
19	*CDH1*	16	2649	63,647
20	*MAP2K4*	12	1233	64,880
21	*PIK3R1*	17	2297	67,177
22	*AR*	9	2783	69,960
23	*APC*	16	8697	78,657
24	*TOP2A*	35	4596	83,253
25	*KRAS*	5	687	83,940
26	*FGFR2*	22	2774	86,714
27	*RB1*	27	2787	89,501

changes in copy number across the genome; and whole-genome bisulfite sequencing, to measure aberrant methylation patterns. A "cancer-like" signal was found in less than 1% of participants who entered the study with no clinical diagnosis of cancer, suggesting the possibility of developing a test with specificity higher than 99%. They showed that major source of false-positive variants is clonal hematopoiesis, a common age-related process that results in variations in the DNA of the white blood cell (WBC) population. Further, optimization of the assay and large-sized validation study are needed to use this technology in cancer screening.

In Seoul National University Hospital, we developed a ctDNA NGS gene panel consisting of 27 genes (Table 16.2). Feasibility study is ongoing using patients' blood sample who are planned to receive neoadjuvant chemotherapy with stage II/III breast cancer.

The critical issue of screening in asymptomatic unselected populations is overtreatment that can severely worsen quality of life, such as seen in the cases of thyroid cancer and prostate cancer. And a further paradox could arise for those cancers detected that have no curative treatment.

16.3 Biomarkers for Prognosis and Needs for Chemotherapy in ER-Positive Breast Cancer

Since the pivotal study published by Sorlie and Perou in 2000 about "Molecular portraits of breast cancer" using microarray and gene expression profiling of breast cancer [5], we have known that there must be important information of patients' long-term clinical outcome printed in the primary tumor. Now there are commercially available multigene expression signatures in breast cancer aiming to identify patients with disease of sufficiently good prognosis to allow the safe omission of adjuvant chemotherapy: MammaPrint (70-gene signature), Veridex 76-gene, Oncotype DX (21-gene signature), Breast Cancer Index (HoxB13:IL17BR, Theros™), Genomic grade index (MapQuantDx), PAM50 (Prosigna™), etc. Despite differences in the genes that compose each of the signatures, they largely identify the same group of patients as having poor prognosis disease [6], and the unifying characteristic is the high expression of proliferation-related genes for the high-risk group. Almost invariably the signatures classify ER-negative cancers as of poor prognosis disease. Clinicopathologic information such as, tumor size and lymph-node status provide prognostic information that is independent of that offered by prognostic signatures. Of them, 21-gene recurrence scores (Oncotype DX) have level I evidence, and incorporated in the NCCN guideline and also recommended in the ASCO guideline. In a recent publication of the TAILORx trial using the 21-gene assay, adjuvant endocrine therapy and chemoendocrine therapy had similar efficacy in women with hormone-receptor-positive, HER2-negative, axillary node-negative breast cancer who had a midrange 21-gene recurrence score, although some benefit of chemotherapy was found in some women 50 years of age or younger [7].

In Seoul National University Hospital, a NGS-based multigene prognostic tool, named Oncofree™ (DCGen, Inc. Seoul, Korea) was developed. It has distinct 149 gene panel for NGS target-gene RNA sequencing. These genes are involved in cell cycle, p53 signaling, DNA replication, and cell proliferation pathways. They are selected from public gene expression database that is highly correlated with 21-gene Recurrence Score. A prognosis prediction model was developed using Artificial Neural Network and Lasso regression analysis in a training set of 250 patients. In a validation set of 93 patients, prediction accuracy of our assay with high vs. low risk of Oncotype DX was 92.5%, and the correlation coefficient was 0.875. In the second validation set of 482 patients who received hormonal therapy and their long-term follow-up data are available, hazard ratio for distant metastasis-free survival of the patients with low vs. high score of our assay was 5.776 (95% CI 3.295–10.126, $p < 0.001$). This assay is the first one developed and

Table 16.3 Summary of assay characteristics commercially available multigene expression signatures in breast cancer

Product	Oncofree™	Oncotype DX	MammaPrint	Prosigna	Endopredict
Service company	DCGen, Korea	Genomic Health, USA	Agendia, USA	NanoString Technologies, USA	Myriad Genetics, USA
Number of genes	149	21	70	58	11
Sample type	FFPE	FFPE	FFPE/Fresh	FFPE	FFPE
Regulatory approval	N/A	CLIA	FDA cleared for centralized lab testing	FDA cleared for decentralized testing	CE marking for decentralized testing
Technology	NGS RNA-seq	RT-PCR	Microarray	nCounter	RT-PCR

tested in Asian country and the only one in the world using NGS technology. It is promising because it can decrease the assay cost significantly (Table 16.3).

16.4 Biomarkers for Selection of Therapy in Metastatic Breast Cancer

As our understanding of breast cancer improves, and our treatment options continue to expand, it is critical to recognize the tremendous heterogeneity in breast cancer that requires us to tailor treatments more effectively to spare patients from overwhelming toxic effects and costs. After the introduction of NGS technology, it was postulated that somatic and germline mutations in a number of genes would be a rich source of biomarkers to drive new treatment pathways. As a result of different international initiatives such as The Cancer Genome Atlas (TCGA) or the International Cancer Genome Consortium (ICGC), the use of NGS has helped define the genomic landscape of early stage breast cancer. These studies have revealed the high level of tumor heterogeneity for each breast tumor that consists of several molecular subsets, which are driven by distinct molecular alterations, indicating that tumors could be treated according to their individual molecular landscape.

Targetable genomic alterations in breast cancer are listed in Table 16.2. These alterations can be detected by use of pan-cancer NGS panel or breast cancer-specific panel. SNUH FIRST panel is a pan-cancer panel (v3.1). It can detect SNV/Indel/CNV for 183 genes including fusion change for 23 genes. Total target region is 1.95 Mb. It is now commercialized and used in practice through Molecular Tumor Board of SNUH. In addition to the pan-cancer panel, we developed a breast cancer-specific NGS panel (SNUH breast cancer panel) consisting of 121 genes that were reported to have high frequency of somatic mutation or gene amplification in TCGA data and METABRIC data. Targetable genes are considered with priority in the gene selection.

One of the most important actionable genes is *ESR1* mutation. Several studies have investigated the genomic landscape of breast cancer from early to metastatic disease, identifying *ESR1* mutations as one of the genomic alterations that mediate resistance to aromatase inhibitors (AI). *ESR1* mutations are rarely found in primary tumor but occur in 10–30% of ER-positive metastatic breast cancer that are resistant to AIs, and lead to ligand-independent activation of the ER. Whether *ESR1* mutations are present as a minor subclone when the cancer arises or are acquired during the treatment are still unknown. The best-understood mutations are localized in the ligand-binding domain (LBD) of *ESR1* with the common mutant alleles being Y537S, Y537N, Y537C, and D538G. Tamoxifen and fulvestrant can inhibit these mutant forms, but at higher drug concentrations that may not be achievable clinically. New antiestrogens that have activity against this *ESR1* mutant breast cancer are under development. Recent clinical results also showed that circulating tumor DNA (ctDNA)-based *ESR1* mutation analysis is more useful [8].

Another actionable mutation is *ERBB2* somatic mutation in patients with HER2 nonamplified breast cancer. These ERBB2/HER2-activating mutations increase tumor growth in vitro and in xenograft models. The frequency of this mutation in primary breast cancer was 1.6%. The two most common mutations were L755S and del 755–759. Neratinib, which is an irreversible pan-HER tyrosine kinase inhibitor was shown to be active in all *ERBB2* mutant forms. Clinical trials are undergoing to explore the efficacy of neratinib in breast cancer with *ERBB2* mutation.

PARP (poly ADP [adenosine diphosphate] ribose polymerase) inhibitors have also shown promise in triple-negative, *BRCA*-associated breast cancer. PARP1 is an enzyme involved in the process of base excision repair, which fixes single-strand DNA breaks. When PARP is inhibited, the cell is largely dependent on *BRCA1*- and *BRCA2*-dependent homologous recombination. Thus, in patients with germline *BRCA1* or *BRCA2* mutation, PARP inhibition will likely result in cell death. Patients with other newly discovered germline mutations that affect DNA repair such as, *PALB2*, *ATM*, *CHK2*, and *RAD51* mutations may also be sensitized to PARP inhibition.

In Seoul National University, we did both whole-exome and whole-transcriptome sequencing of 78 normal-paired primary breast cancer. We used a novel systems biology approach to identify driver mutations escalating the risk of metastasis [9]. As a result, we identified driver mutations in *ADPGK, NUP93, PCGF6, PKP2,* and *SLC22A5*, which are verified to enhance cancer cell migration and prompt metastasis with in vitro experiments. These novel somatic mutations may be used for therapeutic target or for identifying patients who are likely to develop distant metastasis. We also tried to identify recurrent fusion genes from data of 120 patients' whole-transcriptome sequencing using three different fusion-detecting tools (deFuse, Chimerascan, and TopHatFusion) [10]. Notably, a novel read-through fusion, *EEF1DP3-FRY*, was identified and validated in 6.7% (8/120) of the breast cancer samples. This off-frame fusion results in early truncation of the *FRY* gene, which plays a key role in the structural integrity during mitosis.

Another issue using the metastatic tissue sample for the NGS gene analysis is the availability of suitable biospecimen. We compared the sensitivity of fine-needle aspiration (FNA) with gross surgical sampling (GSS) from surgical specimens for the detection of somatic mutations in breast cancer using whole-exome sequencing (WES) [11]. In this study, we showed that FNA is feasible for the collection of tumor samples sufficient for WES analysis and that the higher purity obtained using this method may make it more reliable for genomic studies. This information is valuable to decide biopsy method for the future study design incorporating metastatic tumor sequencing (Table 16.4).

16.5 Biomarkers for Immunotherapy in HER2-Positive and Triple-Negative Breast Cancer

Tumor-associated antigens, such as HER-2 and Mucin 1 (MUC1), are observed in the breast cancer. These antigens have been the successful targets of new drug development for cancer vaccine and monoclonal antibody over the past decade, which have been translated into tumor-specific immune responses and are proven to be clinically beneficial.

By recent advancements in cancer therapy using novel mechanisms involving cancer mutations and the body's immune system, many successes in immunotherapy have been in melanoma, renal cancer, lung cancer, and others that have traditionally been known to be immunogenic. Breast cancer is also immunogenic and immunotherapy becomes a promising new field in breast cancer therapies.

Immunohistochemistry, gene expression profiling, and RNA sequencing have been used to assess the immunogenicity of breast cancer. Recent advances in genomics allow the detection of new targets that underlie immunogenicity in breast cancer. Immunogenicity of breast cancer is evaluated by the assessment of its antigenicity and antigenicity is evaluated by assessing its mutagenicity. Mutational load, the average number of somatic mutations per cancer cell, is associated with antigenicity and is lower in breast cancer compared with other tumors such as melanoma or lung cancer. However, the differences exist between different subtypes of breast cancer; TNBC has the highest mutational load compared with HR-positive breast cancers [12] and high-mutational load is associated with better prognosis in TNBC and HER2+ breast cancer compared with low-mutational load in breast cancer. High-mutational load is associated with high rates of immunotherapeutic antigens, which predict better survival and response to checkpoint inhibitors [13].

PD-L1 is one of the targets for immunotherapy and PD-L1 expression is different among breast cancer subtypes. Data from TCGA have confirmed higher PD-L1 mRNA expression in TNBC than nonTNBC and PD-L1 is not detected in normal breast tissue but is expressed in approximately 20% to 30% of TNBC. Analysis of gene expression profiles of TNBC identified six distinct subtypes and an immune-modulatory subtype was characterized by high expression of immune-related genes

Table 16.4 Targetable genomic alterations in breast cancer

Gene	Alteration	Frequency (%)	Candidate drug	Level of evidence for the target
Growth factor receptors				
ERBB2	Amplifications mutations	>10	HER2 inhibitor	13
FGF3	Amplifications	5–10	FGFR inhibitor	4
FGFR1	Amplifications	5–10	FGFR inhibitor	2
FGFR2	Amplifications	1–5	FGFR inhibitor	2
IGF1R	Amplifications	1–5	IGFR inhibitor	4
EGFR	Amplifications	1–5	EGFR inhibitor	2
PI3K/AKT/mTOR				
PIK3CA	Amplifications mutations	>10	PI3K inhibitor	1–2
PIK3R1	Mutations	1–5	Not known	4
PTEN	Mutations deletions	5–10	AKT inhibitor	3
AKT1	Amplifications mutations	1–5	AKT inhibitor	2
AKT2	Amplifications	1–5	AKT inhibitor	2
AKT3	Amplifications	1–5	AKT inhibitor	4
INPP4B	Deletions	1–5	AKT inhibitor	NA
MEK pathway				
NF1	Mutations	1–5	MEK inhibitor	2c
KRAS	Amplifications	1–5	MEK inhibitor	2c
BRAF	Amplifications	1–5	MEK inhibitor	2c
JNK pathway				
MAP2K4	Mutations deletions	5–10	Not known	NA
MAP3K1	Mutations deletions	5–10	Not known	NA
GPS2	Mutations	1–5	Not known	NA
Cell cycle				
CCND1	Amplifications	>10	CDK4 inhibitor	4

(continued)

Table 16.4 (continued)

Gene	Alteration	Frequency (%)	Candidate drug	Level of evidence for the target
CDKN2A	Deletions	5	Not known	NA
CDKN1B	Alterations	1–5	Not known	NA
CDK4	Amplifications	1–5	CDK4 inhibitor	4
Rb	Mutations deletions	5–10	Resistance to CDK4 inhibitor	3
DNA repair				
BRCA1	Mutations deletions	1–5	PARP inhibitor	1
Gene	Alteration	Frequency (%)	Candidate drug	Level of evidence for the target
BRCA2	Mutations deletions	1–5	PARP inhibitor	1
ATM	Mutations	1–5	PARP inhibitor	3
ATR	Mutations	1–5	PARP inhibitor	3
MDM2	Amplifications	1–5	MDM2 inhibitor	4
P53	Mutations	>10	Not known	NA
ER signaling				
ESR1	Mutations amplifications translocations	>10% in metastatic ER+ MBC resistant to endocrine therapy	Not known	2
GATA3	Mutations	5–10	Endocrine therapy	3
FoxA1	Mutations	1–5	Endocrine therapy	3
Epigenetics				
KMT2C	Mutations	5–10	Drug targeting epigenetics	4
KMT2B	Mutations	1–5	Drug targeting epigenetics	4
KDM6A	Mutations	1–5	Drug targeting epigenetics	4
SETD2	Mutations	1–5	Drug targeting epigenetics	4

(continued)

Table 16.4 (continued)

Gene	Alteration	Frequency (%)	Candidate drug	Level of evidence for the target
Others				
NOTCH3	Amplifications	1–5	NOTCH inhibitor	4

Arnedos, M. et al. (2015) Precision medicine for metastatic breast cancer—limitations and solutions. *Nat. Rev. Clin. Oncol.* doi:https://doi.org/10.1038/nrclinonc.2015.123

[14]. RNA sequencing showed this subtype to have substantially higher expression of PD-L1, PD-1, and CTLA-4. These and other data provide evidence that there may be a subset of TNBC in which checkpoint inhibitors may have particular efficacy.

With a better understanding of the heterogeneity of TNBC and immune targets, checkpoint inhibitors, vaccines, and immune antagonists could be used as therapeutic options in breast cancer. Large randomized clinical studies of atezolizumab (PD-L1 inhibitor) and pembrolizumab (PD-1 inhibitor) are ongoing in TNBC and SNUH also have participated in clinical trial of PD-L1 inhibitor. Cancer tissue from these studies will clarify the relation of response and resistance to PD-1 and PD-L1. First-line atezolizumab plus nab-paclitaxel improved PFS compared with placebo among patients with metastatic or unresectable locally advanced triple-negative breast cancer, according to interim results from the IMpassion130 trial released. Researchers observed prolonged PFS in both the intention-to-treat population and the PD-L1-positive population. Investigators observed prolonged PFS in the intention-to-treat population and the PD-L1-positive population. The OS analysis is ongoing; however, researchers observed encouraging survival results among patients who are PD-L1 positive.

Human epidermal growth factor receptor 2 (HER2)-positive breast cancer is generally associated with high levels of tumor infiltrating lymphocytes (TILs), and tumors with high levels of TILs have better outcomes on HER2-targeted therapy and chemotherapy. While resistance to trastuzumab is associated with poor immune responses, preclinical data indicate that trastuzumab resistance can be overcome by adding immune checkpoint blockades to antiHER2 therapy. At the 2017 San Antonio Breast Cancer Symposium, the results of the phase Ib/II PANACEA study were presented, which evaluated the combination of pembrolizumab and trastuzumab in patients with HER2-positive metastatic breast cancer who had progressed on a prior trastuzumab-based therapy. Metastatic HER2+ breast cancer in heavily pretreated patients is poorly immunogenic. Therefore, future directions of immunotherapy in metastatic HER2+ breast cancer should focus on combinations with effective antiHER2 therapy, particularly in patients with low TIL metastases.

Many clinical trials of immunotherapy are ongoing in adjuvant or metastatic setting of TNBC and HER2+ breast cancer. Immunotherapies have shown great success already in treating other cancers such as melanoma, but their progress for breast cancer has proven more difficult. However, the results of ongoing trials and discovery of response-related genes by NGS could provide a successful therapeutic

Table 16.5 Targetable genomic alterations for immunotherapy in breast cancer

Gene	Coding protein	Role in immune response
PDCD1LG1	PD-L1	Inhibitory
CD276	B7-H3	Inhibitory
SPAG17	SP17	Inhibitory
TNFRSF14	HVEM	Inhibitory
MAGEA9	MAGE-A9	Inhibitory
MAGEA11	MAGE-A11	Inhibitory
MUC1	MUC1	Vaccination
TERT	hTERT	Vaccination
FUT1/2	GLOBO-H	Vaccination

approach in TNBC and HER2+ cancer. Other targeting genes for immunotherapy and vaccination for breast cancer are listed in Table 16.5.

16.6 Future of NGS-Based Biomarkers in Breast Cancer

As genetic information becomes increasingly integrated into clinical practice, there are several limitations to the use of NGS. Variation in results between NGS may be the result of cancer heterogeneity and difference in the number of genes evaluated, extent of coverage within those genes, types of mutations, and limits of detection between NGS analysis. Genetic alterations identified by NGS might not be clinically actionable; detection of mutations does not guarantee therapeutic response. However, rapid increase in global understanding of the cancer genome has enabled us to further refine the molecular classification of cancers based on the combination of genetic and transcriptomic alteration data and trans-omics data (epigenomics, proteomics, and metabolomics). Technical and bioinformatical advances make the NGS technology increasingly more powerful. NGS-based biomarker detection could bring a new paradigm of breast cancer treatment as well as cancer vaccination and realize the true *precision medicine* by classification of cancer and personalized treatments.

References

1. Kurian AW, Antoniou AC, Domchek SM. Refining breast cancer risk stratification: additional genes, additional information. Am Soc Clin Oncol Educ Book. 2016;35:44–56.
2. Ricker C, Culver JO, Lowstuter K, Sturgeon D, Sturgeon JD, Chanock CR, et al. Increased yield of actionable mutations using multi-gene panels to assess hereditary cancer susceptibility in an ethnically diverse clinical cohort. Cancer Genet. 2016;209(4):130–7.
3. Susswein LR, Marshall ML. Pathogenic and likely pathogenic variant prevalence among the first 10,000 patients referred for next-generation cancer panel testing. Genet Med. 2016;18(8):823–32.

4. Balmana J, Digiovanni L, Gaddam P, Walsh MF, Joseph V, Stadler ZK, et al. Conflicting interpretation of genetic variants and cancer risk by commercial laboratories as assessed by the prospective registry of multiplex testing. J Clin Oncol Off J Am Soc Clin Oncol. 2016;34 (34):4071–8.
5. Perou CM, Sorlie T, Eisen MB, van de Rijn M, Jeffrey SS, Rees CA, et al. Molecular portraits of human breast tumours. Nature. 2000;406(6797):747–52.
6. Fan C, Oh DS, Wessels L, Weigelt B, Nuyten DS, Nobel AB, et al. Concordance among gene-expression-based predictors for breast cancer. N Engl J Med. 2006;355(6):560–9.
7. Sparano JA, Gray RJ, Makower DF, Pritchard KI, Albain KS, Hayes DF, et al. Adjuvant chemotherapy guided by a 21-gene expression assay in breast cancer. N Engl J Med. 2018;379 (2):111–21.
8. O'Leary B, Hrebien S, Morden JP, Beaney M, Fribbens C, Huang X, et al. Early circulating tumor DNA dynamics and clonal selection with palbociclib and fulvestrant for breast cancer. Nat Commun. 2018;9(1):896.
9. Lee JH, Zhao XM, Yoon I, Lee JY, Kwon NH, Wang YY, et al. Integrative analysis of mutational and transcriptional profiles reveals driver mutations of metastatic breast cancers. Cell Discov. 2016;2:16025.
10. Kim J, Kim S, Ko S, In YH, Moon HG, Ahn SK, et al. Recurrent fusion transcripts detected by whole-transcriptome sequencing of 120 primary breast cancer samples. Genes Chromosomes Cancer. 2015;54(11):681–91.
11. Lee HB, Joung JG, Kim J, Lee KM, Ryu HS, Lee HO, et al. The use of FNA samples for whole-exome sequencing and detection of somatic mutations in breast cancer surgical specimens. Cancer Cytopathol. 2015;123(11):669–77.
12. Vogelstein B, Papadopoulos N, Velculescu VE, Zhou S, Diaz LA Jr, Kinzler KW. Cancer genome landscapes. Science (New York, NY). 2013;339(6127):1546–58.
13. Rizvi NA, Hellmann MD, Snyder A, Kvistborg P, Makarov V, Havel JJ, et al. Cancer immunology. Mutational landscape determines sensitivity to PD-1 blockade in non-small cell lung cancer. Science (New York, NY). 2015;348(6230):124–8.
14. Lehmann BD, Bauer JA, Chen X, Sanders ME, Chakravarthy AB, Shyr Y, et al. Identification of human triple-negative breast cancer subtypes and preclinical models for selection of targeted therapies. J Clin Invest. 2011;121(7):2750–67.

Chapter 17
Liquid Biopsy in Breast Cancer: Circulating Tumor Cells and Circulating Tumor DNA

Tae-Kyung Yoo

Abstract Cancer is associated with gene mutations, and the analysis of tumor-associated mutations is increasingly used for diagnostic, prognostic, and treatment purposes. These molecular landscapes of solid tumors are currently obtained from surgical or biopsy specimens. However, during cancer progression and treatment, selective pressures lead to additional genetic changes as tumors acquire drug resistance. Tissue sampling cannot be performed routinely owing to its invasive nature and a single biopsy only provides a limited snapshot of a tumor, which may fail to reflect spatial and temporal heterogeneity. This dilemma may be solved by analyzing cancer cells or cancer cell-derived DNA from blood samples, called liquid biopsy. Liquid biopsy is one of the most rapidly advancing fields in cancer diagnostics and recent technological advances have enabled the detection and detailed characterization of circulating tumor cells and circulating tumor DNA in blood samples.

Liquid biopsy is an exciting area with rapid advances, but we are still at the starting line with many challenges to overcome. In this chapter we will explore how tumor cells and tumor-associated mutations detected in the blood can be used in the clinic. This will include detection of cancer, prediction of prognosis, monitoring systemic therapies, and stratification of patients for therapeutic targets or resistance mechanisms.

Keywords Breast cancer · Liquid biopsy · Circulating tumor cells · Circulating tumor DNA · Tumor heterogeneity · Precision medicine

T.-K. Yoo (✉)
Department of Surgery, Seoul St. Mary's Hospital, College of Medicine, The Catholic University of Korea, Seoul, Republic of Korea

D.-Y. Noh et al. (eds.), *Translational Research in Breast Cancer*, Advances in Experimental Medicine and Biology 1187,
https://doi.org/10.1007/978-981-32-9620-6_17

17.1 Introduction

Tissue biopsy is a necessity in breast cancer diagnosis, regarded as the gold standard. Along with histologic definition, tissue biopsy also provides identification of important prognostic and predictive factors such as estrogen receptor, progesterone receptor, and human epidermal growth factor receptor-2 (HER2). More recently, genetic profiling of the tumor enables patient stratification for prognostication and prediction of recurrence and resistance to treatment. Cancer treatment is evolving from a one-size-fits-all strategy to a precision medicine strategy, meaning that patient selection is important more than ever before.

Standard tissue biopsy, such as surgical biopsy or image-guided gun biopsy, is an invasive process including many difficulties in its process. Patients suffer from pain during the procedure and potential complications exist, meaning multiple or serial biopsies are impractical. Also, some tumors are anatomically inaccessible for biopsy. Furthermore, standard biopsy only provides a single snapshot of the tumor, which is limited in time and space, not being able to reflect the evolving characteristics of the cancer cells.

The recent advance of next-generation sequencing (NGS) techniques has enabled us to analyze cancer tissue more minutely, revealing the extensive intertumoral and intratumoral heterogeneity [1, 2]. Beyond spatial heterogeneity, temporal heterogeneity also exists as tumors evolve under selection pressure of treatment. However, the limitations of standard biopsy are restraints in evaluating tumor evolution, likely underestimating the complexity of the genomic landscape of the tumor. The concept of liquid biopsy has emerged in the need to observe tumor genetics and dynamics in new ways.

Liquid biopsy in cancer research can be defined as a minimally invasive test done on a sample of body fluid to look for circulating tumor cells (CTCs) and cell-free circulating nucleic acids (especially, circulating tumor DNA (ctDNA) and exosomes) released from the primary tumor and/or metastatic deposits [3, 4]. Blood is the most commonly used body fluid for liquid biopsy approaches. In addition to blood, urine, stool, cerebrospinal fluid (CSF), saliva, pleural fluid, and ascites are potential sources of tumor-derived material. Obtaining a liquid biomarker from body fluids is a quick, minimally invasive procedure that can be easily obtained with minimal pain and risk (Table 17.1). Serial testing and real-time sampling are possible, reflecting treatment responses and temporal heterogeneity. Biologically liquid biopsies are also more likely to represent the whole tumor, reflecting spatial heterogeneity.

The principle sources for liquid biopsies are represented by CTCs, ctDNAs, exosomes, and circulating cell-free nucleic acids (such as, microRNA, mRNA, and long noncoding RNAs). The analysis of liquid biopsy specimens is, however, challenging because CTC count is limited, and ctDNA are fragmented and contaminated with germline cell-free DNA making it hard to isolate tumor-derived genetic material in high quantities with a pure fraction [7]. Thus, highly sensitive assays are needed, and recent technological advances have enabled the detection and detailed

Table 17.1 Comparison between tissue biopsy and liquid biopsy [3–6]

	Tissue biopsy	Liquid biopsy
Advantage	• Histopathological diagnosis and staging • Gold standard for tumor characterization • Validated tissue processing and handling • Prognostic, predictive • Localized sampling of tissue – Specific mutations for target therapy	• Minimally invasive – Minimal pain and risk – Serial testing, real-time sampling is possible • Quick • Comprehensive tissue profile – Reflects tumor heterogeneity
Disadvantage	• Invasive procedure – Pain and risk – Multiple sampling is frequently impractical – Serial testing is difficult – Sometimes anatomically inaccessible • Time-intensive procedure • Not real-time • Localized sampling of tissue – Not always representative of tumor heterogeneity	• Staging not possible • Special processing and handling are needed • Low amounts of ctDNA, CTC → need considerable amount of blood sample • Variations in levels according to cancer type and individual patient • Limited prognostic feature • Predictive value not proven yet

characterization of CTC and ctDNA in blood samples from cancer patients. Liquid biopsy is a very active research field, and despite of important advances, several technical challenges remain to be solved and the clinical utility of liquid biopsy is still under debate [8]. Research on exosomes and cell-free RNA are still premature to seek into their clinical implications.

In this chapter, we will explore the current concepts and future of liquid biopsies from a clinical practice point of view. In particular, CTCs and ctDNA analyses have opened new diagnostic avenues that may change clinical practice in breast cancer, and we will focus on these perspectives.

17.2 Review of Past Studies

The presence of CTCs was first reported by the Australian physician Thomas Ashworth in 1869 from an autopsy, within the blood of a patient with extensive breast cancer [9]. After its first description, several case reports have followed, but only until recently has CTCs become a widespread topic in cancer research [10–12]. The recent development of modern technologic platforms has made it possible to capture and characterize CTCs. In 2004, the CellSearch® system was introduced, and the prognostic value of CTC enumeration was proven in metastatic breast cancer patients [13]. This led to the clearance of the CellSearch® system by the FDA and also was the start of intensive CTC research. The CellSearch® system is still the only medical device currently approved for CTC selection and enumeration in various cancers.

The term of cell-free DNA (cfDNA) was first reported by Mandel and Metais in 1948, referring to fragmented DNA found in the noncellular component of the blood [14]. In healthy individuals, cfDNA are discovered with a concentration of 1–10 mg/mL in plasma [15, 16]. This level is increased under conditions of tissue stress, including exercise, inflammation, surgery, or tissue injury [17]. In 1977, Leon and colleagues reported that cancer patients had a higher level of cfDNA in the serum compared to healthy individuals [18]. Further research was triggered and in 1989, Stroun and colleagues demonstrated that some of these cfDNA in the plasma of cancer patients originate from cancer cells [19]. Specific mutations were soon found from urinary, stool, and sputum samples of various cancer patients [20]. Sorenson and colleagues were the first to report mutated KRAS in the plasma cfDNA of patients with pancreatic cancer in 1994 [21]. The KRAS mutation found in the plasma was identical to that found in the patient's tumor, confirming that the plasma cfDNA originated from the tumor. Mutations in cfDNA are highly specific markers for cancer, and these gave rise to the term of circulating tumor DNA (ctDNA).

17.3 Current Evidence and Concepts

17.3.1 The Biology Behind CTCs and ctDNA

CTCs are tumor cells that are shed into the periphery blood from solid tumors of primary or metastatic sites. The process of the release of CTCs into the bloodstream is not fully understood yet. Whether the process is an active invasion or a passive shedding of cells and whether it is a random process or predetermined by a biologic program is still on debate [22, 23]. Although thousands of cancer cells are released into the circulation, few survive to become a source of metastasis [24]. The half-life of CTCs is short, reported to be only 1–2.4 h in breast cancer patients [25]. Also apoptotic CTCs or fragmented CTCs are frequently found in the bloodstream [23, 26]. Strong evidence exists that CTCs are capable of metastasis, but CTCs have to endure a strong selection process to obtain their target of metastasis formation [27, 28]. It is still unclear of how CTCs contribute to metastatic spread and progression.

The key technical challenge in CTC research is its rarity in the bloodstream, with estimates of just one CTC per ~10^7 white blood cells per milliliter of blood. Vast array of technologies have been developed to isolate CTCs, by enrichment and detection [29–32]. CTC enrichment is the process of capturing CTCs amongst the vast array of normal blood cells. It is achieved using the physical properties of the cells, such as size, density or charge, or biological properties, such as tumor cell surface marker expression. After enrichment, CTCs must be detected to isolate pure

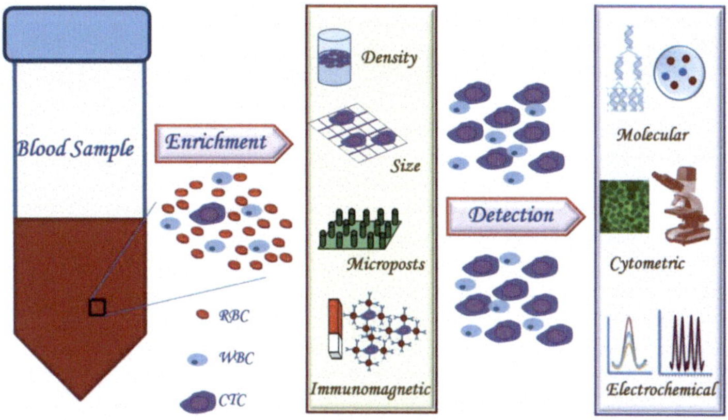

Fig. 17.1 Schematic for the process of enrichment and detection of circulating tumor cells (CTCs) [32]

CTCs from leukocyte contamination. CTCs are detected using immunologic, molecular, or functional assays [33] (Fig. 17.1).

The release of tumor DNA into the blood circulation is from all sources of tumor cells, including primary tumors, metastatic lesions, micrometastasis, and even CTCs. The majority of ctDNA are released passively from necrotic and apoptotic cells in the process of cellular destruction but, active DNA release is also reported [34–36] (Fig. 17.2). However, the biology behind the release of ctDNA into the circulation is still unknown. Once in the circulation, clearance of cfDNA (including ctDNA) is rapid and occurs via the kidneys, liver, and spleen [37]. Observation studies show that the half-life of cfDNA in the circulation is between 16 min and 2.5 h, which enables ctDNA analysis to be considered as a "real-time" snapshot of disease burden [37, 38].

Pharmocological treatments, inflammation, and circardian rhythms are known to influence cfDNA clearance but its mechanism is not entirely understood. In normal physiological conditions, cellular debris, including cfDNA, are cleared by infiltrating phagocytes, but in tumorous conditions clearance is less efficient, increasing the fraction of ctDNA in overall cfDNA [39]. In cancer patients, the fraction of ctDNA in overall cfDNA varies between 0.1% to over 90% [40]. The fraction of patients with detectable ctDNA differs by cancer types. Substantial variability is also observed among patients with the same cancer type, but still has the tendency to be parallel with tumor burden [40].

ctDNA are detected in low levels and its half-life is short, which means specialized approaches are needed to isolate and analyze them. The key issues in detecting ctDNA are the stability of cfDNA itself and contamination of wild-type DNA from lysis of normal blood cells. Plasma must be centrifuged and separated within 1 to 4 hours after blood collection to limit these effects. However, rapid processing has practical challenges and also has the potential of preanalytical variability due to differences in processing time [41, 42]. This prompted the development of

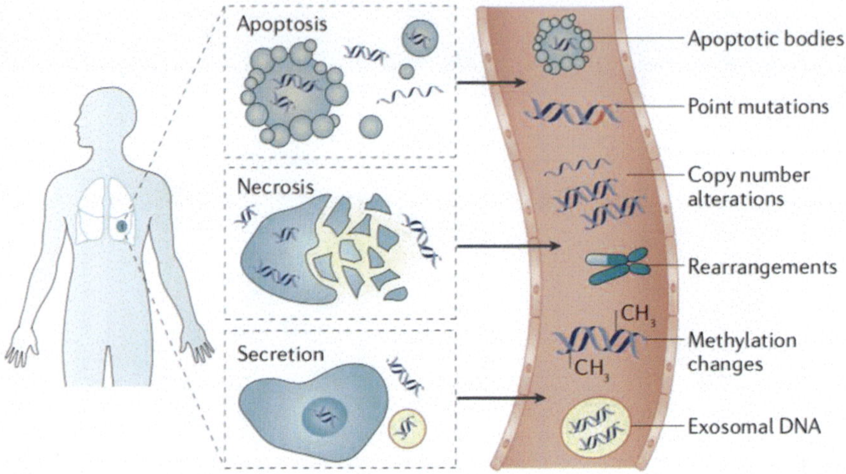

Fig. 17.2 The origins and range of alterations in cell-free DNA [20]

specialized preservative-containing tubes that stabilize cfDNA and intact cells for up to 7–14 days at room temperature [43].

In principle, technologies for mutation detection in ctDNAs can be divided into targeted and untargeted approaches. Targeted approaches aim to detect mutations in a set of predefined genes, whereas untargeted approaches aim to screen the genome and discover new genomic aberrations [17, 23, 44]. Targeted approaches use mutation-specific techniques mainly based on polymerase-chain-reaction (PCR) analysis, such as BEAMing (beads, emulsion, amplification, and magnetics) or droplet digital PCR (ddPCR) analysis [45, 46]. These techniques have high analytical sensitivity, detecting, and quantifying individual point mutations present at allele frequencies of 0.01% or less in ctDNA. However, targeted approaches are only applicable to limited cancer patients where preliminary tumor analysis is already done or only for hotspot mutations (e.g., PIK3CA mutations). NGS methods are mainly used for untargeted approaches which range from whole-genome or whole-exome sequencing to targeted sequencing of a limited gene panel [47, 48]. Untargeted approaches have the main advantage of being applicable to all patients and discovery of novel mutations, but still have limited sensitivity and specificity due to error rate of DNA polymerase and the sequencing reaction. Various techniques are being developed to improve these limits of detection [49, 50].

17.3.2 *Comparison Between CTCs and ctDNA*

Molecular analysis of CTCs and ctDNAs provides distinct but, complementary information (Table 17.2). CTC analysis is not limited to enumeration but can be

Table 17.2 Comparison between CTCs and ctDNA [4, 6, 7, 28, 29]

	Circulating tumor cells	Circulating tumor DNA
Tissue/cell source	Tumors	Apoptotic tumor cells/ necrotic
Isolation	Difficult	Easy
Half-life	1–2.4 h	<1.5 h
Concentration in blood	1–10 CTC/1 mL	30 ng/1 mL
Size	9–30 μm	100–200 bp
Applications		
• Prognostic marker	Yes	Yes
• Predictive marker	Not yet	Not yet
• Potentially addresses spatial and temporal tumor heterogeneity	Yes	Yes
• Detection of somatic mutations, indels, copy-number alterations, and gene fusions	Yes	Yes
• Evaluation of methylation patterns	Yes	Yes
• Analysis of mRNA/ miRNA/lncRNA/RNA splice variants	Yes	Yes
• Analysis of RNA expression	Yes	No
• Cell morphology and functional studies	Yes	No
• In breast cancer	Harvesting difficulties, false-negatives	A few single genes, low rate of hotspot mutations; screening of multiple genes
Advantage	Molecular characterization and functional studies are possible	Relatively stable and easier to detect
Disadvantage	• CTC heterogeneity • Low abundance and fragility • Multiple different technologies for CTC isolation • Lack of validation and qualification of assays (more sensitive technologies and flexibility for characterization are needed) • False-positive and false-negative	• Lack of standardization of techniques • False-positive and false-negative

characterized by DNA, RNA, and proteins. ctDNA analysis is limited to DNA mutations, but has the advantage of easier and more sensitive detection and the potential of reflecting treatment responses more accurately [6, 40, 51].

The analysis of CTC has remarkable depth by allowing analysis of the whole cell. Starting with simple enumeration, characterization by DNA, RNA, and proteins is also possible. Along with the development of single cell technologies, measurements of cancer heterogeneity and subclonal populations are anticipated. Functional studies using ex vivo culture are also expected to allow real-time studies of drug sensitivity and individual therapeutics. However, currently CTC detection is technically challenging, and its concentration is very low [52]. In contrast, ctDNA analysis has the notable attribute of ease of collection and high-throughput analysis. ctDNA genotyping is expected to be rapid, economic, and reliable for clinical application. However, the limitation of ctDNA analysis is its restriction of DNA mutations.

Currently CTC and ctDNA approaches are competing biomarkers. The information obtained through these approaches is different but also complementary. Synergistic, not competitive, applications are expected in the future of clinical oncology. A possible plot is using ctDNA analysis for disease burden monitoring and limited molecular analysis. When increased disease burden is recognized, CTC analysis for comprehensive characterization of tumor DNA, RNA, and protein can help to optimize treatment selection [53].

17.3.3 Clinical Applications in Breast Cancer

Many studies have illustrated the potential of liquid biopsy approaches to determine its prognostic and predictive value, establish a tumor's genomic profile, monitor treatment response and quantify minimal residual disease, and assess treatment resistant. However, research on CTC and ctDNA analysis is still at its starting point and up to present status, there are currently no approved applications in clinical practice for breast cancer patients. Nevertheless, recent studies demonstrate promising results and ongoing research holds expectation for the future of CTCs and ctDNAs for clinical application (Fig. 17.3).

17.3.4 Screening and Early Detection of Cancer

In the early stage, breast cancer is confined to the breast and locoregional lymph nodes, presenting with limited tumor burden. Consequently, CTCs or ctDNAs are likely to be present at a low concentration in the blood. The presence of CTCs in early breast cancer range from 9.4 to 48.6% from previous studies [54–57]. The detection rate is still too low to replace current protein biomarkers or to be considered as a screening tool. Although the Cellsearch® system is established as the gold standard of CTC analysis in metastatic breast cancer, it is still a matter of debate on how to detect CTCs in early breast cancer.

The potential of ctDNA detection as a screening process is suggested in recent preliminary studies. In a prospective study of 29 early breast cancer patients, Beaver

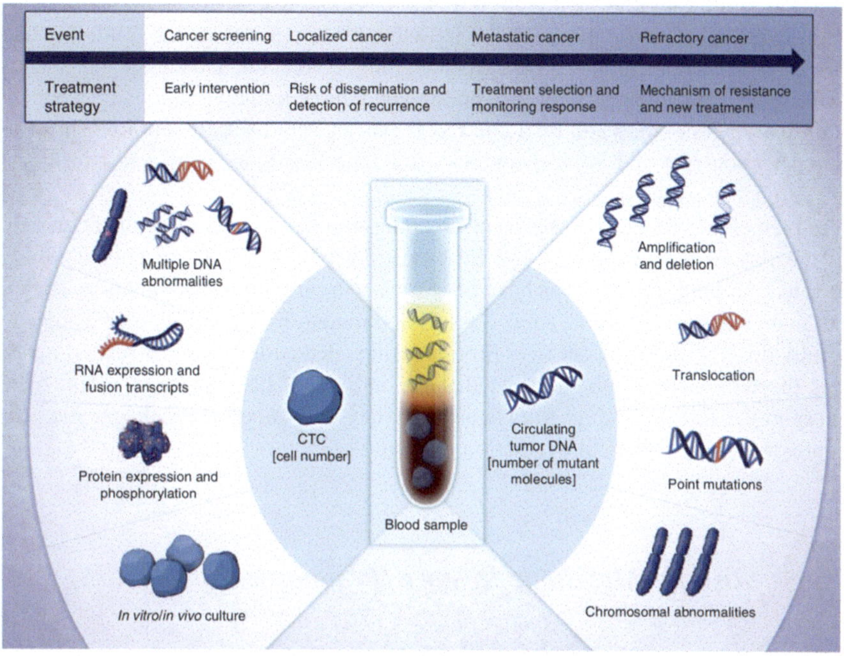

Fig. 17.3 The clinical applications of CTC and ctDNA in breast cancer [52]

and colleagues analyzed presurgery plasma samples for PIK3CA mutations [58]. Among the 29 patients, ten had PIK3CA mutations in their tumor, and were detected in plasma samples with 93.3% sensitivity and 100% specificity. Whereas this approach was performed by matching with primary tumor mutations, Phallen and colleagues applied an untargeted approach using deep sequencing (~30,000×) of 58 genes in 200 cancer patients [59]. Among the 45 breast cancer patients who participated in this study, 56% were detected through this method, without any significant difference according to cancer stage (stage I 67%, stage II 59%, stage III 46%).

A clinical study on cancer screening requires large study population and long follow-up times. An alternative strategy to speed up this process would be to focus on patients with high risk of developing cancer. An ongoing French prospective study (CirCA01) is an example of this strategy, testing the screening value of TP53 ctDNA detection in BRCA carriers [60]. After recruiting germline BRCA1 carriers, blood samples will be obtained at every visit to the hospital. Plasma TP53 mutations will be detected from ctDNAs, to evaluate the sensitivity and specificity for detection of any tumor growth (relapse and/or new tumor).

The greatest technical challenge in applying ctDNA as screening tool is the detection of the low amount of ctDNA and the choice of the right panel of cancer-specific genomic aberrations [23]. Unfortunately, the genomic alterations that drive tumor growth in breast cancer are not specific and still unknown, thus untargeted detection techniques may be preferred. In the USA and Korea, the umbrella LUNAR trial is expected to enroll thousands of individuals to demonstrate the feasibility and efficacy of early detection of breast, ovarian, lung, colorectal, and pancreatic cancers [7]. Targeted sequencing assay for genomic and epigenomic variations is used and preliminary results for stage I–III colorectal cancer were recently reported showing 94% detection rate and 94% specificity [61]. The feasibility of this test in breast cancer must be awaited.

Implementing liquid biopsies as a screening tool is quite an attractive approach, but the risk of over-diagnosis and false-positive is a hurdle to be solved. Many precancerous benign conditions have been shown to carry common mutations shared with malignant tumors. Also, cancer-associated mutations occur with increasing age in individuals with no cancer over lifetime. Thus, detection of cancer-related mutations in ctDNA might not indicate that the individual has cancer or might have cancer in the future, leading to extensive anxiety and unnecessary diagnostic procedures with side effects like radiation exposure [23].

17.3.5 Risk for Metastatic Relapse (Prognostic Factor)

The expectations of CTC as a prognostic factor in metastatic breast cancer were raised when Cristofanilli and colleagues published the results of a prospective, multicenter study that enrolled 177 metastatic breast cancers to evaluate the prognostic value of CTCs using the CellSearch® system [13]. Patients with $\geq$5 CTCs per 7.5 mL blood at baseline had a shorter median progression-free survival compared to patients with <5 CTCs (2.7 months vs. 7.0 months, $p < 0.001$). Furthermore, overall survival also differed according to CTC level ($\geq$5 CTCs, 10.1 months vs. <5 CTCs, >18 months; $p < 0.001$). This study led to the FDA approval of the CellSearch® system for metastatic breast cancer in 2007. The same group performed additional follow-up with subsequent CTC evaluation at each follow-up visit, reporting that detection of elevated CTCs at any time during therapy predicts rapid disease progression and mortality in metastatic breast cancer patients [62]. The prognostic significance of CTCs in metastatic breast cancer has been confirmed in the SWOG S0500 randomized trial [63]. The change of CTCs was analyzed in metastatic breast cancer receiving first-line chemotherapy, and overall survival differed according to baseline CTC level and CTC number change after first dose of chemotherapy. Patients with <5 CTCs at baseline had a median overall survival of 34.8 months, patients who had $\geq$5 CTCs at baseline but decreased to less than 5 CTCs had a median survival of 22.9 months and patients who persistently had $\geq$5 CTCs had a median survival of only 13.1 months (p <0.001). Subsequently, the prognostic value of CTC in metastatic breast cancer was proven by many other groups [64–66].

Whereas the treatment is palliative in nature in metastatic breast cancer, the use of liquid biopsies as a prognostic and predictive marker might be more important for patients with early breast cancer whom undergo curative treatment. The prognostic value of CTCs in patients with nonmetastatic breast cancer was suggested in preliminary prospective clinical trials [55, 67–70]. The individual data from these trials were gathered by Janni and colleagues for a pooled analysis of 3173 patients with stages I–III breast cancer [71]. All studies used the CellSearch® system for CTC analysis, and at least one CTC being detected, regardless of the initial blood volume, was assessed as CTC-positive. CTC detection rate was 20.2% and the number of detected CTCs ranged from 1 to 827. The summary estimate for overall survival and disease-free survival hazard ratio (HR) according to the presence of CTCs was 2.444 (95% CI, 1.811–3.298, $p < 0.001$) and 2.080 (95% CI, 1.688–2.563, $p < 0.001$). The prognostic relevance of CTC detection was independent of tumor grade and stage, nodal stage, hormone receptor, and HER2-receptor expression and persisted in any CTC cut-off value from 1–20. Subgroup analysis demonstrated the prognostic value of CTCs varied among breast cancer subtypes also. The clinical validity of CTC detection as a prognostic marker has also been demonstrated in patients undergoing neoadjuvant chemotherapy by Bidard and colleagues [72]. A meta-analysis of individual patient data from 21 studies was performed in which CTC detection by CellSearch® system was performed before treatment initiation. CTC detection rate was 25.2% and detecting two or more CTCs before starting treatment increased the prognostic ability of multivariable prognostic models for overall survival (HR 3.93, 95% CI 2.81–5.45), distant disease-free survival (HR 3.73, 95% CI 2.82–4.90), and locoregional relapse-free interval (HR 3.02, 95% CI 1.88–4.75).

Alongside with CTCs, ctDNA detection has also been investigated as a prognostic factor in both advanced and early breast cancer. Whereas the data on CTCs are mainly focused on data from the CellSearch® system, the methods for ctDNA detection have various technical differences. Also, ctDNA studies are reported with relatively limited sample sizes.

In metastatic breast cancer patients, the largest study about the prognostic role of ctDNA detection is the data from the BOLERO-2 clinical trial [73]. This phase III study randomized patients to exemestane plus placebo or exemestane plus everolimus. A total of 541 patients had baseline plasma samples and ddPCR was performed to analyze for the two most frequent mutations in ESR1 (Y537S and D538G). ESR1 mutation from ctDNA was detected in 28.2% of the patients, and both mutations were associated with shorter overall survival (wild-type, 32.1 months, 95% CI 28.09–36.40 months; both mutations, 15.5 months, 95% CI 10.87–27.43 months). In contrary of detecting specific mutations, cfDNA tumor fraction can also be considered as a prognostic factor. Stover and colleagues performed low coverage whole-genome sequencing of cfDNA from metastatic triple-negative breast cancer patients to determine cfDNA tumor fraction [74]. A total of 164 patients were evaluated and cfDNA tumor fraction was determined in 96.3% of them. A cfDNA tumor fraction threshold of $\geq 10\%$ was associated with significantly worse metastatic survival (median, 6.4 vs. 15.9 months) and remained significant independent of clinicopathologic factors (HR 2.14, 95% CI 1.4–3.8, $p < 0.001$).

The prognostic role of ctDNA in early breast cancer patients is demonstrated in relatively small sample studies. In a prospective study of 147 early breast cancer patients, Garcia and colleagues detected loss of heterozygosity (six markers) and TP53 mutations from plasma DNA using PCR and Sanger sequencing [75]. Among them, 42.9% (61/142) were detected of molecular changes, and these patients presented with poor OS and DFS compared to negative cases. Oshiro and colleagues used ddPCR assay to detect PIK3CA mutations among early breast cancer patients [76]. PIK3CA mutations were detected in 110 primary cancers and 23% of these patients had corresponding mutations in ctDNA analysis. Patients with a high level of mutant ctDNA exhibited significantly shorter recurrence-free survival and overall survival rates compared to patients with low or no mutant ctDNA [76]. Most recently, Garcia-Murillas and colleagues analyzed two prospective ctDNA sample collection studies (the ChemoNEAR study and the Plasma DNA study), recruiting 170 early breast cancer patients [77]. In blood samples obtained at diagnosis before any treatment, ctDNA was detected in 41 of 80 patients (51.2%), at a median allele frequency of 0.36%. Detection of ctDNA at diagnosis was associated with poor relapse-free survival (HR 5.8, 95% CI 1.2–27.1). A prospective study for stages II–III invasive HER2-positive or triple-negative breast cancer patients is undergoing to evaluate the predictive value of ctDNA in patients undergoing neoadjuvant therapy [78]. A total of 229 patients are planned to be enrolled and survival analysis is also planned, expecting to add-on data for the prognostic significance of ctDNA detection in early breast cancer patients.

The prognostic value of liquid biopsies in early breast cancer might be limited, as a sample of the tumor itself is usually available and provides valuable prognostic information [79]. However, stratification of patients into high-risk and low-risk groups would enable adjuvant therapy to be given to patients who are likely to benefit more [20]. Under this concept, the on-going TREAT-CTC trial is a randomized phase II trial to evaluate the efficacy of additional trastuzumab in HER2-negative breast cancer patients with detectable CBC after completion of adjuvant therapy [80]. The usefulness of liquid biopsy in treatment stratification will be dealt with in detail in the later part of this chapter.

17.3.6 Early Detection of Recurrence

The detection of CTC or ctDNA during surveillance of early breast cancer patients after curative therapy can be considered as a biomarker for early detection of recurrence. Garcia-Murillas and colleagues performed mutation tracking using personalized tumor-specific ddPCR assay for 144 early breast cancer patients with 210 trackable mutations [77, 81]. After a median follow-up of 36.3 months, molecular residual disease was detected in 29 patients which was highly prognostic (HR 17.4, 95% CI 6.3–47.8). The median lead time between ctDNA detection and relapse was 10.7 months (95% CI 8.1–19.1 months). These results were consistently demonstrated in all major breast cancer subtypes. Similar results were demonstrated in the interim analysis of the EBLIS study [82]. In this multicenter, prospective cohort study, breast cancer patients completed of adjuvant therapy but considered high risk for relapse were enrolled and obtained of serial plasma samples. Among the 18 patients who relapsed, plasma ctDNA was detected in 89% (16 patients) with a median lead time of 8.9 months (range 14–721 days). The presence of ctDNA in postsurgical plasma samples or follow-up samples was all associated with poorer prognosis (postsurgical, HR 11.8, 95% CI 4.3–32.5; follow-up, HR 35.8, 95% CI 8.0–161.3).

Larger validation studies will be needed to further clarify the validity of ctDNA monitoring in early breast cancer. Also, clinical trials will be needed to determine the clinical utility of liquid biopsies for early detection of molecular recurrence by means of intervening with treatment according to CTC or ctDNA detection.

17.3.7 Real-Time Monitoring of Therapies in Metastatic Breast Cancer

During treatment for metastatic breast cancer, the patient and physician's most significant concern is whether the disease has progressed. Currently, imaging studies are applied to evaluate treatment response, but they are often noninformative or slow to reflect progression. The issue of radiation exposure related to imaging studies is also a hazard. On the other hand, liquid biopsies are noninvasive, feasible for repetitive sampling and respond to treatments instantly. Treatment monitoring is one of the most promising clinical utility of liquid biopsies in advanced cancer patients. However, perceiving progression before change of clinical symptoms may not prolong survival or quality of life, which will be needed to be investigated in future studies with any biomarkers, including liquid biopsies.

As mentioned before, the prognostic value of CTC in metastatic breast cancer is not only related to its count at baseline but also related to CTC count change after initiating a new systemic therapy [13]. Patients who had a high CTC count ($\geq$5 CTC per 7.5 mL, CellSearch®) before treatment initiation and persisted with a high count after initiating a new systemic therapy performed with the worse survival. This poor prognostic outcome presumably reflects resistance to the therapy. This assumption was the rationale of the SWOG 0500 trial, hypothesizing that when patients failed to reduce CTCs to less than five per 7.5 mL by first follow-up after starting a new first-line chemotherapy, an early change to an alternative chemotherapy regimen might benefit patient survival [63]. However, this strategy did not improve overall survival or even progression-free survival. A more effective treatment than standard chemotherapy will be needed for these patients, with consideration of participation in prospective trials of novel therapies.

The on-going CirCe01 trial is another attempt in changing chemotherapy in patients with persistently elevated CTC count after one cycle of chemotherapy [73, 83]. An additional idea is that the CTC test must be repeated at every initiation of a new treatment to show clinical improvement. Metastatic breast cancer patients starting a third line of chemotherapy will be randomized between the standard arm and CTC-arm. In the CTC-arm, CTC count change will be checked after the first cycle of every new therapy. If CTC count decreases to <5/7.5 mL, treatment will be maintained and managed by standard clinical/radiological tools. If CTC count fails to decrease, treatment will be changed and evaluated by CTC count again. The primary outcome is overall survival, with a medico-economic study as a coprimary endpoint. In patients with chemo-resistant tumor, chemotherapy change will be quick and gives support to discontinuation of chemotherapies and start of palliative care, whereas, a subgroup of patients will benefit by finding effective therapy quickly.

The short half-life of cfDNA in circulation can be advantageous for measuring real-time tumor burden in response to therapy. Dawson and colleagues collected serial plasma specimens from 30 metastatic breast cancer patients, to compare radiographic imaging with ctDNA, CA15-3, and CTCs assay [51]. The dynamic change in ctDNA levels correlated well with tumor burden, performing better compared to CA15-3 and CTCs. Treatment response was also detected earliest by the ctDNA level change. This proof-of-principle study demonstrated the possibility of ctDNA as a real-time monitoring biomarker. O'Leary and colleagues underwent a retrospective analysis of samples from the PALOMA-3 trial, analyzing the predictive value of early ctDNA change in metastatic breast cancer [84]. A relative change in PIK3CA ctDNA level from baseline to 15 days of treatment was strongly predictive to sensitivity to palbociclib, a CDK 4/6 inhibitor. This data supports trials testing the hypothesis that a change in treatment strategy based on early ctDNA dynamics may improve outcome, by switching treatment regimen for patients with inadequate ctDNA suppression.

17.3.8 Real-Time Monitoring of Treatment Response in Neoadjuvant Therapy

Neoadjuvant chemotherapy is a standard treatment for patients with locally advanced breast cancer. Recently its application has widened to early breast cancer for tumor downsizing to allow breast-conserving surgery. However, the monitoring of response to neoadjuvant therapy is not easy, with limited accuracy of radiologic studies. A repeated biopsy is also impracticable in clinical practice, not only because of the patient's discomfort but also due to tumor shrinkage. CTC and ctDNAs have a short half-life in the bloodstream, so changes in these levels are expected to be observed earlier than radiologic images. This approach can overcome the problems of current monitoring tools and allows real-time monitoring of tumor burden.

The clinical validity of CTCs for response monitoring in neoadjuvant therapy has not been validated yet. Bidard and colleagues performed a meta-analysis in nonmetastatic breast cancer patients treated by neoadjuvant chemotherapy to assess the clinical validity of CTC detection [72]. In this meta-analysis, a total of 2156 patients from 16 centers and 21 studies were collected. CTC detection ($\geq$1 CTC) before neoadjuvant treatment was related to a slightly lower rate of pathological complete response compared to patients with no CTC (17.4% vs. 24.2%, $p = 0.01$). However, this was not significant after multivariable logistic regression analysis. Also, CTC detection of other cut-offs or time points had no association with pathological complete response.

The correlation between ctDNA level change and response to neoadjuvant therapy was investigated in two studies. Kim and colleagues enrolled 20 breast cancer patients undergoing neoadjuvant chemotherapy [85]. Among them, ctDNA were collected from 15 patients and serial sampling was done at diagnosis, after the 1st cycle of neoadjuvant chemotherapy and before and after surgery. Targeted ultra-deep sequencing of 82 genes was performed of the plasma DNAs. In two patients, ctDNA disappeared after the 1st cycle of neoadjuvant chemotherapy, and both patients achieved a pathologic complete response. Also, the amount of ctDNA correlated with residual cancer volume detected by breast MRI. Riva and colleagues also performed a similar study with triple-negative breast cancer patients [86]. Customized ddPCR assays were used to track TP53 mutations for 46 patients. TP53 mutations were identified in 40 tumor tissues. Only one patient had increased ctDNA level after the first cycle of treatment, and this was the only patient who progressed during neoadjuvant chemotherapy. A slow decrease of ctDNA level during neoadjuvant chemotherapy was also strongly associated with shorter survival. These two studies suggest the possibility of using ctDNA level change as a tool for early response evaluation during neoadjuvant chemotherapy. A prospective study is undergoing to validate this concept, currently enrolling 229 HER2-positive or triple-negative breast cancer patients planning neoadjuvant therapy (NCT02743910) [78]. The results of this study will give us more clues to the role of ctDNA in real-time monitoring of neoadjuvant therapy.

17.3.9 Stratification and Therapeutic Intervention

Blood-based stratification of targeted therapies in clinical intervention trials is one of the most anticipating roles for CTC and ctDNA analysis. Many clinical trials are planned or on-going to prove the clinical utility of blood-based stratification, mainly in metastatic diseases. We discuss some studies based on CTC and ctDNA analysis that will exemplify this issue.

The concept of using CTC enumeration for treatment guidance is used in the STIC CTC METABREAST clinical trial [87]. Baseline CTC count is an independent prognostic marker in metastatic breast cancer and is hypothesized to be a better criterion in choosing treatment regimen in this study. This large phase III trial randomizes 996 hormone receptor-positive metastatic breast cancer patients between the clinician choice and CTC count-driven choice. In the CTC arm, patients with $\geq$5 CTC/7.5 mL will receive chemotherapy whereas patients with a CTC count lower than 5 will undergo endocrine therapy as first line therapy. The primary endpoint is progression-free survival to prove the noninferiority of the CTC arm. The results are anticipated, hoping to demonstrate the clinical utility of baseline CTC count in metastatic breast cancer patients.

CTCs can be exploited to investigate the presence of drug targets as more-comprehensive molecular characterization gets possible. In this regard, clinical trials using HER2 phenotyping of CTCs for treatment stratification is a starting point of liquid biopsy-based therapeutic intervention. In Greece, Georgoulias and colleagues performed a single-center phase II study of 75 women with HER2-negative early breast cancer and detectable CTCs after adjuvant chemotherapy [88]. These women were randomized between six cycles of trastuzumab or observation for a primary endpoint of 3-year DFS. Double staining for HER2+ was performed in 57 patients and 51 (90%) of them had CK+/HER2+ CTCs. The trastuzumab arm had significantly lower CTC count after trastuzumab administration compared to the observation arm along with a significantly reduced risk of relapse. In contrary, the multicentric phase II CirCe T-DM1 study failed in proving the efficacy of T-DM1 in HER2-negative metastatic breast cancer patients with HER2-amplified CTCs [89]. A total of 155 heavily pretreated metastatic breast cancer patients were screened for HER2-amplified CTC. Among them 14 patients had HER2-amplified CTCs and after treatment of T-DM1, only one patient presented with partial response. The DETECT III trial is designed with a similar concept, screening HER2-negative metastatic breast cancer patients for HER2-positive CTCs, to be randomized between standard therapy or standard therapy plus lapatinib [90]. A total of 282 patients are planned to be enrolled for a primary endpoint of PFS. The results are still anticipated.

Assessment of clinical utility of ctDNA analysis for treatment stratification is mainly demonstrated by specific point mutations. In a prospective-retrospective analysis, plasma ESR1 mutations were assessed in baseline plasma samples from the SoFEA and PALOMA3 trial [91]. Multiplex ddPCR assay was used to analyze seven most common ESR1 mutations. The SoFEA trial compared exemestane vs. fulvestrant vs. fulvestrant with anastrozole in a population previously sensitive to aromatase inhibitors, resulting in no significant difference in its primary endpoint of progression-free survival. However, ctDNA analysis demonstrated that patients with plasma ESR1 mutations had improved PFS after taking fulvestrant compared with exemestane (HR 0.52, 95% CI 0.30–0.92), whereas patients with plasma wildtype ESR1 had similar PFS after both treatments. These results provided the first evidence of potential clinical utility of plasma ESR1 mutation analysis in selecting endocrine therapy regimen. Unfortunately, plasma ESR1 mutation analysis did not prove as a predictive factor for CKD4/6 inhibitors in the PALOMA-3 trial dataset. The BOLERO-2 trial dataset was also analyzed for plasma ESR1 mutations, but also failed to prove any stratification role for everolimus [73].

Prospective trials are needed to assess the clinical utility of ctDNA screening for treatment stratification in metastatic breast cancer, which will be demonstrated by the ongoing multiple parallel cohort phase II clinical trial, plasmaMATCH trial from the UK [92, 93]. Patients will be screened for hotspot mutations in ESR1, HER2, AKT1, and PIK3CA, with HER2 copy number assessment using ddPCRctDNA assays. Patients with mutations identified will enter the matching treatment cohort; ESR1—extended dose fulvestrant 500 mg every 2 weeks, HER2—neratinib ± fulvestrant, AKT1—AZD5363 ± fulvestrant. The study will screen over 1000 women, expecting to enter approximately 20% of these patients into treatment cohorts. The trial is aiming to provide proof of principle efficacy for designated targeted therapies using objective response rate as the primary endpoint.

17.3.10 Monitoring of Resistance and Tumor Heterogeneity

The challenge of precision medicine is the eventual emergence of acquired resistance [92]. Under selective pressure of therapy, acquired resistance develops gradually within the population of tumor cells. Tumor subclones that conceal preexisting resistance alterations emerge and dominate the population of the tumor. These resistant subclones may coexist in the same lesion or in distinct metastatic sites [17]. Therefore, a single-lesion tumor biopsy can underestimate the molecular heterogeneity present. However, multiregional and repeated metastatic tumor biopsies are impractical due to its complications and costs. In contrast, analysis of liquid biopsies is a less-invasive tool for the identification of molecular alterations and is also effective as CTCs and ctDNAs are shed from tumor cells throughout the body.

The key in using liquid biopsies to evaluate tumor heterogeneity is to show detection of multiple unique resistance alterations from different metastatic sites in liquid biopsy samples. Murtaza and colleagues presented extensive analysis of multiple tumor samples and plasma samples from one patient during treatment with sequential targeted therapies over a 3-year clinical course [94]. ctDNA analysis from plasma samples reflected the size and activity of distinct tumor subclones. For example, during lapatinib treatment, a rapid increase in several mutations exclusive to the chest mass was observed in plasma samples, coinciding with disease progression seen on imaging at this site. ctDNA analysis also identified an actionable hotspot mutation in PIK3CA, that was not detected in tumor biopsies, but was detected with an allele frequency of 3.5% at the time of progression on trastuzumab and tamoxifen. After lapatinib treatment started, the plasma levels dropped to 1.1% and then became undetectable.

Tumor heterogeneity limits treatment response rates, especially after tumor progression or relapse. Exposure to targeted therapy can lead to selection of a specific molecular phenotype that may be the molecular target of other drugs. Detection of this selective pressure of therapy can lead to the choice of sequential target drugs. In principle, tracking the emergence of resistance-associated genetic aberrations could be applied to provide the early initiation of alternate therapies before progression or relapse is detected by clinical or radiological examination [79].

The results from Murtaza et al study is from a single patient and needs confirmation in a larger cohort of patients with multiregional biopsies and serial plasma samples. Molecular treatment stratification and tracking of resistant clones in patients treated with targeted therapies may inform the choice of targeted treatments for individual patients. Integration of real-time ctDNA analysis into clinical trials and eventually into standard clinical management heralds a new era for precision cancer medicine.

17.4 Future Research Direction

Liquid biopsies are promising tools for precision cancer medicine. However, to date most studies are proof of concept studies and it is still a matter of speculation to what extent liquid biopsies will replace tumor biopsies in the future. More solid clinical data are needed for liquid biopsies to change clinical practice. There are many limitations to overcome and these will be the direction of future researches.

The major limitation for further clinical application of CTC assays is the low detection rate in current detection technologies. The only FDA-approved test for CTC assessment is the CellSearch® system which has been proven of its prognostic value in breast cancer. However, the detection rate of CTCs using CellSearch® in stage I–III early breast cancer is only 20% [71]. Novel CTC detection methods are being developed to enrich and detect CTC more efficiently presenting with detection rate 100-fold higher compared to previous methods [95]. However, further methods have not been approved for routine clinical use because of the limited benefit of CTCs in treatment-decision making. This reflects the methodological problems related to the nature of CTCs, especially their heterogeneity and diverse metastatic potential, leading to limited clinical significance. Development of novel technology and extended validation would be needed to overcome this barrier.

Recently, CTC research shows a trend of shifting from CTC enumeration to a more detailed molecular and functional characterization of single CTCs [28, 95]. Only a limited number of CTCs are captured in most CTC assays and it is important to expand the isolated CTCs in order to perform subsequent functional analyses. After isolating proliferative and viable CTCs, in vivo models can be used to investigate the functions of these cells. The use of patient-derived CTCs for an ex vivo functional study of chemotherapeutic efficacy monitoring is an appealing approach for immediate treatment decision regarding drug resistance. Current technology on CTCs does not differentiate between apoptotic and viable CTCs. An emerging approach to identify viable cells is detecting protein secreted, released or shed by functional single epithelial cancer cells [96]. RNA extraction from CTCs ispossible and high throughput technology, such as NGS, has made it possible to analyze whole genomes and transcriptomes of individual CTCs [97].

One of the major concerns in ctDNA assays is the lack of standardization of techniques [7, 79]. This lack of standardization extends to each step in the process starting from preanalytical variability; which material will be used (plasma versus serum), what collecting tube to use, what optimal time period between blood draws and processing is needed. Techniques used for the quantification of tumor-associated genetic mutations, for example, ddPCR, NGS, BEAMing, must be defined also.

Analytical variabilities will include intrinsic PCR errors and technological errors related to NGS platforms. Spatial and temporal tumor heterogeneity is needed to be taken into account as biological variabilities. Another obstacle is the fact that it is challenging to determine the clinical sensitivities of ctDNA assays owing to variability among clinical studies. The tumor stages and types assessed, the sample-processing techniques and targeted molecular alterations differ across different studies. Improving assay sensitivity is also important as rare molecular alterations must be detected to anticipate drug resistance.

Interpretation of clinical studies are also hindered owing to the fact that the dynamic biology of CTC and ctDNA release is poorly understood [23]. ctDNA mainly represents the genome of dying cells, but cancer progression and therapy resistance are driven by viable tumor cells. Thus, the time point of blood sampling during the course of treatment will be important in discovering genetic alterations from resistant tumor cell clones. Moreover, it is unclear whether all tumor subclones contribute proportionally to ctDNA or CTC pools, or whether biological factors, such as tumor vascularity or metabolic activity, influence their representations in the bloodstream. Studies about the origin, biology, and dynamics of CTCs and ctDNAs are important as clinical trials aim to interpret liquid biopsy assays in response to clinical treatment.

The integration of liquid biopsy assays into clinical practice will only be possible when the clinical utility is demonstrated in interventional clinical trials. Randomized clinical intervention studies in which therapy decisions are based on liquid biopsy analysis, investigating the effect on survival outcome are needed. Currently there are no liquid biopsy assays that have proven clinical utility in breast cancer. Only in nonsmall cell lung cancer has liquid biopsy entered into clinical practice. The European Medicine Agency (EMA) and US FDA have approved diagnostic kits that detect EGFR mutations in plasma ctDNA for blood-based companion diagnostics of erlotinib, an EGFR inhibitor. The detection rate of EGFR mutations from plasma ctDNA had comparable accuracy to Sanger sequencing of DNA from tumor tissue specimens, established from large clinical trials [98, 99].

Liquid biopsies have great potential to be applied in oncology clinical practice. Proof-of-concept studies show that liquid biopsies are promising research tools for drug development, and for the study of tumor heterogeneity and clonal evolution. Despite the extremely high level of current enthusiasm, there is still little evidence of clinical validity and clinical utility to deploy liquid biopsies in routine clinical practice. Clear understanding of the biological limitations of CTC and ctDNA assays is needed and robust research is needed to enable development of clinical practice recommendations. Over time, it is likely that evidence will emerge to better assess the clinical validity and utility of liquid biopsies and eventually achieve widespread use of CTC and ctDNA assays in routine clinical practice.

17.5 Summary

1. The bench
   More research about the origin, biology, and dynamics of CTCs and ctDNAs is needed to understand them and apply liquid biopsies in the clinic.
2. Translation
   Recent technological advances have enabled the detection and detailed characterization of CTCs and ctDNAs, but many hurdles are left to be cleared.
3. The bedside
   Current clinical studies are only proof-of-concept studies and there is still little evidence of clinical validity and utility to apply liquid biopsies in clinical practice. Comprehensive clinical trials are needed.

References

1. Gerlinger M, Rowan AJ, Horswell S, Math M, Larkin J, Endesfelder D, et al. Intratumor heterogeneity and branched evolution revealed by multiregion sequencing. N Engl J Med. 2012;366(10):883–92.
2. Shah SP, Roth A, Goya R, Oloumi A, Ha G, Zhao Y, et al. The clonal and mutational evolution spectrum of primary triple-negative breast cancers. Nature. 2012;486(7403):395–9.
3. Merker JD, Oxnard GR, Compton C, Diehn M, Hurley P, Lazar AJ, et al. Circulating tumor DNA analysis in patients with cancer: American Society of Clinical Oncology and College of American Pathologists Joint Review. J Clin Oncol. 2018;36(16):1631–41.
4. Wang J, Chang S, Li G, Sun Y. Application of liquid biopsy in precision medicine: opportunities and challenges. Front Med. 2017;11(4):522–7.
5. Arneth B. Update on the types and usage of liquid biopsies in the clinical setting: a systematic review. BMC Cancer. 2018;18(1):527.
6. Eigeliene N, Saarenheimo J, Jekunen A. Potential of liquid biopsies for breast cancer screening, diagnosis, and response to treatment. Oncology. 2019;96(3):115–24.
7. Siravegna G, Marsoni S, Siena S, Bardelli A. Integrating liquid biopsies into the management of cancer. Nat Rev Clin Oncol. 2017;14(9):531–48.
8. Mader S, Pantel K. Liquid biopsy: current status and future perspectives. Oncol Res Treat. 2017;40(7-8):404–8.
9. Ashworth TR. A case of cancer in which cells similar to those in the tumours were seen in the blood after death. Aust Med J. 1869;14:146.
10. Engell HC. Cancer cells in the circulating blood; a clinical study on the occurrence of cancer cells in the peripheral blood and in venous blood draining the tumour area at operation. Acta Chir Scand Suppl. 1955;201:1–70.
11. Seronie-Vivien S, Mery E, Delord JP, Fillola G, Tkaczuk J, Voigt JJ, et al. Carcinocythemia as the single extension of breast cancer: report of a case and review of the literature. Ann Oncol. 2001;12(7):1019–22.
12. Myerowitz RL, Edwards PA, Sartiano GP. Carcinocythemia (carcinoma cell leukemia) due to metastatic carcinoma of the breast: report of a case. Cancer. 1977;40(6):3107–11.
13. Cristofanilli M, Budd GT, Ellis MJ, Stopeck A, Matera J, Miller MC, et al. Circulating tumor cells, disease progression, and survival in metastatic breast cancer. N Engl J Med. 2004;351(8):781–91.
14. Mandel P, Metais P. Les acides nucléiques du plasma sanguin chez l'Homme. Comp Rendus Seances Soc Biol Filiales. 1948;142(3-4):241–3.

15. Dennin RH. DNA of free and complexed origin in human plasma: concentration and length distribution. Klin Wochenschr. 1979;57(9):451–6.
16. Fournie GJ, Gayral-Taminh M, Bouche JP, Conte JJ. Recovery of nanogram quantities of DNA from plasma and quantitative measurement using labeling by nick translation. Anal Biochem. 1986;158(2):250–6.
17. Corcoran RB, Chabner BA. Application of cell-free DNA analysis to cancer treatment. N Engl J Med. 2018;379(18):1754–65.
18. Leon SA, Shapiro B, Sklaroff DM, Yaros MJ. Free DNA in the serum of cancer patients and the effect of therapy. Cancer Res. 1977;37(3):646–50.
19. Stroun M, Anker P, Maurice P, Lyautey J, Lederrey C, Beljanski M. Neoplastic characteristics of the DNA found in the plasma of cancer patients. Oncology. 1989;46(5):318–22.
20. Wan JCM, Massie C, Garcia-Corbacho J, Mouliere F, Brenton JD, Caldas C, et al. Liquid biopsies come of age: towards implementation of circulating tumour DNA. Nat Rev Cancer. 2017;17(4):223–38.
21. Sorenson GD, Pribish DM, Valone FH, Memoli VA, Bzik DJ, Yao SL. Soluble normal and mutated DNA sequences from single-copy genes in human blood. Cancer Epidemiol Biomark Prev. 1994;3(1):67–71.
22. Pantel K, Speicher MR. The biology of circulating tumor cells. Oncogene. 2015;35:1216.
23. Alix-Panabieres C, Pantel K. Clinical applications of circulating tumor cells and circulating tumor DNA as liquid biopsy. Cancer Discov. 2016;6(5):479–91.
24. Allard WJ, Matera J, Miller MC, Repollet M, Connelly MC, Rao C, et al. Tumor cells circulate in the peripheral blood of all major carcinomas but not in healthy subjects or patients with nonmalignant diseases. Clin Cancer Res. 2004;10(20):6897–904.
25. Meng S, Tripathy D, Frenkel EP, Shete S, Naftalis EZ, Huth JF, et al. Circulating tumor cells in patients with breast cancer dormancy. Clin Cancer Res. 2004;10(24):8152–62.
26. Méhes G, Witt A, Kubista E, Ambros PF. Circulating breast cancer cells are frequently apoptotic. Am J Pathol. 2001;159(1):17–20.
27. Powell AA, Talasaz AH, Zhang H, Coram MA, Reddy A, Deng G, et al. Single cell profiling of circulating tumor cells: transcriptional heterogeneity and diversity from breast cancer cell lines. PLoS One. 2012;7(5):e33788.
28. Kowalik A, Kowalewska M, Gozdz S. Current approaches for avoiding the limitations of circulating tumor cells detection methods-implications for diagnosis and treatment of patients with solid tumors. Transl Res. 2017;185:58–84.
29. Ignatiadis M, Lee M, Jeffrey SS. Circulating tumor cells and circulating tumor DNA: challenges and opportunities on the path to clinical utility. Clin Cancer Res. 2015;21(21):4786–800.
30. Yap TA, Lorente D, Omlin A, Olmos D, de Bono JS. Circulating tumor cells: a multifunctional biomarker. Clin Cancer Res. 2014;20(10):2553–68.
31. Krebs MG, Metcalf RL, Carter L, Brady G, Blackhall FH, Dive C. Molecular analysis of circulating tumour cells-biology and biomarkers. Nat Rev Clin Oncol. 2014;11(3):129–44.
32. Arya SK, Lim B, Rahman ARA. Enrichment, detection and clinical significance of circulating tumor cells. Lab Chip. 2013;13(11):1995–2027.
33. Alix-Panabieres C, Pantel K. Challenges in circulating tumour cell research. Nat Rev Cancer. 2014;14(9):623–31.
34. Jahr S, Hentze H, Englisch S, Hardt D, Fackelmayer FO, Hesch RD, et al. DNA fragments in the blood plasma of cancer patients: quantitations and evidence for their origin from apoptotic and necrotic cells. Cancer Res. 2001;61(4):1659–65.
35. Stroun M, Lyautey J, Lederrey C, Olson-Sand A, Anker P. About the possible origin and mechanism of circulating DNA apoptosis and active DNA release. Clin Chim Acta. 2001;313 (1-2):139–42.
36. Anker P, Stroun M, Maurice PA. Spontaneous release of DNA by human blood lymphocytes as shown in an in vitro system. Cancer Res. 1975;35(9):2375–82.
37. Lo YM, Zhang J, Leung TN, Lau TK, Chang AM, Hjelm NM. Rapid clearance of fetal DNA from maternal plasma. Am J Hum Genet. 1999;64(1):218–24.

38. Yao W, Mei C, Nan X, Hui L. Evaluation and comparison of in vitro degradation kinetics of DNA in serum, urine and saliva: a qualitative study. Gene. 2016;590(1):142–8.
39. Pisetsky DS, Fairhurst AM. The origin of extracellular DNA during the clearance of dead and dying cells. Autoimmunity. 2007;40(4):281–4.
40. Bettegowda C, Sausen M, Leary RJ, Kinde I, Wang Y, Agrawal N, et al. Detection of circulating tumor DNA in early- and late-stage human malignancies. Sci Transl Med. 2014;6 (224):224ra24.
41. El Messaoudi S, Rolet F, Mouliere F, Thierry AR. Circulating cell free DNA: preanalytical considerations. Clin Chim Acta. 2013;424:222–30.
42. Swinkels DW, Wiegerinck E, Steegers EA, de Kok JB. Effects of blood-processing protocols on cell-free DNA quantification in plasma. Clin Chem. 2003;49(3):525–6.
43. Alidousty C, Brandes D, Heydt C, Wagener S, Wittersheim M, Schafer SC, et al. Comparison of blood collection tubes from three different manufacturers for the collection of cell-free DNA for liquid biopsy mutation testing. J Mol Diagn. 2017;19(5):801–4.
44. Heitzer E, Ulz P, Geigl JB. Circulating tumor DNA as a liquid biopsy for cancer. Clin Chem. 2015;61(1):112–23.
45. Hindson BJ, Ness KD, Masquelier DA, Belgrader P, Heredia NJ, Makarewicz AJ, et al. High-throughput droplet digital PCR system for absolute quantitation of DNA copy number. Anal Chem. 2011;83(22):8604–10.
46. Diehl F, Li M, He Y, Kinzler KW, Vogelstein B, Dressman D. BEAMing: single-molecule PCR on microparticles in water-in-oil emulsions. Nat Methods. 2006;3(7):551–9.
47. Adalsteinsson VA, Ha G, Freeman SS, Choudhury AD, Stover DG, Parsons HA, et al. Scalable whole-exome sequencing of cell-free DNA reveals high concordance with metastatic tumors. Nat Commun. 2017;8(1):1324.
48. Murtaza M, Dawson SJ, Tsui DW, Gale D, Forshew T, Piskorz AM, et al. Non-invasive analysis of acquired resistance to cancer therapy by sequencing of plasma DNA. Nature. 2013;497(7447):108–12.
49. Newman AM, Lovejoy AF, Klass DM, Kurtz DM, Chabon JJ, Scherer F, et al. Integrated digital error suppression for improved detection of circulating tumor DNA. Nat Biotechnol. 2016;34 (5):547–55.
50. Kinde I, Wu J, Papadopoulos N, Kinzler KW, Vogelstein B. Detection and quantification of rare mutations with massively parallel sequencing. Proc Natl Acad Sci U S A. 2011;108 (23):9530–5.
51. Dawson SJ, Tsui DW, Murtaza M, Biggs H, Rueda OM, Chin SF, et al. Analysis of circulating tumor DNA to monitor metastatic breast cancer. N Engl J Med. 2013;368(13):1199–209.
52. Haber DA, Velculescu VE. Blood-based analyses of cancer: circulating tumor cells and circulating tumor DNA. Cancer Discov. 2014;4(6):650–61.
53. Kidess E, Jeffrey SS. Circulating tumor cells versus tumor-derived cell-free DNA: rivals or partners in cancer care in the era of single-cell analysis? Genome Med. 2013;5(8):70.
54. Maltoni R, Gallerani G, Fici P, Rocca A, Fabbri F. CTCs in early breast cancer: a path worth taking. Cancer Lett. 2016;376(2):205–10.
55. Lucci A, Hall CS, Lodhi AK, Bhattacharyya A, Anderson AE, Xiao L, et al. Circulating tumour cells in non-metastatic breast cancer: a prospective study. Lancet Oncol. 2012;13(7):688–95.
56. Schindlbeck C, Andergassen U, Hofmann S, Juckstock J, Jeschke U, Sommer H, et al. Comparison of circulating tumor cells (CTC) in peripheral blood and disseminated tumor cells in the bone marrow (DTC-BM) of breast cancer patients. J Cancer Res Clin Oncol. 2013;139(6):1055–62.
57. Bidard FC, Mathiot C, Delaloge S, Brain E, Giachetti S, de Cremoux P, et al. Single circulating tumor cell detection and overall survival in nonmetastatic breast cancer. Ann Oncol. 2010;21 (4):729–33.
58. Beaver JA, Jelovac D, Balukrishna S, Cochran RL, Croessmann S, Zabransky DJ, et al. Detection of cancer DNA in plasma of patients with early-stage breast cancer. Clin Cancer Res. 2014;20(10):2643–50.

59. Phallen J, Sausen M, Adleff V, Leal A, Hruban C, White J, et al. Direct detection of early-stage cancers using circulating tumor DNA. Sci Transl Med. 2017;9:403.
60. Circulating tumor DNA and follow-up of BRCA1 mutation carriers (CirCa 01). Available from https://ClinicalTrials.gov/show/NCT02608346.
61. Kim S-T, Raymond VM, Park JO, Zotenko E, Park YS, Schultz M, et al. Combined genomic and epigenomic assessment of cell-free circulating tumor DNA (ctDNA) improves assay sensitivity in early-stage colorectal cancer (CRC). Cancer Res. 2019;79(13):916.
62. Hayes DF, Cristofanilli M, Budd GT, Ellis MJ, Stopeck A, Miller MC, et al. Circulating tumor cells at each follow-up time point during therapy of metastatic breast cancer patients predict progression-free and overall survival. Clin Cancer Res. 2006;12(14 Pt 1):4218–24.
63. Smerage JB, Barlow WE, Hortobagyi GN, Winer EP, Leyland-Jones B, Srkalovic G, et al. Circulating tumor cells and response to chemotherapy in metastatic breast cancer: SWOG S0500. J Clin Oncol. 2014;32(31):3483–9.
64. Pierga JY, Hajage D, Bachelot T, Delaloge S, Brain E, Campone M, et al. High independent prognostic and predictive value of circulating tumor cells compared with serum tumor markers in a large prospective trial in first-line chemotherapy for metastatic breast cancer patients. Ann Oncol. 2012;23(3):618–24.
65. Wallwiener M, Hartkopf AD, Baccelli I, Riethdorf S, Schott S, Pantel K, et al. The prognostic impact of circulating tumor cells in subtypes of metastatic breast cancer. Breast Cancer Res Treat. 2013;137(2):503–10.
66. Bidard FC, Peeters DJ, Fehm T, Nole F, Gisbert-Criado R, Mavroudis D, et al. Clinical validity of circulating tumour cells in patients with metastatic breast cancer: a pooled analysis of individual patient data. Lancet Oncol. 2014;15(4):406–14.
67. Franken B, de Groot MR, Mastboom WJ, Vermes I, van der Palen J, Tibbe AG, et al. Circulating tumor cells, disease recurrence and survival in newly diagnosed breast cancer. Breast Cancer Res. 2012;14(5):R133.
68. Ignatiadis M, Kallergi G, Ntoulia M, Perraki M, Apostolaki S, Kafousi M, et al. Prognostic value of the molecular detection of circulating tumor cells using a multimarker reverse transcription-PCR assay for cytokeratin 19, mammaglobin A, and HER2 in early breast cancer. Clin Cancer Res. 2008;14(9):2593–600.
69. Pierga JY, Bidard FC, Mathiot C, Brain E, Delaloge S, Giachetti S, et al. Circulating tumor cell detection predicts early metastatic relapse after neoadjuvant chemotherapy in large operable and locally advanced breast cancer in a phase II randomized trial. Clin Cancer Res. 2008;14 (21):7004–10.
70. Rack B, Schindlbeck C, Juckstock J, Andergassen U, Hepp P, Zwingers T, et al. Circulating tumor cells predict survival in early average-to-high risk breast cancer patients. J Natl Cancer Inst. 2014;106:5.
71. Janni WJ, Rack B, Terstappen LW, Pierga JY, Taran FA, Fehm T, et al. Pooled analysis of the prognostic relevance of circulating tumor cells in primary breast cancer. Clin Cancer Res. 2016;22(10):2583–93.
72. Bidard FC, Michiels S, Riethdorf S, Mueller V, Esserman LJ, Lucci A, et al. Circulating tumor cells in breast cancer patients treated by neoadjuvant chemotherapy: a meta-analysis. J Natl Cancer Inst. 2018;110(6):560–7.
73. Chandarlapaty S, Chen D, He W, Sung P, Samoila A, You D, et al. Prevalence of ESR1 MUTATIONS in cell-free DNA and outcomes in metastatic breast cancer: a secondary analysis of the BOLERO-2 clinical trial. JAMA Oncol. 2016;2(10):1310–5.
74. Stover DG, Parsons HA, Ha G, Freeman SS, Barry WT, Guo H, et al. Association of cell-free DNA tumor fraction and somatic copy number alterations with survival in metastatic triple-negative breast cancer. J Clin Oncol. 2018;36(6):543–53.
75. Garcia JM, Garcia V, Silva J, Pena C, Dominguez G, Sanchez A, et al. Extracellular tumor DNA in plasma and overall survival in breast cancer patients. Genes Chromosomes Cancer. 2006;45 (7):692–701.

76. Oshiro C, Kagara N, Naoi Y, Shimoda M, Shimomura A, Maruyama N, et al. PIK3CA mutations in serum DNA are predictive of recurrence in primary breast cancer patients. Breast Cancer Res Treat. 2015;150(2):299–307.
77. Garcia-Murillas I, Chopra N, Comino-Mendez I, Beaney M, Tovey H, Cutts RJ, et al. Assessment of molecular relapse detection in early-stage breast cancer. JAMA Oncol. 2019;5 (10):1473–8.
78. Monitoring plasma tumor DNA in early-stage breast cancer.
79. Crowley E, Di Nicolantonio F, Loupakis F, Bardelli A. Liquid biopsy: monitoring cancer-genetics in the blood. Nat Rev Clin Oncol. 2013;10(8):472–84.
80. Ignatiadis M, Rack B, Rothe F, Riethdorf S, Decraene C, Bonnefoi H, et al. Liquid biopsy-based clinical research in early breast cancer: the EORTC 90091-10093 Treat CTC trial. Eur J Cancer. 2016;63:97–104.
81. Garcia-Murillas I, Schiavon G, Weigelt B, Ng C, Hrebien S, Cutts RJ, et al. Mutation tracking in circulating tumor DNA predicts relapse in early breast cancer. Sci Transl Med. 2015;7 (302):302ra133.
82. Coombes RC, Page K, Salari R, Hastings RK, Armstrong A, Ahmed S, et al. Personalized detection of circulating tumor DNA antedates breast cancer metastatic recurrence. Clin Cancer Res. 2019;25(14):4255–63.
83. Bidard F-C, Fehm T, Ignatiadis M, Smerage JB, Alix-Panabières C, Janni W, et al. Clinical application of circulating tumor cells in breast cancer: overview of the current interventional trials. Cancer Metastasis Rev. 2013;32(1-2):179–88.
84. O'Leary B, Hrebien S, Morden JP, Beaney M, Fribbens C, Huang X, et al. Early circulating tumor DNA dynamics and clonal selection with palbociclib and fulvestrant for breast cancer. Nat Commun. 2018;9(1):896.
85. Kim JY, Park D, Son DS, Nam SJ, Kim SW, Jung HH, et al. Circulating tumor DNA shows variable clonal response of breast cancer during neoadjuvant chemotherapy. Oncotarget. 2017;8 (49):86423–34.
86. Riva F, Bidard FC, Houy A, Saliou A, Madic J, Rampanou A, et al. Patient-specific circulating tumor DNA detection during neoadjuvant chemotherapy in triple-negative breast cancer. Clin Chem. 2017;63(3):691–9.
87. Pierga J-Y, Baffert S, Hajage D, Brain E, Armanet S, Simondi C, et al. Abstract 2410: circulating tumor cells to guide the choice between chemotherapy and hormone therapy as first line treatment for metastatic breast cancer patients: the STIC CTC METABREAST trial. Cancer Res. 2013;73(8):2410.
88. Georgoulias V, Bozionelou V, Agelaki S, Perraki M, Apostolaki S, Kallergi G, et al. Trastuzumab decreases the incidence of clinical relapses in patients with early breast cancer presenting chemotherapy-resistant CK-19mRNA-positive circulating tumor cells: results of a randomized phase II study. Ann Oncol. 2012;23(7):1744–50.
89. Berger F, Bidard F-C, Pierga J-Y, Sablin MP, Cottu P, Neffati S, et al. 117PAnti-HER2 therapy efficacy in HER2-negative metastatic breast cancer with HER2-amplified circulating tumor cells: results of the CirCe T-DM1 trial. Ann Oncol. 2017;28:5.
90. Polasik A, Schramm A, Friedl T, Rack B, Trapp E, Fasching P, et al. Abstract OT3-04-02: DETECT III and IV – individualized CTC-based therapy of metastatic breast cancer. Cancer Res. 2017;77(4):4.
91. Fribbens C, O'Leary B, Kilburn L, Hrebien S, Garcia-Murillas I, Beaney M, et al. Plasma ESR1 mutations and the treatment of estrogen receptor-positive advanced breast cancer. J Clin Oncol. 2016;34(25):2961–8.
92. Garraway LA, Janne PA. Circumventing cancer drug resistance in the era of personalized medicine. Cancer Discov. 2012;2(3):214–26.
93. Turner N, Bye H, Kernaghan S, Proszek P, Fribbens C, Moretti L, et al. The plasmaMATCH trial: A multiple parallel cohort, open-label, multi-centre phase II clinical trial of ctDNA screening to direct targeted therapies in patients with advanced breast cancer (CRUK/15/010). Cancer Res. 2018;78(4):6.

94. Murtaza M, Dawson SJ, Pogrebniak K, Rueda OM, Provenzano E, Grant J, et al. Multifocal clonal evolution characterized using circulating tumour DNA in a case of metastatic breast cancer. Nat Commun. 2015;6:8760.
95. Hong B, Zu Y. Detecting circulating tumor cells: current challenges and new trends. Theranostics. 2013;3(6):377–94.
96. Soler A, Cayrefourcq L, Mazel M, Alix-Panabieres C. EpCAM-independent enrichment and detection of viable circulating tumor cells using the EPISPOT assay. Methods Mol Biol. 1634;2017:263–76.
97. Shaw JA, Guttery DS, Hills A, Fernandez-Garcia D, Page K, Rosales BM, et al. Mutation analysis of cell-free DNA and single circulating tumor cells in metastatic breast cancer patients with high circulating tumor cell counts. Clin Cancer Res. 2017;23(1):88–96.
98. Mok T, Wu YL, Lee JS, Yu CJ, Sriuranpong V, Sandoval-Tan J, et al. Detection and dynamic changes of EGFR mutations from circulating tumor DNA as a predictor of survival outcomes in NSCLC patients treated with first-line intercalated erlotinib and chemotherapy. Clin Cancer Res. 2015;21(14):3196–203.
99. Karachaliou N, Mayo-Casas C, Queralt C, de Aguirre I, Melloni B, Cardenal F, et al. Association of EGFR L858R mutation in circulating free DNA with survival in the EURTAC trial. JAMA Oncol. 2015;1(2):149–57.

Chapter 18
Current Biomarkers for Precision Medicine in Breast Cancer

Soo kyung Ahn and So-Youn Jung

Abstract Breast cancer has become the prototypical solid tumor where targets have been identified within the tumor allowing for personalized approach for systemic therapy. Biomarkers are beginning to play an important role in preparing the way for precision treatment. Mandatory biomarkers for every newly diagnosed case of breast cancer are estrogen receptors and progesterone receptors in selecting patients for endocrine treatment and HER2 for identifying patients likely to benefit from antiHER2 therapy. Although methodological problems exist in the determination of Ki67, because of its clearly established clinical value, wide availability, and low costs relative to the available multianalyte signatures, Ki67 may be used for determining prognosis, especially if values are low or high. Also, the androgen receptor (AR) pathway is emerging as a potential therapeutic target in breast cancer. AR-targeted treatments for breast cancer are in development and have shown promising preliminary results. While, most established biomarkers in breast cancer require tissue samples, serum tumor markers are easily accessible and require a less invasive procedure. Among them, tissue polypeptide-specific antigen (TPS), a specific epitope structure of a peptide in serum associated with human cytokeratin 18, is linked to the proliferative activity of tumors. TPS may be a valuable and independent prognostic biomarker for breast cancer.

In order to accelerate progress towards precision treatment for women with breast cancer, we need additional predictive biomarker, especially for enhancing the positive predictive value for endocrine and antiHER2 therapies, as well as biomarkers for predicting response to specific forms of chemotherapy.

S. k. Ahn (✉)
Breast and Thyroid Center, Department of Surgery, Kangnam Sacred Heart Hospital, Hallym University, Seoul, South Korea

S.-Y. Jung
Center for Breast Cancer, National Cancer Center, Goyang-si, South Korea
e-mail: goje1@ncc.re.kr

D.-Y. Noh et al. (eds.), *Translational Research in Breast Cancer*, Advances in Experimental Medicine and Biology 1187,
https://doi.org/10.1007/978-981-32-9620-6_18

Keywords Breast cancer · Biomarker · Estrogen receptor · Progesteron receptor · Human epidermal growth factor receptor 2 · Ki-67 · Androgen receptor · Tissue polypeptide-specific antigen

18.1 Introduction

Following a diagnosis of breast cancer, the most immediate challenges in patient management are the determination of prognosis and identification of the most appropriate adjuvant therapy. While, prognostic biomarker predicts the risk of disease recurrence, predictive biomarker helps identify upfront those patients that are likely to respond or be resistant to specific therapies.

Traditionally, determining patient outcome was based on a series of histopathological and clinical criteria such as the number of lymph node metastasis, tumor size, and tumor grade. Although these factors all supply independent prognostic information in newly diagnosed breast cancer, it is widely accepted that these factors alone are inadequate for optimum management, especially as we move towards the era of precision treatment.

Consequently, in recent years, an enormous amount of research has been devoted to the discovery and validation of molecular biomarkers for breast cancer. This aim of article is to discuss mandatory biomarkers for breast cancer which are used in current clinics.

18.2 Estrogen and Progesterone Receptor (ER and PR)

In the early 1970s, Jensen and coworkers [1] discovered the presence of ER in extracts of primary breast cancers and showed that over half of the women expressing ER in their tumor responded to the then available forms of hormone therapy (i.e., ovariectomy, adrenalectomy, hypophysectomy), while patients lacking the receptor generally failed to benefit. This study was one of the first to show the importance of a biomarker in guiding cancer treatment and the first opening of the door for application of precision treatment to patients with breast cancer.

Estrogens are believed to stimulate breast cancer cell growth by associating with regulatory elements in the genome, thereby enhancing the transcription of genes such as MYC and cyclin D (CCND1) [2]. Since estrogens stimulate tumor growth via binding to and activating ER, it was hypothesized that ER status might be used as a predictor of response to endocrine therapy in advanced breast cancer. Meta-analysis showed that 50–60% of ER-positive patients underwent objective response to first-line hormonal therapy; in contrast, only 5–10% of ER-negative tumors responded [3].

The current main use of ER is in identifying patients with early breast cancer for adjuvant treatment with drugs such as selective estrogen receptor modulators (tamoxifen), aromatase inhibitors (AI) (anastrozole, letrozole, or exemestane), LH-RH agonists (leuprolide, goserelin), pure selective estrogen downregulators (SERDS) (fulvestrant), and oophorectomy. All these therapy ultimately targets ER, preventing it from stimulating breast cancer proliferation. Since they act via different mechanisms, resistant to a specific drug does not necessarily result in resistance to related compounds [2]. Thus, different classes of endocrine therapy may be used sequentially for treatment of ER-positive breast cancers. In an overview analysis of randomized trials, administration of adjuvant tamoxifen to ER-positive patients with early breast cancer for about five years reduced recurrence rate by almost 50% [4]. In contrast to ER-positive patients, those with absent or low levels of ER failed to benefit from receiving tamoxifen.

Moreover, the receptor status of metastasis may be more predictive of response. It does not always correlate with that of the primary tumor with approximately 20-30% conversion rate from ER-positive to ER-negative and much less frequently from ER-negative to ER-positive at relapse [5]. Although 74% of patients with ER-positive primary tumors whose recurrent tumors retained ER expression responded to endocrine therapy, only 12% of patients with ER-positive primaries and ER-negative metastases responded. Loss of ER significantly associated with shorter median survival.

Although, ER is routinely used as predictive factor, it can also be used as prognostic biomarker. Women with ER-positive tumors not receiving systemic therapy after surgery have rates of recurrence at 5 years, which area 5–10% lower than in those with ER- negative tumors. However, ER may be a time-dependent variable, and studies with longer follow-up suggest that, with time, different rates of relapse and death significantly diminish and eventually disappear [6]. It is possible therefore that ER status is associated with indolent, slowing growing tumors and less metastatic potential. PR as a prognostic factor in the absence of endocrine therapy is still an area of debate.

Progesterone receptors are normally measured alongside ER. It has been regarded as an indicator of an intact ER signaling axis. Some large nonrandomized studies suggest that the detection of PR, in addition to ER, increases the endocrine therapy predictive impact [7, 8] but evidence from the overview analyses of randomized studies failed to find an independent predictive value [9].

Expert panels therefore recommend measurement of both ER and PR in all newly diagnosed cases of breast cancer [10, 11]. Furthermore, most also recommend measurement of these receptors in recurrent/metastatic lesions when feasible.

18.3 Human Epidermal Growth Factor Receptor 2 (HER2)

The second most commonly described target in breast caner is the HER2 protein. Measurement of HER2 is now mandatory on all new cases of invasive breast cancer and when feasible, also an recurrent/metastatic lesions. HER2 is a member of the human epidermal growth factor family of receptors. The family consists of four transmembrane proteins (HER 1–4) each of which has different properties. Overexpression of HER2 drives tumor growth by constitutive activating the MAPK and PI3K/AKT signaling pathways, which in turn enhances cell proliferation, invasion, and metastasis [12].

There are two common methods used to test for the HER2 status of a breast cancer cell. Immunohistochemistry (IHC) is used to measured as 0, 1+, 2+, or 3+, depending on the percentage of cells staining. IHC 3+ usually corresponds to gene amplification, whereas 0 or 1+ rarely does. Tumors with 2+ expression are usually tested by fluorescent in situ hybridization. Alternatively, the tumor cells can be tested by the fluorescent in situ hybridization method, which directly stains both the HER2 gene and the centromeres on chromosome 17. The HER2 ratio is the expression of the HER2 gene copies/chromosome 17 centromere copies. A ratio $\geq$2.0 is considered amplified.

HER2 gene is amplified or overexpressed in only 15–20% of invasive breast cancer. In Overexpression/amplification of HER2 is a prognostic marker of poor outcome in the absence of adjuvant treatment and an important predictive marker of responsiveness to certain treatments. The HER2 alteration has been associated with an increased rate of metastasis, decreased time to recurrence, and decreased overall survival [13–15]. HER2 is a prognostic marker independent of nodal status, tumor size, grade, and hormone receptor status [16].

Although HER2 was originally proposed as a prognostic biomarker for breast, its current utility is mainly for predicting response to antiHER2 therapy in the neoadjuvant, adjuvant, and advanced disease setting. Currently, four forms of antiHER2 therapy are approved; humanized antibodies directed against the extracellular domain of the HER2 memebrane protein (trastuzumab, pertuzumab, and trastuzumab emtansine) and dual tyrosine kinase inhibitor of EGFR and HER2 (lapatinib). HER2gene overexpression/amplification appears to be necessary for response to all these treatments. Thus, at present only patients that are HER2-positive can receive antiHER2 therapies.

In the last decade, several randomized controlled trials have shown that combined treatment with trastuzumab and chemotherapy is superior to chemotherapy alone in inducing pathological complete response (pCR) in neoadjuvant setting, extending disease-free interval and overall survival in the adjuvant setting and inducing response, increasing progression-free survival, and extending overall survival in the metastatic setting. In the neoadjuvant setting, administration of trastuzumab plus chemotherapy to HER2-positive patients was found to induce pathological complete response in 26–65% of HER2-positive patients compared to 19–27% response rate with chemotherapy alone [17]. In adjuvant setting, administration of trastuzumab in combination with chemotherapeutic drugs decreases recurrence rates by approximately 50% and mortality by about 30%. Overall survival rates at 8–10 years of follow-up are 70–80% [18]. In the metastatic setting, combined administration of trastuzumab plus chemotherapy resulted in response rates of 30–85%, median times to progression periods of 5–18 months, and overall survival peroids of 11–39 months [19]. Ten to 15% of HER2-positive breast cancer patients with advanced disease treated with trastuzumab and chemotherapy derive long-term benefit with progression-free survival periods >3 years [20].

Despite success of antiHER2 therapy in extending overall survival, the vast majority of pateints develop resistance. In an attempt to minimize resistance and enhance response, a number of trials have investigated dual antiHER2 therapy in HER2-posirive patients, especially in the neoadjuvnt and metastatic setting. In the neoadjuvant setting, combined ttreatment with trastuzumab, lapatinib, and chemotherapy led to a superior pCR than trastuzumab and chemotherapy (55.8% vs. 38.4%, $p = 0.0007$) [18]. Similarly, combined treatment with trastuzumab, pertuzumab, and chemotherapy led to significantly better pCR (45.8%) compared to those receiving trastuzumab and chemotherapy (29%) or those receiving pertuzumab and chemotherapy (24%) ($p = 0.01$) [21]. In the metastatic setting, combined treatment with trastuzumab and pertuzumab has been shown to be superior to single agent treatment, also. In the CLEOPATRA trial, administration of trastuzumab, pertuzumab, and docetaxel resulted in a median overall survival of 56.5 months, in contrast to only 40.8 months in the group without pertuzumab (HR, 0.68; $p < 0.001$). Unlike the situation in the neoadjuvant and metastatic settings, dual antiHER2 treatment (i.e., trastuzumab and lapatinib) was not shown to be superior to trastuzumab in the adjuvant setting [22].

As with ER and PR, measurment of HER should now be performed on all newly diagnosed patients with invasive breast cancer and used for selecting for treatment with anti HER2 therapy in the neoadjuvant, adjuvant, and metastatic setting. However, with the increasing use of dual antiHER2 therapies in the adjuvant and metastatic settings, additional biomarkers are now urgently required to identify those patients that do not require the dual antiHER2 treatment. It would also be desirable to identify biomarkers for selecting patients in the neoadjuvant setting for treatment with antiHER2 therapy without any chemotherapy.

18.4 Ki-67

Uncontrolled proliferation is one of the hallmarks of cancer, thought to be prognostic, and has been assessed by a variety of methods. The most common proliferative marker is Ki-67, which is known as a nuclear marker of cell proliferation that is expressed in all phases of the cell cycle except for G0 and early G1 [23]. It was first identified by Gerdes et al. in 1983 in a Hodgkin lymphoma cell line and named after the Kiel University and 67 after the clone number of the antibody able to detect it [24].

Ki-67 expression is typically detected by IHC and reported as Ki-67 index (often reported as "Ki-67"), which represents the percentage of stained tumor cells within the investigated tumor cells. Lack of standardization impacts the analytic validation of Ki-67. International Ki-67 Breast Cancer Working Group was convened to examine data available on Ki-67 as a biomarker in early breast cancer and to propose guideline [25]. Several antibody clones, such as MIB-1, MM-1, Ki-S5, and SP6, have been tested for Ki-67 detection by IHC on formalin-fixed paraffin-embedded (FFPE) tissue sections. The most popular and most widely used antibody is the MIB-1 clone. A multicenter study carried out by the International Ki67 Breast Cancer Working Group concluded that good interlaboratory agreement was achievable using centrally stained core needle biopsies when scores were higher or lower than intermediate scores (i.e., <10% or >20% cell staining) [26].

Ki-67 is associated with several histopathologic factors in breast cancer. Breast cancer with higher histologic grade, higher tumor stage, and nodal metastasis showed higher Ki-67 expression [27–29]. ER status was inversely correlated with Ki-67 [27]. Jung et al. showed that Ki-67 expression was found to be correlated with tumor size, tumor grade, p53 expression, and HER-2 expression ($P < 0.001$), and inversely correlated with ER, PR, and bcl-2 expression ($P < 0.001$) in 1080 Korean breast cancer patients [30]. In addition, Ki-67 level increased significantly with decreasing age in retrospective analysis of 9321 Korean Women [31]. Ki-67 could be used to distinguish between the Luminal A- and B-like [32]. As a clinical "shorthand", tumors are often classified as "luminal A like" or "luminal B-like" based on routine pathology. Luminal A-like tumors are typically low grade, strongly ER/PR+, HER2- and have low proliferative fraction. Luminal-B-like tumors are ER+ but may have variable degrees of ER/PR expression, are higher grade, and have higher proliferative fraction [33].

Many studies have shown that Ki-67 is an important predictive and prognostic marker in breast cancer. In first meta-analysis, Azambuja et al. collected the data of 12,000 patients with 46 studies and concluded that a high Ki-67 confers a higher risk of relapse and a worse survival rate in patients with early breast cancer [34]. The limitation of this analysis is that a discriminant cut-off point was not established, and the majority of the included studies reported hazard ratios (HRs) calculated as a univariate analysis. As a consequence, a strong and true independent prognostic value of Ki-67 could not be established. In other of the largest meta-analysis studies, Petrelli et al. performed a systematic review of the literature which was followed by a meta-analysis of the individual studies [35], In total 41 studies with 64,196 patient, the threshold displaying the strongest prognostic significance for overall survival (OS) was found to be >25% cell staining (HR 2.05; 95% CI, 1.7–2.5; $p < 0.00001$). It shows that a high Ki-67 cut-off level (at least 10%), evaluated using IHC methods, is associated with more than 50% risk of death among patients with early breast cancer, particularly in those with ER+, node-disease, where the risk of death increases by a similar magnitude. In Korean study with 1080 breast cancer patients, Ki-67 (>10%) was statistically significant for both OS and distant metastasis-free survival (DFS) [30].

As a predictive marker, a study of European Institute of Oncology showed that high Ki-67 predicts the benefit from cytotoxic chemotherapy in addition to luminal breast cancer and 1–3 axillary lymph nodes [36]. Nevertheless, other studies showed either a modest predictive value for chemotherapy benefic in node-positive patients [37, 38]. In neoadjuvant setting, high Ki-67 predicted for complete pathological response (pCR) in many studies [34]. Korean study also showed that TNBC with high Ki-67 expression (≥10%) had a higher pCR rate to neoadjuvant chemotherapy than TNBC with low Ki-67 expression [39]. Furthermore, postneoadjuvant chemotherapy Ki-67 also has prognostic power [40, 41]. In GeparTrio study, low Ki-67 patients had a favorable outcome comparable to the pCR group, while high Ki-67 group experienced higher recurrence and death [42].

In the review of clinical guideline for Ki-67 in breast cancer, although the American Society of Clinical Oncology did not recommend Ki-67 use in clinical practice for newly diagnosed breast cancer patients, because of the lack of analytic validity [43], the St. Gallen International Expert Consensus Conference panel agreed that either grading or Ki-67 could be used to distinguish between the Luminal A- and B-like [33]. In European Group on Tumor Markers (EGTM) recommendation, Ki-67 may be used in combination with established prognostic factors for determining prognosis, especially if values are low (e.g., $<10\%$ cell stating) or high (e.g., $>25\%$ cell staining), although methodological problems exist in the determination of Ki-67 [11].

18.5 Androgen Receptor (AR)

Steroid hormones, androgens, and estrogen, are involved in the development and differentiations of normal breast tissue [44]. Androgens are synthesized from cholesterol, and produced by adrenal glands and ovaries in women. Particularly testosterone and dihydrotestosterone (DHT) bind to androgen receptor (AR) and modulate gene transcription [45] (Fig. 18.1). AR is a steroid hormone receptor, encoded by AR gene on the long arm of X-chromosome. When androgens bind AR, AR which is present in the cytoplasm, can translocate to the nucleus and regulates transcription of androgen-responsive genes [47]. In addition, AR can also be activated by nongenomic signaling pathways such as PI3kinase, Akt, m-TOR [48], HER2/HER3 [49], and MAPK signaling pathway [50].

Because of crosstalk with ER, AR has been known to play different roles in breast cancer. In ER+/AR+ breast cancer cell lines, ligand-bound AR binds to estrogen-related element in the nucleus, which leads to cell apoptosis [51], whereas in ER-/AR + breast cancer cell lines, AR binds to androgen-related element in the nucleus, leading to cell proliferation [52]. In ER+ breast cancer cell, the direct interaction between the AR and ERα leads to the inhibition of both transcriptional activity [51]. In other interaction model between ER, PR, and AR, AR showed different role [53]. In ER+/PR+ BC, when AR binds to the ligand, it moves into the nucleus where it competes with ERα and PR to bind to EREs. As a result, it inhibits the estrogen-dependent signal. However, in ER+/PR- breast cancer, ERβ probably acts by downregulating the ERα target gene transcription. Therefore, AR shows a protumorigenic role, enhancing the effect of ERα gene transcription [53].

AR is reported to be expressed in more than 60% of breast cancer and up to 90% of ER+ breast cancer [54]. Clinical observation studies have showed that AR+ breast cancer had better outcome in ER+ cancer patients, but not in ER- tumors [55, 56]. Interestingly, LAR (Luminal Androgen Receptor) subtype in TNBC is

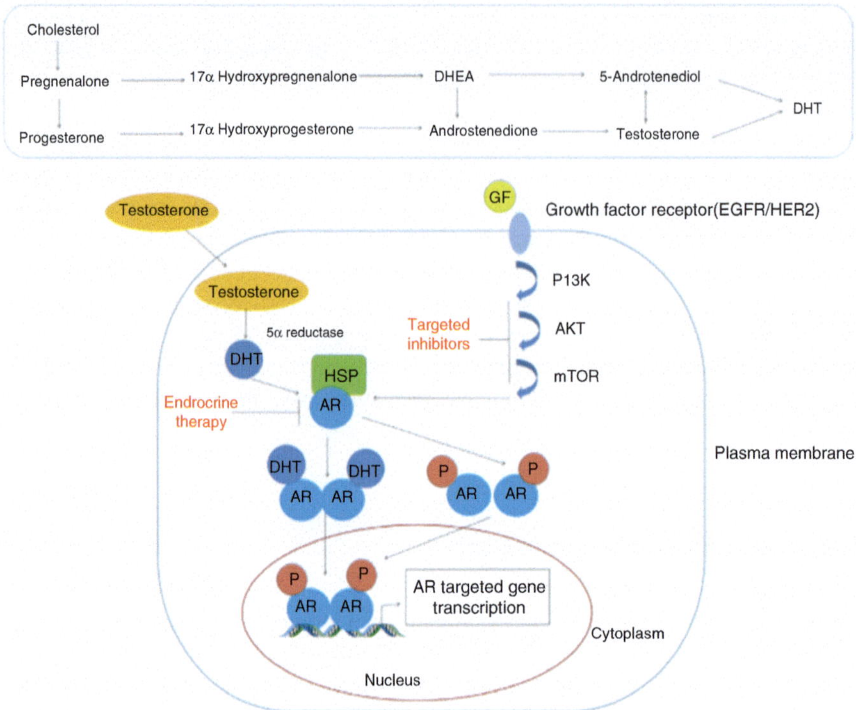

Fig. 18.1 Androgen's role in the breast tissue [46]. The top panel shows the conversion of cholesterol to different steroid hormones while the bottom panel depicts how testosterone diffuses through the plasma membrane and interacts with AR that is sequestered in the cytoplasm by the heat shock proteins (HSPs). Subsequently, AR undergoes a conformational change and is released from HSPs and then translocate to the nucleus due to its intrinsic nuclear localization domain. In the nucleus, AR binds to specific DNA motifs (AREs) wherein it recruits coactivators (not shown) to regulate the gene transcription activities

characterized by overexpression of AR and hyperactivation of this pathway [49, 57]. Compared to the rest of the TNBC subtypes, the LAR subtype seems especially resistant to various chemotherapies and highly responsive to antiandrogens in preclinical studies and clinical trials [58, 59].

AR seems to have associations with resistance of antihormonal therapy in breast cancer patients. Expression micro-arrays and qRT-PCR analysis of cancerous breast tissues have shown increased mRNA levels of AR in tamoxifen-resistant tumors compared to tamoxifen-responsive tumors [60]. Furthermore, in vitro studies of AR-overexpressing MCF-7 cells showed increased resistance to tamoxifen, with tamoxifen having AR-agonistic effects. Treatment with the antiandrogen bicalutamide restored tamoxifen-sensitivity, alluding to the underlying interaction between AR and ERα signaling as a key mechanism regulating the response to tamoxifen [60]. MCF-7 cells with overexpression of both AR and aromatase showed resistance to anastrozole in contrast to the nonAR overexpressing cells

[61]. Recurrent breast cancer tissues showed decreased ER and PR, but increased AR expression, in AI-treated recurrent lesions, suggesting an AR- dependent growth of AI-resistant lesions [62].

As AR targeted therapies, Selective AR modulators (SARM) are a potential treatment option for breast cancer. In the cell line MDA-MB-231, TNBC cells stably expressing wild-type AR, treatment with the selective AR modulator enobosarm showed inhibition of metastasis-promoting paracrine factors such as interleukin-6 and matrix metalloproteinase 13 and subsequent migration and invasion [45]. Clinical trials of selective AR modulators, enobosarm, are ongoing in ER+/AR+ metastatic BC and AR+ TNBC. AR antagonists, Bicalutamide, a nonsteroidal first-generation AR antagonist, interrupts DNA-binding domain binding to the androgen-related element [63]. A phase 2 clinical trial of bicalutamide in breast cancer showed a clinical benefit rate (CBR) at 6 months of 19% (95% CI, 7–39%) and a median progression-free survival duration of 12 weeks (95% CI, 11–22 weeks) but no objective responses [64]. However, acquired mutations in the ligand-binding domain of AR or an increase in AR protein concentration causes resistance to bicalutamide [65]. Enzalutamide, a second-generation AR antagonist, inhibits nuclear translocation, chromatin binding, and interactions with AR coregulators [66]. In a phase 2 study of 75 patients with metastatic AR-positive TNBC, enzalutamide showed a CBR of 35% (95% CI, 24–46%) at 16 weeks, a CBR of 29% (95% CI, 20–41%) at 24 weeks, and median progression-free survival of 14.7 weeks [67]. Although enzalutamide is overall safe and well tolerated, a clinical trial in patients with prostate cancer showed that it was associated with central nervous system adverse events, such as seizures and posterior reversible encephalopathy [68]. A phase 1 study showed no drug interaction between enzalutamide and fulvestrant and between enzalutamide and exemestane [67]. A phase 2 trial of enzalutamide and exemestane is ongoing (NCT02007512). Several other AR antagonists are under development, such as AZD3514 (a selective AR downregulator) [69] and EPI-001 (inhibitor of the AF-1 region in the N-terminal domain of AR) [70]. CYP17A inhibitors, such as abiraterone acetate, orteronel (TAK700), and VT-464 (Viamet), are also currently under investigation in breast cancer. These drugs block androgen production by inhibiting 17α-hydroxylase or 17,20-lyase activity [71].

18.6 Tissue Polypeptide-Specific Antigen (TPS)

Despite numerous studies worldwide, a limited number of single biomarkers have been identified for use in breast cancer management over several years, including estrogen receptor (ER), progesterone receptor (PR), and human epidermal growth factor receptor 2 (HER2). These established markers in breast cancer require tissue samples. The majority of research on cancer prognostic markers to date has focused on tissue, although serum is more readily available than tumor tissue.

Serum tumor markers are easily accessible and require a less invasive procedure than biopsy or surgery. Thus, serum tumor markers that afford independent prognostic information are of significant value. The most widely used serum markers in breast cancer, CA 15-3 and carcinoembryonic antigen (CEA), do not reflect proliferative activity. In contrast, cytokeratin tumor markers measure proliferative activity, one of the most important phenotypic characteristics of tumor aggressiveness, and may thus be more beneficial as a prognostic indicator than the serum tumor markers reported earlier.

The most widely applied cytokeratin tumor markers include tissue polypeptide antigen (TPA), CYFRA 21-1, and tissue polypeptide-specific antigen (TPS). TPA may be effectively applied to estimate cytokeratin 8, 18, and 19 in serum samples [72] which was initially described by Bjorklund and Bjorklund [73]. The group additionally developed a monoclonal antibody (M3) specific for TPA. TPS detects a defined epitope structure on human cytokeratin 18 using the M3 monoclonal antibody, while CYFRA 21-1 measures soluble keratin 19 fragments in the circulation [74].

Tissue polypeptide-specific antigen (TPS) was originally identified in human carcinomas and tumor cell lines using antibodies directed toward insoluble tumor material shown to stain cytoskeletal intermediate filaments in HeLa cells. Intermediate filament types I and II constitute cytokeratins (acidic and basic proteins, respectively). To date, 20 distinct cytokeratins have been identified in the cytoskeleton of epithelial tissue, and further subdivided into types I and II, based on sequence homology. Cytokeratins 1–8 constitute the type II group (53–68 kDa, neutral to basic protein components), while cytokeratins 9–20 constitute the type I group (40–56 kDa, acidic proteins). The cytokeratins are paired into heterodimers, each containing one type I and one type II, which are further organized into filamentous structures via side-by-side alignment to form tetramers and higher cytokeratin polymers with coiled-coil dimeric structures through further end-to-end associations [75].

Tissue polypeptide antigen is proposed to be immunologically related to a mixture of nonepidermal cytokeratins 8, 18, and 19. Earlier monoclonal mapping of a fraction of tissue polypeptide antigen revealed the presence of 35 antigenic determinants. Two epitopes were shown to be related to tumor cell activity. Monoclonal antibodies against these epitope structures were raised in mice with human carcinoma preparations. The monoclonal antibody specific for TPS was raised against the M3 epitope of tissue polypeptide antigen that is related to tumor proliferative activity. TPS is a well-documented cytokeratin tumor marker found in various epithelial cell-associated carcinomas, such as breast, ovarian, prostate, and gastrointestinal cancer.

Conflicting results on the value of TPS as a serum tumor marker in breast cancer have been documented to date. Given et al. [76] showed that TPS fails to act as an effective predictive factor in breast cancer, compared to CA 15-3. In patients receiving neoadjuvant chemotherapy, TPS was inversely associated with histologic grade, and only pretreatment CA 15-3 levels were correlated with higher recurrence rate. On the other hand, other published reports suggest that TPS acts as a marker of recurrence and metastasis.

TPS appears to have utility as a marker of recurrence and metastases, according to published reports. O'Hanlon et al. [77] demonstrated that TPS is elevated with disease stage in breast cancer, and levels are significantly higher in patients with loco-regional recurrence and increased to an even greater extent in patients with metastases. Patients with elevated TPS during follow-up were more likely to experience disease progression on further follow-up. In a recent study, Ahn et al. [78] suggested that elevated preoperative serum TPS is associated with poor breast cancer outcomes. The group assayed preoperative serum TPS levels in 1477 breast cancer patients. Age (>45 years), tumor size (>2 cm), nodal metastasis, negative progesterone receptor, and human epidermal growth factor receptor 2 were associated with elevated TPS. Moreover, elevated TPS was related to poor disease-free survival ($p < 0.001$) and overall survival ($p < 0.001$). Preoperative TPS was identified as a significant prognostic marker for survival, especially in luminal A subtype patients. The researchers proposed that highly proliferative tumors expressing elevated preoperative TPS in the luminal A subtype are more aggressive, and result in increased risk of recurrence or death.

Bjorklund et al. [79] conducted a large review including 3000 cases. Compared to CEA, MCA (mucinous carcinoma-associated antigen), and CA15-3, TPS was the only marker that exhibited an immediate decrease when therapy was effective and increases upon inadequate treatment response. Specifically, upon decrease in TPS to normal levels, applied therapy was effective and tumor activity growth was decreased. However, both CEA and CA15-3 remained elevated due to the continued presence of tumor mass.

Additionally, TPS appeared to indicate clinical outcomes (remission, progression) faster than either CA 15-3 or CEA in metastatic breast cancer patients with different types of routine treatments, and combined determination of CA 15-3 and TPS in monitoring therapy in metastatic breast cancer was recommended. In a European multicenter study, TPS, CA15-3, and CEA were serially measured in 129 metastatic breast cancer patients during a six-month treatment period. After 6 months of follow-up, patients were divided into four groups according to the UICC criteria for treatment response. Forty-six patients with a more favorable prognosis (complete remission, partial remission or stable disease) were followed up for an extended period. In 30 of the 46 patients, at least one marker had increased at the end of the 6-month period by at least 25% (TPS in 54%, CA 15-3 in 20%, CEA in 20%). These 30 patients subsequently developed disease progression. Prognostic sensitivity for TPS, CA 15-3, and CEA was 83%, 30%, and 30%, respectively. The combination of TPS and CA 15-3 increased overall sensitivity to 96% [80]. In two retrospective studies, TPS was evaluated as a marker for clinical follow-up of patients subjected to chemotherapy and/or interferon-based immunotherapy. The results suggest that TPS is a sensitive marker with a longer lead time to recurrence than both CA15-3 and CEA. The prognostic information imparted by circulating TPS levels at the beginning of the study before treatment correlated significantly with longer survival times [81]. In a prospective study, Barak et al. [81] evaluated the utility of TPS in predicting response to Taxol administered as second-line treatment in 87 advanced breast cancer patients. TPS, as well as CEA and CA15-3, were measured before, during and after Taxol treatment. The three-marker combination provided higher sensitivity than each single marker. Significant correlations of TPS levels with response and prognosis were observed. Specifically, 29%, 41%, and 60% of the patients showed a decrease of at least 50% in CEA, CA15-3, and TPS, respectively. Survival was significantly correlated with low pretreatment TPS levels. Pre-Taxol levels for TPS and CEA were further analyzed with multivariate Cox regression analysis, where the difference in relative risk was statistically significant only for TPS (2.1 vs. 1). TPS provides important reliable information in advanced breast cancer regarding Taxol treatment efficacy and survival prognosis [82].

A potential problem with TPS is that it is a recognized nonspecific marker. TPS is elevated in inflammatory conditions, particularly liver cirrhosis. In addition, TPS may be markedly elevated at the time of ovulation, and serum TPS levels are altered according to menopausal status [83].

18.7 Challenges for Future Research

Although substantial progress has been made in the identification and validation of prognostic and predictive biomarkers for breast, several major challenges remain. These include identification and validation biomarker for:

- Predicting response to specific forms of chemotherapy
- Identifying patients likely to develop severe chemotherapy-related toxicity
- Predicting response to radiotherapy
- Enhancing positive predictive value of ER and HER2
- Validate biomarkers for selecting patients who do not need extended adjuvant endocrine therapy
- Selecting patients that preferentially benefit from an aromatase inhibitor vis-à-vis tamoxifen or vice-versa
- Selecting pateints likely to particulary benefit from dual-antiHER2 therapy as opposed to single-agent antiHER2 therapy.
- Establish whether patients with equivocal scores should or should not receive antiHER2 therapy
- Impove interlaboratory variation with assay standarization of Ki-67
- Establish an optimum cut-off point or evaluate the use of ki67 as a continous variable
- Establish if different cut-off points of Ki67 are necessary for prognosis and therapy prediction
- Identify significant interaction of AR with other signaling pathways and potential predictive markers for AR-targeted therapies,
- Identify additional biomarkers to increase value of TPS as prognostic marker

18.8 Summary

Breast cancer has led the way in the introduction of prognostic and predictive biomarkers for cancer patients. Over 40 years ago, ER and PR were first introduced for predicting response to endocrine therapy. Twenty years later, HER2 became available for identifying patients likely to benefit from trastuzumab and later to other forms of anti HER2 therapy. Currently, a considerable research is focusing on Ki67, AR, and TPS, with the aim of identifying new prognositc and predictive biomarkers. However, these emerging biomarkers will have to undergo both anlaytical and clinical validation prior to entering clinical use.

References

1. Jensen EV, Block GE, Smith S, Kyser K, DeSombre ER. Estrogen receptors and breast cancer response to adrenalectomy. Natl Cancer Inst Monogr. 1971;34:55–70.
2. Carroll JS. Mechanisms of oestrogen receptor (ER) gene regulation in breast cancer. Eur J Endocrinol. 2016;175(1):R41–9.
3. Hammond ME, Hayes DF, Dowsett M, Allred DC, Hagerty KL, Badve S, et al. American Society of Clinical Oncology/College of American Pathologists guideline recommendations for immunohistochemical testing of estrogen and progesterone receptors in breast cancer. Arch Pathol Lab Med. 2010;134(6):907–22.
4. Davies C, Godwin J, Gray R, Clarke M, Cutter D, et al. Relevance of breast cancer hormone receptors and other factors to the efficacy of adjuvant tamoxifen: patient-level meta-analysis of randomised trials. Lancet. 2011;378(9793):771–84.
5. Kuukasjarvi T, Kononen J, Helin H, Holli K, Isola J. Loss of estrogen receptor in recurrent breast cancer is associated with poor response to endocrine therapy. J Clin Oncol. 1996;14 (9):2584–9.
6. Schmitt M, Thomssen C, Ulm K, Seiderer A, Harbeck N, Hofler H, et al. Time-varying prognostic impact of tumour biological factors urokinase (uPA), PAI-1 and steroid hormone receptor status in primary breast cancer. Br J Cancer. 1997;76(3):306–11.
7. Ravdin PM, Green S, Dorr TM, McGuire WL, Fabian C, Pugh RP, et al. Prognostic significance of progesterone receptor levels in estrogen receptor-positive patients with metastatic breast cancer treated with tamoxifen: results of a prospective Southwest Oncology Group study. J Clin Oncol. 1992;10(8):1284–91.
8. Elledge RM, Green S, Pugh R, Allred DC, Clark GM, Hill J, et al. Estrogen receptor (ER) and progesterone receptor (PgR), by ligand-binding assay compared with ER, PgR and pS2, by immuno-histochemistry in predicting response to tamoxifen in metastatic breast cancer: a Southwest Oncology Group Study. Int J Cancer. 2000;89(2):111–7.
9. Peto R, Davies C, Godwin J, Gray R, Pan HC, et al. Comparisons between different polychemotherapy regimens for early breast cancer: meta-analyses of long-term outcome among 100,000 women in 123 randomised trials. Lancet. 2012;379(9814):432–44.
10. Harris LN, Ismaila N, McShane LM, Hayes DF. Use of biomarkers to guide decisions on adjuvant systemic therapy for women with early-stage invasive breast cancer: American Society of Clinical Oncology Clinical Practice Guideline Summary. J Oncol Pract. 2016;12(4):384–9.
11. Duffy MJ, Harbeck N, Nap M, Molina R, Nicolini A, Senkus E, et al. Clinical use of biomarkers in breast cancer: updated guidelines from the European Group on Tumor Markers (EGTM). Eur J Cancer. 2017;75:284–98.

12. Rimawi MF, Schiff R, Osborne CK. Targeting HER2 for the treatment of breast cancer. Annu Rev Med. 2015;66:111–28.
13. Slamon DJ, Clark GM, Wong SG, Levin WJ, Ullrich A, McGuire WL. Human breast cancer: correlation of relapse and survival with amplification of the HER-2/neu oncogene. Science. 1987;235(4785):177–82.
14. Slamon DJ, Godolphin W, Jones LA, Holt JA, Wong SG, Keith DE, et al. Studies of the HER-2/neu proto-oncogene in human breast and ovarian cancer. Science. 1989;244(4905):707–12.
15. Kallioniemi OP, Holli K, Visakorpi T, Koivula T, Helin HH, Isola JJ. Association of c-erbB-2 protein over-expression with high rate of cell proliferation, increased risk of visceral metastasis and poor long-term survival in breast cancer. Int J Cancer. 1991;49(5):650–5.
16. Press MF, Bernstein L, Thomas PA, Meisner LF, Zhou JY, Ma Y, et al. HER-2/neu gene amplification characterized by fluorescence in situ hybridization: poor prognosis in node-negative breast carcinomas. J Clin Oncol. 1997;15(8):2894–904.
17. Dent S, Oyan B, Honig A, Mano M, Howell S. HER2-targeted therapy in breast cancer: a systematic review of neoadjuvant trials. Cancer Treat Rev. 2013;39(6):622–31.
18. Hicks M, Macrae ER, Abdel-Rasoul M, Layman R, Friedman S, Querry J, et al. Neoadjuvant dual HER2-targeted therapy with lapatinib and trastuzumab improves pathologic complete response in patients with early stage HER2-positive breast cancer: a meta-analysis of randomized prospective clinical trials. Oncologist. 2015;20(4):337–43.
19. Loibl S, Gianni L. HER2-positive breast cancer. Lancet. 2017;389(10087):2415–29.
20. Park HS, Sohn J, Kim SI, Park S, Park HS, Gho SG, et al. Effects of hormone receptor status on the durable response of trastuzumab-based therapy in metastatic breast cancer. Breast Cancer Res Treat. 2017;163(2):255–62.
21. Gianni L, Pienkowski T, Im YH, Roman L, Tseng LM, Liu MC, et al. Efficacy and safety of neoadjuvant pertuzumab and trastuzumab in women with locally advanced, inflammatory, or early HER2-positive breast cancer (NeoSphere): a randomised multicentre, open-label, phase 2 trial. Lancet Oncol. 2012;13(1):25–32.
22. Swain SM, Baselga J, Kim SB, Ro J, Semiglazov V, Campone M, et al. Pertuzumab, trastuzumab, and docetaxel in HER2-positive metastatic breast cancer. N Engl J Med. 2015;372(8):724–34.
23. Gerdes J, Lemke H, Baisch H, Wacker HH, Schwab U, Stein H. Cell cycle analysis of a cell proliferation-associated human nuclear antigen defined by the monoclonal antibody Ki-67. J Immunol. 1984;133(4):1710–5.
24. Gerdes J, Schwab U, Lemke H, Stein H. Production of a mouse monoclonal antibody reactive with a human nuclear antigen associated with cell proliferation. Int J Cancer. 1983;31(1):13–20.
25. Dowsett M, Nielsen TO, A'Hern R, Bartlett J, Coombes RC, Cuzick J, et al. Assessment of Ki67 in breast cancer: recommendations from the International Ki67 in Breast Cancer working group. J Natl Cancer Inst. 2011;103(22):1656–64.
26. Leung SCY, Nielsen TO, Zabaglo L, Arun I, Badve SS, Bane AL, et al. Analytical validation of a standardized scoring protocol for Ki67: phase 3 of an international multicenter collaboration. NPJ Breast Cancer. 2016;2:16014.
27. Inwald EC, Klinkhammer-Schalke M, Hofstadter F, Zeman F, Koller M, Gerstenhauer M, et al. Ki-67 is a prognostic parameter in breast cancer patients: results of a large population-based cohort of a cancer registry. Breast Cancer Res Treat. 2013;139(2):539–52.
28. Buxant F, Anaf V, Simon P, Fayt I, Noel JC. Ki-67 immunostaining activity is higher in positive axillary lymph nodes than in the primary breast tumor. Breast Cancer Res Treat. 2002;75 (1):1–3.
29. Park D, Karesen R, Noren T, Sauer T. Ki-67 expression in primary breast carcinomas and their axillary lymph node metastases: clinical implications. Virchows Arch. 2007;451(1):11–8.
30. Jung SY, Han W, Lee JW, Ko E, Kim E, Yu JH, et al. Ki-67 expression gives additional prognostic information on St. Gallen 2007 and Adjuvant! Online risk categories in early breast cancer. Ann Surg Oncol. 2009;16(5):1112–21.

31. Kim J, Han W, Jung SY, Park YH, Moon HG, Ahn SK, et al. The value of Ki67 in very young women with hormone receptor-positive breast cancer: retrospective analysis of 9,321 Korean women. Ann Surg Oncol. 2015;22(11):3481–8.
32. Cheang MC, Chia SK, Voduc D, Gao D, Leung S, Snider J, et al. Ki67 index, HER2 status, and prognosis of patients with luminal B breast cancer. J Natl Cancer Inst. 2009;101(10):736–50.
33. Curigliano G, Burstein HJ, Gnant M, Dubsky P, Loibl S, et al. De-escalating and escalating treatments for early-stage breast cancer: the St. Gallen International Expert Consensus Conference on the Primary Therapy of Early Breast Cancer 2017. Ann Oncol. 2017;28(8):1700–12.
34. de Azambuja E, Cardoso F, de Castro G, Colozza M, Mano MS, Durbecq V, et al. Ki-67 as prognostic marker in early breast cancer: a meta-analysis of published studies involving 12,155 patients. Br J Cancer. 2007;96(10):1504–13.
35. Petrelli F, Viale G, Cabiddu M, Barni S. Prognostic value of different cut-off levels of Ki-67 in breast cancer: a systematic review and meta-analysis of 64,196 patients. Breast Cancer Res Treat. 2015;153(3):477–91.
36. Criscitiello C, Disalvatore D, De Laurentiis M, Gelao L, Fumagalli L, Locatelli M, et al. High Ki-67 score is indicative of a greater benefit from adjuvant chemotherapy when added to endocrine therapy in luminal B HER2-negative and node-positive breast cancer. Breast. 2014;23(1):69–75.
37. Penault-Llorca F, Andre F, Sagan C, Lacroix-Triki M, Denoux Y, Verriele V, et al. Ki67 expression and docetaxel efficacy in patients with estrogen receptor-positive breast cancer. J Clin Oncol. 2009;27(17):2809–15.
38. Dumontet C, Krajewska M, Treilleux I, Mackey JR, Martin M, Rupin M, et al. BCIRG 001 molecular analysis: prognostic factors in node-positive breast cancer patients receiving adjuvant chemotherapy. Clin Cancer Res. 2010;16(15):3988–97.
39. Keam B, Im SA, Lee KH, Han SW, Oh DY, Kim JH, et al. Ki-67 can be used for further classification of triple-negative breast cancer into two subtypes with different response and prognosis. Breast Cancer Res. 2011;13(2):R22.
40. Luporsi E, Andre F, Spyratos F, Martin PM, Jacquemier J, Penault-Llorca F, et al. Ki-67: level of evidence and methodological considerations for its role in the clinical management of breast cancer: analytical and critical review. Breast Cancer Res Treat. 2012;132(3):895–915.
41. Denkert C, Loibl S, Muller BM, Eidtmann H, Schmitt WD, Eiermann W, et al. Ki67 levels as predictive and prognostic parameters in pretherapeutic breast cancer core biopsies: a translational investigation in the neoadjuvant GeparTrio trial. Ann Oncol. 2013;24(11):2786–93.
42. von Minckwitz G, Schmitt WD, Loibl S, Muller BM, Blohmer JU, Sinn BV, et al. Ki67 measured after neoadjuvant chemotherapy for primary breast cancer. Clin Cancer Res. 2013;19(16):4521–31.
43. Harris L, Fritsche H, Mennel R, Norton L, Ravdin P, Taube S, et al. American Society of Clinical Oncology 2007 update of recommendations for the use of tumor markers in breast cancer. J Clin Oncol. 2007;25(33):5287–312.
44. Dimitrakakis C, Bondy C. Androgens and the breast. Breast Cancer Res. 2009;11(5):212.
45. Narayanan R, Coss CC, Dalton JT. Development of selective androgen receptor modulators (SARMs). Mol Cell Endocrinol. 2017;59(1):1–31.
46. Majumder A, Singh M, Tyagi SC. Post-menopausal breast cancer: from estrogen to androgen receptor. Oncotarget. 2017;8(60):102739–58.
47. Gao W, Bohl CE, Dalton JT. Chemistry and structural biology of androgen receptor. Chem Rev. 2005;105(9):3352–70.
48. Foradori CD, Weiser MJ, Handa RJ. Non-genomic actions of androgens. Front Neuroendocrinol. 2008;29(2):169–81.
49. Lehmann BD, Bauer JA, Chen X, Sanders ME, Chakravarthy AB, Shyr Y, et al. Identification of human triple-negative breast cancer subtypes and preclinical models for selection of targeted therapies. J Clin Invest. 2011;121(7):2750–67.

50. Garay JP, Karakas B, Abukhdeir AM, Cosgrove DP, Gustin JP, Higgins MJ, et al. The growth response to androgen receptor signaling in ERalpha-negative human breast cells is dependent on p21 and mediated by MAPK activation. Breast Cancer Res. 2012;14(1):R27.
51. Panet-Raymond V, Gottlieb B, Beitel LK, Pinsky L, Trifiro MA. Interactions between androgen and estrogen receptors and the effects on their transactivational properties. Mol Cell Endocrinol. 2000;167(1-2):139–50.
52. Robinson JL, Macarthur S, Ross-Innes CS, Tilley WD, Neal DE, Mills IG, et al. Androgen receptor driven transcription in molecular apocrine breast cancer is mediated by FoxA1. EMBO J. 2011;30(15):3019–27.
53. Karamouzis MV, Papavassiliou KA, Adamopoulos C, Papavassiliou AG. Targeting androgen/estrogen receptors crosstalk in cancer. Trends Cancer. 2016;2(1):35–48.
54. Li W, O'Shaughnessy J, Hayes D, Campone M, Bondarenko I, Zbarskaya I, et al. Biomarker associations with efficacy of abiraterone acetate and exemestane in postmenopausal patients with estrogen receptor-positive metastatic breast cancer. Clin Cancer Res. 2016;22(24):6002–9.
55. Secreto G, Venturelli E, Meneghini E, Greco M, Ferraris C, Gion M, et al. Testosterone and biological characteristics of breast cancers in postmenopausal women. Cancer Epidemiol Biomark Prev. 2009;18(11):2942–8.
56. Secreto G, Meneghini E, Venturelli E, Cogliati P, Agresti R, Ferraris C, et al. Circulating sex hormones and tumor characteristics in postmenopausal breast cancer patients. A cross-sectional study. Int J Biol Markers. 2011;26(4):241–6.
57. Burstein MD, Tsimelzon A, Poage GM, Covington KR, Contreras A, Fuqua SA, et al. Comprehensive genomic analysis identifies novel subtypes and targets of triple-negative breast cancer. Clin Cancer Res. 2015;21(7):1688–98.
58. Loibl S, Muller BM, von Minckwitz G, Schwabe M, Roller M, Darb-Esfahani S, et al. Androgen receptor expression in primary breast cancer and its predictive and prognostic value in patients treated with neoadjuvant chemotherapy. Breast Cancer Res Treat. 2011;130 (2):477–87.
59. Masuda H, Baggerly KA, Wang Y, Zhang Y, Gonzalez-Angulo AM, Meric-Bernstam F, et al. Differential response to neoadjuvant chemotherapy among seven triple-negative breast cancer molecular subtypes. Clin Cancer Res. 2013;19(19):5533–40.
60. De Amicis F, Thirugnansampanthan J, Cui Y, Selever J, Beyer A, Parra I, et al. Androgen receptor overexpression induces tamoxifen resistance in human breast cancer cells. Breast Cancer Res Treat. 2010;121(1):1–11.
61. Rechoum Y, Rovito D, Iacopetta D, Barone I, Ando S, Weigel NL, et al. AR collaborates with ERalpha in aromatase inhibitor-resistant breast cancer. Breast Cancer Res Treat. 2014;147 (3):473–85.
62. Fujii R, Hanamura T, Suzuki T, Gohno T, Shibahara Y, Niwa T, et al. Increased androgen receptor activity and cell proliferation in aromatase inhibitor-resistant breast carcinoma. J Steroid Biochem Mol Biol. 2014;144(Pt B):513–22.
63. Masiello D, Cheng S, Bubley GJ, Lu ML, Balk SP. Bicalutamide functions as an androgen receptor antagonist by assembly of a transcriptionally inactive receptor. J Biol Chem. 2002;277 (29):26321–6.
64. Gucalp A, Tolaney S, Isakoff SJ, Ingle JN, Liu MC, Carey LA, et al. Phase II trial of bicalutamide in patients with androgen receptor-positive, estrogen receptor-negative metastatic Breast Cancer. Clin Cancer Res. 2013;19(19):5505–12.
65. Chen CD, Welsbie DS, Tran C, Baek SH, Chen R, Vessella R, et al. Molecular determinants of resistance to antiandrogen therapy. Nat Med. 2004;10(1):33–9.
66. Tran C, Ouk S, Clegg NJ, Chen Y, Watson PA, Arora V, et al. Development of a second-generation antiandrogen for treatment of advanced prostate cancer. Science. 2009;324 (5928):787–90.
67. Schwartzberg LS, Yardley DA, Elias AD, Patel M, LoRusso P, Burris HA, et al. A phase I/Ib study of enzalutamide alone and in combination with endocrine therapies in women with advanced breast cancer. Clin Cancer Res. 2017;23(15):4046–54.

68. Loriot Y, Miller K, Sternberg CN, Fizazi K, De Bono JS, Chowdhury S, et al. Effect of enzalutamide on health-related quality of life, pain, and skeletal-related events in asymptomatic and minimally symptomatic, chemotherapy-naive patients with metastatic castration-resistant prostate cancer (PREVAIL): results from a randomised, phase 3 trial. Lancet Oncol. 2015;16 (5):509–21.
69. Loddick SA, Ross SJ, Thomason AG, Robinson DM, Walker GE, Dunkley TP, et al. AZD3514: a small molecule that modulates androgen receptor signaling and function in vitro and in vivo. Mol Cancer Ther. 2013;12(9):1715–27.
70. Brand LJ, Olson ME, Ravindranathan P, Guo H, Kempema AM, Andrews TE, et al. EPI-001 is a selective peroxisome proliferator-activated receptor-gamma modulator with inhibitory effects on androgen receptor expression and activity in prostate cancer. Oncotarget. 2015;6 (6):3811–24.
71. Toren PJ, Kim S, Pham S, Mangalji A, Adomat H, Guns ES, et al. Anticancer activity of a novel selective CYP17A1 inhibitor in preclinical models of castrate-resistant prostate cancer. Mol Cancer Ther. 2015;14(1):59–69.
72. Weber K, Osborn M, Moll R, Wiklund B, Luning B. Tissue polypeptide antigen (TPA) is related to the non-epidermal keratins 8, 18 and 19 typical of simple and non-squamous epithelia: re-evaluation of a human tumor marker. EMBO J. 1984;3(11):2707–14.
73. Bjorklund B, Bjorklund V. Antigenicity of pooled human malignant and normal tissues by cyto-immunological technique; presence of an insoluble, heat-labile tumor antigen. Int Arch Allergy Appl Immunol. 1957;10(3):153–84.
74. Bodenmuller H, Donie F, Kaufmann M, Banauch D. The tumor markers TPA, TPS, TPACYK and CYFRA 21-1 react differently with the keratins 8, 18 and 19. Int J Biol Markers. 1994;9 (2):70–4.
75. Coulombe PA, Omary MB, et al. 'Hard' and 'soft' principles defining the structure, function and regulation of keratin intermediate filaments. Curr Opin Cell Biol. 2002;14(1):110–22.
76. Given M, Scott M, Mc Grath JP, Given HF. The predictive of tumour markers CA 15-3, TPS and CEA in breast cancer recurrence. Breast. 2000;9(5):277–80.
77. O'Hanlon DM, Kerin MJ, O'Boyle C, Grimes H, Given HF. Tissue polypeptide specific antigen (TPS) in breast cancer--an initial evaluation. Eur J Surg Oncol. 1996;22(1):38–41.
78. Ahn SK, Moon HG, Ko E, Kim HS, Shin HC, Kim J, et al. Preoperative serum tissue polypeptide-specific antigen is a valuable prognostic marker in breast cancer. Int J Cancer. 2013;132(4):875–81.
79. Schuurman JJ, Bong SB, Einarsson R. Determination of serum tumor markers TPS and CA 15-3 during monitoring of treatment in metastatic breast cancer patients. Anticancer Res. 1996;16(4B):2169–72.
80. Van Dalen A, Barak V, Cremaschi A, Gion M, Molina R, Namer M, et al. The prognostic significance of increasing marker levels in metastatic breast cancer patients with clinically complete remission, partial remission or stable disease. Int J Biol Markers. 1998;13(1):10–5.
81. Barak V, Kalickman I, Nisman B, Farbstein H, Fridlender ZG, Baider L, et al. Changes in cytokine production of breast cancer patients treated with interferons. Cytokine. 1998;10 (12):977–83.
82. Barak V, Goike H, Panaretakis KW, Einarsson R. Clinical utility of cytokeratins as tumor markers. Clin Biochem. 2004;37(7):529–40.
83. Inaba N, Fukasawa I, Okajima Y, Ota Y, Tanaka K, Matsui H, et al. Immunoradiometrical measurement of tissue polypeptide specific antigen (TPS) in normal, healthy, nonpregnant and pregnant Japanese women. Asia Oceania J Obstet Gynaecol. 1993;19(4):459–66.

Chapter 19
The Potential Predictors in Chemotherapy Sensitivity

Eun-Kyu Kim and Hee-Chul Shin

Abstract Monitoring of patient and tumor during chemotherapy is important to determine whether the chemotherapy is effective to the patient. Variants affect drug enzyme activities and altered enzyme activities can be potential predictors for chemotherapeutic agents including cyclophosphamide and paclitaxel. Response to chemotherapy is primarily based on somatic mutations but germline variants may predict cancer cell sensitivity to chemotherapeutic agents. Furthermore, patient's genetic variation of immune system was reported to be associated with drug response and toxicity. Recently, the somaric and germilne genomic variation influences the pharmacokinetics of chemotherapy and these variation can be biomarkers for chemotherapy.

Keywords Breast oncology · Biomarkers · Cancer cell sensitivity · Pharmarcogenetic · Chemotherapy

19.1 Introduction

Monitoring of patient condition and tumor burden during chemotherapy is important to determine whether the chemotherapy is effective to the patient. Currently, monitoring includes periodic assessment of patient symptoms, physical examination, laboratory studies, imaging studies, and serum tumor markers. Tumor markers including CEA, CA15-3, and CA 27.29 are elevated in tumor progression, but may also be elevated in another condition such as benign ovarian cysts, benign breast disease, and benign liver disease. Furthermore, the test of these tumor markers is not reliable for diagnosing cancer or as a screening test for early detection of cancer. Most of the tumor markers do not result in a high level in early stage. However, they may be helpful in the metastatic setting. Tumor markers correlate

E.-K. Kim (✉) · H.-C. Shin
Department of Surgery, Seoul National University Bundang Hospital, Seoul, South Korea

D.-Y. Noh et al. (eds.), *Translational Research in Breast Cancer*, Advances in Experimental Medicine and Biology 1187,
https://doi.org/10.1007/978-981-32-9620-6_19

well with clinical disease course in 60–70% of patients in metastatic setting. There are few data on the use of these serum biomarkers and careful interpretation in context with of other clinical and radiologic findings is required.

The introduction of genome-wide microarray analysis of gene expression led to the recognition of the intrinsic molecular subtypes of breast cancer: luminal A, luminal B, HER2-enriched, and basal-like [1]. Furthermore, each subtype of breast cancer was associated with different prognosis, a poor prognosis for the basal-like subtype and a significant difference in long-term outcome for the luminal A and luminal B [2]. Since then, several RNA-based multigene assays, including Onco*type* Dx, MammoPrint, Prosigna, BCI, EndoPredict, etc., have been introduced in the clinical practice to categorize ER-positive breast cancer into different risk groups of recurrence. Based on the results of Oncotype Dx, the multigene assay for breast cancer, breast cancer patients with low recurrence score had very low recurrence rate with endocrine therapy alone and with high recurrence score had a large benefit from chemotherapy [3, 4]. Patients in the low-risk category by BCI, EndoPredict, or Prosigna also have shown to have extremely low risk of distant late recurrence. These assays each showed ability to provide added prognostic information and are most helpful in patients who are classified in the low-risk category for whom chemotherapy could be avoided. While the application of these multigene assays led to a change in recommendation of adjuvant chemotherapy, the application of assays limited to ER positive and early stage of breast cancer. Non-ER positive breast cancer and advanced or recurrent breast cancer had different biology with early-stage ER-positive breast cancer. An understanding of tumor biology is needed to set treatment strategy.

Given the limitation of conventional measures, novel approaches to detect disease progression and response have been proposed. It has been proposed that the measurement of circulating tumor cells (CTCs) may predict prognosis and response to chemotherapy. In a prospective study, the number of CTCs at the time of treatment initiation was found to be an independent predictor of prognosis. In addition, continued elevation of CTCs at follow-up after initiation of first-line therapy was associated with treatment failure [5, 6]. Recently, pharmacogenetics attempts to predict treatment response using gene analysis. The patient's genomes (germline) and the tumor genomes (somatic) are relevant with cancer. Variation in these genomes can influence the patient's risk of developing cancer and prognosis. Furthermore, these variations can influence the response of chemotherapy and toxicity of chemotherapy. It is critically important that patients receive effective chemotherapy and avoid treatment-related morbidity and sometimes mortality. The Cancer Genome Atlas (TCGA) catalogued the somatic genomes of many tumor types including breast cancer [7]. This study identified the genetic variations that can cause oncogenic transformation and defined a number of pathways for effective cancer treatment [8].

19.2 Drug Pharmacokinetic Pharmacogenetic

There are a few notable pharmacokinetic pharmacogenetic associations for breast cancer drug.

Cyclophosphamide is one of the most commonly used chemotherapeutic agent in breast cancer. Cyclophosphamide is prodrug requiring enzymatic bioactivation. The main active metabolite is 4-hydroxycyclophosphamide. Several cytochrome P450 (CYP) enzymes have been reported to mediate this reaction. Roy et al. found that CYP2B6 metabolized cyclophosphamide in vitro study [9]. Xie et al. found that ciprofloxacin suppressed gene expression of CYP2C11 and CYP3A1 in mRNA level and the metabolic ratio was significantly lower in animals treated with ciprofloxacin compared with control group, which suggested CYP2C11 and CYP3A1 altered the pharmacokinetics of cyclophosphamide in animal study [10]. Griskevicius et al. found that 4-hydroxylation of cyclophosphamide had significant correlation with CYP2C19 activity in human liver microsomes [11]. Previous studies have analyzed the effect of single nucleotide polymorphisms (SNPs) on cyclophosphamide bioactivation or efficacy. Xie et al. reported the genotype of CYP2B6 G516T variant allele influences cyclophosphamide clearance about twice compared with the wild-type gene [12]. In a Japanese study, they found that the homozygotes of CYP2B6*6 (Q172H and K262R) showed higher clearance and shorter half-life of cyclophosphamide than heterozygotes and homozygotes of CYP2B6*1. On the other hand, SNPs of the CYP2B6 gene including g.−2320 T > C, g.-750 T > C (5′-flanking region), g.15582C > T (intron 3), or g.18492 T > C (intron 5) had decreased cyclophosphamide 4-hydroxylation [13]. Another study showed that patients with CYP3A4 *1B*/*1A genotype had significantly worse disease-free survival (DFS) than those who were CYP3A4 *1A/*1A wild-type [14]. Haruoun et al. reported that CYP2B6 *5/*6, *6/*9, or *6/*6 haplotypes were associated with a significantly shorter time to recurrence of the disease in patients receiving cyclophosphamide therapy [15].

Paclitaxel which is used for ovarian cancer, breast cancer, lung cancer, and other types of solid tumor cancer is metabolized in the liver by CYP2C8 and CYP3A4 and transported by P-glycoprotein. The main toxicities are neuropathy and neutropenia. Non-synonymous CYP2C8 variants with decreased paclitaxel metabolite activity compared with wild-type have been reported [16]. Bergmann et al. studied 93 women with ovarian cancer treated with paclitaxel. They reported that patients with CYP2C8*3 were associated with 11% lower clearance of unbound paclitaxel [17]. However, large analyses including 270 paclitaxel-treated patients have failed to replicate this association between genetic variability and paclitaxel clearance [18]. Recently, the association between genetic variation and paclitaxel-induced neuropathy has been reported. A Genome-wide association study identified SNP in FGD4 was associated with paclitaxel-induced neuropathy [19]. Based on these studies, we can hypotheses that reduced enzyme activity leads a poorer outcome. Variants that affect these enzyme activities can be potential predictors for a certain type of drug.

19.3 Cancer Cell Sensitivity

Response to chemotherapy is primarily based on the somatic (tumor) genetics. Somatic genome is associated with the sensitivity of the cancer cell to the particular mechanism of action of drugs. Chemotherapeutic agents have a variety of mechanism of action including damaging DNA, disruption of microtubule function, anti-estrogenic effect, and HER2 targeting agents. Variants that affect the signaling pathway or the target of drug could dictate sensitivity of these drugs. These variants can be validated by comparing treatment response in genetically modified cancer cells or animal models. The typical retrospective research to identify variants relevant to the mechanism of drug is limited. For example, paclitaxel has been used with a putative mechanism of disruption of microtubule function causing mitotic arrest [20]. However, a recent study reported that mitotic arrest was not responsible for the efficacy of paclitaxel but a new mechanism of action that chromosome missegregation on multipolar spindles was [21] Similarly, the mechanism of action for trastuzumab continues to be debated. Our limited understating of drug mechanism precludes effective selection of candidate genes associated with sensitivity of chemotherapy. During past few decades, the cellular biology and oncology have tremendously evolved with the development of genomics. Drugs with specific mechanisms which are vulnerable to cancer cell are under development. Some of these mechanisms exist in germline genome including *BRCA*. These germline pharmacogenic biomarkers can be candidates of drug targets.

The BRCA1/2 genes are very well known for susceptibility to several tumors including breast and ovarian cancer. The BRCA1/2 genes are responsible for homologous recombination, the repair pathway of damaged DNA. Germline BRCA variation increases cancer risk because loss of homologous recombination increases DNA replication error. If BRCA 1/2 is damaged by a BRCA mutation, damaged DNA is not repaired properly, and this increases the risk for cancer [22]. Furthermore, the predominant allele of BRCA1/2 has a normal tumor suppressive function whereas BRCA1/2 mutation causes a loss of function of tumor suppressive function, which induces an increased risk of cancer, especially breast and ovarian cancer [23]. The importance of BRCA mutations are not only cancer risk but also informative of cancer prognosis, and prediction of treatment effectiveness [24].

When germline BRCA genes are mutated, cells are unable to perform homologous recombination and repair damaged DNA that can eventually cause cancer. The function of Poly(ADP-ribose) polymerase (PARP) is to assist the repair of single-strand DNA breaks: base-excision repair. When drugs that inhibit PARP cause multiple double-strand breaks in cancer cell that lacks homologous recombination, these double-strand breaks cannot be efficiently repaired, leading to the cell death. In preclinical study, BRCA mutant cell lines are highly sensitive to PARP inhibition [25]. Clinical trials of the PARP inhibitor olaparib showed positive proof for breast cancer patients with BRCA mutation [26]. In randomized phase III trial with metastatic breast cancer patients with germline BRCA mutation and HER2-negative, olaparib showed a progression-free survival benefit compared with conventional chemotherapy [27]. Based on this trial, olaparib is approved for metastatic breast cancer patients with germline BRCA mutation and HER2-negative. Olaparib proves the potential efficacy of agents designed to target cell vulnerabilities caused by germline genetic variation.

Possible strategy for breast cancer that cannot perform DNA repair is to use a DNA-damaging agent such as platinum. In retrospective studies, BRCA mutations are biomarkers of effectiveness of platinum containing regimens [28, 29]. Several studies reported that variants associated with DNA repair predict sensitivity to DNA-damaging agents. The survival rate was significantly different depending on the ERCC1 genotype in non-small-cell lung cancer and breast cancer patients treated with platinum-based chemotherapy [30, 31]. In meta-analysis, polymorphism of ERCC1/2 was associated with response and survival rate in oxaliplatin-treated gastric and colorectal cancer patients [32]. Non-small-cell lung cancer patients with polymorphisms in the XRCC1 and XPG gene had higher response rate to platinum-based chemotherapy and had longer disease-free survival and overall survival [33–35]. Gallagher et al. reported that germline single nucleotide polymorphisms (SNPs) in IL1B, CCND1, and PARD6B genes were associated with response of uroepithelial carcinoma to platinum-based chemotherapy [36]. Although there are relatively little data for these genes and response in breast cancer specifically, the sensitivity to platinum-based chemotherapy can be theoretically generalized regardless of tumor types.

There are other examples of germline genetic variants that may predict cancer cell sensitivity to drug. TEKT4 germline variations are reported to be associated with the mechanism of resistance to paclitaxel. Tektin4 encoded by TEKT4 associates with tubulin in doublet microtubules and helped stabilize these structures. The expression of variant TEKT4 deregulates the microtubule stability, antagonizes the paclitaxel-induced stabilizing effect of microtubules, and increases paclitaxel resistance [37]. Another study has shown that the polymorphisms of NQO2 and GSTM1 may affect chemotherapy sensitivity in breast cancer patients treated with cyclophosphamide or anthracycline-based regimens [38].

19.4 Immune System Activation

The previous subsections described genetic variations that influence the amount of active drug that reaches the cancer call and the senility of the cancer cell to the drug. Recently, there has been a huge progress in understating of patient's immune system. Some rare treatment-related reactions were not previously explainable but now can be predicted based on patient's genotype. One example is the germline variation of the HLA system. Recently, the germline variation in the HLA system was reported to be associated with treatment-related hypersensitivity reactions [39, 40]. Also, the genetic variations of HLA system were associated with lapatinib-induced hepatotoxicity [41, 42]. These results demonstrate that the response to immune activation can be varied according to the patient's genome.

Despite limited understanding of the interaction between the immune system and the cancer, the immune therapy is likely to be the next evolution in cancer treatment. There is a large amount of knowledge about the intercell signaling and immune system activation. With this information, candidate genes for pharmacogenetic biomarker can be developed. Pharmacogenetic predictors of breast cancer response to immunotherapy are now under development.

In HER2-positive breast cancer, HER2-directed therapy including trastuzumab is the standard practice. Trastuzumab works through antibody-dependent cell cytotoxicity as well as inhibition of HER2 dimerization and prevention of cellular signaling. Antibody-dependent cell cytotoxicity occurs when monoclonal antibody attaches on one end to HER2 and the other end with the effector cell of the immune system. Several effector cells of the immune system bind to the Fc fragment of antibodies including natural killer cells, dendritic cells, and macrophages. This interaction activates the effector cell, which signals other immune cells to locate cancer cells expressing the antigen and destroy cancer cells. Binding of the effector cells to trastuzumab occurs via the fragment-c gamma receptor (FcγR) [43]. FcγR has several subtypes including non-synonymous polymorphism of *FCGR*. There were several reports that the *FCGR* polymorphisms predict efficacy of trastuzumab [44, 45]. However, another prospective study showed that FCGR genotypes and trastuzumab efficacy was not associated in HER2-positive breast cancer [46].

Other relevant pharmacogenetic biomarkers of immune therapy are likely to be found in the germline genome. Immunotherapy includes Programmed cell death-1 (PD-1) inhibitors, such as nivolumab, which was approved in malignant melanoma [47]. Nivolumab showed clinical efficacy in non-small-cell lung cancer and renal cell carcinoma is currently being tested in many tumor types including breast cancer (NCT02129556).

19.5 Conclusions and Further Research

The genomic variation influences the pharmacokinetics of chemotherapy. However, the discovery, validation, and translation of such biomarkers for chemotherapy have limited the clinical usefulness in prediction of breast cancer response. Further studies are required for concentration of active metabolites of prodrugs to find which genomic variations are likely to be clinically useful. Biomarkers of efficacy for chemotherapy may be associated with somatic genome, but some of these originate in the germline genome. The predictors of chemotherapy and immunotherapy are likely to exist in the patient's genome. Systematic analysis of germline genetics and biomarkers of immune activation will ensure efficient discovery and validation of biomarkers in well-designed retrospective and prospective analyses. A more detailed study for selecting and identifying candidate genes or variants would be instrumental for pharmacogenetic analyses. Development of cellular and animal models for genetic variation on pharmacokinetics, cancer cell sensitivity, and effector cell activation would be able to validate the pharmacogenetic discoveries for clinical translation. As treatment strategy for cancer cell has changed from carpet bombing to precision targeting, the age of somatic genome may well be the age of germline genome.

References

1. Perou CM, Sorlie T, Eisen MB, van de Rijn M, Jeffrey SS, Rees CA, et al. Molecular portraits of human breast tumours. Nature. 2000;406(6797):747–52.
2. Pau Ni IB, Zakaria Z, Muhammad R, Abdullah N, Ibrahim N, Aina Emran N, et al. Gene expression patterns distinguish breast carcinomas from normal breast tissues: the Malaysian context. Pathol Res Pract. 2010;206(4):223–8.
3. Sparano JA, Gray RJ, Makower DF, Pritchard KI, Albain KS, Hayes DF, et al. Prospective validation of a 21-gene expression assay in breast Cancer. N Engl J Med. 2015;373 (21):2005–14.
4. Paik S, Tang G, Shak S, Kim C, Baker J, Kim W, et al. Gene expression and benefit of chemotherapy in women with node-negative, estrogen receptor-positive breast cancer. J Clin Oncol. 2006;24(23):3726–34.
5. Cristofanilli M, Budd GT, Ellis MJ, Stopeck A, Matera J, Miller MC, et al. Circulating tumor cells, disease progression, and survival in metastatic breast cancer. N Engl J Med. 2004;351 (8):781–91.
6. Cristofanilli M, Hayes DF, Budd GT, Ellis MJ, Stopeck A, Reuben JM, et al. Circulating tumor cells: a novel prognostic factor for newly diagnosed metastatic breast cancer. J Clin Oncol. 2005;23(7):1420–30.
7. Cancer Genome Atlas N. Comprehensive molecular portraits of human breast tumours. Nature. 2012;490(7418):61–70.
8. Chmielecki J, Meyerson M. DNA sequencing of cancer: what have we learned? Annu Rev Med. 2014;65:63–79.
9. Roy P, Yu LJ, Crespi CL, Waxman DJ. Development of a substrate-activity based approach to identify the major human liver P-450 catalysts of cyclophosphamide and ifosfamide activation based on cDNA-expressed activities and liver microsomal P-450 profiles. Drug Metab Dispos. 1999;27(6):655–66.
10. Xie HJ, Broberg U, Griskevicius L, Lundgren S, Carlens S, Meurling L, et al. Alteration of pharmacokinetics of cyclophosphamide and suppression of the cytochrome p450 genes by ciprofloxacin. Bone Marrow Transplant. 2003;31(3):197–203.
11. Griskevicius L, Yasar U, Sandberg M, Hidestrand M, Eliasson E, Tybring G, et al. Bioactivation of cyclophosphamide: the role of polymorphic CYP2C enzymes. Eur J Clin Pharmacol. 2003;59(2):103–9.
12. Xie H, Griskevicius L, Stahle L, Hassan Z, Yasar U, Rane A, et al. Pharmacogenetics of cyclophosphamide in patients with hematological malignancies. Eur J Pharm Sci. 2006;27 (1):54–61.
13. Nakajima M, Komagata S, Fujiki Y, Kanada Y, Ebi H, Itoh K, et al. Genetic polymorphisms of CYP2B6 affect the pharmacokinetics/pharmacodynamics of cyclophosphamide in Japanese cancer patients. Pharmacogenet Genom. 2007;17(6):431–45.
14. Gor PP, Su HI, Gray RJ, Gimotty PA, Horn M, Aplenc R, et al. Cyclophosphamide-metabolizing enzyme polymorphisms and survival outcomes after adjuvant chemotherapy for node-positive breast cancer: a retrospective cohort study. Breast Cancer Res. 2010;12(3):R26.

15. Haroun F, Al-Shaar L, Habib RH, El-Saghir N, Tfayli A, Bazarbachi A, et al. Effects of CYP2B6 genetic polymorphisms in patients receiving cyclophosphamide combination chemotherapy for breast cancer. Cancer Chemother Pharmacol. 2015;75(1):207–14.
16. Bahadur N, Leathart JB, Mutch E, Steimel-Crespi D, Dunn SA, Gilissen R, et al. CYP2C8 polymorphisms in Caucasians and their relationship with paclitaxel 6alpha-hydroxylase activity in human liver microsomes. Biochem Pharmacol. 2002;64(11):1579–89.
17. Bergmann TK, Brasch-Andersen C, Green H, Mirza M, Pedersen RS, Nielsen F, et al. Impact of CYP2C8*3 on paclitaxel clearance: a population pharmacokinetic and pharmacogenomic study in 93 patients with ovarian cancer. Pharmacogenomics J. 2011;11(2):113–20.
18. de Graan AJ, Elens L, Smid M, Martens JW, Sparreboom A, Nieuweboer AJ, et al. A pharmacogenetic predictive model for paclitaxel clearance based on the DMET platform. Clin Cancer Res. 2013;19(18):5210–7.
19. Baldwin RM, Owzar K, Zembutsu H, Chhibber A, Kubo M, Jiang C, et al. A genome-wide association study identifies novel loci for paclitaxel-induced sensory peripheral neuropathy in CALGB 40101. Clin Cancer Res. 2012;18(18):5099–109.
20. De Brabander M, Geuens G, Nuydens R, Willebrords R, De Mey J. Taxol induces the assembly of free microtubules in living cells and blocks the organizing capacity of the centrosomes and kinetochores. Proc Natl Acad Sci U S A. 1981;78(9):5608–12.
21. Zasadil LM, Andersen KA, Yeum D, Rocque GB, Wilke LG, Tevaarwerk AJ, et al. Cytotoxicity of paclitaxel in breast cancer is due to chromosome missegregation on multipolar spindles. Sci Transl Med. 2014;6(229):229ra43.
22. Friedenson B. The BRCA1/2 pathway prevents hematologic cancers in addition to breast and ovarian cancers. BMC Cancer. 2007;7:152.
23. O'Donovan PJ, Livingston DM. BRCA1 and BRCA2: breast/ovarian cancer susceptibility gene products and participants in DNA double-strand break repair. Carcinogenesis. 2010;31 (6):961–7.
24. Bolton KL, Chenevix-Trench G, Goh C, Sadetzki S, Ramus SJ, Karlan BY, et al. Association between BRCA1 and BRCA2 mutations and survival in women with invasive epithelial ovarian cancer. JAMA. 2012;307(4):382–90.
25. Bryant HE, Schultz N, Thomas HD, Parker KM, Flower D, Lopez E, et al. Specific killing of BRCA2-deficient tumours with inhibitors of poly(ADP-ribose) polymerase. Nature. 2005;434 (7035):913–7.
26. Tutt A, Robson M, Garber JE, Domchek SM, Audeh MW, Weitzel JN, et al. Oral poly (ADP-ribose) polymerase inhibitor olaparib in patients with BRCA1 or BRCA2 mutations and advanced breast cancer: a proof-of-concept trial. Lancet. 2010;376(9737):235–44.
27. Robson M, Im SA, Senkus E, Xu B, Domchek SM, Masuda N, et al. Olaparib for metastatic breast Cancer in patients with a Germline BRCA mutation. N Engl J Med. 2017;377(6):523–33.
28. Cass I, Baldwin RL, Varkey T, Moslehi R, Narod SA, Karlan BY. Improved survival in women with BRCA-associated ovarian carcinoma. Cancer. 2003;97(9):2187–95.
29. Alsop K, Fereday S, Meldrum C, de Fazio A, Emmanuel C, George J, et al. BRCA mutation frequency and patterns of treatment response in BRCA mutation-positive women with ovarian cancer: a report from the Australian ovarian Cancer study group. J Clin Oncol. 2012;30 (21):2654–63.
30. Isla D, Sarries C, Rosell R, Alonso G, Domine M, Taron M, et al. Single nucleotide polymorphisms and outcome in docetaxel-cisplatin-treated advanced non-small-cell lung cancer. Ann Oncol. 2004;15(8):1194–203.
31. Palomba G, Atzori F, Budroni M, Ombra M, Cossu A, Sini M, et al. ERCC1 polymorphisms as prognostic markers in T4 breast cancer patients treated with platinum-based chemotherapy. J Transl Med. 2014;12:272.
32. Yin M, Yan J, Martinez-Balibrea E, Graziano F, Lenz HJ, Kim HJ, et al. ERCC1 and ERCC2 polymorphisms predict clinical outcomes of oxaliplatin-based chemotherapies in gastric and colorectal cancer: a systemic review and meta-analysis. Clin Cancer Res. 2011;17(6):1632–40.

33. Jin ZY, Zhao XT, Zhang LN, Wang Y, Yue WT, Xu SF. Effects of polymorphisms in the XRCC1, XRCC3, and XPG genes on clinical outcomes of platinum-based chemotherapy for treatment of non-small cell lung cancer. Genet Mol Res. 2014;13(3):7617–25.
34. Li L, Wan C, Wen FQ. Polymorphisms in the XRCC1 gene are associated with treatment response to platinum chemotherapy in advanced non-small cell lung cancer patients based on meta-analysis. Genet Mol Res. 2014;13(2):3772–86.
35. Hu W, Pan J, Zhao P, Yang G, Yang S. Genetic polymorphisms in XPG could predict clinical outcome of platinum-based chemotherapy for advanced non-small cell lung cancer. Tumour Biol. 2014;35(6):5561–7.
36. Gallagher DJ, Vijai J, Hamilton RJ, Ostrovnaya I, Iyer G, Garcia-Grossman IR, et al. Germline single nucleotide polymorphisms associated with response of urothelial carcinoma to platinum-based therapy: the role of the host. Ann Oncol. 2013;24(9):2414–21.
37. Jiang YZ, Yu KD, Peng WT, Di GH, Wu J, Liu GY, et al. Enriched variations in TEKT4 and breast cancer resistance to paclitaxel. Nat Commun. 2014;5:3802.
38. Yu KD, Huang AJ, Fan L, Li WF, Shao ZM. Genetic variants in oxidative stress-related genes predict chemoresistance in primary breast cancer: a prospective observational study and validation. Cancer Res. 2012;72(2):408–19.
39. McCormack M, Alfirevic A, Bourgeois S, Farrell JJ, Kasperaviciute D, Carrington M, et al. HLA-A*3101 and carbamazepine-induced hypersensitivity reactions in Europeans. N Engl J Med. 2011;364(12):1134–43.
40. Pavlos R, Mallal S, Phillips E. HLA and pharmacogenetics of drug hypersensitivity. Pharmacogenomics. 2012;13(11):1285–306.
41. Spraggs CF, Budde LR, Briley LP, Bing N, Cox CJ, King KS, et al. HLA-DQA1*02:01 is a major risk factor for lapatinib-induced hepatotoxicity in women with advanced breast cancer. J Clin Oncol. 2011;29(6):667–73.
42. Schaid DJ, Spraggs CF, McDonnell SK, Parham LR, Cox CJ, Ejlertsen B, et al. Prospective validation of HLA-DRB1*07:01 allele carriage as a predictive risk factor for lapatinib-induced liver injury. J Clin Oncol. 2014;32(22):2296–303.
43. Sondermann P, Huber R, Oosthuizen V, Jacob U. The 3.2-a crystal structure of the human IgG1 fc fragment-fc gammaRIII complex. Nature. 2000;406(6793):267–73.
44. Varchetta S, Gibelli N, Oliviero B, Nardini E, Gennari R, Gatti G, et al. Elements related to heterogeneity of antibody-dependent cell cytotoxicity in patients under trastuzumab therapy for primary operable breast cancer overexpressing Her2. Cancer Res. 2007;67(24):11991–9.
45. Tamura K, Shimizu C, Hojo T, Akashi-Tanaka S, Kinoshita T, Yonemori K, et al. FcgammaR2A and 3A polymorphisms predict clinical outcome of trastuzumab in both neoadjuvant and metastatic settings in patients with HER2-positive breast cancer. Ann Oncol. 2011;22(6):1302–7.
46. Hurvitz SA, Betting DJ, Stern HM, Quinaux E, Stinson J, Seshagiri S, et al. Analysis of Fcgamma receptor IIIa and IIa polymorphisms: lack of correlation with outcome in trastuzumab-treated breast cancer patients. Clin Cancer Res. 2012;18(12):3478–86.
47. Tsai KK, Daud AI. Nivolumab plus ipilimumab in the treatment of advanced melanoma. J Hematol Oncol. 2015;8:123.

Chapter 20
Hormone Resistance

Jonghan Yu

Abstract Hormone therapy is a major therapy for hormone receptor-positive breast cancer that improves survival. However, despite these hormone treatments, there are de novo or acquired resistance of breast cancer. Many studies revealed these resistance mechanisms, which are related to hormonal receptors including low expression or mutation of estrogen receptor alpha(ERα), co-factors and progesterone receptor, and with activation of growth signaling pathways such as PIK3A/Akt/mTOR pathway or cell cycle pathway. To overcome endocrine resistance based on these mechanisms, there have been many efforts in clinical studies of new agents which are representative of steroidal selective estrogen receptor down-regulator, cyclin-dependent kinase (CDK) 4/6 inhibitors, inhibitors of the PI3K/AKT/mTOR Pathway and histone deacetylase (HDAC) Inhibitors. Our studies at LBCB focused the endocrine resistance in young age and showed that age under 35 years is poor prognostic factor on not only single-center data but also Korean Breast Cancer Registry Data and that women with hormone receptor-positive breast cancer who were younger than 35 years of age had less response to anti-hormonal therapy. Also, a study for gene expression in hormone receptor-positive breast cancer at a very young age (<35) revealed that *e*xpression of cell cycle-related genes increased higher than that of premenopausal women in their forties. There have been a lot of studies and clinical trials to investigate the mechanisms of resistance to endocrine treatment and to overcome them with new drugs. However, many still do not know the precise mechanism of recurrence of breast cancer after endocrine treatment. In particular, the identification of the mechanism of endocrine resistance in young

J. Yu (✉)
Breast Division, Department of Surgery, Samsung Medical Center, Seoul, South Korea

Department of Surgery, Sungkyunkwan University School of Medicine, Seoul, South Korea

D.-Y. Noh et al. (eds.), *Translational Research in Breast Cancer*, Advances in Experimental Medicine and Biology 1187,
https://doi.org/10.1007/978-981-32-9620-6_20

women, and the combination of drugs and clinical trials to overcome this require much effort.

Keywords Breast neoplasm · Hormones · Resistance · Age · Young

Hormone therapy is a major therapy for hormone receptor-positive breast cancer that improves not only disease-free survival but also overall survival (OS). From tamoxifen, aromatase inhibitors and ovarian ablation (GnRH agonist, oophorectomy, and ovarian radiation) have been used as hormone therapy. However, despite these hormone treatments, there are cases of recurrence of breast cancer. Any patient with hormone receptor-positive tumors do not respond to endocrine treatment (de novo resistance) or those who responded to endocrine treatment initially become the refractory to the treatment later (acquired resistance). Moreover, hormone receptor-positive breast cancer does not lower its risk compared with recurrent hormone receptor-negative breast cancer after 5 years. This recurrence pattern is the basis for a decade of hormone therapy.

In this section, we review the basic mechanisms and clinical factors related to the resistance to hormone therapy, and also describe the studies in LBCB that have been conducted in relation to this.

20.1 Bench: Molecular Mechanism and Conquest of Endocrine Therapy Resistance

20.1.1 Hormone Receptor

20.1.1.1 Estrogen Receptor (ER)

ERα low expression: lack of ERα expression is the primary mechanism for de novo endocrine resistance.

ERα mutation (ESR1 mutation): The mutation of the ESR1 gene, which matches the estrogen receptor, activates estrogen receptor function with or without estrogen, and induces the expression of genes related to cell proliferation. Therefore, endocrine treatment, especially the treatment of postmenopausal breast cancer in a way (aromatase inhibitor(AI)-treated breast cancer) that lowers estrogen level, is not effective in breast cancer with ESR1 gene mutation, resulting in endocrine resistance.

Cofactors: In order to activate estrogen receptors, various cofactors are involved, and their response to antihormonal therapy may vary depending on their action and degree. Typical cofactors activate the estrogen receptor-related pathway through its mechanism of action so that inhibitors to these can be used to overcome endocrine resistance.

20.1.1.2 Progesterone Receptor (PR)

PR, estrogen-related receptor, is expressed in about 50% of ER+ breast cancer. ER+/PR+ breast cancer is generally more responsive to endocrine treatment than ER+/PR- breast cancer. PR- in ER+ breast cancers was able to serve as a poor predictor of endocrine treatment outcome [1]. Previous study showed that PR and Her1-3 status could be a predictor of early recurrence in ER+ tamoxifen-treated breast cancer [2]. So, more studies for relation of PR with growth factor activities are needed to solve the resistance on endocrine treatment and to overcome the endocrine-resistance breast cancer.

20.1.2 Growth Signaling Pathway

20.1.2.1 RTK (GF) Signaling Pathway (PIK3A/Akt/mTOR Pathway)

If SERM or SERD block the estrogen receptor-related pathway, another growth factor-related RTK signaling pathway may be activated at the opposite end. The most representative pathway is the PIK3A/Akt/mTOR pathway. Many molecules targeting Akt and mTOR have been developed and undergoing clinical trials. In particular, mTOR inhibitors have already been shown to be effective in recurrence or metastasis of hormone receptor-positive breast cancer in clinical trials and have been used for treatment with exemestane and combination therapies. Many candidate drugs targeting PIK3A and Akt are currently in clinical trials.

20.1.2.2 Cell-Cycle Regulators

Another pathway that increases expression when estrogen receptor activation is blocked is the cell-cycle pathway. Several regulators have been identified and inhibitors that target them are currently being used in clinical trials and others being in clinical trials. In particular, the CDK4/6 inhibitors (palbociclib, ribociclib, abemaciclib, etc.) are now being used as second-line aromatase inhibitors or GnRH agonists and AI in recurrent or metastatic hormone receptor positive breast cancer. In particular, clinical trials showed that the addition of these agents extended the progression-free survival (PFS) by more than two times compared with the use of antihormonal agents alone.

20.2 Bed: Clinical Trials—Overcoming Endocrine Resistance

There have been many efforts and new drugs for overcoming the endocrine resistance. We will classify them according to the mechanism.

20.2.1 *Fulvestrant*

Fulvestrant is a steroidal selective estrogen receptor down-regulator that blocks ER and degrades its function. This drug was given intramuscularly and did not show superior results when compared with conventional tamoxifen and anastrozole at a dose of 250 mg [3–6].

It is known that the dosage of 250 mg once a day for the first time after loading with 500 mg reaches the concentration for 250 mg for 3–6 months within 28 days [7]. A loading dose fulvestrant alone showed similar median time to progression (TTP) in the EFFECT trial compared with exemestane in postmenopausal breast cancer patients who progressed in taking nonsteroidal aromatase inhibitors [8]. The results of SOFEA and FACT trial, which compared the loading dose fulvestrant in combination with an aromatase inhibitor with fulvestrant alone or with AI alone, did not show superior results in acquired resistance to prior endocrine therapy [9, 10]. However, SWOG 0226 trial involving tamoxifen therapy with approximately 40% with de novo metastatic disease and 60% without prior adjuvant therapy, fulvestrant–anastrozole combination, showed better median time progression-free survival than anastrozole alone or sequential anastrozole and fulvestrant [11]. CONFIRM trial comparing this use with 250 mg showed high progression-free survival(PFS) in the high-dose group (500 mg) in postmenopausal patients with recurrent breast cancer in whom previous endocrine therapy had failed [12]. Subsequent data analysis also showed a median overall survival (OS) of 4.1 months longer in the high-dose group [13].

20.2.2 *CDK 4/6 Inhibitors*

The CDK 4/6 inhibitors inhibit cell growth by stopping the cell cycle. Here are studies showing the combination of CDK 4/6 inhibitor and AI for postmenopausal women with metastatic breast cancer. The CDK 4/6 inhibitors inhibit cell growth by stopping the cell cycle. PALOMA-1 and PALOMA-2 trials have shown that combination of palbociclib and letrozole improves median PFS compared with letrozole alone [14, 15]. The MONALEESA-2 trial showed that the combination of ribociclib and letrozole is better than letrozole alone [16]. The PALOMA-3 trial showed that the combination of palbociclib and fulvestrant was more than twice as likely to improve PFS as compared with fulvestrant alone. In addition, luteinizing hormone-releasing hormone agonist goserelin was added to premenopausal women, and the results showed the same high PFS [17].

Studies using a variety of CDK 4/6 inhibitors have been conducted. There is the study of the use of ribociclib–fulvestrant which included patients with advanced breast cancer who had progressed on only 1 prior line of endocrine therapy (MONALEESA-3 trial). MONARCH-2, -3 trials are about abemaciclib in combination with fulvestrant or a nonsteroidal AI for patients with pretreated HR-positive breast cancer [18].

20.2.3 Inhibitors of the PI3K/AKT/mTOR Pathway

The PI3K/AKT/mTOR signaling pathway is a very important pathway in many diverse cellular processes. Therefore, aberrations of this pathway have been implicated in cancer development and resistance to cancer treatment [19]. However, these aspects have developed the new therapeutic modalities to treat breast cancer with endocrine resistance.

Inhibition of mTOR activation has been often involved in cancer-cell resistance to treatment [20]. In BOLERO-2 trial, everolimus in combination with steroidal AI (exemestane) showed significantly better PFS in postmenopausal patients who had progressed on prior nonsteroidal AIs, compared with AI alone [21]. Furthermore, in the phase II TAMRAD study, tamoxifen–everolimus was assessed in postmenopausal patients who had progressed on prior nonsteroidal AIs. Combination arm was better than tamoxifen alone in time to progression (TTP) and OS [22]. In the most recent phase II study (PRECOG 0102), the addition of everolimus to high-dose fulvestrant, compared with fulvestrant–placebo, doubled the median PFS in postmenopausal metastatic breast cancer resistant to AI therapy [23].

Alterations in the PI3k/AKT pathway are frequently associated with resistance to endocrine therapy in breast cancer. Somatic mutations in the PI3K catalytic subunit p110α(PIK3CA) are the most common genetic alterations in that pathway [24]. The results of the pan-PI3K inhibitor (buparlisib) with fulvestrant in BELLE-3 trial and BELLE-2 trial are waiting. In the phase III SOLAR-1 trial, alpelisib, an α-specific PI3K inhibitor, in combination with fulvestrant in patients with disease progression on prior AI therapy is ongoing. Another ongoing phase III trial, SANDPIPER, is combining taselisib, another α-specific PI3K inhibitor, with fulvestrant in postmenopausal patients with *PIK3CA*-mutant who progressed on prior AIs.

20.2.4 Histone Deacetylase (HDAC) Inhibitors

The repression of ER is affected by HDAC at a transcriptional level. This is a potential mechanism of resistance. Inhibitors of HDAC therefore potentially offer a way to overcome endocrine resistance. So, the efficacy of adding a HDAC inhibitor (entinostat, vorinostat) to AI therapy in women whose breast cancer has progressed is being evaluated (NCT00828854, NCT01720602 at http://ClinicalTrials.gov).

20.3 LBCB Studies Related with Young Age Breast Cancer

20.3.1 Bed

The study for Korean breast cancer patients also showed the same result as that of previous western study and that age under 35 years is poor prognostic factor independently by multivariate analysis on single center data (Fig. 20.1) and Korean Breast Cancer Registry Data (Fig. 20.2) [25, 26].

The analysis for relation between age at diagnosis and death revealed that hazard ratio was increased by 5% according to decreasing of 1 year from 35 years in contrast to that there was no significant change of hazard ratio in patients over 35 years (Fig. 20.3) [27].

Women with hormone receptor-positive breast cancer who were younger than 35 years of age had a worse prognosis than women with hormone receptor-positive

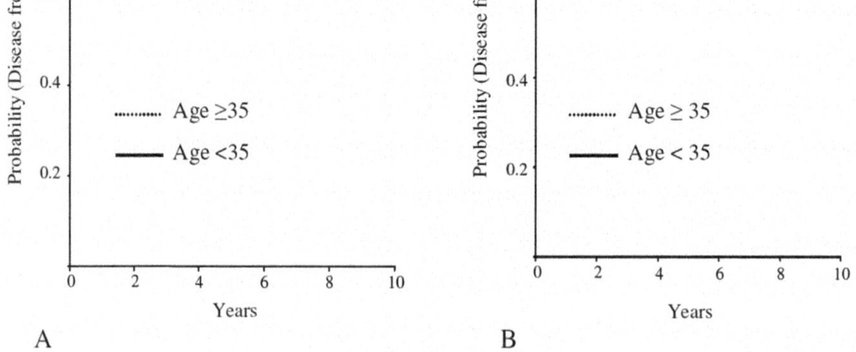

Fig. 20.1 (**a**) Disease-free survival curves for women <35 vs. ≥35 years old. Patients younger than 35 had significantly worse outcomes than their older counterparts ($p < 0.001$). (**b**) Overall survival curves showing patients younger than 35 had significantly worse outcomes than their older counterparts ($p = 0.002$)

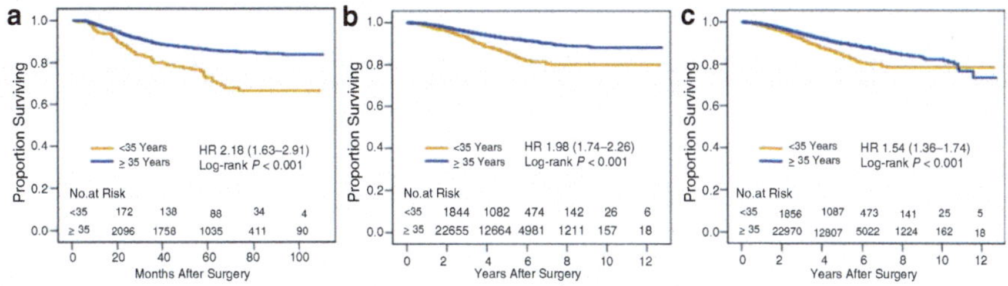

Fig. 20.2 Survival curves for younger (<35 years) and older (≥35 years) patients. (**a**) Recurrence-free survivals for the SNUHBCC database. (**b**) Breast cancer-specific survivals for the KBCR database. (**c**) Overall survivals for the KBCR database

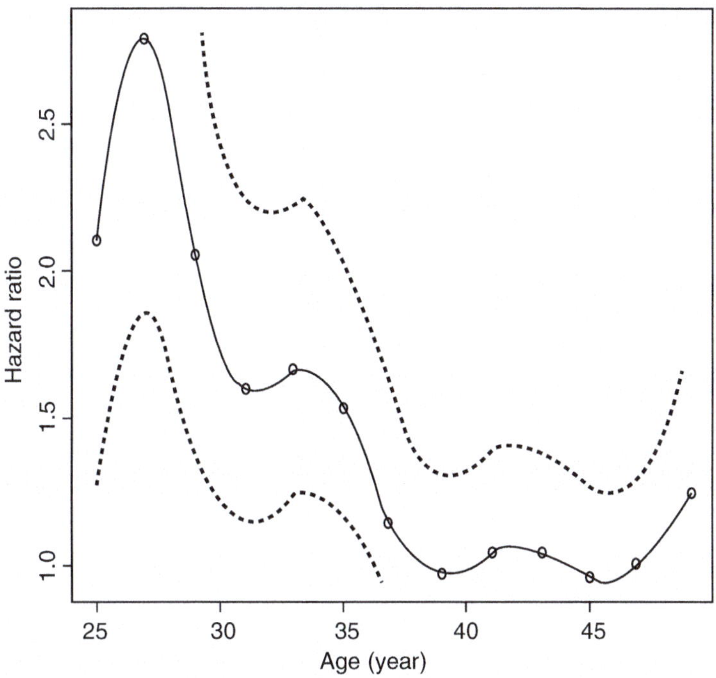

Fig. 20.3 Plot of the relationship between breast cancer onset age and hazard ratio

breast cancer in their forties of the same premenopausal age and had less response to antihormonal therapy (Fig. 20.4) [28].

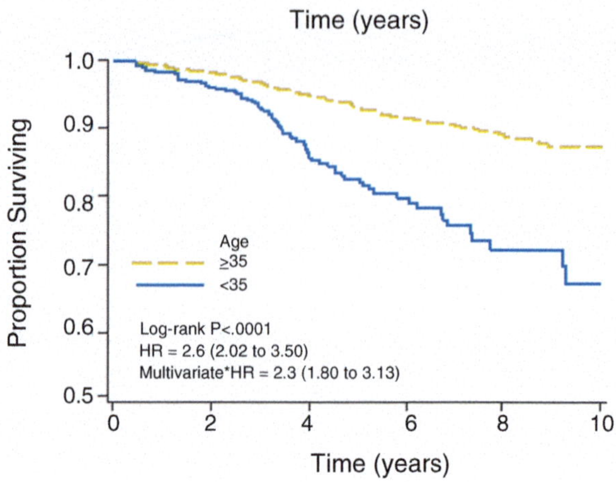

Fig. 20.4 Breast cancer-specific survival according to age in adjuvant hormone therapy when hormone receptor status is unknown or positive

20.3.2 Bench to Bed: Translational Area in LBCB

20.3.2.1 Study for Gene Expression in Hormone Receptor-Positive Breast Cancer with Very Young Age (<35)

Expression of cell cycle-related genes through cDNA microarray was increased in breast cancer in women younger than 35 years of age compared with premenopausal women in their forties. Based on this, 40 genes were selected, which were associated with the cell cycle gene, CCNB1 (Table 20.1). In silico validation based on the expression of these 40 gene set, the prognosis was poor when the expression of these 40 gene set was high (Fig. 20.5). In the future, it is necessary to validate the expression in breast cancer tissues under 35 years old and breast cancer tissues in women in their forties.

20.4 Conclusion

There are a lot of studies and clinical trials to investigate the mechanisms of resistance to endocrine treatment and to overcome them with new drugs. However, many still do not know the precise mechanism of recurrence of breast cancer after endocrine treatment. In particular, the identification of the mechanism of endocrine resistance in young women and the combination of drugs and clinical trials to overcome this require much effort.

Table 20.1 40 genes correlated with CCNB1

Gene	Correlation coeff.	Gene	Correlation coeff.
CCNB1	1	NDC80	0.702598
DEPDC1B	0.775522	UBE2C	0 701318
BTJB1B	0.770129	FAM83D	0.695056
CKS2	0.754076	PLK4	0.69184
PBK	0.750199	CDCA5	0.687702
CDK1	0.745293	KIF2C	0.687533
MELK	0.743334	NCAPG	0.684262
SKA3	0.740616	HJURP	0.683499
CCNB2	0.739845	PCNA	0.68234
GINS1	0.736509	TOP2A	0.681719
KIF11	0.730844	NEK2	0.679521
DLGAP5	0.729363	BIRC5	0.673604
PTTG1	0.726934	NUF2	0.666893
MAD2L1	0.720674	TTK	0.662272
KIF15	0.718614	CCDC99	0.658729
FBXO5	0.712902	KIF23	0.6573
TPX2	0.711182	CENPF	0.655939
SPC25	0.71081	CCNA2	0.654745
MYBL2	0.709569	PLK1	0.654105
BUB1	0.708197	AURKA	0 645461

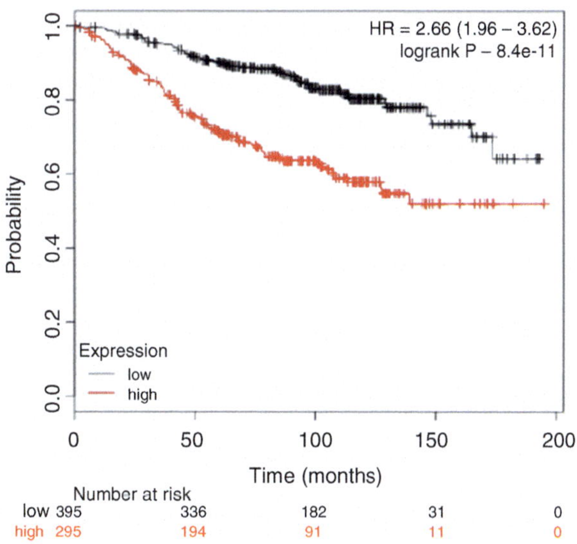

Fig. 20.5 Kaplan–Meier Plotter by using 40 gene set related with CCNB1 gene in hormone-positive breast cancer

References

1. Bardou VJ, et al. Progesterone receptor status significantly improves outcome prediction over estrogen receptor status alone for adjuvant endocrine therapy in two large breast cancer databases. J Clin Oncol. 2003;21(10):1973–9.
2. Tovey S, et al. Can molecular markers predict when to implement treatment with aromatase inhibitors in invasive breast cancer? Clin Cancer Res. 2005;11(13):4835–42.
3. Osborne CK, et al. Double-blind, Randomized trial comparing the efficacy and tolerability of fulvestrant versus anastrozole in postmenopausal women with advanced breast cancer progressing on prior endocrine therapy: results of a North American trial. J Clin Oncol. 2002;20(16):3386–95.
4. Howell A, et al. Comparison of fulvestrant versus tamoxifen for the treatment of advanced breast cancer in postmenopausal women previously untreated with endocrine therapy: a multinational, double-blind, randomized trial. J Clin Oncol. 2004;22(9):1605–13.
5. Howell A, et al. Fulvestrant, formerly ICI 182,780, is as effective as anastrozole in postmenopausal women with advanced breast cancer progressing after prior endocrine treatment. J Clin Oncol. 2002;20(16):3396–403.
6. Vergote I, Robertson JFR. Fulvestrant is an effective and well-tolerated endocrine therapy for postmenopausal women with advanced breast cancer: results from clinical trials. Br J Cancer. 2004;90:S11–4.
7. Robertson JFR, et al. Pharmacokinetic profile of intramuscular fulvestrant in advanced breast cancer. Clin Pharmacokinet. 2004;43(8):529–38.
8. Chia S, et al. Double-blind, randomized placebo controlled trial of fulvestrant compared with exemestane after prior nonsteroidal aromatase inhibitor therapy in postmenopausal women with hormone receptor-positive, advanced breast cancer: results from EFECT. J Clin Oncol. 2008;26 (10):1664–70.
9. Johnston SR, et al. Fulvestrant plus anastrozole or placebo versus exemestane alone after progression on non-steroidal aromatase inhibitors in postmenopausal patients with hormone-receptor-positive locally advanced or metastatic breast cancer (SoFEA): a composite, multicentre, phase 3 randomised trial. Lancet Oncol. 2013;14(10):989–98.
10. Bergh J, et al. FACT: an open-label randomized phase III study of fulvestrant and anastrozole in combination compared with anastrozole alone as first-line therapy for patients with receptor-positive postmenopausal breast cancer. J Clin Oncol. 2012;30(16):1919–25.
11. Mehta RS, et al. Combination anastrozole and fulvestrant in metastatic breast cancer. N Engl J Med. 2012;367(5):435–44.
12. Di Leo A, et al. Results of the confirm phase III trial comparing fulvestrant 250 mg with fulvestrant 500 mg in postmenopausal women with estrogen receptor-positive advanced breast cancer. J Clin Oncol. 2010;28(30):4594–600.
13. Di Leo A, et al. Final overall survival: fulvestrant 500 mg vs 250 mg in the randomized confirm trial. JNCI. 2014;106:1.
14. Finn RS, et al. The cyclin-dependent kinase 4/6 inhibitor palbociclib in combination with letrozole versus letrozole alone as first-line treatment of oestrogen receptor-positive, HER2-negative, advanced breast cancer (PALOMA-1/TRIO-18): a randomised phase 2 study. Lancet Oncol. 2015;16(1):25–35.
15. Finn RS, et al. Palbociclib and letrozole in advanced breast cancer. N Engl J Med. 2016;375 (20):1925–36.
16. Hortobagyi GN, et al. Ribociclib as first-line therapy for HR-positive, advanced breast cancer. N Engl J Med. 2016;375(18):1738–48.
17. Turner NC, Bartlett CH, Cristofanilli M. Palbociclib in hormone-receptor-positive advanced breast cancer reply. N Engl J Med. 2015;373(17):1672–3.

18. Dickler MN, et al. MONARCH 1, a phase II study of abemaciclib, a CDK4 and CDK6 inhibitor, as a single agent, in patients with refractory HR+/HER2(-) metastatic breast cancer. Clin Cancer Res. 2017;23(17):5218–24.
19. Vivanco I, Sawyers CL. The phosphatidylinositol 3-kinase AKT pathway in human cancer. Nat Rev Cancer. 2002;2(7):489–501.
20. Jiang BH, Liu LZ. Role of mTOR in anticancer drug resistance: perspectives for improved drug treatment. Drug Resist Updat. 2008;11(3):63–76.
21. Baselga J, et al. Everolimus in postmenopausal hormone-receptor-positive advanced breast cancer. N Engl J Med. 2012;366(6):520–9.
22. Bachelot T, et al. Randomized phase II trial of everolimus in combination with tamoxifen in patients with hormone receptor-positive, human epidermal growth factor receptor 2-negative metastatic breast cancer with prior exposure to aromatase inhibitors: a GINECO study. J Clin Oncol. 2012;30(22):2718–24.
23. Kornblum NS, et al. PrECOG 0102: a randomized, double-blind, phase II trial of fulvestrant plus everolimus or placebo in post-menopausal women with hormone receptor (HR)-positive, HER2-negative metastatic breast cancer (MBC) resistant to aromatase inhibitor (AI) therapy. Cancer Res. 2017;2017:77.
24. Koboldt DC, et al. Comprehensive molecular portraits of human breast tumours. Nature. 2012;490(7418):61–70.
25. Han WS, et al. Young age: an independent risk factor for disease-free survival in women with operable breast cancer. BMC Cancer. 2004;2004:4.
26. Kim EK, et al. Prognostic significance of young age (<35 years) by subtype based on ER, PR, and HER2 status in breast cancer: a nationwide registry-based study. World J Surg. 2011;35 (6):1244–53.
27. Han W, Kang S, Soc KBC. Relationship between age at diagnosis and outcome of premenopausal breast cancer: age less than 35 years is a reasonable cut-off for defining young age-onset breast cancer. Breast Cancer Res Treat. 2010;119(1):193–200.
28. Ahn SH, et al. Poor outcome of hormone receptor-positive breast cancer at very young age is due to tamoxifen resistance: nationwide survival data in Korea - a report from the Korean Breast Cancer Society. J Clin Oncol. 2007;25(17):2360–8.

Part V
Managing High Risk Women

Chapter 21
High-Risk Population Based on BC Risk Factors

Sue K. Park and Keun-Young Yoo

Abstract Breast cancer (BC) is the second leading cause of female cancers worldwide in 2018, followed by lung cancer, and the fifth fatal cancer, followed by lung, colorectal, gastric, and liver cancers. The incidence and mortality rates of breast cancer in Western women have been shown to decrease for a long period of time, while the incidence and mortality rates of Asian women are rapidly increasing. The incidence and mortality rates of BC in Western women have been changing to a recent decrease from a fluctuation in rates for a long time, while in Asian women, the incidence and mortality rates have increased rapidly. The secular changes in rates are mainly related to medical advancement in treatment or diagnosis for BC, and preventive management and policy in each country, but also to the change of risk factors in the population.

In this chapter, we briefly review the epidemiologic characteristics of breast cancer reported so far and summarize the results for various risk factors of breast cancer. Moreover, we summarize the potential for risk modification in high-risk population of breast cancer with various risk factors.

Keywords Breast neoplasm · Epidemiology · Risk factors · Risk modification · Prevention

S. K. Park (✉)
Department of Preventive Medicine, Seoul National University College of Medicine, Seoul, South Korea

Cancer Research Institute, Seoul National University, Seoul, South Korea
e-mail: suepark@snu.ac.kr

K.-Y. Yoo
Department of Preventive Medicine, Seoul National University College of Medicine, Seoul, South Korea

Graduate School of Cancer Science and Policy, National Cancer Center, Goyang-si, Gyeonggi-do, South Korea

D.-Y. Noh et al. (eds.), *Translational Research in Breast Cancer*, Advances in Experimental Medicine and Biology 1187,
https://doi.org/10.1007/978-981-32-9620-6_21

21.1 Introduction

Breast cancer (BC) is the second leading cause of cancer among women worldwide, followed by lung cancer. The rates of BC can be mostly attributed to changes in environmental factors such as westernization of lifestyles, dietary intake, and the changes of reproductive factors. Family history and genetic predisposition, including BRCA1 and 2 mutations, are also important risk factors for BC. BC with a family history of BC or ovarian cancer, early BC diagnosed before age 40, or other cancers that may be caused by BRCA mutations, since it is highly probable to have a genetic predisposition, it is necessary to consult with experts on whether they are subject to genetic testing such as BRCA1, 2 mutations, etc.

Finding the epidemiologic features and risk factors of BC is important for predicting the probability of individual BC development and establishing guidelines for BC prevention and intervention. In this chapter, we will look at the risk factors of BC, BC risk assessment models, and BC prevention methods based on BC risk factors.

21.2 Epidemiology of BC

In 2018, BC incidence rates are 46.3 per 100,000 women and more than two million new BC cases ($N = 2,088,849$) of 18,078,957 cancer cases worldwide occurred. BC has geographical variation in incidence rates and mortality rates (Fig. 21.1) [1, 2].

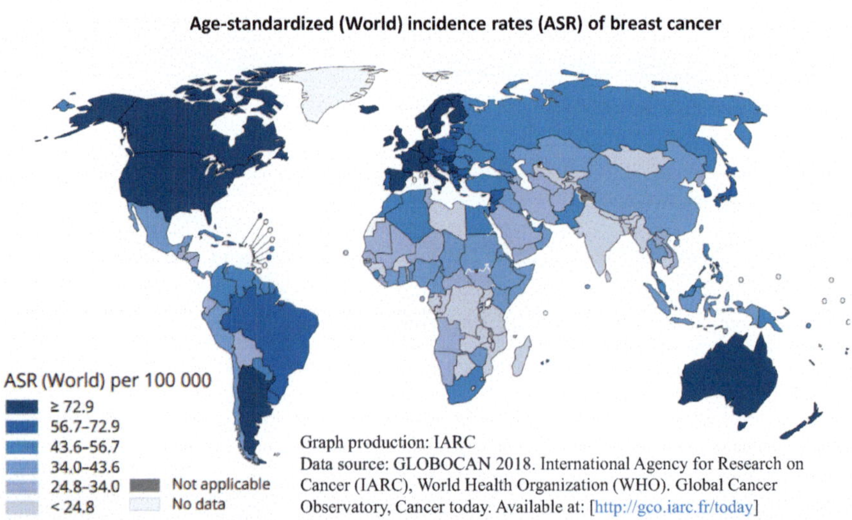

Fig. 21.1 Geographical variation in age-standardized (World) incidence rates (ASIR) of BC

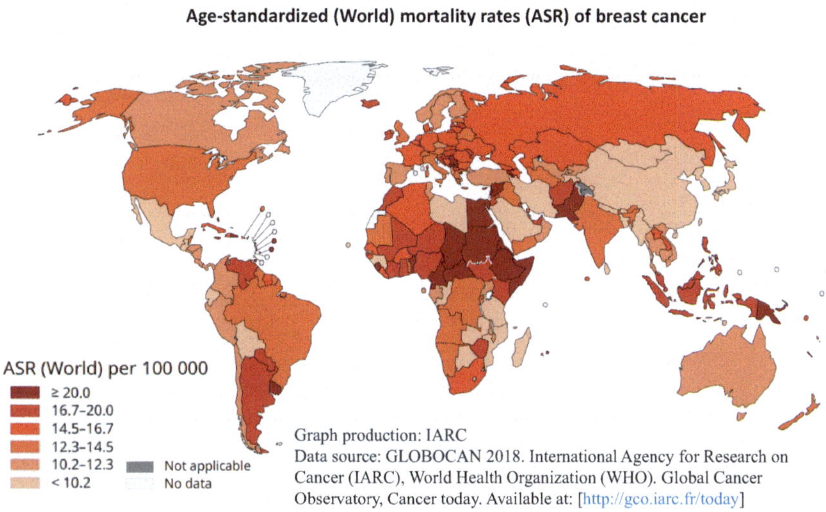

Fig. 21.2 Geographical variation in age-standardized (World) mortality rates (ASMR) of BC

The highest incidence rates were found among women in Oceania, North America, most of western and northern Europe but mortality rates in those regions were low, while the lowest incidence rates were found among those in middle and Eastern Africa but the highest mortality rates area were found. Although BC is the most common cancer among most Asian women as well as Western women, BC incidence in Asian women is still low compared to Western women in 2012.

The mortality rates of BC were 13.0 per 100,000 women in the world in 2018, followed by lung, colorectal, gastric, liver cancers, and 626,679 (6.6%) BC deaths occurred among total 9,555,027 deaths. BC also has geographical variation in mortality rates (Fig. 21.2) [1, 3].

Over the past two decades, the mortality rates of BC have continued to increase in Asian countries, but mortality has declined in Western countries.

The 5-year survival rates of BC in Korea and Japan are similar to those in USA (Korea, 92.7% in 2012–2016; Japan, 91.1% in 2006–2008; USA, 91.1% in 2006–2010). Therefore, it is expected that BC mortality rate will slow down and then return to a declining trend in the future in Japan and Korea [4, 5, 6].

The incidence and mortality rates of BC have been increasing steadily in Asian women over the past two decades, whereas the incidence rates have been decreasing or very slightly increasing pattern and the mortality rates have been dramatically decreasing in Western women, except brazilian women (Figs. 21.3 and 21.4) [2, 3]. The secular changes in rates are mainly related to medical advancement in treatment or diagnosis for BC, and preventive management and policy in each country, but also to the change of risk factors in the population.

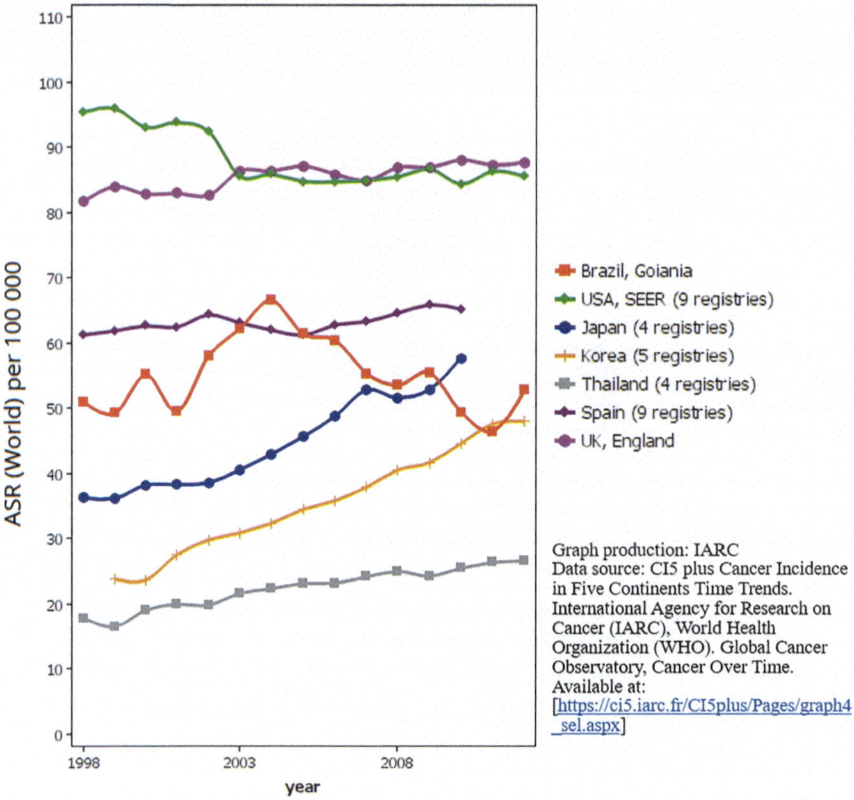

Fig. 21.3 Secular trend in age-standardized (World) incidence rates (ASIR) of BC

21.3 Risk Factors of BC

The BC is defined as multifactorial disease, including hormonal factors, genetic factors, family history, medications, personal diseases, environmental factors including internal environmental factors such as lifestyle, dietary factors, and external environmental factors such as occupational exposures, pesticides, pollutants, etc. Among them, the exposure of cumulative sex hormones (major: estrogen and progesterone, and minor: testosterone) is known to be the most important factor of BC.

The International Agency for Research for Cancer (IARC) in the World Health Organization (WHO) selected exogenous synthetic sex hormones (including estrogen–progesterone (E-P) combined postmenopausal hormone replacement therapy (HRT), E-P combined oral contraceptives, and diethylstilbestrol (DES)) as carcinogenic to BC with sufficient evidence for the human body (Table 21.1) [7].

The risk of BC increases gradually with longer use of HRT in current or recent users (recent users defined as past users within 5 years from BC diagnosis). Current

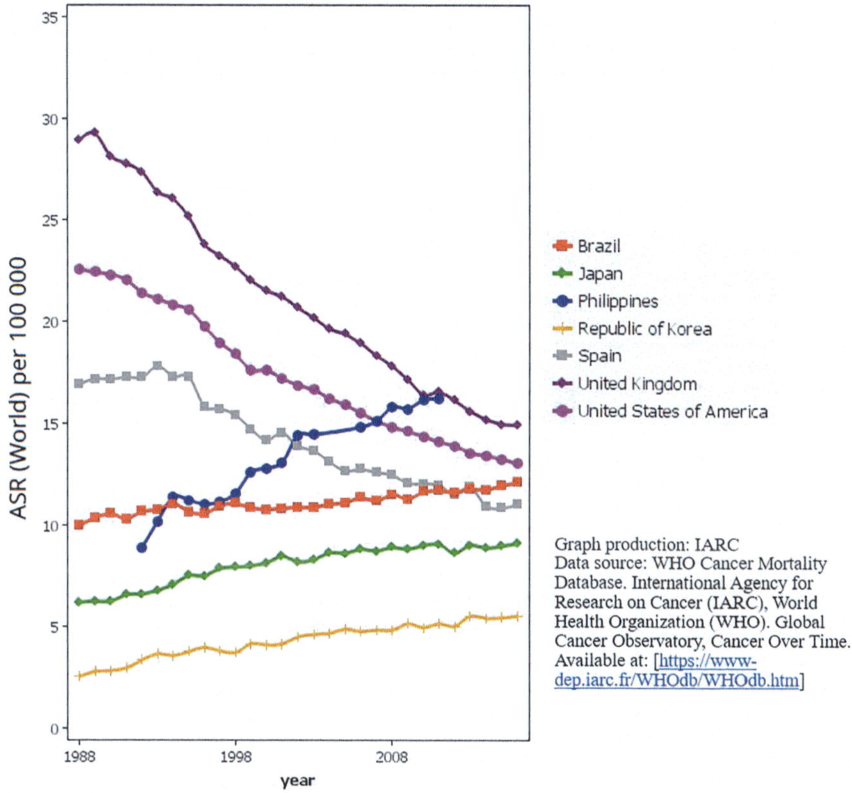

Fig. 21.4 Secular trend in age-standardized (World) mortality rates (ASMR) of BC

users of combined HRT are associated with at least 1.5 times higher risk for BC compared to nonusers, which is consistently observed in the Women's Health Initiative (WHI) clinical trial and its extended cohort study. The risk of BC among past users are near RR = 1 and even excess risk among current users disappear after 2 years from the last use. E-only HRT, selected as group 2A carcinogenic agent to BC by the IARC (probable carcinogen in human) [7], increases BC risk by 1.3-fold.

Ever use of oral contraceptives (OC), relative to nonuse, has very low risk of BC (1.1-fold). Total current users have 1.2-fold higher risk of BC. Current users who use OC for 1–4 years slightly increases BC risk by 1.3-fold and increasing duration of OC use correlates increasing BC risk, while recent users who use OC for at least 5–9 years have at same BC risk (1.3-fold). There was no correlation between duration of use and risk of BC in non-recent past users. Women who have started OC use (age < 20) are at a moderately increased risk (RR = 1.5) for BC.

Diethylstilbestrol (DES) is a legendary drug used in the past that relates to subsequent BC in users and vaginal clear cell carcinoma in users' daughters [7]. It was developed as a synthetic estrogen in 1938 and was approved by the US Food and Drug Administration (FDA) in 1947 for the treatment of threatening or habitual

Table 21.1 Environmental risk factors for BC

	'Sufficient evidence' in human carcinogen (IARC) [7]	Strong evidence in 'convincing' or 'probable' causal relation (WCRF/AICR) [8]
BC risk increased	Alcoholic drinks E-P combined HRT E-P combined contraceptives Diethylstilbestrol (DES) x- or γ-radiation	Alcoholic drinks Tall height Body fatness throughout adulthood (measured by BMI, WC, WHR) [in postmenopausal women] Adult weight gain[a] [in postmenopausal women] Greater birth weight [in premenopausal women]
BC risk decreased		Lactation Body fatness at age 18–30 Vigorous physical activity Physical activity (total, recreational, occupational, and household activity) [in postmenopausal women]

[a]The results were associated with reduced risk of premenopausal breast cancer in the meta-analysis of the WCRF/AICR. The results were consistent among Western women but among Asian women, were rather opposite, showing increased risk

abortions. However, its use was reduced after two studies reported no efficacy in the prevention of miscarriage, premature birth, and preeclampsia in 1953. Nevertheless, it had been continually used in the USA and Europe until early and late 1970s, respectively. DES-exposed women relative to non-exposed women had a slightly increased risk of BC (RR = 1.4); and excess risk was observed at least 20 years after DES administration. DES was not used in women before in Asian countries including Korea and Japan.

The risk of individual BC increases with age due to the lifetime effects of female hormones and the exposure of environmental factors to female hormones. Therefore, women's age is an important demographic factor because not only female hormones but also the related risk factors are affected by age (Table 21.2). Family history of BC among families with first or second degree relatives, accounting for approximately 6–19% of all BC patients, is associated with increased risk for BC, and as the number of BC family history increases, the risk of BC increases (Table 21.2). In the SEBCS (Seoul BC Study), a population-based case–control study composed of about 5000 BC cases and 6500 controls, the family history of BC among families at first and second relatives is observed in 7–10% of cases and 2–3% of controls and it is associated with 1.5–2.3 fold higher risk for BC in prior studies [9].

Hereditary BC caused by specific genes. The best known of these is the genes from BRCA1 and 2 mutations. Although the prevalence of BRCA1 and BRCA2 gene in the general population is rare (<0.1%), women who have BRCA1 and 2 mutations have increased risk of BC, hereditary breast-ovarian cancer syndromes, as well as increase risk of BRCA-relating cancers such as pancreatic, colorectal, and larynx cancers. The lifetime risk of BC in women with BRCA 1/2 mutations is

Table 21.2 Individual predisposing or precipitating risk factors of BC

Factors	Individual risk factors
Age	Age increase
Benign breast status	Benign breast diseases Proliferative diseases without atypia Proliferative diseases with atypia Dense breast on mammography (Fibroglandular breast tissue)
Past BCs	Breast carcinoma in situ Triple negative BC
Familial factors	Family history (FH) of BC FH of BC among families of first degree relatives FH of BC among families of first/second degree relatives The number of family members with BC FH
Genetic factors	High penetrance genes (very rare–rare prevalence and high risk) BRCA1, BRCA2: Major in hereditary breast and ovarian cancer (HBOC) syndrome Tumor suppressors such as TP53, CDH1, STK11, PTEN, NBS1 Moderate penetrance genes (rare prevalence and moderate risk) DNA repair genes such as ATM, CHEK2, RAD50, FANCJ, ATR Low penetrance genes (common prevalence and low risk using polygenic risk score (PRS)) FGFR2, LSP1, MAP3K1, TGFB1, TOX3, VEGF, PGR, KRAS, etc.

substantially increased compared to the general population regardless of ethnic groups [10, 11, 12]. High penetrance genes including BRCA1/2 mutations, and moderate and low penetrance genes for BC (Table 21.2) [10, 11], will be described in detail in the next chapters.

Benign breast diseases are also risk factors for BC under pathologic classification and radiologic classification. Dense breast showing fibroglandular breast tissue, found in mammograms as a radiological classification, is associated with increasing BC risk (Table 21.2). Of pathologically benign epithelial breast diseases (which are classified into three categories such as non-proliferative breast disease including breast cysts, apocrine change, epithelial calcifications, and mild hyperplasia, similar terms of fibrocystic disease, chronic cystic mastitis, and mammary dysplasia, non-atypical breast proliferation, and atypical hyperplasia), non-atypical breast proliferation and atypical hyperplasia are associated with BC risk (Table 21.2). The BC risk progressively increases from non-atypical breast proliferation to atypical hyperplasia. According to BC subtype, both non-atypical breast proliferation and atypical hyperplasia are associated with only ER + BC subtype.

Women with breast carcinoma in situ (BCIS) are at higher risk of subsequent invasive BC relative to general population. In the analysis by BC molecular subtypes, triple negative BC (TNBC) subtype has an elevated risk of subsequent invasive BC, relative to other subtypes.

Table 21.3 Reproductive risk factors of BC

Factors	Individual risk factors
Menstrual history	Earlier menarche Later age at menopause
Pregnancy, delivery history	Later age at first full-term pregnancy Nullipara Higher number of parity[a]
Breastfeeding history	Breastfeeding[a] Longer duration of breastfeeding[a]
Surgical histories	Oophorectomy[a] Hysterectomy (regardless of oophorectomy)[a]

[a]Risk decreased

The distribution of reproductive factors in women with BC will change to longer life-time exposure to estrogen and progesterone. Thus, theoretically, earlier menarche and later menopause may be associated with a higher risk of BC, while factors such as pregnancy, childbirth, and breastfeeding, which interfere with repeated female hormone exposure, are associated with lower risk of BC (Table 21.3).

Women's early menarche and late menopause are associated with an increased risk of BC. The first delivery of baby at late age increases the risk of BC. Parous women have a reduced risk of BC, relative to nulliparous women; and as the number of live births increases, the risk of BC decreases gradually. Most reproductive risk factors commonly show much stronger association with ER+ subtypes [13]. But there are a few results for BC subtypes, such as luminal A, B, HER2-enrinched, and TNBC, up to date and less consistent across the studies.

As the duration of breastfeeding increases, the risk of BC decreases gradually. The World Cancer Research Fund/American Institute for Cancer Research (WCRF/AICR) categorizes that breastfeeding is a preventable risk factor with probable evidence in causal relation with BC (Table 21.1) [8]. The BC risk per 5-month breastfeeding decreases 2%.

Premenopausal women taking BSOH (bilateral salpingooophorectomy with hysterectomy) and even only hysterectomy without oophorectomy have a 20–40% reduced risk of BC. The effect is strongly pronounced at earlier age (age < 45) but is not observed at old postmenopausal ages.

The IARC categorizes ionizing radiation exposure as a carcinogenic agent with sufficient evidence for human BC (Table 21.1) [7]. Radiation therapy due to specific cancers or diseases taking repeated radiation therapy in children and adolescent before puberty increases BC risk, compared to general population. The evidence of diagnostic radiation exposures, such as CT, before puberty, is not clearly confirmed up to date. Thus, research for the hazards of the repeated diagnostic radiation exposures before puberty should be further conducted.

The IARC, WHO and the WCRF/AICR, the two accredited official bodies that assess causal links to cancer, have been already reporting the bad effect by higher alcohol intakes in relation to cancer (Table 21.1) [7]. BC risk for women who drink alcohol is 10–20% higher than women who do not drink. Among women who drink alcohol, women who drink alcohol 10 g/day have an excess risk of about 10%. For use of this information, we can estimate the BC risk increase by alcohol dose using the excess risk. If a glass contains 8 grams of alcohol in Korea, the BC risk is 8% higher for women who drink 2 glasses/day than for women who drink 1 glass/day (In Korea, 1 glass of Beer (= 200 mL of Beer; 1 glass of Soju = 50 mL of Soju) contains 8 g of alcohol (= 10 mL of alcohol)). The risk of BC by heavy alcohol drinking is increased by nearly 50%.

The WCRF/AICR classifies that excess body fatness and its increasing change in postmenopausal women are a convincing risk factor for BC (Table 21.1) [8]. Overweight (25–29.9 kg/m^2) and obese ($\geq$30 kg/m^2) postmenopausal women are at increasing BC risk relative to those with normal BMI (<25 kg/m^2). The higher the BMI, the higher the risk of BC is in postmenopausal women only, especially only women with no HRT. In premenopausal women, the higher the BMI, the lower BC risk was shown in Western premenopausal women. However, in Asian premenopausal women, the decreasing BC risk by higher BMI is not clearly demonstrated.

Increased abdominal fatness, like the direction in association with BMI, is associated with an increased risk of BC in postmenopausal women and a reduced risk of BC in premenopausal women. Adult weight gain is only associated with an increased risk of BC risk in postmenopausal women; but weight gain at age 18–30 is associated with decreased risk of BC in both pre- and post-menopausal women.

Increasing women's height is associated with an increased risk of BC, regardless of menopausal status. The greater the weight at birth, the greater the likelihood of BC when it becomes an adult, which is seen only in premenopausal women.

Physically inactive or low active women are at higher risk for BC, relative to highly active postmenopausal women [8]. Higher total physical activity (any physical activities including household, occupational, walking, moderate, or vigorous physical activity) relative to no physical activity or low physical activity is associated with lower risk of BC (at least 10% decreased risk). The vigorous physical activity has a reduced risk for BC in both pre- and post-menopausal women.

Cigarette smoking is classified as a carcinogenic agent by the IARC but it is a limited carcinogen in the carcinogenic classification for BC (with limited evidence in human studies but confirmed evidence in experimental in vivo and in vitro studies) [7]. The BC risk of past smokers and current smokers is known to be 8–10% higher than that of nonsmokers, and women who start smoking before the first delivery may have a BC risk as high as 20%.

As the other risk factors of BC, the IARC suggests several limited carcinogenic agents for BC such as digoxin, shiftwork (circadian disruption), polychlorinated biphenyls (PCBs), and ethylene oxide.

21.4 BC Prevention Recommendations for High-Risk Population of Breast Cancer based on risk factors

Based on risk factors for BC, the risk-based intervention method is a noninvasive method that can be used to prevent BC as well as high-risk individuals. Although further studies are needed because there are few clinical trials for lifestyle modification and intervention with high risk of developing BC, the following suggests possible lifestyle modification based on the evidence of BC risk factors in observational studies.

1. Risk modification for the risk factors with "Sufficient evidence" or "Strong evidence (convincing or probable)"

   (a) *Control of obesity and overweight*

   Overweight and obesity, abdominal fatness, and adult weight gains are associated with an increased risk for BC in postmenopausal women. Although body fatness or weight gain in premenopausal women or young women is effective in reducing the risk of BC for a while, it is not clearly observed in Asian women. Moreover, the risk of BC in women increases with age. Therefore, we should encourage women to maintain optimal weight when considering women's entire lifespan and to do risk modification for preventing overweight and obesity.

   (b) *Recommended for high physical activity*

   Although total physical activity (occupational, household, walking, etc.) has limited evidence for premenopausal BC risk, it has been reported to reduce the risk of only postmenopausal BC. Vigorous intensity physical activity can reduce BC risk in both premenopausal and postmenopausal women. Vigorous physical activity is defined as physical activity that requires a large amount of effort and causes rapid breathing and a substantial increase in heart rate, including running, walking/climbing briskly up a hill, fast cycling, aerobics, fast swimming, competitive sports (i.e., football, volleyball, hockey, basketball), heavy shoveling/digging ditches, and carrying/moving heavy loads (>20 kg), etc.

   Although there is no evidence of minimal exercise frequency and duration or intensity to prevent BC, moderate to vigorous physical activity should be recommended to women.

   (c) *Strongly recommended for breastfeeding*

   Breastfeeding is modifiable and probable preventable factors in the evidence evaluation of the WCRF/AICR. Breastfeeding has the other beneficial effect, such as decreased risk for ovarian cancer, and decreased postpartum weight and blood pressure. Therefore, breastfeeding should be strongly recommended to all women. The WHO recommends exclusive breastfeeding (not-combined milk-feeding) at least for the first 6 months and more continual breastfeeding up to 2 years or beyond.

(d) *Limitations on alcohol drinking*

The WCRF/AICR reported that there is no minimum threshold for alcohol drinking in female BC risk and the risk continues to increase with increasing dose. Drinking alcohol of 10 g increases about 10% BC, regardless of types of alcohol drinking and various ethnic groups. Therefore, we should encourage women to limit alcohol consumption to prevent BC.

(e) *Individualized recommendation to restrict radiation exposures*

Low-dose ionizing radiation is still arguable for whether it has a nonharmful effect by homeostasis or harmful effect. But repeated low-dose exposure to radiation or radiotherapy, especially during early ages (childhood or adolescents), can increase the risk of BC. It is suggested as the Group 1 carcinogen in human with sufficient evidence by the IARC. It is not possible to fully protect from inevitable repeated radiation exposure before puberty. Annual radiation exposure doses of individuals should be monitored.

(f) *Individualized recommendation to balanced use of oral contraceptives and postmenopausal HRT*

The use of E-P combined HRT in postmenopausal women without hysterectomy can increase risk for BC and cardiovascular disease relative to nonuse. But it can prevent bone mineral loss and fracture and improve metabolic profile in women if HRT is started under the age of 60 years.

The use of estrogen-only HRT in postmenopausal women with hysterectomy does not increase the risk for BC; but it still increase the risk for ovarian and endometrial cancers. It is debatable for whether E-only HRT is safe for hysterectomized postmenopausal women because hysterectomy itself partly contributes to reduce risk of BC.

Although OC has the drawback of slightly increasing BC risk, it has lots of beneficial effects, such as prevention of unwanted pregnancy several cancers (including endometrial, ovarian, and colon cancers), and treatment effect for some diseases (including postmenopausal syndrome, endometriosis, etc.).

It is therefore necessary to make individualized optimal clinical decisions taking into account of the balance between the risk and benefits for the use of postmenopausal HRT and premenopausal OC.

2. Risk modification for healthy living and risk factors that are limited evidence

(a) *Control of cigarette smoking*

Although smoking has been reported to increase the incidence of premenopausal BC, it is still controversial because the evidence in Asian women is not confirmed due to low smoking prevalence in Asian women. Nonetheless, BC risk of female smokers should be warned.

(b) *Maintaining healthy eating habits and choosing healthy foods*

The WCRF/AICR meta-analyzed the association of various foods and diets with BC risk. Although the evidence of the underlying causality of BC is weak, it is necessary to encourage healthy eating (such as consuming a lot of vegetables and fruits, and eating less red meats and processed meats), in terms of preventing obesity and maintaining hormone balance.

3. The impact of risk modification

   The US Preventive Service Task Force (USPSTF, https://uspreventiveservicestaskforce.org/uspstf/) recommends risk assessment and genetic counseling, including genetic testing if indicated, to high-risk women, where high-risk women means those with a personal or family history of breast, ovarian, tubal, or peritoneal cancer, who have an ancestry with breast cancer susceptibility 1 and 2 (BRCA1/2) gene mutations. In the case of the risk assessment tool, it is the joint score generated by the various risk factors including familial risk described above. The more exposure to risk factors, the higher the scores, which means that breast cancer is likely to develop in the future. In the case of behavior modification for breast cancer prevention, it is a part that needs to be further researched in order to generate the evidence for the population area, but if the risk factors of individuals are well understood and exposure to risk factors is reduced, it can be predicted that the incidence of breast cancer will decrease in the future have. Therefore, the impact of prevention for risk intervention is here. For women at increased risk for BC in risk assessment, the USPSTF recommends chemoprevention by SERM (selective estrogen receptor medication) (Grade B). Moreover, the USPSTF strongly recommends intensive and multicomponent behavioral interventions for women with BMI $\geq$30 kg/m^2 (Grade B), which is also important in preventing BC because obesity is a strong risk factor for postmenopausal BC.

21.5 Conclusion

There are various alleged risk factors for BC, such as sex hormone relating factors such as exogenous hormones including postmenopausal HRT, oral contraceptives, and endogenous hormonal changes including reproductive-pregnancy-related factors, lifestyle factors such as overweight/obesity, physical activity, alcohol consumption, cigarette smoking, environmental factors such as radiation exposure, shiftwork, PCBs, etc. These alleged risk factors explain only about 40–50% of BC etiology. Of the remaining half, 5–10% are familial and/or genetic predispositions including BRCA1, 2 mutations, yet 30–40% still are not known yet. The still unknown risk factors appear to be related to genetic–environmental interactions, gene–gene interactions, and proteomics and metabolic studies.

Clear understanding of the risk factors for BC is essential for risk modification and intervention for prevention of BC in patients as well as healthy general women. Therefore, we should be aware of BC risk factors and be prepared to recommend individualized risk modification and intervention methods based on this information.

Further Reading

1. International Agency for Research on Cancer (IARC), World Health Organization (WHO). Global cancer observatory. Cancer today. http://gco.iarc.fr/.
2. International Agency for Research on Cancer (IARC), World Health Organization (WHO). GI5 plus: cancer Incidence in five continents. Online analysis. http://ci5.iarc.fr/CI5plus/Pages/online.aspx.
3. International Agency for Research on Cancer (IARC), World Health Organization (WHO). WHO cancer mortality database. Online analysis. http://www-dep.iarc.fr/WHOdb/WHOdb.htm.
4. Noone AM, Howlader N, Krapcho M, Miller D, Brest A, Yu M, Ruhl J, Tatalovich Z, Mariotto A, Lewis DR, Chen HS, Feuer EJ, Cronin KA, editors. SEER Cancer statistics review, 1975–2015. Bethesda, MD: National Cancer Institute. Based on November 2017 SEER data submission, posted to SEER website, April 2018
5. Monitoring of cancer incidence in Japan–survival 2006–2008 report (center for Cancer Control and Information Services, National Cancer Center, 2016) [Japanese].
6. Korea National Cancer Center. 2016' Cancer registry statistics. http://www.ncc.re.kr/cancerStatsView.ncc?bbsnum=459&searchKey=total&searchValue=&pageNum=1.
7. International Agency for Research on Cancer (IARC), World Health Organization (WHO). IARC monographs on the identification of carcinogenic hazards to humans. Volumes 1–123. Last update: 25 March 2019. https://monographs.iarc.fr/agents-classified-by-the-iarc/.
8. World Cancer Research Fund (WCRF), American Institute for Cancer Research (AICR), Continuous Update Project (CUP). Breast cancer: how diet, nutrition, and physical activity affect breast cancer risk. Last update: 2018. https://www.wcrf.org/dietandcancer/breast-cancer.
9. Park B, Ma SH, Shin A, Chang MC, Choi JY, Kim SW, Han W, Noh DY, Ahn SH, Kang DH, Yoo KY, Park SK. Korean risk assessment model for BREAST CANCER risk prediction. PLoS One. 2013;8:e76736.
10. Foulkes WD. Inherited susceptibility to common cancers. N Engl J Med. 2008;359:2143–53.
11. Kobayashi H, Ohno S, Sasaki Y, Matsuura M. Hereditary breast and ovarian cancer susceptibility genes (review). Oncol Rep. 2013;30:1019–29.
12. Park B, Dowty JG, Ahn C, Win AK, Kim SW, Lee MH, Lee JW, Kang E, Hopper JL, Park SK. BREAST CANCER risk for Korean women with germline mutations in BRCA1 and BRCA2. Breast Cancer Res Treat. 2015;152:659–65.
13. Park B, Choi JY, Sung HK, Ahn C, Hwang Y, Jang J, Lee J, Kim H, Shin HR, Park S, Han W, Noh DY, Yoo KY, Kang D, Park SK. Attribution to heterogeneous risk factors for BREAST CANCER subtypes based on hormone receptor and human epidermal growth factor 2 receptor expression in Korea. Medicine (Baltimore). 2016;95:e3063.

Chapter 22
Breast Cancer-Related Low Penetrance Genes

Daehee Kang and Ji-Yeob Choi

Abstract Susceptibility genes involved in disease etiology and prognosis are categorized into two groups: high penetrance genes (i.e., *BRCA1*, *CHEK2*, *ATM*, etc.) and low penetrance genes (i.e., NATs, GSTs, CYPs, etc., and variants identified by genome-wide association studies). Since low penetrance genes have high population attributable risk, the usefulness of those genes to research on breast cancer prevention is not small. In this chapter, the previous studies on low-penetrance genetic susceptibility through a candidate gene approach and genome-wide association of breast cancer were summarized. The contribution of low-penetrance susceptibility genes to the breast cancer risk prediction models will also be discussed on the utility in clinical or public health application.

Keywords Genetic susceptibility · Low-penetrance genes · High-penetrance genes · Genome-wide association study · Polygenic risk score · Risk assessment · Prediction model

22.1 Genetic Susceptibility of Breast Cancer

Indicators of genetic susceptibility to breast cancer can be grouped into two categories: high susceptibility loci and low penetrance [1] (Table 22.1). Penetrance is defined by the proportion of individuals in a population with a genetic variant who develop the disease associated with that variant. High penetrance genes are usually caused by some mutation in one or a few cells and these mutations then lead to the onset of a disease state, such as the malignant transformation of the affected cell. Among the recognized susceptibility loci, genes such as BRCA1/2 and p53 mutations are widely known as major susceptibility genes in breast cancer, and research focuses on aspects of breast cancer cluster ability in high-risk families. Overall,

D. Kang (✉) · J.-Y. Choi
Seoul National University, Seoul, South Korea
e-mail: dhkang@snu.ac.kr

D.-Y. Noh et al. (eds.), *Translational Research in Breast Cancer*, Advances in Experimental Medicine and Biology 1187,
https://doi.org/10.1007/978-981-32-9620-6_22

Table 22.1 Characteristics of two categories of susceptibility genes (modified from [2])

Penetrance	High	Low
Frequency	Rare	Common (<1%)
Family history	High	Low
Population attributable risk	Low	High
Role of environmental exposure	Secondary and variable	Critical
G–E interaction	Low	High
Study subjects	Family	Population
Study type	Linkage	Association
Role for disease development	Necessary and sufficient condition	Neither necessary nor sufficient condition
Genes	Recognized	Putative
Example	*BRCA1/2*	6q25

5–10% of all breast cancer patients have a family history [3] and it was reported that 22.3% of patients with a family history of breast cancer had a BRCA mutation in a survey of BRCA mutations in Koreans [4].

Common single-nucleotide polymorphisms (SNPs) are referred to as low-penetrant, as risk alleles typically confer modest risk. Low penetrance genes in which somatic mutations are rarely if ever seen, and genetic variation is found throughout the population at these loci. These polymorphic genes may be involved in risk as either homozygotes or heterozygotes vs. wild type, considering the most common allele arbitrary. Genes involved in carcinogen metabolism including NATs, GSTs, CYPs, and others are observed in breast tissue in putative susceptibility loci. They are interacting with environmental risk factors, and many of the population have variations in these genes. Thus, the low-penetrance susceptibility genes are important in understanding the basis of both individual differences in susceptibility and the mechanisms of gene–environment interactions in cancer [1].

22.2 Hypothesis-Driven Candidate SNPs

Before Genome-wide association studies (GWAS) has become a growing body of results in the risk of breast cancer, candidate-gene association studies were the most prevalent type of investigation to identify common breast-cancer susceptibility alleles. Earlier genetic epidemiology studies have investigated a specific number, typically a few down to several hundreds, of candidate genes located throughout the genome. Selected common SNP in genes involved in the metabolism of carcinogens (activation, detoxification) and genes involving DNA repair, cell cycle control, and nutrient metabolism are widely studied to discover the role of these genes on breast carcinogenesis.

Candidate gene studies were often producing non-reproducible results due to lack of proper study designs (e.g., small sample size, mutant allele frequency in different ethnic groups, etc.). The first reported SNP associations were often the largest and the subsequent investigators reported smaller or nonsignificant associations when larger studies were undertaken and more genetic material was available [5]. In the review of Zhang et al. [6], meta-analyses were done for 279 genetic variants in 128 candidate genes or chromosomal loci that had at least three data sources published before Feb, 2010. Whereas most genetic variants assessed in previous candidate-gene studies showed no association with breast cancer risk in meta-analyses, 14 variants in nine genes (strong for ten variants in six genes (*ATM, CASP8, CHEK2, CTLA4, NBN*, and *TP53*), moderate for four variants in four genes (*ATM, CYP19A1, TERT*, and *XRCC3*)) had evidence for an association (Table 22.2).

The survival of breast cancer patients is largely influenced by tumor characteristics, such as TNM stage, tumor grade, and hormone receptor status. The studies of SNPs on prognosis are fewer than those of the association of risk because of difficulty to follow-up the patients and define the event or response. However, there is growing evidence that inherited genetic variation might affect the disease prognosis and response to treatment. The most promising candidate gene approach on breast cancer prognosis is the prediction of chemotherapy response according to the SNPs of transporter genes and the hazards of recurrence or death. Kim et al. [7] reviewed the studies of the genetic polymorphisms of the ATP-binding cassette (ABC) and solute carrier (SLC) genes as the subfamilies of transporters and the prognosis of various cancers published from January 2000 to December 2016 as showing the summary of the studies of associations between the genetic polymorphisms of transporters and breast cancer prognosis. Although *ABCB1* rs1045642 ($C > T$) was associated with poor PFS ($HR = 1.33$, 95% CI: 1.07–1.64) overall, the result of meta-analysis limited to breast cancer did not find a significant association. Table 22.3 summarizes the association of variants of transporter genes (including ABCs and SLCs) and breast cancer prognosis.

22.3 Genome-Wide Association Study (GWAS)

GWAS, a hypothesis-free study design to associate complex disease to particular genotypes, were succeeded in breast cancer. They offer a more efficient strategy for identifying disease genes and overcoming bias in the more traditional candidate gene approach. The statistical power to detect associations between DNA variants and a trait depends on the experimental sample size, the distribution of effect sizes of (unknown) causal genetic variants that are segregating in the population, the frequency of those variants, and the linkage disequilibrium between observed genotyped DNA variants and the unknown causal variants (reviewed in [12]). GWAS have identified SNPs associated with breast cancer risk [13–29] (Table 22.4). After one of the very first large GWAS reported five significant loci

Table 22.2 Genetic variants with an association with breast cancer risk in meta-analysis (adopted from [6])

Gene	Variant	Comparison[a]	Freq (%)	Studies	Cases	Controls	OR (95% CI)	*P*-value	*P*-value for heterogeneity	I^2
Strong evidence of genetic variants associated with breast cancer risk										
ATM	Glu1978X	Carriers vs noncarriers	0.05	4	6593	3793	4.56 (1.35–15.42)	0.015	1.000	0%
CASP8	rs1045485 (Asp302His)	C vs G	13.29	17	18,382	19,419	0.89 (0.85–0.93)	4.65×10^{-8}	0.992	0%
CASP8	rs6723097 (A35438C)	A vs C	36.33	3	2610	3040	1.16 (1.07–1.25)	1.91×10^{-4}	0.997	0%
CHEK2	IVS2 + 1G > A	Carriers vs noncarriers	0.39	5	9970	7526	3·07 (2.03–4.63)	9.82×10^{-8}	0.707	0%
CHEK2	rs17879961 (Ile157Thr)	Carriers vs noncarriers	4.19	8	13,311	10,817	1.52 (1.31–1.77)	4.76×10^{-8}	0.324	14%
CHEK2	Deletion	Carriers vs noncarriers	0.30	5	10,543	8447	2.53 (1.61–3.97)	6.33×10^{-5}	0.419	0%
CHEK2	1100delC	Carriers vs noncarriers	0.49	47	41,791	50,910	3.10 (2.59–3.71)	$<10^{-20}$	0.315	8%
CTLA4	rs231775 (Thr17Ala)	A vs G	38.54	3	2214	2288	1.25 (1.14–1.37)	1.59×10^{-6}	0.676	0%
NBN	657del5	Carriers vs noncarriers	0.36	7	7082	9504	2.42 (1.54–3.80)	1.18×10^{-4}	0.736	0%
TP53	rs17878362 (16 bp Del/Ins)	Insertion vs deletion	15.40	12	2961	3496	1.15 (1.04–1.26)	0.007	0.520	0%
Moderate evidence of genetic variants associated with breast cancer risk										
ATM	rs1800057 (Pro1054Arg)	(CG + GG) vs CC	5.06	9	4998	6122	1.20 (1.01–1.44)	0.038	0.466	0%
CYP19A1	$(TTTA)_{10}$	R10 vs R7	1.76	13	7979	8564	1.53 (1.05–2.22)	0.027	0.044	45%
XRCC3	rs861539 (Thr241Met)	T vs C	10.98	3	1283	1120	1.32 (1.08–1.06)	0.007	0.855	0%

TERT	rs2853669 (T-244C)	C vs T	27.99	4	4553	5319	0.76 (0.64–0.91)	0.002	–	22%
Genetic variants with no association with breast cancer risk, in meta-analyses with at least 10,000 cases and 10,000 controls										
ADH1B	rs1042026 (A19107G)	G vs A	28.93	9	11,381	15,573	0.99 (0.95–1.03)	0.617	0.375	7%
ATM	rs1800054 (Ser49Cys)	(CG + GG) vs CC	2.37	16	16,682	20,729	1.16 (0.95–1.41)	0.138	0.064	38%
AURKA	rs2273535 (Phe31Ile)	A vs T	31.96	16	19,709	24,646	1.03 (0.98–1.09)	0.277	0.001	61%
BID	rs8190315 (Ser10Gly)	(GG + AG) vs AA	3.41	11	13,783	14,272	1.05 (0.87–1.27)	0.607	0.093	38%
BRCA1	rs1799950 (Gln356Arg)	C vs T	7.72	9	11,280	19,210	1.00 (0.86–1.15)	0.949	0.001	70%
BRCA2	rs144848 (Asn372His)	G vs T	27.37	21	21,906	27,399	1.01 (0.98–1.04)	0.547	0.410	4%
CASP10	rs13010627 (Val410Ile)	A vs G	6.07	28	29,904	32,870	1.02 (0.95–1.09)	0.609	0.005	46%
CASP8	rs3834129 (−652 6 N del)	Del vs non-del	43.41	16	13,254	13,639	0.96 (0.90–1.03)	0.233	0.001	62%
CCND1	rs9344 (Pro241Pro)	A vs G	50.53	14	12,846	13,118	1.04 (0.99–1.08)	0.115	0.179	26%
CDKN1A	rs1801270 (Ser31Arg)	A vs C	7.73	20	22,003	29,324	1.05 (0.95–1.15)	0.329	0.000	68%
COMT	rs4680 (Val158Met)	A vs G	47.01	41	27,433	34,787	0.98 (0.95–1.02)	0.339	0.022	33%
CYP17A1	rs743572 (T-34C)	C vs T	40.90	42	25,596	32,480	1.02 (0.99–1.05)	0.239	0.308	9%
CYP19A1	rs10046 (C132810T)	C vs T	48.27	8	12,122	17,607	1.03 (0.97–1.10)	0.279	0.023	57%
CYP1A1	rs1048943 (Ile462Val)	G vs A	8.44	27	12,332	17,182	1.06 (0.95–1.20)	0.299	0.000	64%
CYP1A1	rs4646903 (T3801C)	C vs T	19.36	26	10,568	14,542	1.00 (0.91–1.09)	0.956	0.000	61%
CYP1B1	rs10012 (Arg48Gly)	G vs C	28.63	9	10,821	12,597	1.03 (0.98–1.07)	0.255	0.511	0%

(continued)

Table 22.2 (continued)

Gene	Variant	Comparison[a]	Freq (%)	Studies	Cases	Controls	OR (95% CI)	*P*-value	*P*-value for heterogeneity	I^2
CYP1B1	rs1056827 (Ala119Ser)	T vs G	28.46	10	10,576	11,536	1.04 (0.97–1.11)	0.242	0.081	41%
CYP1B1	rs1800440 (Asn453Ser)	G vs A	17.48	11	11,311	13,410	0.99 (0.92–1.07)	0.826	0.098	38%
ERCC2	rs1799793 (Asp312Asn)	A vs G	32.99	22	13,994	13,868	0.98 (0.92–1.05)	0.635	0.000	67%
ERCC4	rs744154 (G6068C)	C vs G	27.24	28	29,136	31,799	1.00 (0.97–1.02)	0.882	0.492	0%
ESR2	rs1256049 (Val328Val)	A vs G	7.28	9	13,331	17,820	1.02 (0.94–1.09)	0.689	0.313	15%
ESR2	rs4986938 (G39A)	A vs G	34.33	10	13,346	19,153	0.97 (0.94–1.01)	0.104	0.739	0%
HSD17B1	rs605059 (Ser312Gly)	G vs A	47.25	11	13,987	17,066	0.98 (0.95–1.01)	0.196	0.480	0%
ICAM5	rs1056538 (Val301Ile)	T vs C	38.29	19	19,484	24,474	0.99 (0.95–1.03)	0.428	0.043	39%
IL6	rs1800795 (G-174C)	C vs G	38.50	9	10,885	18,602	1.02 (0.97–1.08)	0.545	0.294	17%
LIG4	rs1805386 (Asp568Asp)	C vs T	17.44	8	10,068	11,140	0.96 (0.91–1.02)	0.179	0.393	5%
MDM2	rs2279744 (14 + 309 T > G)	G vs T	36.27	24	14,180	13,223	1.03 (0.98–1.08)	0.249	0.097	29%
MTHFR	rs1801131 (Glu429Ala)	C vs A	24.80	24	13,131	16,813	0.98 (0.94–1.03)	0.482	0.074	31%
NAT2	Acetylation phenotype	Fast vs slow	45.03	30	10,745	12,497	0.98 (0.92–1.05)	0.603	0.066	30%
NUMA1	rs3750913 (Ala794Gly)	(CC + CG) vs GG	5.63	16	16,182	18,908	1.08 (0.93–1.26)	0.332	0.008	52%
PGR	rs1042838 (Val660Leu)	T vs G	14.48	28	31,672	37,579	1.02 (0.98–1.07)	0.300	0.027	37%

PGR	rs10895068 (G331A)	A vs G	5.13	8	13,544	17,547	1.05 (0.97–1.15)	0.252	0.283	19%
PTGS2	rs5275 (T8473C)	C vs T	32.94	7	10,907	14,091	1.03 (0.98–1.07)	0.238	0.390	5%
PTGS2	rs5277 (Val102Val)	G vs C	15.04	3	10,583	12,607	0.97 (0.87–1.08)	0.598	0.027	72%
SHBG	rs6259 (Asp356Asn)	A vs G	12.28	7	10,092	12,663	0.98 (0.91–1.04)	0.452	0.321	14%
SOD2	rs4880 (Val16Ala)	C vs T	47.31	31	26,976	35,015	1.01 (0.97–1.05)	0.583	0.001	49%
TGFB1	rs1800469 (C-509 T)	T vs C	34.85	11	12,125	15,273	1.00 (0.94–1.05)	0.889	0.056	44%
TGFB1	rs1800470 (Leu10Pro)	C vs T	40.30	32	20,125	27,269	1.01 (0.98–1.06)	0.461	0.049	31%
TNF	rs361525 (A-417G)	A vs G	4.82	30	31,996	34,887	1.01 (0.95–1.06)	0.851	0.479	0%
TP53	rs1042522 (Arg72Pro)	C vs G	29.63	52	31,484	35,113	0.98 (0.94–1.03)	0.446	0.000	62%
VDR	rs1544410 (G63980A)	A vs G	37.22	22	11,377	13,572	0.97 (0.93–1.03)	0.311	0.048	36%
VDR	rs2228570 (Met1Arg/Lys/Thr)	T vs C	37.64	19	12,349	16,707	1.05 (0.98–1.12)	0.159	0.000	67%
XRCC1	rs1799782 (Arg194Trp)	T vs C	8.50	20	10,414	10,796	0.98 (0.88–1.09)	0.682	0.012	47%
XRCC2	rs3218536 (Arg188His)	G vs A	7.78	15	17,932	18,738	0.96 (0.90–1.02)	0.192	0.298	14%
XRCC3	rs1799796 (A17893G)	G vs A	32.88	6	10,870	12,263	1.00 (0.92–1.08)	0.906	0.003	73%

Moderate linkage disequilibrium (LD) was found between *ESR1* rs3020314 and rs1801132; high LD was found between *CASP8* rs6435074 and rs6723097; perfect LD was found between *TP53* rs12947788 and rs12951053. *OR* odds ratio, *C* cytosine, *G* guanine, *A* adenine, *R* repeat, *T* thymine, *bp* base pair, *Del* deletion, *Ins* insertion

Minor allele frequency for common variants, or population frequency of test group for rare variants

Assessment of cumulative epidemiological evidence for *CHEK2* rs17879961 was done among northern and eastern Europeans

[a]Allelic contrast for common variants, or genetic comparison for rare variants except for *TERT* (recessive genetic model)

Table 22.3 Summary of the associations between genetic polymorphisms of transporter genes and breast cancer prognosis (adopted from [7])

First author, year	Clinical trial	Regimen	No. of patients	Country	Gene	SNP	Endpoints
Bray, 2010 [8]	N	Cyclophosphamide, doxorubicin	230	UK	*ABCB1*	rs2032582	HR = 4.8 (1.1–21.6) for OS HR = 4.3 (1.3–14.5) for PFS
Ji, 2012 [9]	Y	TA/TAC, FAC	153	China	*ABCB1*	rs1045642	HR = 0.639 (0.338–1.208) for DFS
Lee, 2014 [10]	Y	Gemcitabine, paclitaxel	85	Korea	*SLC28A3*	rs7867504	HR = 2.646 (1.12–6.28) for OS
Kim, 2015 [11]	Y	Docetaxel, doxorubicin	216	Korea	*ABCB1*	rs1045642	HR = 0.223 (0.054–0.972) for OS
						rs1128503	HR = 1.168 (0.543–2.510) for OS
						rs2032582	HR = 0.688 (0.335–1.256) for OS
Kim, 2018 [7]	N	Cyclophosphamide, doxorubicin	1338	Korea	*ABCB1*	rs1202172	HR = 1.81 (1.34–2.43) for DFS HR = 1.42 (0.93–2.18) for OS

Abbreviations: *OS* overall survival, *PFS* progression-free survival, *DFS* disease-free survival

Table 22.4 Summary of the breast cancer susceptibility loci identified by a GWAS approach (adopted from [30])

Study	Year	SNP	Locus	Genes[d]	OR[e]	*P*-value
Easton et al. [16]	2007	rs889312	5q11.2[b,c]	Intergenic	1.13	7.00×10^{-20}
		rs13281615	8q24.21[b,c]	*CASC21, CASC8*	1.08	5.00×10^{-12}
		rs2981582	10q26.13[c]	*FGFR2*	1.26	2.00×10^{-76}
		rs3817198	11p15.5[b,c]	*LSP1*	1.07	3.00×10^{-9}
		rs3803662	16q12.1[c]	*CASC16*	1.2	1.00×10^{-36}
Stacey et al. [25]	2007	rs13387042	2q35[b,c]	Intergenic	1.2	1.30×10^{-13}
Stacey et al. [26]	2008	rs10941679	5p12[c]	Intergenic	1.19	2.90×10^{-11}
Zheng et al. [29]	2009	rs2046210	6q25.1[b,c]	Intergenic	1.29	2.00×10^{-15}
Ahmed et al. [13]	2009	rs4973768	3p24.1[b,c]	*SLC4A7*	1.11	4.10×10^{-23}
		rs6504950	17q22[c]	*STXBP4*	0.95	1.40×10^{-8}
Thomas et al. [27]	2009	rs11249433	1p11.2[c]	*EMBP1*	1.16	6.74×10^{-18}
		rs999737	14q24.1[b,c]	*RAD51B*	0.94	1.74×10^{-7}
Turnbull et al. [28]	2010	rs3757318	6q25.1[b,c]	*CCDC170*	1.3	2.90×10^{-6}
		rs1562430	8q24.21[b]	*CASC21, CASC8*	1.17	5.80×10^{-7}
		rs1011970	9p21.3[c]	*CDKN2B*	1.09	2.50×10^{-8}
		rs2380205	10p15.1	Intergenic	0.94	4.60×10^{-7}
		rs10995190	10q21.2[b,c]	*ZNF365*	0.86	5.10×10^{-15}
		rs704010	10q22.3[c]	*ZMIZ1*	1.07	3.70×10^{-9}
		rs909116	11p15.5[b]	*TNNT3*	1.17	7.30×10^{-7}
		rs614367	11q13.3[c]	Intergenic	1.15	3.20×10^{-15}
Antoniou et al. [31]	2010	rs8170	19p13.11[b]	*BABAM1*	1.26[f]	2.30×10^{-9}
		rs2363956	19p13.11[b]	*ANKLE1*	0.84[f]	5.50×10^{-9}
Fletcher et al. [32]	2011	rs9383938	6q25.1[b]	*ESR1*	1.18	1.41×10^{-7}
		rs865686	9q31.2[b,c]	Intergenic	0.89	1.75×10^{-10}
Cai et al. [33]	2011	rs10822013	10q21.2[b]	*ZNF365*	1.12	5.87×10^{-9}
Ghoussaini et al. [34]	2012	rs10771399	12p11.22[c]	Intergenic	0.85	2.70×10^{-35}
		rs1292011	12q24.21[c]	Intergenic	0.92	4.30×10^{-19}
		rs2823093	21q21.1[c]	Intergenic	0.94	1.10×10^{-12}
Siddiq et al. [24]	2012	rs17530068	6q14.1[c]	Intergenic	1.12	1.10×10^{-9}
		rs2284378	20q11.22	*RALY*	1.08	1.30×10^{-6}
Long et al. [22]	2012	rs9485372	6q25.1[b]	*TAB2*	0.9	3.86×10^{-12}
Kim et al. [20]	2012	rs13393577	2q34	*ERBB4*	1.53	8.80×10^{-14}
Michailidou et al. [35]	2013	rs616488	1p36.22	*PEX14*	0.94	2.00×10^{-10}
		rs11552449	1p13.2	*DCLRE1B*	1.07	1.80×10^{-8}
		rs4849887	2q14.2	Intergenic	0.91	3.70×10^{-11}
		rs2016394	2q31.1[b]	Intergenic	0.95	1.20×10^{-8}
		rs1550623	2q31.1[b]	Intergenic	0.94	3.00×10^{-8}
		rs16857609	2q35[b]	*DIRC3*	1.08	1.10×10^{-15}
		rs6762644	3p26.1	*ITPR1*	1.07	2.20×10^{-12}
		rs12493607	3p24.1[b]	*TGFBR2*	1.06	2.30×10^{-8}

(continued)

Table 22.4 (continued)

Study	Year	SNP	Locus	Genes[d]	OR[e]	*P*-value
		rs9790517	4q24	*TET2*	1.05	4.20×10^{-8}
		rs6828523	4q34.1	*ADAM29*	0.9	3.50×10^{-16}
		rs10472076	5q11.2[b]	Intergenic	1.05	2.90×10^{-8}
		rs1353747	5q11.2[b]	*PDE4D*	0.92	2.50×10^{-8}
		rs1432679	5q33.3	*EBF1*	1.07	2.00×10^{-14}
		rs11242675	6p25.3	Intergenic	0.94	7.10×10^{-9}
		rs204247	6p23	Intergenic	1.05	8.30×10^{-9}
		rs720475	7q35	*ARHGEF5*	0.94	7.00×10^{-11}
		rs9693444	8p12	Intergenic	1.07	9.20×10^{-14}
		rs6472903	8q21.11[b]	*CASC9*	0.91	1.7×10^{-17}
		rs2943559	8q21.11[b]	*HNF4G*	1.13	5.7×10^{-15}
		rs11780156	8q24.21[b]	Intergenic	1.07	3.4×10^{-11}
		rs10759243	9q31.2[b]	Intergenic	1.06	1.2×10^{-08}
		rs7072776	10p12.31[b]	Intergenic	1.07	4.30×10^{-14}
		rs11814448	10p12.31[b]	Intergenic	1.26	9.30×10^{-16}
		rs7904519	10q25.2	*TCF7L2*	1.06	3.10×10^{-8}
		rs11199914	10q26.12	Intergenic	0.95	1.90×10^{-8}
		rs3903072	11q13.1	Intergenic	0.95	8.60×10^{-12}
		rs11820646	11q24.3	Intergenic	0.95	1.10×10^{-9}
		rs12422552	12p13.1	Intergenic	1.05	3.70×10^{-8}
		rs17356907	12q22	Intergenic	0.91	1.80×10^{-22}
		rs11571833	13q13.1	*BRCA2*	1.26	4.90×10^{-8}
		rs2236007	14q13.3	*PAX9*	0.93	1.70×10^{-13}
		rs2588809	14q24.1[b]	*RAD51B*	1.08	1.40×10^{-10}
		rs941764	14q32.11	*CCDC88C*	1.06	3.70×10^{-10}
		rs17817449	16q12.2[b]	*FTO*	0.93	6.40×10^{-14}
		rs13329835	16q23.2	*CDYL2*	1.08	2.10×10^{-16}
		rs527616	18q11.2[b]	Intergenic	0.95	1.60×10^{-10}
		rs1436904	18q11.2[b]	*CHST9*	0.96	3.20×10^{-8}
		rs4808801	19p13.11[b]	*ELL*	0.93	4.60×10^{-15}
		rs3760982	19q13.31	Intergenic	1.06	2.10×10^{-10}
		rs132390	22q12.2	*EMID1*	1.12	3.10×10^{-9}
		rs6001930	22q13.1	*MKL1*	1.12	8.80×10^{-19}
Cai et al. [36]	2014	rs4951011	1q32.1b	*ZC3H11A*	1.09	8.82×10^{-9}
		rs10474352	5q14.3	Intergenic	1.09	1.67×10^{-9}
		rs2290203	15q26.1	*PRC1*	1.08	4.25×10^{-8}
Milne et al. [37]	2014	rs1053338	3p14.1	*ATXN7*	1.07	1.00×10^{-8}
		rs6964587	7q21.2	*AKAP9*	1.05	2.00×10^{-10}

[a]Independent associated variant
[b]Locus mapped by more than one independent variant
[c]Locus replicated in Michailidou et al. [32] at a GWAS significance level
[d]Name of the gene where the variant lies (intronic, exonic, or at 5' or 3' UTR regions). Note that not always the gene where the variant is placed is the one affected by the causal variant within the associated locus
[e]Per allele OR
[f]Breast cancer risk for *BRCA1* mutation carrier

associated with breast cancer risk among 26,258 cases and 26,894 control in three-stage in 2007 [16], 78 new loci have been identified (reviewed in [30]).

There have been studies limited to GWAS in breast cancer survival. Several studies reported the associations of breast cancer risk loci with breast cancer survival and identified little overlap between the breast cancer risk SNPs and the SNPs with associated with breast cancer prognosis [38, 39]. Guo et al. [40] conducted a large meta-analysis of studies in populations of European ancestry and identified rs148760487 at 2q24.2 associated with breast cancer-specific survival in all breast cancer (HR = 1.75, 95% CI = 1.39–2.20, $P = 1.44 \times 10^{-6}$) and rs2059614 at 11q24.2 associated with breast cancer survival in ER-negative case patients (HR = 1.95, 95% CI = 1.55–2.47, $P = 1.91 \times 10^{-8}$).

Kim et al. [20] conducted a three-stage GWAS in Korean women (6322 cases and 5897 controls) in Seoul Breast Cancer Study (SEBCS) in Table 22.4. They not only confirmed previously identified loci in Europeans or Chinese populations or both but also found rs13393577 at 2q34/*ERBB4* as a new breast cancer susceptibility variant with combined odds ratios (95% CI) of 1.53 (1.37–1.70) (combined *P* for trend = 8.8×10^{-14}). SEBCS is a multicenter-based case–control study and case–cohort study on breast cancer [7, 41–45] from four major teaching hospitals and community health screening programs in Seoul between 2001 and 2007. In a case–cohort design of SEBCS, a two-stage GWAS on disease-free survival (DFS) in breast cancer stratified by tumor subtypes based on hormone receptor and human epidermal growth factor receptor 2 was conducted. Rs166870 and rs10825036 were consistently associated with DFS in the HR+ HER2- and HR- HER2-breast cancer subtypes, respectively ($P_{rs166870} = 2.88 \times 10^{-7}$ and $P_{rs10825036} = 3.54 \times 10^{-7}$ in the combined set). When patients were classified by the recursive partitioning analysis (RPA) in each subtype, genetic factors contributed significantly to differentiating the high risk group associated with DFS in breast cancer (Table 22.5) [46].

22.4 Use of Polygenic Risk Score for Individual Risk Assessment

With an increasing number of genetic susceptibility loci being identified for breast cancer, it is critical to examine whether genetic information could have utility in clinical or public health applications. The individual risks conferred by GWAS-discovered loci are low but their combined effects, when summarized as a polygenic risk score (PRS) are useful for population-based risk stratification [47]. Possible applications include risk stratified prevention and screening strategies targeted to susceptible subgroups of the population at elevated risk, or conversely defining subgroups at a low risk that would benefit least from interventions [48]. Mavaddat et al. [49] developed and validated. PRS among Europeans with 313 SNPs. While the odds ratio for overall disease per 1 standard deviation was 1.61 (95%CI: 1.57–1.65) with the area under receiver-operator curve (AUC) = 0.630 (95%CI: 0.628–0.651), the lifetime risk of overall breast cancer in the top centile of the PRSs

Table 22.5 Associations between different combined groups of clinical and genetic factors and disease-free survival (DFS) among breast cancer patients (adopted from [46])

	Discovery set			Replication set		
	HR[a]	(95% CI)	*P*	HR[a]	(95% CI)	*P*
Group by RPA among HR+ HER2-breast cancer patients						
Group 1: TNM stage 0-II and rs166870$_{CC + CT}$	1.00	Ref.	1.18×10^{-8}	1.00	Ref.	2.08×10^{-5}
Group 2: TNM stage 0-II and rs166870$_{TT}$	5.52	(2.00–15.28)		2.01	(0.90–4.47)	
Group 3: TNM stage III and rs166870$_{CC + CT}$	3.61	(2.29–5.68)		3.07	(0.64–14.83)	
Group 4: TNM stage III and rs166870$_{TT}$	10.50	(1.43–77.06)		7.26	(2.95–17.88)	
Group by RPA among HR- HER2-breast cancer patients						
Group1: rs10825036$_{TT + TG}$	1.00	Ref.	2.35×10^{-4}	1.00	Ref.	2.60×10^{-2}
Group2: rs10825036$_{GG}$	3.45	(1.78–6.67)		2.17	(1.10–4.28)	

Abbreviations: *DFS* disease-free survival, *HR* hazard ratio, *CI* confidence interval, *RPA* recursive partitioning analysis, *HR* hormone receptor, *HER2* human epidermal growth factor receptor 2
[a]Cox proportional hazard model adjusted for age and recruiting center, additional TNM stage for group by tumor subtypes and selected SNPs

was 32.6%. Compared with women in the middle quintile, those in the highest 1% of risk had 4.37- and 2.78-fold risks and those in the lowest 1% of risk had 0.16- and 0.27-fold risks, of developing ER-positive and ER-negative disease, respectively.

SNP profiles could be added to existing individual risk models developed by known risk factors including demographical, lifestyle factors, reproductive, and family history. The addition of PRS substantially improved existing breast cancer risk prediction models including age at menarche, parity, age at first birth, combined MHT, body mass index, benign breast disease, alcohol intake, smoking, and family history of breast cancer in first-degree relatives [48, 50, 51]. For example, Garcia-Closas et al. [48] showed questionnaire-based risk factors and mammographic breast density could identify 5.6% of the population at moderate-to-high risk that would account for 14.9% of the cases for 50-year-old women in the population. The 76-SNP PRS by itself could identify 4.0% of the population at moderate-to-high risk, capturing 9.6% of the cancers. When combining the 76-SNP PRS with questionnaire-based risk factors and density, one could identify 8.5% of the population capturing 24.5% of the cancers. This could increase to 10.2% of the population capturing 32.2% of cases for the improved PRS. Maas et al. [51] evaluated combined risk stratification utility of common low penetrant SNPs and epidemiologic risk factors in the Breast and Prostate Cancer Cohort Consortium (BPC3) and in the 2010 National Health Interview Survey. For women in the highest decile of risk owing to nonmodifiable factors with PRS, those who had low BMI, did not drink or smoke, and did not use MHT had risks comparable to an average woman in the general population. The model can identify subsets of the population at an elevated risk that would benefit most from risk-reduction strategies based on altering modifiable factors.

The analysis of gene–environment interaction (G×E) may hold the key for further understanding the etiology of breast cancer and identification of the certain high-risk population. Based on GWAS data, wide-range of types of environmental data, and the design of consortiums of multiple studies, the methodologies of G×E studies have been suggested [52, 53]. As reviewed in [54], several comprehensive large-scale GxE studies conducted, however, associations between common variants and breast cancer risk are only weakly modified by environmental factors.

22.5 Future Research Direction

The GWAS is used to detect associations between common variants with low penetrance and breast cancer risk or prognosis. The primary goal of them is to better understand the biology of disease, and a better understanding will lead to prevention or better prognosis. GWASs have been successfully implemented for defining the role of genes and the environment in breast cancer risk, assisting in risk prediction (enabling preventive and personalized medicine). Personalized preventive research will have a pivotal role in future medicine particularly, in individual risk assessment using genetic and nongenetic information. In order to achieve this goal, well-designed epidemiologic studies are required to provide comprehensive preventive medical care [55].

The next steps will need to include the assessment of variants with lower frequencies and smaller effect sizes interacting with environmental factors. GWASs to date have been based on SNP arrays designed to tag common variants in the genome. These arrays do not cover all genetic variants in the population, and most GWASs to date have been conducted on individuals of European descent, although there is a growing number of studies on populations of Asian and African ancestry. It would seem natural that future GWASs will be based on fine mapping or whole genome sequence to identify the causal variant across ethnicities and understand functional mechanisms (reviewed in [12]). These will necessitate even larger cohorts of breast cancer patients, as well as the development of new statistical methods, to comprehensively evaluate combinations of variants conferring low to moderate increases in risk.

22.6 Summary

Understanding the role of low-penetrance susceptibility genes on breast cancer development leads us to improve the usefulness of the polygenic risk score combined with already known risk factors to clinical practice and preventive research in the future.

References

1. Newman B, Millikan RC, King MC. Genetic epidemiology of breast and ovarian cancers. Epidemiol Rev. 1997;19(1):69–79.
2. Caporaso N. Selection of candidate genes for population studies. IARC Sci Publ. 1999;148:23–36.
3. Goldberg JI, Borgen PI. Breast cancer susceptibility testing: past, present and future. Expert Rev Anticancer Ther. 2006;6(8):1205–14.
4. Kang E, Seong MW, Park SK, Lee JW, Lee J, Kim LS, et al. The prevalence and spectrum of BRCA1 and BRCA2 mutations in Korean population: recent update of the Korean Hereditary Breast Cancer (KOHBRA) study. Breast Cancer Res Treat. 2015;151(1):157–68.
5. Bracken MB, Ferris FL, Ott J, Barnstable C, Hoh J. Genomewide association studies. In: Rebbeck TR, Ambrosone CB, Shields PG, editors. Molecular epidemiology: applications in cancer and other human diseases. New York: Informa Healthcare; 2008. p. 225–38.
6. Zhang B, Beeghly-Fadiel A, Long J, Zheng W. Genetic variants associated with breast-cancer risk: comprehensive research synopsis, meta-analysis, and epidemiological evidence. Lancet Oncol. 2011;12(5):477–88.
7. Kim JE, Choi J, Park J, Park C, Lee SM, Park SE, et al. Associations between genetic polymorphisms of membrane transporter genes and prognosis after chemotherapy: meta-analysis and finding from Seoul Breast Cancer Study (SEBCS). Pharmacogenomics J. 2018;18(5):633–45.
8. Bray J, Sludden J, Griffin MJ, Cole M, Verrill M, Jamieson D, et al. Influence of pharmacogenetics on response and toxicity in breast cancer patients treated with doxorubicin and cyclophosphamide. Br J Cancer. 2010;102(6):1003–9.
9. Ji M, Tang J, Zhao J, Xu B, Qin J, Lu J. Polymorphisms in genes involved in drug detoxification and clinical outcomes of anthracycline-based neoadjuvant chemotherapy in Chinese Han breast cancer patients. Cancer Biol Ther. 2012;13(5):264–71.
10. Lee SY, Im SA, Park YH, Woo SY, Kim S, Choi MK, et al. Genetic polymorphisms of SLC28A3, SLC29A1 and RRM1 predict clinical outcome in patients with metastatic breast cancer receiving gemcitabine plus paclitaxel chemotherapy. Eur J Cancer. 2014;50(4):698–705.
11. Kim HJ, Im SA, Keam B, Ham HS, Lee KH, Kim TY, et al. ABCB1 polymorphism as prognostic factor in breast cancer patients treated with docetaxel and doxorubicin neoadjuvant chemotherapy. Cancer Sci. 2015;106(1):86–93.
12. Visscher PM, Wray NR, Zhang Q, Sklar P, McCarthy MI, Brown MA, et al. 10 years of GWAS discovery: biology, function, and translation. Am J Hum Genet. 2017;101(1):5–22.
13. Ahmed S, Thomas G, Ghoussaini M, Healey CS, Humphreys MK, Platte R, et al. Newly discovered breast cancer susceptibility loci on 3p24 and 17q23.2. Nat Genet. 2009;41 (5):585–90.
14. Antoniou AC, Kuchenbaecker KB, Soucy P, Beesley J, Chen X, McGuffog L, et al. Common variants at 12p11, 12q24, 9p21, 9q31.2 and in ZNF365 are associated with breast cancer risk for BRCA1 and/or BRCA2 mutation carriers. Breast Cancer Res. 2012;14(1):R33.
15. Cox A, Dunning AM, Garcia-Closas M, Balasubramanian S, Reed MW, Pooley KA, et al. A common coding variant in CASP8 is associated with breast cancer risk. Nat Genet. 2007;39 (3):352–8.
16. Easton DF, Pooley KA, Dunning AM, Pharoah PD, Thompson D, Ballinger DG, et al. Genome-wide association study identifies novel breast cancer susceptibility loci. Nature. 2007;447 (7148):1087–93.
17. Gaudet MM, Kirchhoff T, Green T, Vijai J, Korn JM, Guiducci C, et al. Common genetic variants and modification of penetrance of BRCA2-associated breast cancer. PLoS Genet. 2010;6(10):e1001183.
18. Gold B, Kirchhoff T, Stefanov S, Lautenberger J, Viale A, Garber J, et al. Genome-wide association study provides evidence for a breast cancer risk locus at 6q22.33. Proc Natl Acad Sci U S A. 2008;105(11):4340–5.

19. Haiman CA, Chen GK, Vachon CM, Canzian F, Dunning A, Millikan RC, et al. A common variant at the TERT-CLPTM1L locus is associated with estrogen receptor-negative breast cancer. Nat Genet. 2011;43(12):1210–4.
20. Kim HC, Lee JY, Sung H, Choi JY, Park SK, Lee KM, et al. A genome-wide association study identifies a breast cancer risk variant in ERBB4 at 2q34: results from the Seoul Breast Cancer Study. Breast Cancer Res. 2012;14(2):R56.
21. Lambrechts D, Truong T, Justenhoven C, Humphreys MK, Wang J, Hopper JL, et al. 11q13 is a susceptibility locus for hormone receptor positive breast cancer. Hum Mutat. 2012;33 (7):1123–32.
22. Long J, Cai Q, Sung H, Shi J, Zhang B, Choi JY, et al. Genome-wide association study in east Asians identifies novel susceptibility loci for breast cancer. PLoS Genet. 2012;8(2):e1002532.
23. Murabito JM, Rosenberg CL, Finger D, Kreger BE, Levy D, Splansky GL, et al. A genome-wide association study of breast and prostate cancer in the NHLBI's Framingham Heart Study. BMC Med Genet. 2007;8(Suppl 1):S6.
24. Siddiq A, Couch FJ, Chen GK, Lindstrom S, Eccles D, Millikan RC, et al. A meta-analysis of genome-wide association studies of breast cancer identifies two novel susceptibility loci at 6q14 and 20q11. Hum Mol Genet. 2012;21(24):5373–84.
25. Stacey SN, Manolescu A, Sulem P, Rafnar T, Gudmundsson J, Gudjonsson SA, et al. Common variants on chromosomes 2q35 and 16q12 confer susceptibility to estrogen receptor-positive breast cancer. Nat Genet. 2007;39(7):865–9.
26. Stacey SN, Manolescu A, Sulem P, Thorlacius S, Gudjonsson SA, Jonsson GF, et al. Common variants on chromosome 5p12 confer susceptibility to estrogen receptor-positive breast cancer. Nat Genet. 2008;40(6):703–6.
27. Thomas G, Jacobs KB, Kraft P, Yeager M, Wacholder S, Cox DG, et al. A multistage genome-wide association study in breast cancer identifies two new risk alleles at 1p11.2 and 14q24.1 (RAD51L1). Nat Genet. 2009;41(5):579–84.
28. Turnbull C, Ahmed S, Morrison J, Pernet D, Renwick A, Maranian M, et al. Genome-wide association study identifies five new breast cancer susceptibility loci. Nat Genet. 2010;42 (6):504–7.
29. Zheng W, Long J, Gao YT, Li C, Zheng Y, Xiang YB, et al. Genome-wide association study identifies a new breast cancer susceptibility locus at 6q25.1. Nat Genet. 2009;41(3):324–8.
30. Fachal L, Dunning AM. From candidate gene studies to GWAS and post-GWAS analyses in breast cancer. Curr Opin Genet Dev. 2015;30:32–41.
31. Antoniou AC, Wang X, Fredericksen ZS, McGuffog L, Tarrell R, Sinilnikova OM, et al. A locus on 19p13 modifies risk of breast cancer in BRCA1 mutation carriers and is associated with hormone receptor-negative breast cancer in the general population. Nat Genet. 2010;42 (10):885–92.
32. Fletcher O, Johnson N, Orr N, Hosking FJ, Gibson LJ, Walker K, et al. Novel breast cancer susceptibility locus at 9q31.2: results of a genome-wide association study. J Natl Cancer Inst. 2011;103(5):425–35.
33. Cai Q, Long J, Lu W, Qu S, Wen W, Kang D, et al. Genome-wide association study identifies breast cancer risk variant at 10q21.2: results from the Asia breast Cancer consortium. Hum Mol Genet. 2011;20(24):4991–9.
34. Ghoussaini M, Fletcher O, Michailidou K, Turnbull C, Schmidt MK, Dicks E, et al. Genome-wide association analysis identifies three new breast cancer susceptibility loci. Nat Genet. 2012;44(3):312–8.
35. Michailidou K, Hall P, Gonzalez-Neira A, Ghoussaini M, Dennis J, Milne RL, et al. Large-scale genotyping identifies 41 new loci associated with breast cancer risk. Nat Genet. 2013;45 (4):353–61, 61e1-2.
36. Cai Q, Zhang B, Sung H, Low SK, Kweon SS, Lu W, et al. Genome-wide association analysis in East Asians identifies breast cancer susceptibility loci at 1q32.1, 5q14.3 and 15q26.1. Nat Genet. 2014;46(8):886–90.

37. Milne RL, Burwinkel B, Michailidou K, Arias-Perez JI, Zamora MP, Menendez-Rodriguez P, et al. Common non-synonymous SNPs associated with breast cancer susceptibility: findings from the Breast Cancer Association Consortium. Hum Mol Genet. 2014;23(22):6096–111.
38. Barrdahl M, Canzian F, Lindstrom S, Shui I, Black A, Hoover RN, et al. Association of breast cancer risk loci with breast cancer survival. Int J Cancer. 2015;137(12):2837–45.
39. Pirie A, Guo Q, Kraft P, Canisius S, Eccles DM, Rahman N, et al. Common germline polymorphisms associated with breast cancer-specific survival. Breast Cancer Res. 2015;17:58.
40. Guo Q, Schmidt MK, Kraft P, Canisius S, Chen C, Khan S, et al. Identification of novel genetic markers of breast cancer survival. J Natl Cancer Inst. 2015;107(5):djv081.
41. Choi JY, Lee KM, Park SK, Noh DY, Ahn SH, Chung HW, et al. Genetic polymorphisms of SULT1A1 and SULT1E1 and the risk and survival of breast cancer. Cancer Epidemiol Biomark Prev. 2005;14(5):1090–5.
42. Choi JY, Lee KM, Park SK, Noh DY, Ahn SH, Yoo KY, et al. Association of paternal age at birth and the risk of breast cancer in offspring: a case control study. BMC Cancer. 2005;5:143.
43. Han W, Kang D, Lee JE, Park IA, Choi JY, Lee KM, et al. A haplotype analysis of HER-2 gene polymorphisms: association with breast cancer risk, HER-2 protein expression in the tumor, and disease recurrence in Korea. Clin Cancer Res. 2005;11(13):4775–8.
44. Song N, Choi JY, Sung H, Chung S, Song M, Park SK, et al. Heterogeneity of epidemiological factors by breast tumor subtypes in Korean women: a case-case study. Int J Cancer. 2014;135 (3):669–81.
45. Chung S, Park SK, Sung H, Song N, Han W, Noh DY, et al. Association between chronological change of reproductive factors and breast cancer risk defined by hormone receptor status: results from the Seoul breast Cancer Study. Breast Cancer Res Treat. 2013;140(3):557–65.
46. Song N, Choi JY, Sung H, Jeon S, Chung S, Park SK, et al. Prediction of breast cancer survival using clinical and genetic markers by tumor subtypes. PLoS One. 2015;10(4):e0122413.
47. Chatterjee N, Shi J, Garcia-Closas M. Developing and evaluating polygenic risk prediction models for stratified disease prevention. Nat Rev Genet. 2016;17(7):392–406.
48. Garcia-Closas M, Gunsoy NB, Chatterjee N. Combined associations of genetic and environmental risk factors: implications for prevention of breast cancer. J Natl Cancer Inst. 2014;106 (11):dju305.
49. Mavaddat N, Michailidou K, Dennis J, Lush M, Fachal L, Lee A, et al. Polygenic risk scores for prediction of breast cancer and breast cancer subtypes. Am J Hum Genet. 2019;104(1):21–34.
50. Zhang X, Rice M, Tworoger SS, Rosner BA, Eliassen AH, Tamimi RM, et al. Addition of a polygenic risk score, mammographic density, and endogenous hormones to existing breast cancer risk prediction models: a nested case-control study. PLoS Med. 2018;15(9):e1002644.
51. Maas P, Barrdahl M, Joshi AD, Auer PL, Gaudet MM, Milne RL, et al. Breast cancer risk from modifiable and nonmodifiable risk factors among white women in the United States. JAMA Oncol. 2016;2(10):1295–302.
52. Gauderman WJ, Mukherjee B, Aschard H, Hsu L, Lewinger JP, Patel CJ, et al. Update on the state of the science for analytical methods for gene-environment interactions. Am J Epidemiol. 2017;186(7):762–70.
53. McAllister K, Mechanic LE, Amos C, Aschard H, Blair IA, Chatterjee N, et al. Current challenges and new opportunities for gene-environment interaction studies of complex diseases. Am J Epidemiol. 2017;186(7):753–61.
54. Rudolph A, Chang-Claude J, Schmidt MK. Gene-environment interaction and risk of breast cancer. Br J Cancer. 2016;114(2):125–33.
55. Song M, Lee HW, Kang D. The potential application of personalized preventive research. Jpn J Clin Oncol. 2014;44(11):1017–24.

Chapter 23
Rare Coding Variants Associated with Breast Cancer

Mi-Ryung Han

Abstract Breast cancer is the most common invasive cancer in females worldwide and in Asian countries. Common variants found by genome-wide association studies (GWAS) only explain approximately 16% of the heritability of breast cancer: therefore, it is important to examine rare/low-frequency variants in GWAS-identified loci which may also contribute to breast cancer risk. Previous studies have reported that genetic variants with lower allele frequency are more likely to be functional than common variants in coding regions. In future studies, the contribution of observed rare variants will be estimated more clearly when additive and recessive genetic variants will be investigated using sequencing technology, eQTL studies, and improved statistical methods in large samples.

Keywords Breast cancer · Rare coding variant · Genome-wide association studies (GWAS)

23.1 Introduction

Genome-wide association studies (GWAS) have identified novel and known loci associated with breast cancer risk. Although GWAS continue to reveal new associations, each newly associated variant has a smaller effect size and contributes only marginally to the cumulative variation of complex diseases. This suggests that GWAS of population-based subjects may be reaching the limits of their ability to reveal genetic variation underlying complex traits. Then, a question has arisen whether additional forms of genetic variation, such as rare variants with large individual effects, could contribute to the heritability of complex traits such as breast cancer.

M.-R. Han (✉)
Division of Life Sciences, College of Life Sciences and Bioengineering, Incheon National University, Incheon, South Korea
e-mail: genetic0309@inu.ac.kr

D.-Y. Noh et al. (eds.), *Translational Research in Breast Cancer*, Advances in Experimental Medicine and Biology 1187,
https://doi.org/10.1007/978-981-32-9620-6_23

23.1.1 Impact of Genome-Wide Association Studies

In the last 10 years, GWAS have been extremely successful in mapping susceptibility loci for complex diseases and quantitative traits [1]. As of 20 February 2015, the National Human Genome Research Institute's (NHGRI) GWAS catalog listed 2111 publications and 15,396 single nucleotide polymorphisms (SNPs) that showed significant or suggestive association with one or more of over 900 different phenotypes, including disease states, drug responses, behavioral traits, and physiological measures [2]. The associations found by GWAS implicated many genes that were not considered a priori to be good candidates for the traits of interest. Thus, GWAS have made an important contribution in finding many novel variants in many clinically relevant phenotypes.

So far, association studies of individual common variants are often referred to as GWAS since GWAS systematically evaluate common variants, typically with a minor allele frequency (MAF) $> 5\%$. In contrast, association studies of sets of rare variants in coding regions are often referred to as exome- or whole genome-sequencing studies. GWAS are designed to detect associations through linkage disequilibrium (LD) between genotyped (or imputed) common SNP markers and unknown causal variants. There has been impressive increase in the number of common susceptibility loci identified via GWAS, and this has made us take an important step forward in our understanding of cancer biology. The rate of discovery of new susceptibility loci for cancer through GWAS has increased dramatically. For example, one of the very first large GWAS has found five significant loci to be associated with breast cancer risk in 2007 [3]. Since then, more than 180 new loci have been identified through genome-wide approaches [4–9].

One of the important findings through GWAS is that the majority of risk variants and their proxies are located in non-protein-coding sequences. The etiologic mechanisms at noncoding susceptibility loci have also been found using epigenetic information such as chromatin histone modifications. For instance, Rhie et al. conducted functional characterization of 71 breast cancer susceptibility loci and they found only 21 SNPs in exon region among 1005 SNPs in LD with the index SNPs ($r^2 \geq 0.5$) [10]. They found 76 SNPs in predicted transcription start-site regions and 921 SNPs in putative enhancers at 60 of the 71 breast cancer risk loci [10]. GWAS have also discovered pleiotropic associations, defined as a single genotype or locus of the genome being associated with risk of different cancers [3]. This association has also been found between cancer and non-cancer phenotypes, for example, endometrial and prostate cancers and type 2 diabetes at *HNF1B* gene on 17q12 [11, 12]. Even though we already know that cancers generally evolve from a common sequence of events such as proliferation and altered DNA repair capacity, GWAS have started to suggest common mechanisms of carcinogenesis or disease susceptibility pathways across different disease phenotypes. So far, GWAS have delivered meaningful biologically relevant knowledge since the combination of large sample sizes (meta-analysis) and stringent significance testing have discovered a large number of replicable associations between complex traits and genetic variants

[13, 14]. A number of variants or different variants at the same loci have been found to be associated with the same disease in different ethnic groups. This implies that combination of multiple variants with small effect sizes can predict disease status in independent samples. Therefore, GWAS have led to huge advances in genetic research area by discovering the role of known cancer pathways and unknown biological significance of noncoding regions of the genome involved in common diseases and other complex traits.

23.1.2 Limitations of GWAS

Despite the success of GWAS in identifying common variants that contribute to complex diseases, the majority of genetic variants contributing to disease remain unknown. The GWAS field focused on the simple common disease-common variant (CDCV) hypothesis which argues that genetic variations with appreciable frequencies in the population at large, but relatively low "penetrance," are the major contributors to genetic susceptibility to common diseases [15]. As an alternative to CDCV, common disease rare variant (CDRV) hypothesis has been proposed since common diseases could be influenced by numerous rare or low-frequency variants with large effects on disease risk [15]. At least part of the "missing heritability" might be explained by a cumulative effect of multiple rare variants (MAF $< 1\%$). This "missing heritability" from GWAS has been issued since the variance contributed by the causal variants would be higher than the variance explained by the associated genotyped SNP, because the genotyped SNPs will not tag the causal variants with great precision. The source of "missing heritability" remains unclear, and it is unlikely to be captured in current GWAS which focus on common variants.

The importance of rare and common variants is one of the topics that leads an intense debate. Some researchers suggested "synthetic associations" where association signals detected for common variants could, in fact, be caused by rare variants with large effects (Odds Ratio $\sim$ 10) [16]. Recently, Saunders et al. revealed evidence for the nature of causal variation at GWAS hits in the *HOXB13* gene and their contribution to the heritability of prostate cancer [17]. They found synthetic associations by fine mapping the *HOXB* region and detected common variants tagging a rare coding allele [18]. Although examples of synthetic associations cannot explain all GWAS results, if rare variants influencing a disease are disproportionately located at the same loci as the common variants already identified, then targeted resequencing of GWAS regions in large samples could be fruitful in discovering causal rare variants.

One of the limitations of current GWAS technology is its limited chip design to detect rare, low-frequency variants. In order to overcome this limitation, tag-SNP analyses have been increased using a genotype imputation method in which data analysis is not restricted to SNPs that have been experimentally genotyped. Siu et al. revealed that GWAS coverage of rare variants was still inadequate despite using improved chips designed to detect them [19]. They found that the quality of imputed low-frequency and rare variants is generally lower than that for common variants [19]. Also, it has been estimated that previous GWAS have found less than 20% of all independent GWAS-detectable SNPs in chronic diseases that have been recorded in the NHGRI Catalog of Published GWAS [20]. However, recently, the Haplotype Reference Consortium (HRC) creates a large reference panel of human haplotypes by combining together sequencing data from multiple cohorts (http://www.haplotype-reference-consortium.org/). Their first release in early summer 2015 will consist of 64,976 haplotypes at 39,235,157 SNPs, all with an estimated minor allele count of $\geq$5 from 32,914 samples. With this large reference panel, we can extend the reach of imputation into low-frequency variants and improve imputation accuracy for both common and rare variants. We would expect that future GWAS can potentially detect more SNPs through improved coverage with increased sample sizes.

GWAS is based on the theory that a causal, functional variant is located on a haplotype, and therefore a marker allele in LD with the causal variant (proxy SNP) will show an association with a disease. However, GWAS have identified only a small number of the causal variants for recently identified genetic loci, which interpret only a small portion of the genetic contribution to diseases [16, 18, 21, 22]. Most variants identified through GWAS are noncoding and located in intronic or intergenic regions. Although causal variants can be identified, the ability to interpret their biological role in a genome is still limited by incomplete knowledge of noncoding regulatory elements, their unknown function in the cellular states and processes, and their mechanisms of action.

In addition, reproducibility of GWAS findings is crucial to provide convincing statistical evidence of novel associations and to rule out associations due to biases [23]. However, GWAS sometimes do not replicate across different populations or ethnic groups [24]. There are several reasons for this non-replication including false positives of the original observations, insufficient power of the follow-up studies, true etiologic heterogeneity in subsequent studies, and differences in design or trait definitions [23]. Large replication studies in different populations are required in order to validate whether the same association is commonly found in human populations regardless of the differences in environmental and genetic factors.

In medical genetics, the ultimate goal is to identify causal functional variants and explain the biological mechanisms through which they exert their effects on disease. In order to fill out gap between GWAS findings and identification of causal variants, new approaches to isolate and define causal variants are necessary to investigate genetic variants that affect disease. These new methods, including improved imputation algorithms for rare variants, would explain the "missing heritability" issue of the GWAS.

23.1.3 Genotype Imputation

In addition to the sequencing technology, imputed SNP analysis has been widely used in the post-GWAS era especially when many studies are combined (meta-analysis) in efforts to find associations that are too small to be detectable in any single study. Imputation is useful when not all studies used the same genotyping platform, and Hidden Markov Model (HMM) that describes the haplotype pair as an imperfect mosaic of the other haplotypes is widely used for fast and very large-scale SNP imputation in a number of programs [25, 26]. Imputation can also be used to examine rare variants associated with complex traits. For example, recent study identified novel associations between rare variants in *APP* gene and Alzheimer's disease and between rare variants in *PDX1* gene and T2D through sequencing the whole genomes of 2630 Icelanders, followed by imputation into large sets of GWAS data [27, 28].

23.1.4 Gene Regulatory Effects of GWAS SNPs

It has been increasingly suggested that SNPs associated with complex traits are more likely to be expression quantitative trait loci (eQTLs) which is a region of the genome harboring a genetic variant contributing to gene expression variation. Currently, eQTL data in multiple tissues have been made publicly available, and it becomes possible to investigate if any of the variants within the association have transcriptional effects through association mapping (eQTL mapping) of variable transcription levels among individuals [29, 30]. Recently, gene expression eQTL studies using direct sequencing of mRNA (RNA-seq) have emerged due to known problems with the hybridization method of arrays and the decrease in cost of RNA-seq [31–33]. RNA-seq can detect expression at the gene, exon, transcript, and coding DNA sequence levels unlike microarray technology which is limited to the gene level for most arrays and the exon level for specially designed exon arrays.

It has been shown that GWAS signals are enriched with eQTL variants in a tissue-specific manner, providing insight into biology of transcription regulation [34, 35]. For example, eQTL analyses of 15 previously reported breast cancer risk loci resulted in the discovery of three variants (at 2q35 (*IGFBP5*), 5q11 (*C5orf35*), and 16q12 (*TOX3*)) that are significantly associated with transcript levels [36]. For rare variant studies using cis-eQTL mapping, Cheng et al. discovered rare variants associated with autism spectrum disorders in the GWAS candidate gene (*SEMA5A*) [37]. It is important to use appropriate eQTL data since some eQTL data come from a tissue or cell line of limited pathophysiological relevance to the condition of interest.

Rapid advances of genotyping technologies built on GWAS have made it possible to discover a large number of genetic variants at low cost. There should be a careful consideration of utilizing many available resources elucidating the role of common and rare variants in diseases and complex traits. Although imputation methods has been suggested with increased reference genome, challenges remain with imputation techniques such as distinguishing between missing data for biological reasons and those arising from sampling variation. By combining information from multiple sources and new statistical approaches specifically designed to study rare alleles, we will be able to uncover the genetic architecture of complex traits including breast cancer.

23.2 Review of Past Studies

23.2.1 Current Status of Genetic Research on Breast Cancer

Breast cancer is the most common malignancy among women in the United States and many other countries around the world [38]. It is a complex disease in which genetic factors play an important role [39, 40]. In the 1990s, the two major susceptibility genes for breast cancer, *BRCA1* [41] and *BRCA2* [42], were identified through family-based linkage studies. Due to the limitation of linkage studies which aimed at identifying rare and high-risk disease-associated mutations based on multiple individuals in a family, a large number of candidate gene studies were conducted over the following decade. Candidate gene approaches have focused on selecting genes based on their known biological function and aimed at identifying moderate and low-penetrance alleles believed to be responsible for the remaining familial risk. Several DNA repair genes including *ATM* [43], *CHEK2* [44], *BRIP1* [45], and *PALB2* [46] and an apoptosis gene, *CASP8* [47, 48], have been implicated in susceptibility to breast cancer. However, the majority of reported SNP associations in candidate genes could not be replicated.

Extensive genetic studies have identified high-penetrance genes (*BRCA1*, *BRCA2*, *PTEN*, and *TP53*), moderate-penetrance genes (*CHEK2*, *ATM*, *BRIP1*, *PALB2*, *RAD51C*, *STK11*, *CDH1*, *RAD50*, and *NBN*), and more than 180 low-penetrance loci that contribute to the risk of breast cancer over the past 20 years [4, 6, 39, 49–51]. It has been shown that pathogenic mutations in the *BRCA1* and *BRCA2* genes are associated with a 10- to 20-fold increased risk of breast cancer which corresponds to a cumulative risk of breast cancer by age 70 years of 55–65% for *BRCA1* mutation carriers and 45–47% for *BRCA2* mutation carriers [52]. Recently, it has been reported that female *PTEN* mutation carriers have an 85% lifetime risk of developing breast cancer with 50% penetrance by 50 years of age [53]. These findings were subsequently confirmed by two other studies [54, 55]. Mutations in the *TP53* gene are associated with at least a ten-fold increased risk of breast cancer and account for 2–7% of early-onset breast cancer [56, 57]. It is estimated that the cumulative risk of breast cancer by 70 years is approximately 14% for women who carry *CHEK2 1100delC*, and a subsequent meta-analysis based on 29,154 cases and 37,064 controls from 25 case–control studies reported a significant association between *CHEK2 1100delC* heterozygotes and breast cancer risk with OR (95% CI) of 2.75 (2.25–3.36) [58, 59]. Similarly, the approximate risk of breast cancer is 15% for those who carry *ATM* mutations [60]. It is estimated that the eight confirmed high and moderate-penetrance genes (*BRCA1*, *BRCA2*, *PTEN*, *TP53*, *CHEK2*, *ATM*, *BRIP1*, and *PALP2*), explain approximately 20% of the familial risk of breast cancer [61].

Since 2005, GWAS have made an important contribution to find many novel variants for human diseases that were not found by the candidate gene approach. GWAS are designed to detect associations through linkage disequilibrium (LD) between genotyped (or imputed) common SNP markers and unknown causal variants. Approximately 180 common genetic susceptibility loci for breast cancer risk have been found, including those identified in studies among Asian women [4, 9, 49, 62, 63].

In 2008, the Asia Breast Cancer Consortium (ABCC) has been initiated, a GWAS in East Asians to search for novel genetic susceptibility loci for breast cancer risk. Over the years, this consortium has grown into a large collaboration involving cases and controls recruited in studies conducted in multiple Asian countries [8]. Using data generated from ABCC, Dr. Wei Zheng's group from Vanderbilt University have identified ten novel susceptibility loci for breast cancer risk [4, 6, 8, 64–68], and many of these loci were subsequently replicated in studies of European descendants [4, 8, 64, 69]. Recently, Han et al. (author of this chapter) identified two novel breast cancer susceptibility loci in Ease Asians using ABCC data [70]. We conducted a two-stage genome-wide association study (GWAS) including 14,224 cases and 14,829 controls of East Asian women to search for novel genetic susceptibility loci for breast cancer. SNPs in two loci (1p22.3 near the *LMO4* gene and 21q22.12 near the *LINC00160* gene) were found to be associated with breast cancer risk at the genome-wide significance level [70]. Association of SNP rs12118297 at 1p22.3 was replicated in another study, DRIVE GAME-ON Consortium, including 16,003 cases and 41,335 controls of European ancestry. Functional annotation using the ENCODE data indicates that rs12118297 at 21q22.12 might be located in a repressed element and locus 21q22.12 may affect breast cancer risk through regulating *LINC00160* expressions and interaction with estrogen receptor signaling. Our findings provide additional insights into the genetics of breast cancer.

Despite the recent success of GWAS, the majority of the genetic component of many complex traits remains unexplained. In addition, although the statistical evidence for an association between SNP and breast cancer risk is overwhelming, the biologically relevant variants and the mechanism by which they lead to increased risk are unknown and require further genetic and functional characterization. As rare variants have been comparatively less well-studied than common variants, attention has shifted to identifying additional risk factors.

23.2.2 Breast Cancer Susceptibility: The Role of Rare Variants

GWAS are designed to evaluate common genetic variants, typically with a MAF > 0.05; therefore, examining only a portion of the genomic landscape of complex traits. GWAS identified more than 100 common genetic susceptibility loci associated with breast cancer so far; however, these loci collectively explain approximately 16% of the heritability of breast cancer [51]. It is reasonable to assume that most common and highly penetrant susceptibility genes have already been discovered for breast cancer. Currently, many studies are investigating rare (MAF < 0.01) variants which have been more challenging to assess.

23.2.3 Missing Heritability

More than 20 years ago, the identification of the two high-penetrance genes in breast cancer, *BRCA1* and *BRCA2*, launched a sustained effort to uncover new genes explaining the "missing heritability" in the disease. The best known high or moderate-penetrance genes include *BRCA1*, *BRCA2*, *TP53*, *PTEN*, *STK11*, *PALB2*, and *ATM*, and these genes globally account for around 35% of the familial breast cancer cases [71]. Many explanations, such as rare variants, epistatic interactions, gene–environment interactions, structural variants, heritable epigenetic factors, parent-of-origin effects, or inflated heritability estimates have been proposed to illustrate the "missing heritability" that the GWAS loci and high-penetrance genes could not explain [72–75]. The major debates over the nature of the genetic contribution to individual susceptibility to common complex diseases are common disease-common variant (CDCV) and common disease rare variant (CDRV) hypotheses. The CDCV hypothesis argues that genetic variations with appreciable frequencies in the population at large, but relatively low penetrance (or the probability that a carrier of the relevant variants will express the disease), are the major contributors to genetic susceptibility to common diseases [15]. CDRV argues that multiple rare DNA sequence variants, each with relatively high penetrance, could account for the genetic variance in disease susceptibility [15].

Many investigators have tried the alternative CDRV hypothesis. Pritchard argued that the notion that multiple, very recent rare variations contributing to disease arising in the last two centuries is more consistent with human population pathobiology than the notion that older, common variations are contributing to disease [76]. This is because rare variants are often evolved from more recent mutations and subjected to less natural selection. Leal pointed out that rare variants, although individually rare, are collectively frequent, and even though their effect sizes are greater than those observed for common variants, they are not large enough to produce familial aggregation [75]. In this light, reports on the frequency of human alleles and their likely "functional" or phenotypic effects suggest that rare coding variants are enriched for functional importance [77]. We are in the era of investigating rare variants that might play an important role in explaining the "missing heritability" of complex traits including breast cancer.

23.2.4 Rare Variants Associated with Breast Cancer and Other Diseases

It has been increasingly recognized that the "missing heritability" for breast cancer could be partially explained by low-frequency (MAF 0.01–0.05) and rare (MAF < 0.01) variants. There is strong evidence that rare genetic variation is important in breast cancer predisposition [78]. In the 1990s, genome-wide linkage analysis and positional cloning led to the identification of the DNA repair genes *BRCA1* and *BRCA2*, and rare mutations of those genes in noncoding region confer substantial risks to breast cancer [78]. More recently, through case–control resequencing studies of candidate genes, several rare coding variants have been shown to be associated with breast cancer risk such as *ERBB2*, *CHEK2*, *ATM*, *BRIP1*, *PALB2*, *RAD51C*, *RAD51D*, and *PPM1D* genes [79–85]. Rare protein-truncating variant (PTV) mutations in the p53-inducible protein phosphatase gene *PPM1D* are associated with predisposition to breast cancer [81]. In addition, a known moderate susceptibility indel variant (*CHEK2 1100delC*) and a catalog of 11 rare variants in other genes (*FANCM*, *WNT8A*, *MAPKAP1*, *TNFSF8*, *PTPRF*, *UBA3*, *AXIN1*, *TIMP3*, *SLBP*, *CNTROB*, and *S1PR3*), presenting signs of association with breast cancer, were identified through whole-exome sequencing [71].

23.3 Current Evidence and Concepts

Recently, multiple papers reported that low-frequency or rare variants in GWAS loci have been identified for other diseases through target sequencing or fine mapping [86–88]. Beaudoin et al. have used a targeted sequencing approach in 200 ulcerative colitis cases and 150 healthy controls, all of French Canadian descent, to study 55 genes in regions associated with ulcerative colitis [86]. They found significant association with rare non-synonymous variants in both *IL23R* and *CARD9*, previously identified from sequencing of Crohn's disease loci, as well as a novel association in *RNF186* [86]. Fine mapping of GWAS loci associated with low-density lipoprotein cholesterol also led to the discovery of several low-frequency or rare variants [87]. In addition, Johansen et al. reported that an accumulation of rare variants is present in GWAS-identified genes and that these contribute to the heritability of complex traits among individuals at the extreme of a lipid phenotype [88]. These studies support the hypothesis that rare coding variants in GWAS loci may contribute to breast cancer risk.

Zhang et al. recently investigated rare missense/nonsense variants with MAF $\leq$ 0.05 located in flanking 1 Mb of each of the index SNP in 67 GWAS loci from the Shanghai Breast Cancer Study including 3472 cases and 3595 controls [89]. Notably, five rare variants in different genes (*BRCA2*, *EDEM1*, *EFEMP2*, and *FBXO18*) were associated with breast cancer risk at *P*-value <0.01 [89]. Han et al. (author of this chapter) found two novel missense variants with minor allele frequency (MAF) < 0.01 that were associated with breast cancer risk: rs201870990 (Val498Met) in the *ANO1* gene and rs139163400 (Ile2029Thr) in the *ZFYVE26* gene [90]. Compared to Zhang's study, we included an increased number of Chinese (5766 cases and 5703 controls) and investigated other ethnic groups, European Americans (2204 cases and 5240 controls) and African Americans (1034 cases and 1053 controls) as well. We performed more comprehensive functional and eQTL analyses to prioritize candidate genes in the 1 Mb regions flanking the breast cancer GWAS loci using three major databases (the Cancer Genome Atlas (TCGA) [63], the Genotype-Tissue Expression (GTEx) [91], and Molecular Taxonomy of Breast Cancer International Consortium (METABRIC) [92]), and assessed rare recessive variants in addition to additive models. With increased number of populations and improved statistical methods, we had more power to detect rare variants associated with breast cancer risk compared with Zhang's study.

For rare coding variant studies, it is important to use appropriate eQTL data, statistical method, and algorithms for treatment of confounding factors. These are explained in below paragraphs.

23.3.1 eQTL Analysis

GWAS have identified thousands of variants that are associated with complex traits and diseases. However, because most variants are noncoding and located in intronic or intergenic regions, it is difficult to identify causal genes. Polymorphisms associated with messenger RNA (mRNA) levels are typically referred to as eQTLs. eQTLs have provided key insights into genes and pathways as well as the genetic architecture of gene expression [36]. Several eQTL-mapping studies have shown that disease-predisposing variants often affect the gene expression levels of nearby genes (cis-eQTLs) [93–95]. Cis-acting regulation is due to DNA variation that directly influences the transcription process in an allele-specific manner. Alternatively, trans-acting regulation affects the gene expression by modifying the activity (or abundance) of the factors that regulate the gene [96]. Regarding rare variant studies, Cheng et al. discovered rare variants associated with autism spectrum disorders in the GWAS candidate gene (*SEMA5A*) using cis-eQTL mapping [37]. Recently, eQTL analyses of 15 previously reported breast cancer risk loci resulted in the discovery of three variants (at 2q35 (*IGFBP5*), 5q11 (*C5orf35*), and 16q12 (*TOX3*)) that are significantly associated with transcript levels [36].

The eQTL approach is valuable when causal variants exert remote regulatory effects on genes whose coding regions lie outside the region of association, and this approach has potential to find candidate genes and their functional variants. To investigate rare variants in the eQTL genes might be particularly informative since the associated rare variants for complex diseases will be more facile to evaluate for functional impact.

23.3.2 Statistical Issues and Functional Annotation of Rare Variants

The standard approach in GWAS to testing for association between genetic variants and complex traits is a single-variant test under an additive genetic model. However, the single-marker-based analysis on each of the rare variants will lead to severe loss of power due to the low frequency of rare variants. To address this issue, researchers tried to evaluate cumulative effects of multiple variants in a biologically relevant region, such as a gene, instead of testing the effects of single variants which is commonly done in GWAS. Several methods for testing association by combining rare variants have already been developed [97–101]. Recently, Lee et al. provided a systematic review of recently developed methods for rare-variant association test [99]. They suggested that omnibus tests that combine different tests can provide an attractive alternative for balancing power and robustness since it is hard to have a test that is optimal for all scenarios [99]. In addition to these methods that have been developed for population-based rare-variant analysis, several statistical methods have also been released in the last 3 years for family-based rare-variant analysis [102–105]. Family-based studies enable us to collect multiple copies of rare variants in smaller sample sizes and powerful for studying de novo mutations.

One of the major challenges for rare-variant analysis includes limited available information for prioritizing and annotating functional variants, which is important for grouping variants for multi-marker tests and interpreting results. There are a variety of computational resources available to annotate DNA sequence variants for both coding and noncoding variants (e.g., PolyPhen-2, SIFT, VEP, ENCODE, FANTOM5, RegulomeDB, etc.). Using these tools, rare variants can be prioritized for a group-based analysis, and most coding variants that are probably detrimental, including nonsense, splice site, frameshift, and stop-gain/stop-loss, are selected. However, researchers are currently investigating strategies to catalog all loss-of-function alleles in the human genome and to distinguish missense variants between phenotypically active and neutral alleles as population genetic theory and empirical observations showed that even functional missense variants will mostly have small effect sizes [106–108].

23.3.3 Treatment of Confounding

Population stratification refers to differences in allele frequencies between cases and controls due to systematic differences in ancestry rather than association of genes with disease. In GWAS, population stratification is a major confounding factor for case–control association studies and can result in false-positive associations since the association found could be due to the underlying structure of the population and not a disease-associated locus [109, 110]. Therefore, population stratification can be confounders depending on which data people used in their GWAS.

When analyzing rare variants, it is especially important to adequately control for population substructure since rare variants tend to have occurred more recently and therefore have greater population diversity than common variants. Figure 23.1 shows that the rarer a genetic variant is within a population, the less likely it is to be found in all ethnic groups [111]. If a GWAS-identified genetic marker is linked to a mixture of common and rare causal alleles, some of the rare ones are likely to differ in frequency in different populations, or even be completely absent in some populations [111]. In GWAS, principal component analysis (PCA) and linear mixed models are commonly used to adjust for population stratification [112].

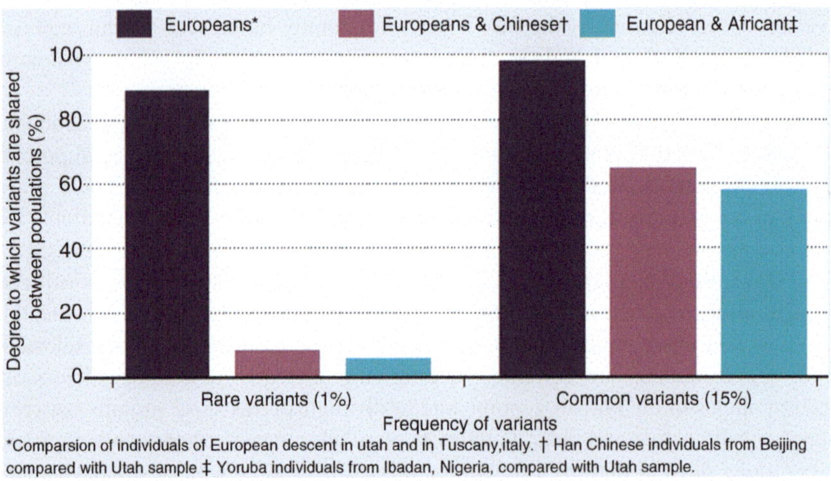

Fig. 23.1 Rare alleles more likely population-specific (100 people were sampled from each population). Figure reprinted from Bustamante et al. Genomics for the world. Nature 2011;475 (7355):163–5 [16]

23.4 Future Research Direction

Due to many successful results from GWAS, researchers are able to use resources of GWAS-identified loci associated with breast cancer. Studies previously evaluating rare coding variants associated with breast cancer have been limited to their sample sizes. However, it remains possible that rare variants in GWAS-identified genes may contribute significantly to breast cancer risk [86–88, 113].

If a rare variant is predicted to have a functional effect according to several functional prediction algorithms, further biological validation is required to prove any suspected functional effect. Specifically, LOF variants are expected to be found at lower frequencies in the genome due to evolutionary pressure which results in an enrichment for false positives among such variants [106, 114]. Therefore, proper biological validation of these variants is especially important.

Although the classic dominant inheritance model is still useful for rare variant evaluation, recessive patterns of compound heterozygotes (CH) of rare variants can also expose the function altering effects of rare variants. For validation of CH findings and explanation of the functional effect of rare variants, family-based sequencing studies will serve as valuable resources. Therefore, further studies including experimental validations are necessary to explain rare variant findings in the genetics of breast cancer.

23.5 Summary

From GWAS results, researchers are able to investigate rare variants associated with breast cancer risk using various statistical methods and eQTL studies. It is now important to examine rare variants as other studies have proven that rare coding variants in GWAS loci contribute to breast cancer risk. However, researchers should pay attention to their study design and statistical power since rare variant studies require large sample sizes for detecting low-frequency ($MAF < 0.01$ or 0.001) ones.

Funding This research was supported by Incheon National University Research Grant in 2019.

References

1. Visscher PM, Wray NR, Zhang Q, Sklar P, McCarthy MI, Brown MA, Yang J. 10 years of GWAS discovery: biology, function, and translation. AJHG. 2017;101:5–22.
2. Welter D, MacArthur J, Morales J, Burdett T, Hall P, Junkins H, et al. The NHGRI GWAS catalog, a curated resource of SNP-trait associations. Nucleic Acids Res. 2014;42(D1): D1001–6.

3. Easton DF, Pooley KA, Dunning AM, PDP P, Thompson D, Ballinger DG, et al. Genome-wide association study identifies novel breast cancer susceptibility loci. Nature. 2007;447 (7148):1087–93.
4. Cai Q, Zhang B, Sung H, Low S-K, Kweon S-S, Lu W, et al. Genome-wide association analysis in East Asians identifies breast cancer susceptibility loci at 1q32.1, 5q14.3 and 15q26.1. Nat Genet. 2014;46(8):886–90.
5. Ghoussaini M, Fletcher O, Michailidou K, Turnbull C, Schmidt MK, Dicks E, et al. Genome-wide association analysis identifies three new breast cancer susceptibility loci. Nat Genet. 2012;44(3):312–8.
6. Cai Q, Long J, Lu W, Qu S, Wen W, Kang D, et al. Genome-wide association study identifies breast cancer risk variant at 10q21.2: results from the Asia breast cancer consortium. Hum Mol Genet. 2011;20(24):4991–9.
7. Thomas G, Jacobs KB, Kraft P, Yeager M, Wacholder S, Cox DG, et al. A multistage genome-wide association study in breast cancer identifies two new risk alleles at 1p11.2 and 14q24.1 (*RAD51L1*). Nat Genet. 2009;41(5):579–84.
8. Zheng W, Long J, Gao Y-T, Li C, Zheng Y, Xiang Y-B, et al. Genome-wide association study identifies a new breast cancer susceptibility locus at 6q25. Nat Genet. 2009;41(3):324–8.
9. Michailidou K, Lindström S, Dennis J, Beesley J, Hui S, Kar S, et al. Association analysis identifies 65 new breast cancer risk loci. Nature. 2017;551(7678):92–4.
10. Rhie SK, Coetzee SG, Noushmehr H, Yan C, Kim JM, Haiman CA, et al. Comprehensive functional annotation of seventy-one breast cancer risk loci. PLoS One. 2013;22:e63925.
11. Spurdle AB, Thompson DJ, Ahmed S, Ferguson K, Healey CS, O'Mara T, et al. Genome-wide association study identifies a common variant associated with risk of endometrial cancer. Nat Genet. 2011;43(5):451–4.
12. Kasper JS, Liu Y, Giovannucci E. Diabetes mellitus and risk of prostate cancer in the health professionals follow-up study. Int J Cancer. 2009;124(6):1398–403.
13. Zou L, Zhong R, Lou J, Lu X, Wang Q, Yang Y, et al. Replication study in Chinese population and meta-analysis supports association of the 11q23 locus with colorectal cancer. PLoS One. 2012;18:e45461.
14. Long J, Zhang B, Signorello LB, Cai Q, Deming-Halverson S, Shrubsole MJ, et al. Evaluating genome-wide association study-identified breast cancer risk variants in African-American women. PLoS One. 2013;8(4):e58350.
15. Schork NJ, Murray SS, Frazer KA, Topol EJ. Common vs. rare allele hypotheses for complex diseases. Curr Opin Genet Dev. 2009;19(3):212–9.
16. Graham RR, Kyogoku C, Sigurdsson S, Vlasova IA, Davies LRL, Baechler EC, et al. Three functional variants of IFN regulatory factor 5 (IRF5) define risk and protective haplotypes for human lupus. Proc Natl Acad Sci. 2007;104(16):6758–63.
17. Rare Variants Create Synthetic Genome-Wide Associations. 2018. http://journals.plos.org/plosbiology/article?id=10.1371/journal.pbio.1000294
18. Saunders EJ, Dadaev T, Leongamornlert DA, Jugurnauth-Little S, Tymrakiewicz M, Wiklund F, et al. Fine-mapping the HOXB region detects common variants tagging a rare coding allele: evidence for synthetic Association in Prostate Cancer. PLoS Genet. 2014;10(2): e1004129.
19. Siu H, Zhu Y, Jin L, Xiong M. Implication of next-generation sequencing on association studies. BMC Genomics. 2011;12:322.
20. Lindquist KJ, Jorgenson E, Hoffmann TJ, Witte JS. The impact of improved microarray coverage and larger sample sizes on future genome-wide association studies. Genet Epidemiol. 2013;37(4):383–92.
21. Visscher PM, Brown MA, McCarthy MI, Yang J. Five years of GWAS discovery. Am J Hum Genet. 2012;90(1):7–24.
22. Sigurdsson S, Nordmark G, Göring HHH, Lindroos K, Wiman A-C, Sturfelt G, et al. Polymorphisms in the tyrosine kinase 2 and interferon regulatory factor 5 genes are associated with systemic lupus erythematosus. Am J Hum Genet. 2005;76(3):528–37.

23. Kraft P, Zeggini E, Ioannidis JPA. Replication in genome-wide association studies. Stat Sci Rev J Inst Math Stat. 2009;24(4):561–73.
24. Nebert DW, Zhang G, Vesell ES. From human genetics and genomics to pharmacogenetics and pharmacogenomics: past lessons, future directions. Drug Metab Rev. 2008;40 (2):187–224.
25. MaCH: using sequence and genotype data to estimate haplotypes and unobserved genotypes. 2018. https://www.ncbi.nlm.nih.gov/pmc/articles/PMC3175618/.
26. Stephens M, Scheet P. Accounting for decay of linkage disequilibrium in haplotype inference and missing-data imputation. Am J Hum Genet. 2005;76(3):449–62.
27. Steinthorsdottir V, Thorleifsson G, Sulem P, Helgason H, Grarup N, Sigurdsson A, et al. Identification of low-frequency and rare sequence variants associated with elevated or reduced risk of type 2 diabetes. Nat Genet. 2014;46(3):294–8.
28. Jonsson T, Atwal JK, Steinberg S, Snaedal J, Jonsson PV, Bjornsson S, et al. A mutation in APP protects against Alzheimer's disease and age-related cognitive decline. Nature. 2012;488 (7409):96–9.
29. Yang T-P, Beazley C, Montgomery SB, Dimas AS, Gutierrez-Arcelus M, Stranger BE, et al. Genevar: a database and Java application for the analysis and visualization of SNP-gene associations in eQTL studies. Bioinformatics. 2010;26(19):2474–6.
30. Stranger BE, Montgomery SB, Dimas AS, Parts L, Stegle O, Ingle CE, et al. Patterns of cis regulatory variation in diverse human populations. PLoS Genet. 2012;8(4):e1002639.
31. Verdugo RA, Farber CR, Warden CH, Medrano JF. Serious limitations of the QTL/microarray approach for QTL gene discovery. BMC Biol. 2010;8:96.
32. Westra H-J, Franke L. From genome to function by studying eQTLs. Biochim Biophys Acta (BBA) - Mol Basis Dis. 2014;1842(10):1896–902.
33. Majewski J, Pastinen T. The study of eQTL variations by RNA-seq: from SNPs to phenotypes. Trends Genet. 2011;27(2):72–9.
34. Using eQTL weights to improve power for genome-wide association studies: a genetic study of childhood asthma. 2018. https://www.ncbi.nlm.nih.gov/pmc/articles/PMC3668139/.
35. Linking disease associations with regulatory information in the human genome. 2018. http://genome.cshlp.org/content/22/9/1748.long.
36. Li Q, Seo J-H, Stranger B, McKenna A, Péer I, La Framboise T, et al. A novel eQTL-based analysis reveals the biology of breast cancer risk loci. Cell. 2013;152(3):633–41.
37. eQTL mapping approach reveals that rare variants in the SEMA5A regulatory network impact autism risk. Hum Mol Genet. 2018. https://academic.oup.com/hmg/article/22/14/2960/754868.
38. Siegel RL, Miller KD, Jemal A. Cancer statistics, 2017. CA Cancer J Clin. 2017;67:7–30. https://doi.org/10.3322/caac.21387/full.
39. Zhang B, Beeghly-Fadiel A, Long J, Zheng W. Genetic variants associated with breast-cancer risk: comprehensive research synopsis, meta-analysis, and epidemiological evidence. Lancet Oncol. 2011;12(5):477–88.
40. Ghoussaini M, Pharoah PDP, Easton DF. Inherited genetic susceptibility to breast cancer: the beginning of the end or the end of the beginning? Am J Pathol. 2013;183(4):1038–51.
41. Miki Y, Swensen J, Shattuck-Eidens D, Futreal PA, Harshman K, Tavtigian S, et al. A strong candidate for the breast and ovarian cancer susceptibility gene BRCA1. Science. 1994;266 (5182):66–71.
42. Wooster R, Bignell G, Lancaster J, Swift S, Seal S, Mangion J, et al. Identification of the breast cancer susceptibility gene BRCA2. Nature. 1995;378(6559):789–92.
43. Renwick A, Thompson D, Seal S, Kelly P, Chagtai T, Ahmed M, et al. ATM mutations that cause ataxia-telangiectasia are breast cancer susceptibility alleles. Nat Genet. 2006;38 (8):873–5.
44. The CHEK2-Breast Cancer Consortium. Low-penetrance susceptibility to breast cancer due to CHEK2*1100delC in noncarriers of BRCA1 or BRCA2 mutations. Nat Genet. 2002;31 (1):55–9.

45. Seal S, Thompson D, Renwick A, Elliott A, Kelly P, Barfoot R, et al. Truncating mutations in the Fanconi anemia J gene BRIP1 are low-penetrance breast cancer susceptibility alleles. Nat Genet. 2006;38(11):1239–41.
46. Rahman N, Seal S, Thompson D, Kelly P, Renwick A, Elliott A, et al. PALB2, which encodes a BRCA2-interacting protein, is a breast cancer susceptibility gene. Nat Genet. 2007;39 (2):165–7.
47. Lin W-Y, et al. Identification and characterization of novel associations in the CASP8/ ALS2CR12 region on chromosome 2 with breast cancer risk. Hum Mol Genet. 2018;24 (1):285–98. https://doi.org/10.1093/hmg/ddu431.
48. Cox A, et al. A common coding variant in CASP8 is associated with breast cancer risk. Nat Genet. 2018;39(3):352–8. https://doi.org/10.1038/ng1981.
49. Zheng W, Zhang B, Cai Q, Sung H, Michailidou K, Shi J, et al. Common genetic determinants of breast-cancer risk in east Asian women: a collaborative study of 23 637 breast cancer cases and 25 579 controls. Hum Mol Genet. 2013;22(12):2539–50.
50. Long J, Shu X-O, Cai Q, Gao Y-T, Zheng Y, Li G, et al. Evaluation of breast cancer susceptibility loci in Chinese women. Am Soc Prev Oncol. 2010;19(9):2357–65.
51. Michailidou K, Beesley J, Lindstrom S, Canisius S, Dennis J, Lush MJ, et al. Genome-wide association analysis of more than 120,000 individuals identifies 15 new susceptibility loci for breast cancer. Nat Genet. 2015;47(4):373–80.
52. Chen S, Parmigiani G. Meta-analysis of BRCA1 and BRCA2 penetrance. J Clin Oncol. 2007;25(11):1329–33.
53. Tan M-H, Mester JL, Ngeow J, Rybicki LA, Orloff MS, Eng C. Lifetime cancer risks in individuals with germline PTEN mutations. Clin Cancer Res. 2012;18(2):400–7.
54. Bubien V, Bonnet F, Brouste V, Hoppe S, Barouk-Simonet E, David A, et al. High cumulative risks of cancer in patients with PTEN hamartoma tumour syndrome. J Med Genet. 2013;50 (4):255–63.
55. Nieuwenhuis MH, Kets CM, Murphy-Ryan M, Yntema HG, Evans DG, Colas C, et al. Cancer risk and genotype–phenotype correlations in PTEN hamartoma tumor syndrome. Fam Cancer. 2014;13(1):57–63.
56. Lalloo F, Varley J, Moran A, Ellis D, O'Dair L, Pharoah P, et al. BRCA1, BRCA2 and TP53 mutations in very early-onset breast cancer with associated risks to relatives. Eur J Cancer. 2006;42(8):1143–50.
57. Walsh T, Casadei S, Coats KH, Swisher E, Stray SM, Higgins J, et al. Spectrum of mutations in BRCA1, BRCA2, CHEK2, and TP53 in families at high risk of breast cancer. JAMA. 2006;295(12):1379–88.
58. CHEK2 Breast Cancer Case-Control Consortium. CHEK2*1100delC and susceptibility to breast cancer: a collaborative analysis involving 10,860 breast cancer cases and 9,065 controls from 10 studies. Am J Hum Genet. 2004;74(6):1175–82.
59. Yang Y, Zhang F, Wang Y, Liu S-C. CHEK2 1100delC variant and breast cancer risk in Caucasians: a meta-analysis based on 25 studies with 29,154 cases and 37,064 controls. Asian Pac J Cancer Prev. 2012;13(7):3501–5.
60. ATM and breast cancer susceptibility. Oncogene. 2018. https://www.nature.com/articles/ 1209873
61. Stratton MR, Rahman N. The emerging landscape of breast cancer susceptibility. Nat Genet. 2018;40:17–22.
62. Ramensky V, Bork P, Sunyaev S. Human non-synonymous SNPs: server and survey. Nucleic Acids Res. 2002;30(17):3894–900.
63. The Cancer Genome Atlas Research Network, et al. The cancer genome atlas pan-cancer analysis project. Nat Genet. 2018;45:1113–20.
64. Long J, Cai Q, Shu X-O, Qu S, Li C, Zheng Y, et al. Identification of a functional genetic variant at 16q12.1 for breast cancer risk: results from the Asia breast cancer consortium. PLoS Genet. 2010;6(6):e1001002.

65. Shi J, Sung H, Zhang B, Lu W, Choi J-Y, Xiang Y-B, et al. New breast cancer risk variant discovered at 10q25 in east Asian women. Cancer Epidemiol Prev Biomark. 2013;22 (7):1297–303.
66. Long J, Delahanty RJ, Li G, Gao Y-T, Lu W, Cai Q, et al. A common deletion in the APOBEC3 genes and breast cancer risk. JNCI J Natl Cancer Inst. 2013;105(8):573–9.
67. Genome-wide association study in East Asians identifies novel susceptibility loci for breast cancer. 2018. http://journals.plos.org/plosgenetics/article?id=10.1371/journal.pgen.1002532
68. Ma X, et al. Pathway analyses identify TGFBR2 as potential breast cancer susceptibility gene: results from a consortium study among Asians. Cancer Epidemiol Biomarkers Prev. 2018;21 (7):1176–84.
69. Xuan D, Li G, Cai Q, Deming-Halverson S, Shrubsole MJ, Shu X-O, et al. APOBEC3 deletion polymorphism is associated with breast cancer risk among women of European ancestry. Carcinogenesis. 2013;34(10):2240–3.
70. Genome-wide association study in East Asians identifies two novel breast cancer susceptibility loci. Hum Mol Genet. 2018. https://academic.oup.com/hmg/article/25/15/3361/2525788
71. Whole exome sequencing suggests much of non-BRCA1/BRCA2 familial breast cancer is due to moderate and low penetrance susceptibility alleles. 2018. http://journals.plos.org/plosone/article?id=10.1371/journal.pone.0055681
72. Using extended genealogy to estimate components of heritability for 23 quantitative and dichotomous traits. 2018. http://journals.plos.org/plosgenetics/article?id=10.1371/journal.pgen.1003520
73. Zuk O, Hechter E, Sunyaev SR, Lander ES. The mystery of missing heritability: genetic interactions create phantom heritability. Proc Natl Acad Sci. 2012;109(4):1193–8.
74. Rare and common variants: twenty arguments. Nat Rev Genet. 2018. https://www.nature.com/articles/nrg3118
75. Eichler EE, Flint J, Gibson G, Kong A, Leal SM, Moore JH, et al. Missing heritability and strategies for finding the underlying causes of complex disease. Nat Rev Genet. 2010;11 (6):446–50.
76. Pritchard JK. Are rare variants responsible for susceptibility to complex diseases? Am J Hum Genet. 2001;69(1):124–37.
77. Gorlov IP, Gorlova OY, Sunyaev SR, Spitz MR, Amos CI. Shifting paradigm of association studies: value of rare single-nucleotide polymorphisms. Am J Hum Genet. 2008;82 (1):100–12.
78. Turnbull C, Rahman N. Genetic predisposition to breast cancer: past, present, and future. Annu Rev Genomics Hum Genet. 2008;9(1):321–45.
79. Frank B, Hemminki K, Wirtenberger M, Bermejo J, Bugert P, Klaes R, et al. The rare ERBB2 variant Ile654Val is associated with an increased familial breast cancer risk. Breast Cancer Res. 2005;7(2):18.
80. McInerney NM, Miller N, Rowan A, Colleran G, Barclay E, Curran C, et al. Evaluation of variants in the CHEK2, BRIP1 and PALB2 genes in an Irish breast cancer cohort. Breast Cancer Res Treat. 2010;121(1):203–10.
81. Ruark E, Snape K, Humburg P, Loveday C, Bajrami I, Brough R, et al. Mosaic PPM1D mutations are associated with predisposition to breast and ovarian cancer. Nature. 2013;493 (7432):406–10.
82. Lu W, Wang X, Lin H, Lindor NM, Couch FJ. Mutation screening of RAD51C in high-risk breast and ovarian cancer families. Fam Cancer. 2012;11(3):381–5.
83. Tavtigian SV, Oefner PJ, Babikyan D, Hartmann A, Healey S, Le Calvez-Kelm F, et al. Rare, evolutionarily unlikely missense substitutions in ATM confer increased risk of breast cancer. Am J Hum Genet. 2009;85(4):427–46.
84. The RAD51D E233G variant and breast cancer risk: population-based and clinic-based family studies of Australian women. SpringerLink. 2018. https://link.springer.com/article/10.1007%2Fs10549-007-9832-0.

85. Rare variants in the ATM gene and risk of breast cancer. Breast Cancer Res. 2018. https://breast-cancer-research.biomedcentral.com/articles/10.1186/bcr2919.
86. Beaudoin M, Goyette P, Boucher G, Lo KS, Rivas MA, Stevens C, et al. Deep resequencing of GWAS loci identifies rare variants in CARD9, IL23R and RNF186 that are associated with ulcerative colitis. PLoS Genet. 2013;9(9):e1003723.
87. Sanna S, Li B, Mulas A, Sidore C, Kang HM, Jackson AU, et al. Fine mapping of five loci associated with Low-density lipoprotein cholesterol detects variants that double the explained heritability. PLoS Genet. 2011;7(7):e1002198.
88. Excess of rare variants in genes identified by genome-wide association study of hypertriglyceridemia. Nat. Genet. 2018. https://www.nature.com/articles/ng.628.
89. Rare coding variants and breast cancer risk: evaluation of susceptibility loci identified in genome-wide association studies. Cancer Epidemiol Biomarkers Prev. 2018. http://cebp.aacrjournals.org/content/23/4/622.long
90. Han, Mi-Ryung. Rare coding variants in GWAS identified loci with breast cancer risk. Doctoral dissertation. Vanderbilt University; 2016.
91. GTEx Consortium. The Genotype-Tissue Expression (GTEx) project. Nat Genet. 2013;45(6):580–5.
92. The genomic and transcriptomic architecture of 2,000 breast tumours reveals novel subgroups. Nature. 2018. https://www.nature.com/articles/nature10983
93. Trans-eQTLs reveal that independent genetic variants associated with a complex phenotype converge on intermediate genes, with a major role for the HLA. 2018. http://journals.plos.org/plosgenetics/article?id=10.1371/journal.pgen.1002197.
94. Understanding mechanisms underlying human gene expression variation with RNA sequencing. Nature. 2018. https://www.nature.com/articles/nature08872.
95. Trait-associated snps are more likely to be eQTLs: annotation to enhance discovery from GWAS. 2018. http://journals.plos.org/plosgenetics/article?id=10.1371/journal.pgen.1000888.
96. Wittkopp PJ, Haerum BK, Clark AG. Evolutionary changes in cis and trans gene regulation. Nature. 2004;430(6995):85–8.
97. Li B, Leal SM. Methods for detecting associations with rare variants for common diseases: application to analysis of sequence data. Am J Hum Genet. 2008;83(3):311–21.
98. Madsen BE, Browning SRA. Groupwise association test for rare mutations using a weighted sum statistic. PLoS Genet. 2009;5(2):e1000384.
99. Lee S, Abecasis GR, Boehnke M, Lin X. Rare-variant association analysis: study designs and statistical tests. Am J Hum Genet. 2014;95(1):5–23.
100. Price AL, Kryukov GV, de BPIW, Purcell SM, Staples J, Wei L-J, et al. Pooled association tests for rare variants in exon-resequencing studies. Am J Hum Genet. 2010;86(6):982.
101. Haplotype-based association analysis via variance-components score test. 2018. https://www.ncbi.nlm.nih.gov/pmc/articles/PMC2265651/.
102. Rare-variant extensions of the transmission disequilibrium test: application to autism exome sequence data. ScienceDirect. 2018. https://www.sciencedirect.com/science/article/pii/S0002929713005697?via%3Dihub.
103. Schifano ED, Epstein MP, Bielak LF, Jhun MA, Kardia SLR, Peyser PA, et al. SNP set association analysis for familial data. Genet Epidemiol. 2012;36(8):797–810.
104. Chen H, Meigs JB, Dupuis J. Sequence kernel association test for quantitative traits in family samples. Genet Epidemiol. 2013;37(2):196–204.
105. Family-based association tests for sequence data, and comparisons with population-based association tests. 2018. https://www.ncbi.nlm.nih.gov/pmc/articles/PMC3778346/.
106. MacArthur DG, Balasubramanian S, Frankish A, Huang N, Morris J, Walter K, et al. A systematic survey of loss-of-function variants in human protein-coding genes. Science. 2012;335(6070):823–8.

107. Kryukov GV, Pennacchio LA, Sunyaev SR. Most rare missense alleles are deleterious in humans: implications for complex disease and association studies. Am J Hum Genet. 2007;80 (4):727–39.
108. Distribution and medical impact of loss-of-function variants in the Finnish founder population. 2018. http://journals.plos.org/plosgenetics/article?id=10.1371/journal.pgen.1004494.
109. Devlin B, Roeder K. Genomic control for association studies. Biometrics. 1999;55 (4):997–1004.
110. Lee S, Wright FA, Zou F. Control of population stratification by correlation-selected principal components. Biometrics. 2011;67(3):967–74.
111. Genomics for the world. Nature. 2018. https://www.nature.com/articles/475163a.
112. Price AL, Zaitlen NA, Reich D, Patterson N. New approaches to population stratification in genome-wide association studies. Nat Rev Genet. 2010;11(7):459–63.
113. Morris AP. Fine mapping of type 2 diabetes susceptibility loci. Curr Diab Rep. 2014;14 (11):549.
114. Loss-of-function variants in the genomes of healthy humans. 2018. https://www.ncbi.nlm.nih.gov/pmc/articles/PMC2953739/.

Chapter 24
Multigene Panel Testing for Hereditary Cancer and Genetic Counseling

Eun-Shin Lee, Jongjin Kim, and Wonshik Han

Abstract As sequencing technology and information of the genomic causes for cancer development expand, multi-gene panel testing for hereditary cancer is increasing in clinical practice. In this chapter, we reviewed the application of multi-gene panel with pre-/post- testing considerations and summarized genetic counseling based on panel testing results in clinical field. In addition, we introduce multi-gene panel for hereditary cancer developed in Seoul National University Hospital.

Keywords Hereditary/familial breast cancer · Breast cancer susceptibility · Multigene panel testing · Next-generation sequencing · High penetrance gene · Genetic counseling · *BRCA1/2* gene mutation

As sequencing technology advances and next-generation sequencing increases with cost effectiveness, the application of assaying large panels of genes, called "multigene panel" or "panel testing", for hereditary cancer risk assessment is becoming commonplace in clinical practice. Gene panel testing simultaneously analyzes a set of genes associated with a specific family cancer phenotype or syndrome of cancer. Gene panel included low to moderate penetrance genes like as *PALB2, ATM, CHEK2, NBN, NF1, RAD50*, and so on as well as high penetrance mutations in *BRCA1/2, TP53, PTEN, STK11*, and *CDH1*, even though the clinical meaning of these genes is not yet completely defined. (Fig. 24.1).

In the early stage of the widespread use with NGS-based multigene panel, Stephen E. Lincoln et al. [1] estimated reliability of the multigene panel testing. They compared between traditional (previously received clinical testing in several

E.-S. Lee · W. Han (✉)
Seoul National University Hospital, Seoul, South Korea
e-mail: hanw@snu.ac.kr

J. Kim
SMG – SNU Boramae Medical Center, Seoul, South Korea

D.-Y. Noh et al. (eds.), *Translational Research in Breast Cancer*, Advances in Experimental Medicine and Biology 1187,
https://doi.org/10.1007/978-981-32-9620-6_24

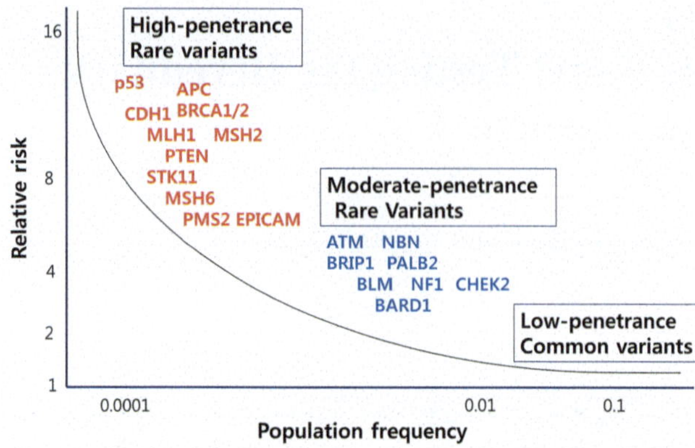

Fig. 24.1 Genetic architecture of relative cancer risk and allele frequency. This figure depicts finding of rare, high-penetrance variants, such as pathogenic mutations in *BRCA1/BRCA2* genes associated with hereditary breast and ovarian cancer, moderate-penetrance variants, and low-penetrance alleles identified in genome-wide association studies

genes including *BRCA 1/2*) and NGS-based multigene panel testing with 29-gene for hereditary breast and ovarian cancer genes in more than 1000 patients. They showed that NGS can achieve high-analytic sensitivity and specificity in comparison with traditional genetic testing methods, even for some technically challenging (e.g., CNVs and large indels) classes of genetic variation that make up a significant fraction of the pathogenic variants in HBOC. Interpretation concordance for BRCA1 and BRCA2 was also high, demonstrating that broadly available resources combined with recent guidelines can produce results similar to those of an established laboratory using a large proprietary database. Furthermore, half (372 of 750) of the variants were in genes other than *BRCA1* or *BRCA2*, and most (607 of 750) of these variants were reported by the previous tests, providing the most unbiased view of sensitivity for the NGS panel (607 of 607 Z 100%; 95% CI, 100% e99.59%). Thus, they concluded gene panels can be a viable replacement for traditional tests in appropriate circumstances. The additional pathogenic variants uncovered by panel testing appeared clinically relevant, albeit with the caveat of identifying many additional VUSs. Another group of research, Nimmi S. Kapoor et al. [2], presented similar result about validation of multigene panel. Multigene panel testing comparing traditional test detected pathogenic *BRCA1/2* mutations at equivalent rates (4.0 vs. 3.6%, $p = 0.86$) with increasing proportion of the VUS. An additional 3.9% ($n = 13$) in nonBRCA pathogenic mutations and 13.4% ($n = 45$) had nonBRCA VUSs identified in patients who underwent panel testing. The most common nonBRCA mutations were in *PALB2*, *CHEK2*, and *ATM* gene. They recommended multigene panel testing for the patients at risk for hereditary breast cancer as a safe, more beneficial, and efficient modality.

Recently, many researchers from various countries have released large-scale result about hereditary cancer risk and multigene panel testing. Fergus J. Couch et al. [3] evaluated the associations between nonBRCA1/2 predisposition genes and breast cancer in over than 65,000 patients. They showed there are a total of 10.2% frequency of pathogenic variants in 21 panel genes including *BRCA1, BRCA2*, syndromic breast cancer genes (*CDH1, PTEN,* and *TP53*), and high or moderate penetrance genes (*ATM, BARD1, CHEK2, PALB2*, and *RAD51D*) and 6.2% frequency of women with breast cancer after exclusion of BRCA1 and BRCA2. This study established several panel genes as high- and moderate-risk breast cancer; most commonly mutated nonBRCA1/2 genes among white women with breast cancer were *CHEK2* (1.73%), *ATM* (1.06%), and *PALB2* (0.87%) and provided estimates of breast cancer risk associated with pathogenic variants in these genes with relative risk from high (OR 7.46 in *PALB2*) to moderate (OR 3.07, 2.78, and 2.16 in *RAD 51D, ATM*, and *CHEK2*, respectively). In another study conducted by Saundra S. Buys et al. [4], the authors analyzed about 35,000 women with 25-gene panel testing and stratified to high risk for hereditary cancer who met NCCN guideline for HBOC testing regarding age at diagnosis and family history of ovary/pancreas cancer or not. Among the women who met NCCN testing criteria, 9.6% (316 of 32,993) had a deleterious mutation, compared with 5.9% (143 of 2416) of those who did not meet NCCN criteria. Nearly one-half of the pathogenic variants (PV) identified during testing were in the *BRCA1* (24.0%) and *BRCA2* (24.4%) genes. An additional 40.9% of the PVs were in other genes associated with breast cancer, including *CHEK2* (11.7%), *ATM* (9.7%), and *PALB2* (9.3%). Other genes on the panel accounted for 10.7% of mutations, including those associated with Lynch syndrome (7.0%).

As the application of multigene panel expands beyond breast cancer, the result on the outcomes of testing to identify inherited risks for colorectal, endometrial, gastric, pancreatic, prostate, and melanoma cancers as well as breast and ovary cancer was reported [5]. In this study, multigene hereditary cancer testing detected >1 pathogenic variants (PVs) in 6.7% of individuals and they showed up to 50% of all clinically significant findings would have been missed by single-syndrome testing.

Now, several companies offer panel tests composed of various cancer susceptibility genes, and it is commercially available to use in clinical practice with the purpose of personalized management for whom had a genetic predisposition to hereditary cancer. Clinicians or even individual oneself who wants the test can choose genetic test services among companies, list of genes, and number of gene-set range from single to dozens of genes. The companies provided the information online including available gene list-associated familial cancer type, clinical meaning of each gene, indications of the test based on individual's risk, cautions of the test, and process to the genetic test for both the medical staff and patients/patients' family members.

There are some issues in multigene panel testing: (1) lack of evidence for clinical application in several genes especially moderate-penetrant genes, which had limited data on the degree of cancer risk and failed to provide guidelines on risk management for carriers of pathogenic variants, (2) not all genes included on available multigene panel are clinically actionable, and (3) increased likelihood of finding variants of unknown significance (VUS). Many reports, previously mentioned, established the finding of a number of VUS with multigene panel testing in large cohort, and it ranged from about 10–70%. Thomas Paul Slavin et al. [6] reported only 6.2% of pathogenic variants in high-risk genes included in the panels (*BRCA1, BRCA2, MSH6, PMS2, TP53, APC*, and *CDH1*). Instead, they identified variants of uncertain significance (VUS) in 42%. They insisted that adequate pretest counseling is more important in anticipation of higher percentages of positive, unexpected, and ambiguous test results including VUSs. Test result ambiguity can be limited by the use of phenotype-specific panels. Furthermore, for pathogenic variants in low and moderate risk genes, the researchers said adequate risk modeling based on the patient's personal and family history of cancer can be better than gene-specific risk. They stressed further research efforts will be needed to better classify variants and reduce clinical ambiguity of multigene panels.

Most important issue among these is clinical validity; the decision to test with multigene panel is focused on identifying a mutation known to be clinically actionable, that is, whether the management of an individual with a risk for hereditary cancer is altered based on the presence or absence of a mutation. Additionally, it needs to determine with discretion which group with a specific condition would get the crucial benefit from the application of multigene panel. LeifW. Ellisen et al. in Massachusetts General Hospital Cancer Center [7] designed interesting research to define the potential clinical effect of multigene panel testing for HBOC in a clinically representative cohort. They evaluated the likelihood of (1) a posttest management change and (2) an indication for additional familial testing, considering gene-specific consensus management guidelines, gene-associated cancer risks, and personal and family history. Among mutation-positive patients, about half (33 [52%] of 63) considered additional disease-specific screening and/or prevention measures beyond those based on personal and family history alone. Furthermore, additional familial testing would be considered for those with first-degree relatives (42 [72%] of 58; 95% CI, 59.8–82.2%) based on potential management changes for mutation-positive relatives. They concluded multigene testing is more likely to alter near-term cancer risk assessment and management recommendations for mutation-affected individuals.

Multigene testing may play a role in individuals with negative result in a single or just two genes but whose personal or familial history reveals suggestive of an inherited susceptibility or developed multiple phenotypes in a family. With all this in mind, the new NCCN committee suggested that multigene panel testing is offered in the context of professional genetic expertise with elaborate pre- and posttest counseling [8].

As the risk of cancer in carriers identified genetic mutations are stratified to several factors, the genetic expertise must evaluate the risk of inherited cancer based on individuals' needs and concerns as well as cancer history of the detailed personal/family/relatives. Based on reliable risk assessment compounding history and genetic results, the expert should provide appropriate guidelines to the carrier with information of lifetime cancer risks, adequate screening test, and risk-reducing procedure. Though a major dilemma regarding multigene testing is that there are limited evidence and a lack of clear guidelines, several countries suggested similar guidelines for managing the care of individuals with predisposition to hereditary cancer (NCCN; United States, NICE; United Kingdom; GC-HBOC–; Germany, eviQ Cancer Treatments Online; Australia, and so on).

As a result, since identification of abnormality in *BRCA1/2* genes has made contribution to the care of hereditary cancer patients and their families, further progress in our understanding of the genetic factors with cancer phenotype still continues. But the penetrance and phenotype of mutations are different among individuals, that is, there are not sufficient data about association between cancer development and detection of a pathogenic mutation. In addition, a negative result from genetic testing even in a large number of genes does not mean an individual has no risk of cancer. It is also another challenge to share information with the patients as well as the interpretation adequately of the result on germline mutations. Furthermore, gene testing can give rise to psychosocial consequences of all individuals and their families and may also have effect on social community. As the genetic test expands, the role of experts is more important; the integrated approach of clinicians and genetic counselors is indispensable. They should carefully access to better clarify counseling and management for the patient and family. The adequate prediction of the risk for hereditary cancer through enough risk assessment process and consideration of the patients' need and concern with regarding the impact on patients and their families of the gene test result should be preceded in pretest counseling. In addition, in the analysis and transmission of the meaning of gene results, they should strive to provide comprehensive conclusions about the risk of cancer development considering the patient's personal and family history and educate tailored risk-reducing guidelines.

24.1 Development and Application of Multigene Panel for Hereditary Cancer in SNUH

24.1.1 Introduction

Though many commercial multiple-gene panels provide genetic information for hereditary cancer risk assessment, there is insufficient information on differences among ethnicities in cancer-susceptible germline mutations, and the assessment of germline mutations in all ethnic groups with clinical data is mandatory especially in Korea and Asia. We applied multiple-gene panel testing to 64 cancer-susceptibility genes to examine the frequency of mutations and to assess the clinical value of NGS-based multiple-gene panel testing in Korean breast cancer patients with clinical features of hereditary breast and ovarian cancer syndrome (HBOC). (Table 24.1).

Table 24.1 Hereditary cancer predisposing genes in the multiple-gene panel test

Gene	Breast	Ovarian	Colorectal	Endometrial	Gastric	Pancreatic	Melanoma	Prostate	Other
ALK			●		●	●			●
APC			●			●			●
ATM	●					●			●
ATR									●
BAP1									
BARD1	●								●
BLM			●						
BMPR1A			●		●	●			●
BRCA1	●	●				●		●	
BRCA2	●	●				●	●	●	
BRIP1	●	●							
CDH1	●		●		●				
CDK4							●		
CDKN2A						●	●		
CHEK2	●		●					●	
EPCAM		●	●	●	●	●			●
FAM175A	●	●							●
FANCA	●								●
FANCB									●
FANCC	●								●
FANCD2									●
FANCE									●
FANCF									●
FANCG									●
FANCI									●
FANCL									●

FH									•
FLCN									•
GSTP1	•								•
HOXB13								•	
KRAS			•		•	•	•		
LIG4									•
MEN1									•
MET									•
MLH1		•	•	•	•	•			•
MRE11A	•								
MSH2		•	•	•	•	•			•
MSH6		•	•	•	•	•			•
MUTYH			•						•
NAT			•						•
NBN	•							•	
NF1									•
PALB2	•					•			
PALLD									
PMS2		•	•	•	•	•			•
PRKAR1A									•
PRSS1					•	•			
PTEN	•		•	•					•
RAD50	•	•							
RAD51	•	•							
RAD51C	•	•							
RAD51D	•	•							
RB1									•

(continued)

Table 24.1 (continued)

Gene	Breast	Ovarian	Colorectal	Endometrial	Gastric	Pancreatic	Melanoma	Prostate	Other
RET									•
SDHB									•
SDHC									•
SDHD									•
SLX4									•
SMAD4									•
SPINK1									•
STK11	•	•	•	•	•	•			•
TP53	•	•	•	•	•	•	•	•	•
VHL	•	•	•						•
XRCC2	•								•

24.1.2 Materials and Methods

The study population included 496 breast cancer patients with the following features of HBOC: (1) diagnosed with breast cancer and another primary cancer; (2) a family history that included at least two cases of breast cancer in first- or second-degree relatives; (3) bilateral breast cancer; or (4) breast cancer diagnosis before the age of 40 years. Of the patients, 349 patients were admitted to Seoul National University Hospital, Korea, and 147 patients were admitted to National Cancer Center, Korea, between 2002 and 2017. The medical records were reviewed and personal and family histories and pathologic data of cancer were recorded. Genomic DNA was extracted from the participants' peripheral blood samples. Our panel included 64 hereditary cancer predisposing genes (*ALK, APC, ATM, ATR, BAP1, BARD1, BLM, BMPR1A, BRCA1, BRCA2, BRIP1, CDH1, CDK4, CDKN2A, CHEK2, EPCAM, FAM175A, FANCA, FANCB, FANCC, FANCD2, FANCE, FANCF, FANCG, FANCI, FANCL, FH, FLCN, GSTP1, HOXB13, KRAS, LIG4, MEN1, MET, MLH1, MRE11A, MSH2, MSH6, MUTYH, NAT, NBN, NF1, PALB2, PALLD, PMS2, PRKAR1A, PRSS1, PTEN, RAD50, RAD51, RAD51C, RAD51D, RB1, RET, SDHB, SDHC, SDHD, SLX4, SMAD4, SPINK1, STK11, TP53, VHL*, and *XRCC2*).

For mutation analysis, 64 gene-containing DNA fragments were enriched by solution-based hybridization capture followed by sequencing with an Illumina NextSeq platform (Illumina, San Diego, CA, USA) with the 150-bp paired end read module. The target region included all coding exons. Capture probes were generated by Celemics, Inc. (Seoul, Korea). The hybridization capture procedure was also performed according to the manufacturer's standard protocol. Genomic DNA was sheared via sonication. Biotynilated RNA oligonucleotide probes were hybridized with sheared DNA. Captured fragments were removed from solution via streptavidin-coated magnetic beads and subsequently eluted. The enriched fragment library was then subjected to polymerase chain reaction (PCR) amplification using primers specific to the linked Illumina adaptors. Resulting libraries were quantified via Agilent 2200 TapeStation before proceeding to Illumina NextSeq platform. All samples were pooled into a single lane on a flow cell and sequenced together. Raw FASTQ files were filtered using Trimmomatic (Version 0.33) and aligned with the genome of reference (GRCh37/hg19) using Burrows-Wheeler Aligner (Version 0.7.10). PCR duplicates, overrepresented sequences, and low-quality reads were removed. Realignments of insertions and deletions were performed using GATK. Reads with mapping quality of 0 were filtered out. If a read was able to be mapped at two different places with an identical percentage, the mapping quality equaled zero. Otherwise, the read was mapped to the most identical region. Variant calling was performed using Samtools (Version 1.1) and Varscan (Version 2.4.0).

Variants were described according to the nomenclature recommendations of the Human Genome Variation Society (http://www.hgvs.org/mutnomen) and classified according to the following American College of Medical Genetics and Genomics recommendations: pathogenic (P), likely pathogenic (LP), variants of unknown significance (VUS), likely benign, and benign/polymorphism [7]. We used online databases, including the Human Gene Mutation Database, the Single Nucleotide Polymorphism Database, the 1000 Genome project, ClinVar, the Sorting Intolerant From Tolerant, Polymorphism Phenotyping-2, and the Korean Reference Genome Database, for in silico prediction of identified variants. Variants classified as P or LP were considered deleterious mutations.

24.1.3 Results

24.1.3.1 Study Population

The clinical characteristics of the patients are shown in Table 24.2. The median age at diagnosis of cancer was 48 years (range, 19–80 years). In these patients, 390 patients (78.6%) had stage I or II disease. More than half of the patients

Table 24.2 Characteristics of patients with and without deleterious mutations

Characteristics	Total (%)	No deleterious mutation (%)	Deleterious mutation (%)	*P*-value (χ^2)
Number of patients	496 (100)	401 (80.8)	95 (19.2)	
Age at diagnosis (years), median (range)	48 (19–80)	49 (19–80)	45 (22–72)	0.027*
Breast cancer stage				
0	32 (6.5)	30 (7.5)	2 (2.1)	0.078
I	209 (42.1)	170 (42.4)	39 (41.1)	
II	181 (36.5)	138 (34.4)	43 (45.3)	
III	62 (12.5)	52 (13.0)	10 (10.5)	
IV	10 (2.0)	10 (2.5)	0 (0)	
Unknown	2 (0.4)	1 (0.2)	1 (1.1)	
Risk factors for HBOC				
Breast cancer with another primary cancer	250 (50.4)	211 (52.6)	39 (41.1)	0.052
Family history of breast cancer (≥2 relatives)	169 (34.1)	131 (32.7)	38 (40.0)	0.187
Bilateral breast cancer	57 (11.5)	41 (10.2)	16 (16.8)	0.075
Breast cancer diagnosis at <40 years old	84 (16.9)	60 (15.0)	29 (30.5)	0.022
two or more risk factors	64 (12.9)	42 (10.5)	22 (23.2)	0.002

*Statistical significance was evaluated by Student's *t* test

($N = 250$, 50.4%) had another primary cancer, including ovarian cancer, stomach cancer, colon cancer, lung cancer, or other malignancy. In all, 169 patients (34.1%) reported that they had two or more first- or second-degree relatives with breast cancer. Fifty-seven patients (11.5%) had synchronous or metachronous bilateral breast cancer, and 84 patients (16.9%) were diagnosed with breast cancer at an age younger than 40 years. Sixty-four patients had two or more risk factors for HBOC (e.g., bilateral breast cancer and breast cancer diagnosis <40 years old).

24.1.3.2 Frequency of Deleterious Mutations

A total of 95 (19.2%) among all 496 patients were found to have deleterious germline mutations of cancer-susceptibility genes. The proportions of risk factors, including breast cancer with another primary cancer, family history of breast cancer, and bilateral breast cancer were also not different between the groups with or without deleterious mutations. However, the proportion of patients with deleterious mutations were higher in patients who were diagnosed with breast cancer at younger than 40 years old than patients with another risk factors ($P = 0.022$). Furthermore, having two or more risk factors for HBOC was also associated with a higher rate of deleterious mutations ($P = 0.001$). Table 24.3 and Fig. 24.2 summarize 48 deleterious mutations found in 95 patients.

Of these patients with deleterious mutations, 60 patients (63.2%) had *BRCA1* (31) and *BRCA 2* (30) mutations. Patients _309 and _502 had 2 BRCA1 mutations, and patient HOPE_57 carried both *BRCA1* and *BRCA2* mutations. In addition, 38 patients (40.0%) had cancer-susceptibility gene mutations other than *BRCA1/2*: 35 patients (36.8%) had nonBRCA1/2 mutations and 3 patients had both a BRCA1/2 mutation and a nonBRCA1/2 mutation (Patient_14 had *BRCA2* and *SPINK1* mutations; Patient_33 had *BRCA2, CDH1,* and *TP53* mutations; and patient_421 had *BRCA1* and *NBN* mutations). Most of the deleterious mutations were found in *CDH1* ($N = 8$, 8.4%), *RAD51* ($N = 7$, 7.4%), *SPINK1* ($N = 6$, 6.3%), *TP53* ($N = 5$, 5.3%), and *NBN* ($N = 3$, 3.2%). The remaining patients had deleterious mutations in *CHEK2, FANCA, MLH1* ($N = 2$ of each, 2.1%), *BRIP1, MRE11A, MSH2,* and *MUTYH* ($N = 1$ of each, 1.1%).

The proportion of deleterious mutations varied according to risk factors. The deleterious mutations were found in 39 of 250 patients (15.6%) who had breast cancer and another primary cancer, 38 of 169 patients (22.5%) who had a family history ($\geq$2 relatives) of breast cancer, 16 of 57 patients (28.1%) who had bilateral breast cancer, and 29 of 84 patients (34.5%) who were diagnosed with breast cancer at younger than 40 years old (Fig. 24.3). Furthermore, the distributions of the cancer-susceptibility genes were different according to risk factors (Fig. 24.4). In breast cancer patients with another primary cancer, BRCA1/2 and nonBRCA1/2 mutations accounted for 52.3% and 47.7% of mutations, respectively. The nonBRCA1/2 mutations comprised *CDH1* (11.4%), *SPINK1* (9.1%), *RAD51* (6.8%), and *TP53* (6.8%) mutations. In breast cancer patients with a family history of breast cancer, 65.8% carried a *BRCA1/2* mutation. In 34.2% of nonBRCA1/2 mutations, 7.9% had

Table 24.3 List of deleterious mutations identified in patients

Gene	Mutation	Transcript	HGVS cDNA	Amino acid change
BRCA1	Frame shift insertion	NM_007294.3	c.3627dupA	p.E1210Rfs
	Nonsense mutation	NM_007294.3	c.4981G > T	p.E1661*
	Nonsense mutation	NM_007294.3	c.5080G > T	p.E1694*
	Frame shift deletion	NM_007297.3	c.1575delA	p.E525Dfs
	Frame shift deletion	NM_007294.3	c.1961delA	p.K654Sfs
	Missense mutation	NM_007294.3	c.5339 T > C	p.L1780P
	Nonsense mutation	NM_007294.3	c.3991C > T	p.Q1331*
	Nonsense mutation	NM_007294.3	c.928C > T	p.Q310*
	Frame shift insertion	NM_007294.3	c.1511dupG	p.K505*
	Frame shift deletion	NM_007294.3	c.923_924delGC	p.S308Kfs
	Frame shift deletion	NM_007294.3	c.3700_3704delGTAAA	p.V1234Qfs
	Nonsense mutation	NM_007294.3	c.5445G > A	p.W1815*
	Nonsense mutation	NM_007294.3	c.390C > A	p.Y130*
	Splice donor variant	NM_007294.3	c.5467 + 1G > A	p.=
BRCA2	Frame shift deletion	NM_000059.3	c.700delT	p.S234Pfs
	Frame shift deletion	ENST00000380152.3	c.3096_3111delAAGATATTGAAGAACA	p.K1032Nfs
	Frame shift insertion	NM_000059.3	c.9253dupA	p.T3085Nfs
	Missense mutation	NM_000059.3	c.8023A > G	p.I2675V
	Nonsense mutation	NM_000059.3	c.1399A > T	p.K467*
	Frame shift deletion	NM_000059.3	c.4092_4093delAT	p.I1364Mfs
	Nonsense mutation	NM_000059.3	c.8140C > T	p.Q2714*
	Nonsense mutation	NM_000059.3	c.8140C > T	p.Q3026*
	Frame shift deletion	NM_000059.3	c.5575_5578delATTA	p.I1859Kfs
	Nonsense mutation	NM_000059.3	c.7480C > T	p.R2494*
	Frame shift deletion	NM_000059.3	c.2798_2799delCA	p.T933Rfs
	Nonsense mutation	NM_000059.3	c.8951C > G	p.S2984*
	Frame shift deletion	NM_000059.3	c.3192_3195delAATT	p.N1066Lfs
	Frame shift deletion	NM_000059.3	c.3744_3747delTGAG	p.S1248Rfs
	Frame shift deletion	NM_000059.3	c.755_758delACAG	p.D252Vfs

BRIP1	Nonsense mutation	NM_032043.2	c.2392C > T	p.R798*
CDH1	Missense mutation	NM_004360.4	c.2494G > A	p.V832M
CHEK2	Nonsense mutation	NM_007194.3	c.409C > T	p.R137*
	Nonsense mutation	NM_001005735.1	c.1684C > T	p.R562*
FANCA	Frame shift deletion	NM_000135.3	c.3720_3724del	p.E1240Dfs
	Frame shift deletion	NM_000135.2	c.2546delC	p.S849Ffs
MLH1	Frame shift insertion	NM_000249.3	c.1758dupC	p.M587Hfs
	Nonsense mutation	ENST00000441265	c.728 T > A	p.Y283*
MRE11A	Missense mutation	NM_005591.3	c.140C > T	p.A47V
MSH2	Frame shift deletion	NM_000251.2	c.229_230delAG	p.S77Cfs
MUTYH	Nonsense mutation	NM_001128425.1	c.55C > T	p.R19*
NBN	Missense mutation	NM_002485.4	c.511A > G	p.I171V
RAD51	Missense mutation	NM_002875.4	c.449G > A	p.R150Q
SPINK1	Missense mutation	NM_003122.4	c.101A > G	p.N34S
TP53	Missense mutation	NM_000546.5	c.566C > T	p.A189V
	Missense mutation	NM_000546.5	c.638G > A	p.R213Q
	Missense mutation	NM_000546.5	c.743G > A	p.R248Q

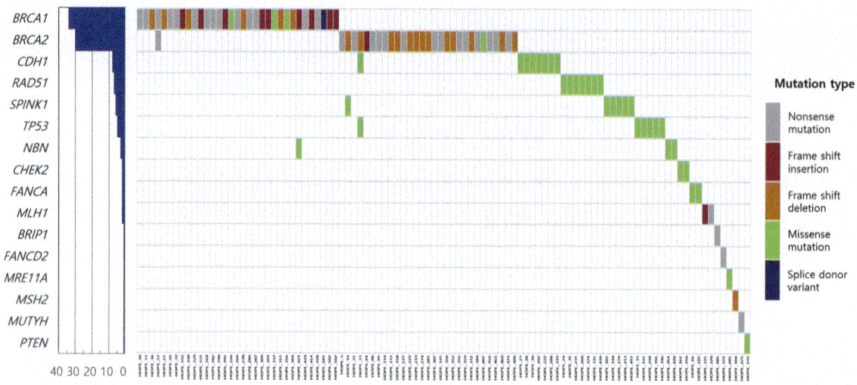

Fig. 24.2 Summary of 48 deleterious mutations in 95 patients

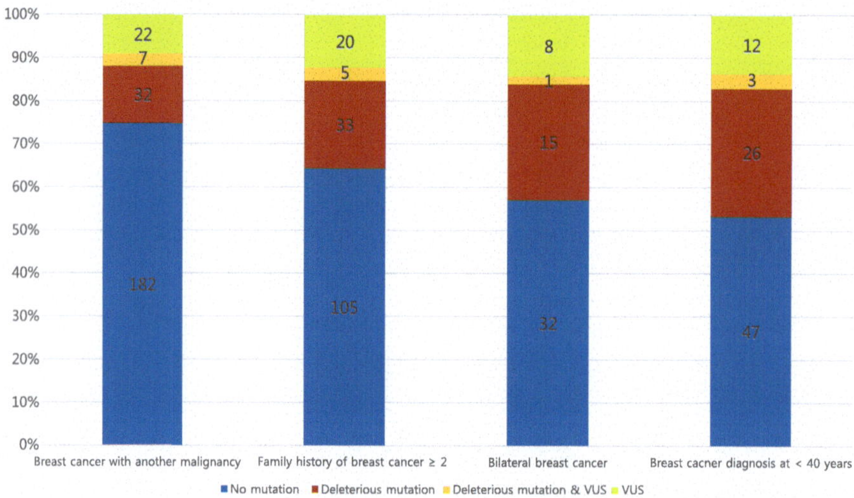

Fig. 24.3 The proportion of deleterious mutations according to risk factors of hereditary

RAD51 and *TP53* mutations and 5.3% had *CDH1* and *SPINK1* mutations. In bilateral breast cancer patients, 68.4% carried a *BRCA1/2* mutation.

Among 31.6% who had nonBRCA1/2 mutations, *CHEK2* (10.5%) was found frequently and 5.3% of patients had *CDH1, TP53, NBN*, and *MRE11A* mutations. In patients diagnosed with breast cancer at younger than 40 years old, 62.1% carried *BRCA1/2* mutations and 37.9% carried nonBRCA1/2 mutations including *RAD51, NBN, CHEK2, CDH1, TP53, PTEN, FANCA*, and *MRE11A* mutations. In 64 hereditary cancer predisposing genes, we found deleterious mutations in 16 genes, including *BRCA1/2*. However, we did not find deleterious mutations in the remaining 48 genes.

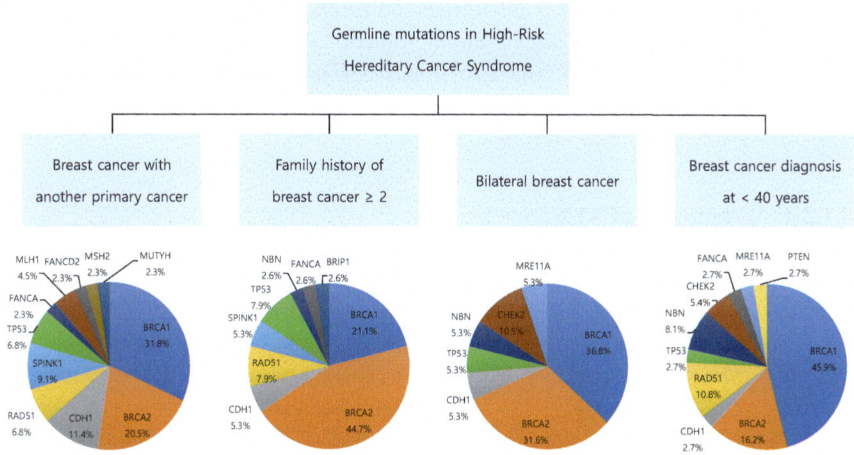

Fig. 24.4 The distributions of the cancer-susceptibility genes according to risk factors of hereditary cancer syndrome

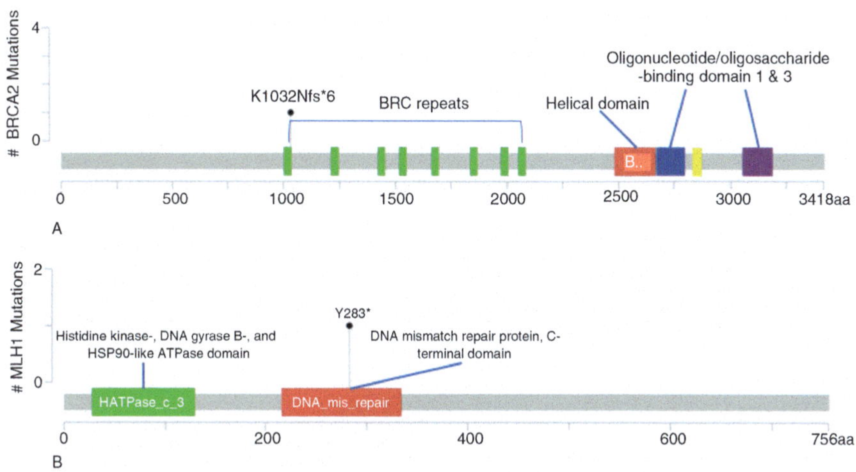

Fig.24.5 (**a**) c.3096_3111del (p. K1032Nfs) in *BRCA2*. (**b**) c.849T>A (p.Y283*) in *MLH1*

24.1.3.3 Novel Deleterious Mutations

We detected two novel deleterious mutations that were not previously reported: c.3096_3111del (p. K1032Nfs) in *BRCA2* and c.849T>A (p.Y283*) in *MLH1*. The p. K1032Nfs mutation in *BRCA2* is identified in patient_468. This mutation encodes a truncated nonfunctional protein in the domain of the BRC repeats, interfering with cellular response to DNA damage (Fig. 24.5a). The p.Y283* mutation in *MLH1* is identified in patient_378 and is also predicted to encode a nonfunctional protein, leading to the disruption of an important functional domain, such as the MutL C-terminal domain (Fig. 24.5b). The impact of both mutations was predicted deleterious mutations in in silico prediction.

24.1.3.4 Frequency of VUS

A total of 333 missense mutations were identified in 64 genes. After in silico prediction by database and bioinformatics analysis to evaluate pathogenicity, most of the missense mutations were classified as benign or likely benign. Mutations with conflicting interpretations of pathogenicity but suspicion of being deleterious were classified as VUS. A total of 20 VUS were identified in 67 patients (13.5%) (Table 24.4). In 15 patients, deleterious mutation and VUS were found concurrently. The proportion of VUS differed among the risk factors for HBOC (Fig. 24.3). VUS was identified in 11.6% of breast cancer patients with another primary cancer, 14.8% of patients with a family history of breast cancer, 15.8% of bilateral breast cancer patients, and 17.0% of patients who were diagnosed with breast cancer younger than 40 years old. Additionally, 13 patients with VUS also had a concurrent deleterious mutation (patient_33, 66, 105, 115, 133, 182, 222, 233, 264, 280, 454, 468, and 501).

Table 24.4 Variants of uncertain significance strongly suspected of being deleterious mutations

Gene	Mutation	Transcript	HGVS cDNA	Amino acid change
ALK	Missense mutation	NM_004304.4	c.3260C > T	p.T1087I
ATR	Missense mutation	NM_001184.3	c.3637A > G	p.S1213G
BLM	Missense mutation	NM_000057.3	c.2371C > T	p.R791C
BRCA1	Missense mutation	NM_007294.3	c.154C > T	p.L52F
	Missense mutation	NM_007294.3	c.3448C > T	p.P1150S
BRCA2	Missense mutation	NM_000059.3	c.7522G > A	p.G2508S
CDH1	Missense mutation	NM_004360.4	c.1018A > G	p.T340A
CHEK2	Missense mutation	NM_001005735.1	c.1240C > T	p.H414Y
FANCD2	Missense mutation	NM_001018115.2	c.2480A > C	p.E827A
FANCD2	Nonsense mutation	NM_001018115.1	c.1318C > T	p.Q440*
FANCE	Missense mutation	NM_021922.2	c.991C > G	p.L331V
FANCI	Missense mutation	NM_001113378.1	c.1111A > G	p.S371G
FH	Missense mutation	NM_000143.3	c.302G > A	p.R101Q
LIG4	Missense mutation	NM_001098268.1	c.2586 T > A	p.H862Q
MSH2	Missense mutation	NM_000251.2	c.14C > A	p.P5Q
	Missense mutation	NM_000251.2	c.1255C > A	p.Q419K
MSH6	Missense mutation	NM_000179.2	c.3772C > G	p.Q1258E
	Missense mutation	NM_000179.2	c.2503C > G	p.Q835E
PALB2	Missense mutation	NM_024675.3	c.2509G > A	p.E837K
PTCH1	Start lost	NM_001083603.2	c.1A > G	p.M1V
TP53	Missense mutation	NM_001126114.2	c.847C > T	p.R283C

24.2 Conclusion

To the best of our knowledge, this is the largest study to include Korean breast cancer patients with clinical features of HBOC and examine the frequency and characteristics of germline mutations in BRCA1/2 and nonBRCA1/2 cancer-susceptibility genes.

We analyzed germline mutations from 496 breast cancer patients of Asian ethnicity with clinical features of HBOC using NGS-based multigene panel testing. Overall, 95 patients (19.2%) were found to carry 48 deleterious germline mutations in 16 cancer-susceptibility genes. The NGS-based multigene panel test improved the detection rates of deleterious mutations and provided a cost-effective cancer risk assessment compared with a gene-by-gene approach.

References

1. Lincoln SE, Kobayashi Y, Anderson MJ, Yang S, Desmond AJ, Mills MA, et al. A systematic comparison of traditional and multigene panel testing for hereditary breast and ovarian cancer genes in more than 1000 patients. J Mol Diagn. 2015;17(5):533–44.
2. Kapoor NS, Curcio LD, Blakemore CA, Bremner AK, McFarland RE, West JG, et al. Multigene panel testing detects equal rates of pathogenic BRCA1/2 mutations and has a higher diagnostic yield compared to limited BRCA1/2 analysis alone in patients at risk for hereditary breast cancer. Ann Surg Oncol. 2015;22(10):3282–8.
3. Couch FJ, Shimelis H, Hu C, Hart SN, Polley EC, Na J, et al. Associations between cancer predisposition testing panel genes and breast cancer. JAMA Oncol. 2017;3(9):1190–6.
4. Buys SS, Sandbach JF, Gammon A, Patel G, Kidd J, Brown KL, et al. A study of over 35,000 women with breast cancer tested with a 25-gene panel of hereditary cancer genes. Cancer. 2017;123(10):1721–30.
5. Rosenthal ET, Bernhisel R, Brown K, Kidd J, Manley S. Clinical testing with a panel of 25 genes associated with increased cancer risk results in a significant increase in clinically significant findings across a broad range of cancer histories. Cancer Genet. 2017;218:58–68.
6. Slavin TP, Niell-Swiller M, Solomon I, Nehoray B, Rybak C, Blazer KR, et al. Clinical application of multigene panels: challenges of next-generation counseling and cancer risk management. Front Oncol. 2015;5:208.
7. Desmond A, Kurian AW, Gabree M, Mills MA, Anderson MJ, Kobayashi Y, et al. Clinical actionability of multigene panel testing for hereditary breast and ovarian cancer risk assessment. JAMA Oncol. 2015;1(7):943–51.
8. Daly MB, Pilarski R, Berry M, Buys SS, Farmer M, Friedman S, et al. NCCN guidelines insights: genetic/familial high-risk assessment: breast and ovarian, version 2.2017. J Natl Compr Canc Netw. 2017;15(1):9–20.
9. Shin HC, Lee HB, Yoo TK, Lee ES, Kim RN, Park B, Yoon KA, Park C, Lee ES, Moon HG, Noh DY. Detection of germline mutations in breast cancer patients with clinical features of hereditary cancer syndrome using a multi-gene panel test. Cancer Res Treat. 2020;52(3): 697–713.

Chapter 25
BRCA and Breast Cancer-Related High-Penetrance Genes

Sang-Ah Han and Sung-Won Kim

Abstract Genetic susceptibility explains 5–10% of all breast cancer cases. High-penetrance breast cancer susceptibility genes deliberate a greater than tenfold relative risk of breast cancer. *BRCA1* and *BRCA2* genes are the most common cause of hereditary breast cancer, and *TP53*, *PTEN*, and *SKT11* (*LKB1*) are rarely present. The prevalence of *BRCA1* and *BRCA2* genetic alterations differ in various ethnic groups. The Korean Hereditary Breast Cancer (KOHBRA) Study, nationwide-scale study, was established to acquire evidence for the accurate risk assessment and management of hereditary breast and ovarian cancer (HBOC) in Korea prospectively since 2007. In this chapter, we review previous research related to hereditary breast cancer and summarize the present concepts and research results centered on the Korean Hereditary Breast Cancer Research at this time.

Keywords Breast cancer · Genetic susceptibility · *BRCA1/2* · *TP53* · *PTEN* · *STK11* · KOHBRA study

25.1 Introduction

Genetic susceptibility is an important risk factor for breast cancer, accounting for 5–10% of all breast cancer [1]. Sporadic breast cancer with no family history accounts for 75–85% of breast cancer, and familial breast cancer caused by exposure to the same environment and risk factors accounts for 10–15% of total breast cancer. Clinically, hereditary breast cancer has an early onset compared with sporadic breast cancer, and they are characterized by bilateral breast cancer and multiple cancers. Most of them are autosomal dominant.

S.-A. Han (✉)
Kyung Hee University, School of Medicine, Seoul, South Korea

S.-W. Kim
Daerim St.Mary's Hospital, Seoul, South Korea

D.-Y. Noh et al. (eds.), *Translational Research in Breast Cancer*, Advances in Experimental Medicine and Biology 1187,
https://doi.org/10.1007/978-981-32-9620-6_25

BRCA1 and *BRCA2* genes are the most common cause of hereditary breast cancer. Since *BRCA1* and *BRCA2* have been identified in 1994 [2] and 1995 [3], respectively, studies have been undertaken on experimental biochemical techniques to identify the function of *BRCA1/2* and related proteins in the biochemical domain and to detect such mutations [4]. Scientists tried to figure out the function of each mutation and its relationship to disease. Epidemiologists researched the prevalence of the genetic mutation in each ethnic group, identified new problematic genetic loci, increasing the risk of disease [5, 6]. They expanded the area of study into gene-gene interactions and gene-environment interactions [5].

The breast cancer susceptibility factors identified to date can be stratified by risk profile into three levels [7]. High-Penetrance breast cancer susceptibility genes confer a greater than tenfold relative risk of breast cancer [8]. At present, discovered high-penetrance genes are *BRCA1*, *BRCA2*, *TP53*, *PTEN*, and *LKB1* [9–11]. *ATM*, *BRIP1*, *CHEK2*, and *PALB2* are intermediate penetrance gene [12–14]. Mutations in these genes are rare and confer a relative risk of breast cancer of 2–4. There is currently strong evidence for the association with breast cancer of diverse low-penetrance loci (rs3803662, rs889312, rs3817198, and rs13281615), which each confers a relative risk of breast cancer of <1.5 [15–17].

In the clinical field, there are *BRCA1/2*, *TP53*, and *PTEN* genes that need to be noted in the medical setting environment because they are frequently found and/or have high penetration rates, and the main medical guidelines involving hereditary breast and ovary cancer syndrome target these genes [8, 18]. Clinical researchers are studying appropriate management, treatment, and prophylactic interventions in a carrier and genetic alteration in mostly *BRCA1/2* associated breast ovarian cancer patients [18].

Though many studies have been active over the last 20 years, most of them are of the Western population. According to previous studies, the prevalence of *BRCA1/2* genetic alterations varies in different ethnicities. The penetrance of *BRCA* mutations is different among ethnic groups as well, and this might be associated with the potential interactions of environmental and genetic backgrounds. In 1995, *BRCA1* mutation was reported in Korea, firstly [19], but few studies of *BRCA1* and *BRCA2* genetic alteration followed until the early 2000s. The opportunity for *BRCA1* and *BRCA2* gene test and preventive management for breast and ovary cancer were unnoticed in Korea.

In 2007, the Korean Hereditary Breast Cancer (KOHBRA) Study, a large, prospective study, was performed to assess the accurate risk and management strategy of hereditary breast and ovarian cancer (HBOC) in Korea [20–23].

In this chapter, we review previous research related to hereditary breast cancer and summarize the present concepts and research results centered on the Korean Hereditary Breast Cancer Research at this time (Fig. 25.1).

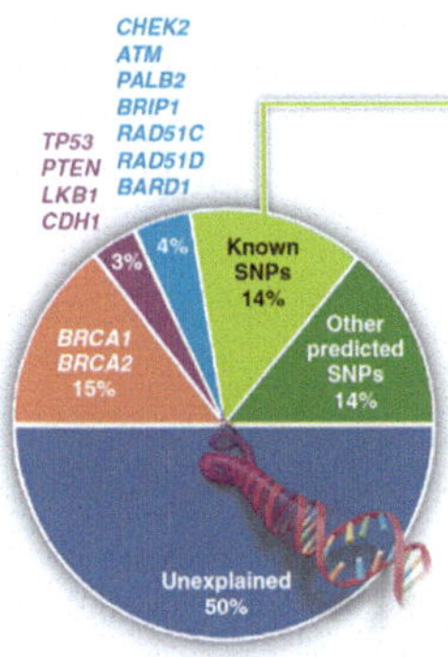

Locus	SNP	Odds ratio
6q14.1	rs17529111	1.97
**BRCA2*	rs11571833	1.44
CCND1	rs75915166	1.38
ESR1	rs3757318	1.33
FGFR2	rs2981579	1.33
CCND1	rs554219	1.33
FGFR2	rs2981582	1.26
**MERIT40*	rs8170	1.26
TERT	rs10069690	1.24
DNAJC1	rs11814448	1.22
CCDN1	rs614367	1.21
MKL1	rs6001930	1.21
MDM4	rs4245739	1.19
ESR1	rs2046210	1.16
HNF4G	rs2943559	1.14
5p12	rs10941679	1.13
12p13.1	rs12422552	1.13
MAP3K1	rs889312	1.12
TCF7L2	rs7904519	1.12
22q12.2	rs132390	1.12
2p24.1	rs12710696	1.11
2q31.1	rs2016394	1.1
SLC4A7	rs4973768	1.1
EBF1	rs1432679	1.1
FTO	rs11075995	1.1
1p11.2	rs11249433	1.09

Locus	SNP	Odds ratio
8q24	rs13281615	1.09
TOX3	rs3803662	1.09
CDYL2	rs13329835	1.09
1p13.2*	rs11552449	1.08
2q35	rs16857609	1.08
RANBP1	rs204247	1.08
ZMIZ1	rs704010	1.08
12q24	rs1292011	1.08
3p26.2	rs6762644	1.07
8p21.1	rs9693444	1.07
8q24.21	rs11780156	1.07
LSP1	rs3817198	1.07
CCDC88C	rs941764	1.07
TET2	rs9790517	1.06
CDKN2A/B	rs1011970	1.06
TGFBR2	rs12493607	1.05
9q31.2	rs10759243	1.05
DNAJC1	rs7072776	1.05
19q13.31	rs3760982	1.05
RAB3C	rs10472076	1.04
ANKRD16	rs2380205	0.98
**CASP8*	rs1045485	0.97
7q35	rs720475	0.96
CHST9	rs1436904	0.96
FTO	rs17817449	0.95
18q11.2	rs527616	0.95

Locus	SNP	Odds ratio
CDCA7	rs1550623	0.94
10q26.12	rs11199914	0.94
COX11	rs6504950	0.94
**SSBP4*	rs4808801	0.94
2q35	rs13387042	0.93
PDE4D	rs1353747	0.93
11q13.1	rs3903072	0.92
11q24.3	rs11820646	0.92
PAX9	rs2236007	0.92
RAD51L1	rs999737	0.92
NRIP1	rs2823093	0.92
PEX14	rs616488	0.91
FOXQ1	rs11242675	0.91
8q21.11	rs6472903	0.91
RAD51L1	rs2588809	0.91
LGR6	rs6678914	0.9
NTN4	rs17356907	0.9
2q14.2	rs4849887	0.89
9q31	rs865686	0.89
ZNF365	rs10995190	0.86
ADAM29	rs6828523	0.84
MERIT40	rs2363956	0.82
TERT	rs2736108	0.77
PTHLH	rs10771399	0.72

* Denotes coding variant

Fig. 25.1 Genetic variants that predispose to breast cancer [17]. The pie chart on the left shows the estimated percentage contribution of mutations in high-penetrance (*BRCA1/2*, *TP53*, *CDH1*, *LKB1*, and *PTEN*) and moderate-penetrance (e.g., *CHEK2*, *ATM*, and *PALB2*) genes and common low-penetrance genetic variants to familial relative risk. Common genetic variants are denoted as SNPs. "Known SNPs" are SNPs associated with breast cancer through GWAS, as listed on the right. The odd ratios refer to the increase (or, in some cases, the reduction) in risk conferred by the rare allele of the variants. "Other predicted SNPs" refer to the estimated contribution of all SNPs, other than known loci, which were selected for replication of breast cancer GWAS [15, 16]

25.2 Review of Past Studies

25.2.1 Five High-Penetrance Genes and Function

25.2.1.1 *BRCA1* and *BRCA2*

BRCA1 gene was found in 1994 on chromosome 17 [2]. *BRCA1* gene consists of 24 exons. BRCA1, the protein product of translation of *BRCA1* gene, consists of 1863 amino acids. *BRCA2* gene was found in 1995 on chromosome 13 [3]. *BRCA2* gene consists of 27 exons. BRCA2 protein consists of 3418 amino acids. Critically, the BRCA1 and BRCA2 proteins are involved in maintaining genomic stability. BRCA1/2 proteins promote repair of double-strand breaks, acting as a tumor suppressor gene. BRCA1 proteins are involved in the early stages of the reaction after damage to DNA, making damage aware, making it easier to get access to the damage, and regulating cell cycle checkpoints [24]. BRCA2 proteins mainly engage in double-helix DNA recovery, and they combine and adjust directly with RAD51, which is essential as a catalyst for homologous recombination [25]. *BRCA1* and *BRCA2* mutations are the most powerful genetic variation responsible for 15% of hereditary breast cancers (HBCs). Flaws in DNA repair associated with the *BRCA1/2* mutations could be used to develop a new targeted therapy approach for cancer in the mutation carrier.

25.2.1.2 BRCA Chronology

In 1971, Henry Lynch first associated hereditary breast and ovarian cancer in the same family [26].

Mary-Claire King demonstrates that a gene on chromosome 17 may be responsible for breast cancers in some families [27].

Mark Skolnick and colleague discovered *BRCA1* gene on chromosome 17, associated with breast and ovarian cancer, in 1994.

Wooster et al. identified *BRCA2* in 1995 [3].

The effectiveness of preventive breast surgery in *BRCA* mutation carriers was shown in 2001 [28, 29], effectiveness of risk-reducing ovarian surgery was documented in 2002 [30]. The safety of lumpectomy and radiation therapy in *BRCA*-related breast cancer cases was proved in 2005 and 2007 [31].

In 2006, the role of preimplantation genetics in preventing transmission of hereditary cancer was reported firstly [32].

Genome-wide association studies of low-risk common genetic variants with very mildly increased risk of breast cancer were published during 2007 and 2008 [15, 16].

In 2010, Susan Domcheck demonstrated that preventive ovarian surgery improves mortality in women with *BRCA* mutations [33]. Genome-wide association study was performed to define "genetic-modifiers" of breast cancer risk in 2010. In 2013, the Myriad *BRCA1* gene patent was overturned in the US supreme court [34].

A series of events in Korea led to changes in *BRCA*-related breast cancer care settings.

National health insurance benefits for *BRCA* testing began by starting reimbursement for familial breast cancer patients in 2005. The KOHBRA (Korean Hereditary Breast Cancer study) I was conducted during 2007–2010. The KOHBRA study II was conducted during 2010–2013. According to the core findings from the KOHBRA study, reimbursement of *BRCA* testing was expanded to nonfamilial high-risk breast cancer patients [35].

25.2.1.3 *TP53*

Li-Fraumeni syndrome (LFS) is a condition that early-onset breast cancer, associated sarcoma and childhood cancer involving the adrenal cortex, brain, and other systems is highly frequent in the family [36]. The *TP53* is a universal tumor suppressor gene that is involved in multiple pathways in a cell, and its genetic defects lead to the development of multiple cancers [37].

While the rate of penetrance is high, the rarity of the condition makes epidemiologic data rare. Recently, Bougeard et al. updated the description of this condition from 1730 French patients and reported that the 322 affected carriers developed 552 tumors, and 43% had developed multiple malignancies. The mean age of first tumor onset was 24.9 years, with 41% have developed a tumor by age 18 [38]. In childhood, the LFS tumor spectrum was characterized by osteosarcomas, adrenocortical carcinomas, CNS tumors, and soft tissue sarcomas (STS) observed in 30%, 27%, 26%, and 23% of the patients, respectively. In adults, the tumor distribution was characterized by the predominance of breast carcinomas observed in 79% of the females, and STS observed in 27% of the patients. This study has confirmed the clinically aggressive behavior of this syndrome and extremely high penetrance [38].

25.2.1.4 *PTEN*

Cowden syndrome is an autosomal dominant inherited condition. It is characterized by multiple hamartomas and benign and malignant tumors of the breast, thyroid, and endometrium. This higher-penetrance clustered disease includes mucocutaneous lesions, macrocephaly, and hamartomatous intestinal polyps. *PTEN* on chromosome 10q was identified as a causative gene through linkage analysis, 12 Cowden syndrome families. *PTEN* gene is translated into lipid phosphatase. Lipid phosphatase has functioned as a tumor suppressor involving in negative regulation of a cell-survival signaling pathway. It is known that cross-talk exists between this *PTEN*-related pathway and Ras-, p53-, and TOR-related pathways [39].

25.2.1.5 *STK11*

Serine/threonine kinase 11 (STK11) is a protein kinase that inhibits cellular proliferation, controls cell polarity, and interacts with the TOR pathway. Deleterious alteration of *STK11* on chromosome 19p is characterized by hamartomatous intestinal polyps, mucocutaneous pigmentation, and increased incidence of several malignancies. The complex of these diseases is called Peutz-Jeghers syndrome. The lifetime risk of breast cancer is also elevated with this syndrome at 15 times than the average population [40].

25.3 Current Evidence and Concepts

25.3.1 KOHBRA Study

Primary aims of KOHBRA Study I (May 2007–May 2010) were to assess the prevalence of *BRCA1* and *BRCA2* mutations in breast cancer patients and their families at elevated risk of HBOC. Secondary aims of the KOHBRA study I were to classify Korean founder mutations and found a *BRCA1/2* mutation carrier cohort. KOHBRA Study II was conducted from June 2010 to May 2013. Primary aims of KOHBRA study II were to identify the clinical and pathological characteristics and prognostic factors of *BRCA*-associated breast cancer and environmental and genetic modifiers of *BRCA* mutations and to develop a Korean BRCA risk prediction model and nationwide genetic counseling network for HBC in Korea [35, 41].

25.3.2 *Inclusion Criteria*

Through the KOHBRA study I and II, 3015 subjects were enrolled between May 2007 and December 2013 from 36 institutions. The eligible subjects for enrollment are as follows: (1) breast cancer patients with a family history of breast or ovarian cancer (familial); (2) breast cancer patients without a family history of breast or ovarian cancer (nonfamilial) who were 40 years and younger at diagnosis, diagnosed with bilateral breast cancer or another primary malignancy, or male; (3) family members of *BRCA1/2* mutation carriers. The risk of carrying a deleterious *BRCA* mutation among these high-risk populations generally satisfies greater than 10%, the classic cutoffs for offering a *BRCA* genetic testing (Fig. 25.2).

25.3.3 *Prevalence of* BRCA *Mutations [35]*

The overall prevalence of *BRCA1/2* mutations was 22.3% in breast cancer patients with a family history of breast or ovarian cancer. Prevalence was recalculated by subgroup according to the strength and type of family history. The prevalence was

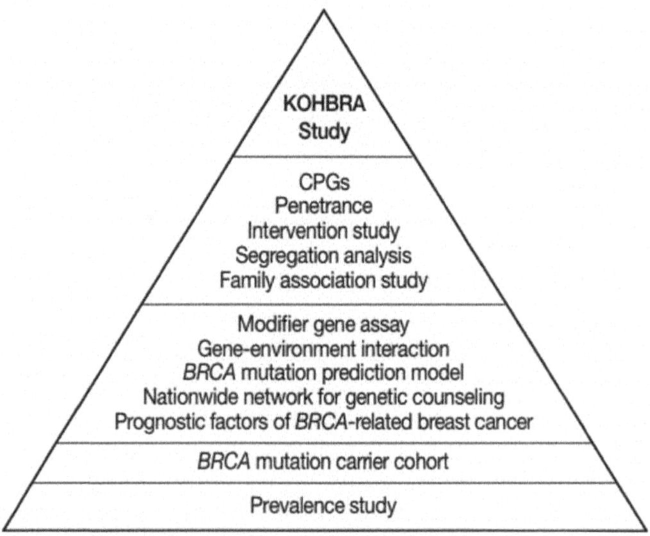

Fig. 25.2 The Korean Hereditary Breast Cancer (KOHBRA) Study [21]. The KOHBRA Study was planned as a 10-year project to develop Korean clinical practice guidelines (CPGs)

Table 25.1 The prevalence of BRCA1/2 mutation in 2403 probands up to 2013 [35]

	Risk	Total number	BRCA1/2 mutation (+)	Prevalence (%)
Breast cancer patients +FH	FH of BC	1085	224	20.6
	FH of OC	102	30	29.4
	FH of BC and OC	41	20	48.8
	Total	1228	274	22.3
Breast cancer patients–FH	Early-onset BC	845	60	7.1
	Bilateral BC	209	34	16.3
	BC and OC in same patient	8	3	37.5
	Multiple organ cancers	74	3	4.1
	Male BC	21	1	4.8
	Risks ≥2	18	3	16.7
	Total	1175	104	8.9

BC breast cancer, *OC* ovary cancer, *FH* family history.

20.6% in patients with a family history of only breast cancer and 29.4% in patients with a family history of only ovarian cancer. In breast cancer patients with a family history of ovarian cancer, mutation prevalence (range, 26.3–100.0%) was very high in all subgroups regardless of type and number of family history of breast cancer. In breast cancer patients without a family history of ovarian cancer, the more the breast cancer family history, the higher the *BRCA1/2* mutation prevalence rate is. The prevalence of *BRCA1/2* mutations according to the number of relatives with breast cancer was 17.8, 30.2, and 43.2% in patients with 1 relative, 2 relatives, and 3 relatives with breast cancer, respectively. There was no statistical difference in mutation prevalence (range, 14.1–21.7%) according to the closest degree of relatives with breast cancer.

The overall prevalence of *BRCA1/2* mutations was 8.9% in nonfamilial breast cancer patients at high risk of HBOC: 7.1% in early-onset breast cancer patients (≤40 years), 16.3% in bilateral breast cancer patients, 37.5% in patients with both breast and ovarian cancer, 4.8% in male breast cancer patients, 4.1% in patients with multi-organ cancer including breast cancer, and 16.7% in patients with two or more of these forms.

In the early-onset breast cancer subsets, *BRCA1/2* mutation rates varied depending on whether other risk factors are present. The age at diagnosis of breast cancer also had a significant impact on the prevalence of this subset (Table 25.1).

In 845 patients without other risks, *BRCA1/2* mutations were observed in 39 of 441 (8.8%) patients who were diagnosed with breast cancer and were less than 35 years old and in 21 of 404 (5.2%) patients who were diagnosed with breast cancer between 35 and 40 years old. In addition, we had further analysis to determine the difference between *BRCA1/2* prevalence according to breast cancer subtype in 441 young breast cancer patients (<35 years) without other risk factors. The rates of *BRCA1/2* mutations showed a difference depending on the presence of the triple-negative subtype. The prevalence in patients with triple-negative breast cancer was 12.5% (13/104), and the rates of *BRCA1/2* mutations in breast cancer patients with non triple-negative subtype and unknown subtype were 7.8% (24/308) and 6.9% (2/29), respectively [35].

Among 91 patients with breast and other cancers, *BRCA1/2* mutations were observed in 2 (3.3%) of 60 patients with thyroid cancer, in 1 of 12 (8.3%) patients with uterine cancer, in 1 of 6 (16.7%) patients with renal cell carcinoma, and in 1 of 1 (100%) patient with osteosarcoma.

25.3.4 *Mutation Spectrum and Founder Mutation in Korea [21, 35]*

From an analysis of the mutation spectra, 63 *BRCA1* and 90 *BRCA2* different mutations, including 44 novel mutations, were identified in 378 index cases (154 *BRCA*1, 221 *BRCA*2, and 3 with both *BRCA1* and *BRCA*2). The c.7480 (p. Arg2494Ter) mutation in *BRCA2* (10.1%) was the most commonly identified in this cohort. Among 345 patients whose mutations were analyzed by both direct sequencing and multiplex ligation-dependent probe amplification, 62 *BRCA1/2* small mutations and only one large genomic deletion (*BRCA1* whole gene deletion) were found (Table 25.2).

25.3.5 *Breast and Ovarian Cancer Risks Associated with* BRCA *Mutations*

BRCA1/2 mutation carriers are 10–20 times more likely to have breast cancer and ovarian cancer than the average population to receive systematic care, including intensive cancer screening surveillance and preventative surgery. The probability of genotype expression into phenotype is defined as the penetrance rate. The risks of breast and ovarian cancers in *BRCA1* and *BRCA2* mutation carriers by the age of 70 years were 57% (95% confidence interval [CI], 47–66%) and 40% (95% CI, 35–46%) for *BRCA1* mutation carriers and 49% (95% CI, 40–57%) and 18% (95% CI, 13–23%) for *BRCA2* mutation carriers, respectively [42]. The penetrance of *BRCA1* and *BRCA2* mutations is different between countries and races. This is because diverse genetic modifiers and environmental influences have combined effects on breast cancer development.

The cumulative risk of breast and ovarian cancers among 61 *BRCA1* and 47 *BRCA2* mutation carrier families is calculated using Kaplan-Meier analyses. The average cumulative risk of breast and ovarian cancers by age 70 years was 72.1% (95% CI, 59.5–84.8%) and 24.6% (95% CI, 0–50.3%) for *BRCA1* carriers and 66.3% (95% CI, 41.2–91.5%) and 11.1% (95% CI, 0–31.6%) for *BRCA2*

Table 25.2 The candidates for the Korean founder mutation ($n = 148$) [21]

	Systemic nomenclature	BIC nomenclature	Effect on amino acid	No. of times observed	%
BRCA2	c.7480C > T	7708C > T	p.Arg2494X	18	12.2
BRCA1	c.390C > A	509C > A	p.Tyr130X	11	7.4
BRCA1	c.5496_5506del11insA	5615_5625del11insA	p.Val1833SerfsX7	11	7.4
BRCA2	c.1399A > T	1627A > T	p.Lys467X	8	5.4
BRCA2	c.3744_3747deiTGAG	33972_3975defTGAG	p.Ser1248ArgfsX10	7	4.7
BRCA2	c.6724_6725delGA	6952_6953delGA	pAsp2242PhefsX2	5	3.4
BRCA1	c.3627_3628insA	3746_3747insA	p.Glu1210ArgfsX9	4	2.7
BRCA1	c.5445G > A	5564G > A	p.Trp1815X	4	2.7
BRCA2	c.5567_5579defTTAA	5804_5807defTTAA	p.lle1859LysfsX3	4	2.7
BRCA1	c.992_994delAGCinsT	1041_1043delAGCinsT	p.Ser308X	3	2.0

BIC breast cancer information core.

carriers, respectively [21]. The results are comparable to those of western studies. This study is limited to a small number of subjects, a high incidence of the proband, short follow-up periods, and large confidence intervals; however, it became clear that Korean *BRCA1/2* carriers also need to be properly managed for the increased risk of breast and/or ovary cancer. KOHBRA study group hopes to complement its limits to produce more conclusive penetrance data of Korean *BRCA1/2* carriers (Table 25.3).

25.3.6 *Breast Cancer Survival in* BRCA1/2 *Mutation Carriers*

Several studies have suggested different answers to the different outcomes for *BRCA1/2*-related breast cancer and sporadic breast cancer.

While breast cancer with a *BRCA1* mutation is reported to have a poorer prognosis than sporadic breast cancer [43], some literature suggests that the prognosis is similar between *BRCA1* related and sporadic [44].

In a large population study, 10-year survival rates between *BRCA1/2* carriers and noncarriers are reported to be similar [45]. Based on this report, breast cancer in *BRCA1/2* carriers is considered a similar prognosis to noncarriers. It might be interpreted by the differences between *BRCA1* and *BRCA2*, the relatively small number of *BRCA* carriers, and the different primary outcomes and follow-up periods for these inconsistent findings.

The KOHBRA study group conducted a meta-analysis to overcome these limitations and see the prognosis for *BRCA1/2*-related cancers.

Through the meta-analysis of 11 studies dealing with mortality and relapse rate in *BRCA1/2* related cancer, overall survival (OS), and disease-free survival (DFS) rates were obtained [46]. *BRCA1*-related cancer had significantly lowered short-term and long-term OS rates than noncarriers (hazard ratio [HR], 1.92 [95% CI, 1.45–2.53]; HR, 1.33 [95% CI, 1.12–1.58]). On the contrary, short-term and long-term OS rates were similar in *BRCA2* mutation carriers and noncarriers (HR, 1.30 [95% CI, 0.95–1.76]; HR, 1.12 [95% CI, 0.86–1.45]). *BRCA1* mutation carriers had a significantly worse short-term DFS rate than noncarriers (HR, 1.54; 95% CI, 1.12–2.12), whereas the short-term DFS rate was similar for *BRCA2* mutation carriers and noncarriers (HR, 1.23; 95% CI, 0.96–1.58). These findings show that *BRCA1*-related cancers have poor short and long-term OS rates and short-term DFS rates, and oncologic outcomes do not vary based on the presence of *BRCA2*.

Table 25.3 Cumulative risk till each age of breast and ovarian cancer among family members with BRCA1/2 mutation carriers [21]

		Breast cancer risk				Ovarian cancer risk			
	Age (year)	Carriers (No.)	Breast cancer (No.)	Cumulative risk (%)	95% Cl (%)	Carriers (No.)	Ovary cancer (No.)	Cumulative risk (%)	95% Cl (%)
BRCA1	21–30	19	1	5.3	0.1–10.4	61	0	0.0	0.0–0.0
	31–40	18	1	10.8	3.6–18.1	54	0	0.0	0.0–0.0
	41–50	13	6	55.4	42.0–68.8	35	2	5.7	0.0–13.4
	51–60	6	1	62.8	49.8–75.9	15	1	12.0	0.0–25.9
	61–70	4	2	72.1	59.5–84.8	7	1	24.6	0.0–50.3
BRCA2	21–30	16	0	0.0	0.0–0.0	47	0	0.0	0.0–0.0
	31–40	13	1	7.7	0.3–15.1	42	0	0.0	0.0–0.0
	41–50	11	2	32.7	16.5–48.8	34	0	0.0	0.0–0.0
	51–60	5	0	32.7	16.5–48.8	17	0	0.0	0.0–0.0
	61–70	5	1	66.3	41.2–91.5	9	1	11.1	0.0–31.6

Cl confidence interval.

25.3.7 Genetic Counseling in Korea and the Influence of KOHBRA Study

During the KOHBRA Study, professional genetic consultants from the headquarters provided genetic counseling to all participants [41]. After the study period, we analyzed practice patterns of HBOC, including genetic counseling, to show that the KOHBRA study provides proper standards guidelines for the management of hereditary breast cancer and improved perception and education of health care providers. However, the problem was that it was difficult to continue providing relevant genetic counseling in Korea because of the absence of certified genetic consultants. The KOHBRA study group deployed standardized genetic counseling systems in Korea, forming genetic counseling networks in conjunction with major hospitals nationwide, publishing genetic counseling textbooks and manuals, and creating a training course and certification under the supervision of the Korean breast cancer society.

25.3.8 Risk Assessment for HBOC in KOREA

Accurate risk measurement as base data is crucial to diagnosing HBOC and implementing its first step, genetic counseling.

Arithmetic and empirical models are being used to predict the probability of individuals having mutations. The most broadly used models are the Myriad II [47], BRCAPRO [48], BOADICEA (Breast and Ovarian Analysis of Disease Incidence and Carrier Estimation Algorithm) [49], and Manchester models [50], which were developed from western population data. BRCAPRO and Myriad II have been validated for various racial groups, and these models have a problem to underestimate the proportion of *BRCA1/2* mutation carriers among Asians [51].

Evaluation of the accuracy of the BRCAPRO and Myriad II models in 236 Korean female breast cancer patients who underwent *BRCA1/2* mutation testing resulted in both models underestimating the overall number of *BRCA1/2* mutations significantly. The observed mutation rate was 19.5%, whereas BRCAPRO predicted 9.0% and Myriad II predicted 5.6% as mutation rate, respectively. It is concluded that western models are inappropriate to find a candidate for the *BRCA* mutation test in Korean [52].

Based on the KOHBRA data of 1600 female participants, Kang et al. developed a mutation prediction model suitable for Koreans.

Logistic regression analysis was used to identify the predictive clinical factors for pathogenic *BRCA1* and *BRCA2* mutations. Familial and nonfamilial models were separately built named KOHCal (KOHBRA BRCA Risk Calculator). Ages at breast cancer diagnosis, bilateral breast cancer, triple-negative breast cancer (TNBC), and the number of relatives with breast or ovarian cancer were included in the familial model. A breast cancer diagnosis at age under 35 years, bilateral breast cancer, both breast and ovarian cancers, and TNBC were included in the nonfamilial model. Using the information input, the estimated probability of *BRCA1/2* mutations and the observed prevalence data were calculated and presented in percent. Internet link to KOHcal was posted on the KOHBRA Study website (www.kohbra.kr) to assist in selection of proper subjects for *BRCA* mutation testing and help in the decision to accept genetic tests in the Korean population.

25.3.9 Carrier Management and Korean CPG Guideline

In 2013, when the fifth Korean clinical practice guideline for Breast cancer was compiled, it was first published jointly with clinical practice guidelines for hereditary breast cancer, making it one of the ultimate goals of the KOHBRA Study's 10-year project. Following the second clinical practice guidelines (CPG) for hereditary breast cancer compiled in conjunction with the seventh Korean clinical practice guideline for Breast cancer in 2015, the third CPG was compiled in 2017, reflecting the latest developments in the NCCN guideline, ASCO guideline, and St. Galen guideline.

Genetic breast cancer accounts for 5% of all breast cancer cases. So rarely do researchers design large-scale studies that are credible enough to be commonly used as a basis for clinical guidance. International major guidelines also reflect evidence level 2–4 not only evidence level 1 for the hereditary breast cancer field. The KOHBRA study has produced basic data about prevalence, penetrance, risk assessment, oncologic outcome, and so on, but present the basic data on the carrier management, especially for risk-reducing options. In Korea, the first case underwent a contralateral risk-reducing mastectomy and RRSO in a *BRCA* mutation carrier with breast cancer was reported in 2008 [53], and the first bilateral risk-reducing double mastectomy in an asymptomatic *BRCA* mutation carrier [54] was reported in 2010. However, chemoprevention using Tamoxifen and RRSO was not widely practiced in Korea. According to the result of an evaluation of factors affecting the decision to undergo RRSO among women with *BRCA1/2* mutations in a single institution, the uptake rate of RRSO was 29.6% among 71 carriers suitable for RRSO [55]. The uptake rate of RRSO in this institution was higher than in other hospitals in Korea, but it was lower than the uptake rates in Western reports. The rate of RRSO was different according to the age of the carrier. The fifth decade of life (52.6%) presents the highest uptake rate. The fourth decade of life (33.3%) and sixth and later decades of life (10.7%) were followed. Person who had breast cancer presented higher RRSO uptake rate (39.2% vs. 5.0%, $p = 0.004$). A person who had a family history of breast or ovarian cancer showed a higher rate of RRSO uptake in univariate analysis.

Age (fourth and fifth decades of life) and personal history of breast cancer were independent factors affecting the uptake of RRSO after multivariate analysis. Therefore, age, personal history of breast cancer, and other factors affecting the decision to undergo RRSO should be closely monitored when genetic counseling is performed. Despite the limitations of the small sample size and the single-institution design, this is the first study to address the RRSO uptake rate and factors affecting the decision to undergo RRSO in *BRCA1/2* carriers in an Asian country.

Even if high level of evidence is a difficult fact to achieve in the hereditary breast cancer field, it is necessary to share the latest knowledge in HBOC and apply it to the Korean care environment.

The latest Korean CPG for HBC centers on *BRCA1/2* mutation as there are few reports about other high penetrance genetic syndrome in Korea. Clinical recommendations are based on KOHBRA data and major international guidelines.

Management options for women with *BRCA* mutations include close surveillance, chemoprevention, and risk-reducing surgery (RRS). According to the NCCN guideline [18], "monthly breast self-examinations beginning at age 18, clinical breast examinations twice annually beginning at age 25, and annual mammography and breast magnetic resonance imaging screening beginning at age 25 are recommended for breast cancer surveillance. Biannual ovarian cancer screening with transvaginal ultrasonography and CA-125 serology beginning at age 35 are recommended for ovarian cancer surveillance. Because ovarian cancer screening is not sufficiently sensitive to detect ovarian cancer at an early stage, the preferred option for ovarian cancer prevention is risk-reducing salpingo-oophorectomy (RRSO). RRSO is recommended for *BRCA* mutation carriers aged between 35 and 40 years (after the completion of childbearing) and reduces the risk of ovarian and breast cancers by 95% and 50%, respectively." In *BRCA2* carrier, RRSO can be delayed until the age of 40–45. RRSO has also been associated with a reduction of all-cause, breast cancer-specific, and ovarian cancer-specific mortality. The NCCN guidelines recommend discussing risk-reducing mastectomy (RRM) with *BRCA1/2* mutation carriers, and reconstructive surgery and psychological consultation should also be considered in the decision-making process for RRM. Chemopreventive agents such as tamoxifen for breast cancer and oral pills for ovary cancer may be considered to reduce cancer risk, and the benefits and risks of these agents should be discussed.

Korean CPG further described that the test subjects might include patients with triple-negative breast cancer before the age of 60 years old base on findings that *BRCA 1/2* mutations in 13.1% of overall patients and 14.5% of patients $\leq$ 60 years in unselected patients [56]. It said the multigene panel could be introduced by attaching a hint that new aspects of care are needed when assessing its efficacy and making clinical applications.

25.4 Future

25.4.1 Collaborative Study

The KOHBRA Study group is participating in IBCCS (International *BRCA1/2* Carrier Cohort Study) and CIMBA (the Consortium of Investigators of Modifiers of *BRCA1/2* to identify epidemiologic factors and genetic modifiers of cancer risk in

BRCA1 and *BRCA2* mutation carriers) in terms of international collaboration. Research in conjunction with KOHBRA and CIMBA has found new genetic susceptibility loci of hereditary breast cancer. KOHBRA Study group starts up Asian BRCA (ABRCA) Consortium as a leading member in 2011. Korea, Malaysia, Hong Kong, Japan, China, Indonesia, and Singapore were initial starting member countries to share knowledge and quality of care about HBOC in Asia. After the annual meeting for 7 years, India, the Philippines, and Vietnam have joined. The ABRCA working groups are collaborating in studies to review the *BRCA* mutation spectrum and founder mutations in Asia and to evaluate the status of genetic counseling and genetic testing for HBOC in Asian countries [57–59]. ABRCA groups are going to assess lifestyle modifiers of breast cancer and estimate the penetrance of *BRCA* mutations in Asian populations.

Collaborative studies represented by IBCCS and CIMBA have enabled the formation of the largest cohort in the limited area of genetic breast cancer across borders and races. Collaborative studies figured out the optimal risk reduction strategy and the clinical effectiveness of each measure, the GWAS (genome-wide association study) uses a large enough cohort sample to find out new susceptibility loci, and different cancer development risk depends on different genetic locus involved. A personalized strategy that knows and approaches an individual's risk correctly forms the basis for selecting the subject of the risk prevention surgery, which is inevitably disruptive when adapting to the wrong target.

Figuring out the genetic potential of the variant unknown significance is among the unknown. This is also a task to be addressed in the future by sharing international cohort data. Finding the best therapeutic agent in the knowledge of its function is already done in the clinical trial and is a representative of the PARP inhibitor.

Already at the point where multigene panels are introduced as a result of the development of genetic technology, understanding the genetic information of the fetus before giving birth and choosing the embryos that have no genetic problems before birth is no longer impossible in technic. With a solution to the complex ethical, moral, and philosophical problems that are introduced in the clinical adoption, many researchers are continuing to implement the development of gene therapy.

25.5 Summary

According to the KOHBRA study, the prevalence of *BRCA1/2* mutation and penetrance were similar to those of the western population. Since risk estimation models of Western underestimate the probability of having genetic alteration, KOHcal is highly recommended in Koreans.

As a result of the KOHBRA study, which has produced data that are unique to Koreans, Korean CPG for HBC is now available for clinical use. However, international cooperative studies are also underway to find solutions to problems that are difficult to solve at the national scale for relatively few study populations. Efforts to apply the breakthroughs in the past decade in the field of genetics into the clinical field and patients will continue.

References

1. Claus EB, Schildkraut JM, Thompson WD, Risch NJ. The genetic attributable risk of breast and ovarian cancer. Cancer. 1996;77(11):2318–24.
2. Miki Y, Swensen J, Shattuck-Eidens D, Futreal PA, Harshman K, Tavtigian S, et al. A strong candidate for the breast and ovarian cancer susceptibility gene BRCA1. Science. 1994;266 (5182):66–71.
3. Wooster R, Bignell G, Lancaster J, Swift S, Seal S, Mangion J, et al. Identification of the breast cancer susceptibility gene BRCA2. Nature. 1995;378(6559):789–92.
4. Gudmundsdottir K, Ashworth A. The roles of BRCA1 and BRCA2 and associated proteins in the maintenance of genomic stability. Oncogene. 2006;25(43):5864–74.
5. Antoniou AC, Easton DF. Models of genetic susceptibility to breast cancer. Oncogene. 2006;25 (43):5898–905.
6. Smith P, McGuffog L, Easton DF, Mann GJ, Pupo GM, Newman B, et al. A genome wide linkage search for breast cancer susceptibility genes. Genes Chromosomes Cancer. 2006;45 (7):646–55.
7. Foulkes WD. Inherited susceptibility to common cancers. N Engl J Med. 2008;359 (20):2143–53.
8. Antoniou A, Pharoah PD, Narod S, Risch HA, Eyfjord JE, Hopper JL, et al. Average risks of breast and ovarian cancer associated with BRCA1 or BRCA2 mutations detected in case series unselected for family history: a combined analysis of 22 studies. Am J Hum Genet. 2003;72 (5):1117–30.
9. Lalloo F, Varley J, Moran A, Ellis D, O'Dair L, Pharoah P, et al. BRCA1, BRCA2 and TP53 mutations in very early-onset breast cancer with associated risks to relatives. Eur J Cancer. 2006;42(8):1143–50.
10. Hobert JA, Eng C. PTEN hamartoma tumor syndrome: an overview. Genet Med. 2009;11 (10):687.
11. Ford D, Easton DF, Stratton M, Narod S, Goldgar D, Devilee P, et al. Genetic heterogeneity and penetrance analysis of the BRCA1 and BRCA2 genes in breast cancer families. Am J Human Genet. 1998;62(3):676–89.
12. C-BC C. Low-penetrance susceptibility to breast cancer due to CHEK2* 1100delC in non-carriers of BRCA1 or BRCA2 mutations. Nat Genet. 2002;31(1):55.
13. Antoniou AC, Casadei S, Heikkinen T, Barrowdale D, Pylkäs K, Roberts J, et al. Breast-cancer risk in families with mutations in PALB2. N Engl J Med. 2014;371(6):497–506.
14. Southey MC, Goldgar DE, Winqvist R, Pylkäs K, Couch F, Tischkowitz M, et al. PALB2, CHEK2 and ATM rare variants and cancer risk: data from COGS. J Med Genet. 2016;53 (12):800–11. https://doi.org/10.1136/jmedgenet-2016-103839.
15. Bahcall OG. iCOGS collection provides a collaborative model. Nat Genet. 2013;45(4):343.
16. Michailidou K, Hall P, Gonzalez-Neira A, Ghoussaini M, Dennis J, Milne RL, et al. Large-scale genotyping identifies 41 new loci associated with breast cancer risk. Nat Genet. 2013;45 (4):353–61.
17. Couch FJ, Nathanson KL, Offit K. Two decades after BRCA: setting paradigms in personalized cancer care and prevention. Science. 2014;343(6178):1466–70.
18. Genetic/familial high-risk assessment: breast and ovarian. 2019. https://www.nccn.org/store/login/login.aspx?ReturnURL=https://www.nccn.org/professionals/physician_gls/pdf/genetics_screening.pdf

19. Oh JH, Noh DY, Choe KJ, Kang SB, Kim LS, Ro MS, et al. Germline mutation of BRCA1 gene in Korean breast and Overian cancer patients. Cancer Res Treat. 1995;27(6):1061–70.
20. Han SA, Park SK, Ahn SH, Son BH, Lee MH, Choi DH, et al. The breast and ovarian cancer risks in Korea due to inherited mutations in BRCA1 and BRCA2: a preliminary report. J Breast Cancer. 2009;12:92–9.
21. Kang E, Kim SW. The korean hereditary breast cancer study: review and future perspectives. J Breast Cancer. 2013;16(3):245–53.
22. Han SA, Kim SW, Kang E, Park SK, Ann SH. The prevalence of BRCA mutations among familial breast cancer patients in Korea: results of the Korean hereditary breast cancer study. Fam Cancer. 2012;12(1):75–81.
23. Son BH, Ahn SH, Kim SW, Kang E, Park SK, Lee MH, et al. Prevalence of BRCA1 and BRCA2 mutations in non-familial breast cancer patients with high risks in Korea: the Korean hereditary breast cancer (KOHBRA) study. Breast Cancer Res Treat. 2012;133(3):1143–52.
24. Moynahan ME, Chiu JW, Koller BH, Jasin M. Brca1 controls homology-directed DNA repair. Mol Cell. 1999;4(4):511–8.
25. Pellegrini L, Yu DS, Lo T, Anand S, Lee M, Blundell TL, et al. Insights into DNA recombination from the structure of a RAD51-BRCA2 complex. Nature. 2002;420(6913):287–93.
26. Lynch HT, Krush AJ. Carcinoma of the breast and ovary in three families. Surg Gynecol Obstet. 1971;133(4):644–8.
27. Friedman LS, Ostermeyer EA, Lynch ED, Szabo CI, Anderson LA, Dowd P, et al. The search for BRCA1. Cancer Res. 1994;54(24):6374–82.
28. Hartmann LC, Sellers TA, Schaid DJ, Frank TS, Soderberg CL, Sitta DL, et al. Efficacy of bilateral prophylactic mastectomy in BRCA1 and BRCA2 gene mutation carriers. J Natl Cancer Inst. 2001;93(21):1633–7.
29. Meijers-Heijboer H, van Geel B, van Putten WL, Henzen-Logmans SC, Seynaeve C, Menke-Pluymers MB, et al. Breast cancer after prophylactic bilateral mastectomy in women with a BRCA1 or BRCA2 mutation. N Engl J Med. 2001;345(3):159–64.
30. Rebbeck TR, Lynch HT, Neuhausen SL, Narod SA. Van't veer L, Garber JE, et al. prophylactic oophorectomy in carriers of BRCA1 or BRCA2 mutations. N Engl J Med. 2002;346 (21):1616–22.
31. Kirova YM, Savignoni A, Sigal-Zafrani B, de La Rochefordiere A, Salmon RJ, This P, et al. Is the breast-conserving treatment with radiotherapy appropriate in BRCA1/2 mutation carriers? Long-term results and review of the literature. Breast Cancer Res Treat. 2010;120(1):119–26.
32. Offit K, Kohut K, Clagett B, Wadsworth EA, Lafaro KJ, Cummings S, et al. Cancer genetic testing and assisted reproduction. J Clin Oncol. 2006;24(29):4775–82.
33. Domchek SM, Friebel TM, Singer CF, Evans DG, Lynch HT, Isaacs C, et al. Association of risk-reducing surgery in BRCA1 or BRCA2 mutation carriers with cancer risk and mortality. JAMA. 2010;304(9):967–75.
34. Supreme court strikes down brca gene patent. 2013. https://abcnews.go.com/Politics/supreme-court-strikes-brca-gene-patent/story?id=19392299
35. Kang E, Seong MW, Park SK, Lee JW, Lee J, Kim LS, et al. The prevalence and spectrum of BRCA1 and BRCA2 mutations in Korean population: recent update of the Korean hereditary breast cancer (KOHBRA) study. Breast Cancer Res Treat. 2015;151(1):157–68.
36. Birch JM, Blair V, Kelsey AM, Evans DG, Harris M, Tricker KJ, et al. Cancer phenotype correlates with constitutional TP53 genotype in families with the li-Fraumeni syndrome. Oncogene. 1998;17(9):1061–8.
37. Prochazkova K, Foretova L, Sedlacek Z. A rare tumor and an ethical dilemma in a family with a germline TP53 mutation. Cancer Genet Cytogenet. 2008;180(1):65–9.
38. Bougeard G, Renaux-Petel M, Flaman JM, Charbonnier C, Fermey P, Belotti M, et al. Revisiting li-Fraumeni syndrome from TP53 mutation carriers. J Clin Oncol. 2015;33 (21):2345–52.
39. Bennett KL, Mester J, Eng C. Germline epigenetic regulation of KILLIN in Cowden and Cowden-like syndrome. JAMA. 2010;304(24):2724–31.

40. Daniell J, Plazzer JP, Perera A, Macrae F. An exploration of genotype-phenotype link between Peutz-Jeghers syndrome and STK11: a review. Fam Cancer. 2018;17(3):421–7.
41. Han SA, Park SK, Ahn SH, Lee MH, Noh DY, Kim LS, et al. The Korean hereditary breast cancer (KOHBRA) study: protocols and interim report. Clin Oncol (R Coll Radiol). 2011;23 (7):434–41.
42. Chen S, Parmigiani G. Meta-analysis of BRCA1 and BRCA2 penetrance. J Clin Oncol. 2007;25 (11):1329–33.
43. Robson ME, Chappuis PO, Satagopan J, Wong N, Boyd J, Goffin JR, et al. A combined analysis of outcome following breast cancer: differences in survival based on BRCA1/BRCA2 mutation status and administration of adjuvant treatment. Breast Cancer Res. 2004;6(1):R8–r17.
44. El-Tamer M, Russo D, Troxel A, Bernardino LP, Mazziotta R, Estabrook A, et al. Survival and recurrence after breast cancer in BRCA1/2 mutation carriers. Ann Surg Oncol. 2004;11 (2):157–64.
45. Rennert G, Bisland-Naggan S, Barnett-Griness O, Bar-Joseph N, Zhang S, Rennert HS, et al. Clinical outcomes of breast cancer in carriers of BRCA1 and BRCA2 mutations. N Engl J Med. 2007;357(2):115–23.
46. Lee EH, Park SK, Park B, Kim SW, Lee MH, Ahn SH, et al. Effect of BRCA1/2 mutation on short-term and long-term breast cancer survival: a systematic review and meta-analysis. Breast Cancer Res Treat. 2010;122(1):11–25.
47. Frank TS, Deffenbaugh AM, Reid JE, Hulick M, Ward BE, Lingenfelter B, et al. Clinical characteristics of individuals with germline mutations in BRCA1 and BRCA2: analysis of 10,000 individuals. J Clin Oncol. 2002;20(6):1480–90.
48. Parmigiani G, Berry D, Aguilar O. Determining carrier probabilities for breast cancer-susceptibility genes BRCA1 and BRCA2. Am J Hum Genet. 1998;62(1):145–58.
49. Antoniou AC, Pharoah PP, Smith P, Easton DF. The BOADICEA model of genetic susceptibility to breast and ovarian cancer. Br J Cancer. 2004;91(8):1580–90.
50. Evans DG, Lalloo F, Wallace A, Rahman N. Update on the Manchester scoring system for BRCA1 and BRCA2 testing. J Med Genet. 2005;42(7):e39.
51. Kurian AW, Gong GD, Chun NM, Mills MA, Staton AD, Kingham KE, et al. Performance of BRCA1/2 mutation prediction models in Asian Americans. J Clin Oncol. 2008;26(29):4752–8.
52. Kang E, Park SK, Yang JJ, Park B, Lee MH, Lee JW, et al. Accuracy of BRCA1/2 mutation prediction models in Korean breast cancer patients. Breast Cancer Res Treat. 2012;134 (3):1189–97.
53. Kim KS, Kim S, Han SA, Kang E, Jeon YT, Ha T-H, et al. Contralateral prophylactic mastectomy and prophylactic Salphingo-oophorectomy in a BRCA1-positive breast cancer patient: a case report. J Breast Cancer. 2008;11(4):218–22.
54. Choi M-Y, Lee JE, Kim S-W, Lee SK, Hur SM, Kim S, et al. Incidental detection of ductal carcinoma in situ of the breast from bilateral prophylactic mastectomy of asymptomatic BRCA2 mutation carrier: a case report. J Breast Cancer. 2010;13(3):311–7.
55. Kim D, Kang E, Hwang E, Sun Y, Hwang Y, Yom CK, et al. Factors affecting the decision to undergo risk-reducing salpingo-oophorectomy among women with BRCA gene mutation. Fam Cancer. 2013;12(4):621–8.
56. Ryu JM, Choi HJ, Kim I, Nam SJ, Kim SW, Yu J, et al. Prevalence and oncologic outcomes of BRCA 1/2 mutations in unselected triple-negative breast cancer patients in Korea. Breast Cancer Res Treat. 2019;173(2):385–95.
57. Kim HC, Lee JY, Sung H, Choi JY, Park SK, Lee KM, et al. A genome-wide association study identifies a breast cancer risk variant in ERBB4 at 2q34: results from the Seoul breast cancer study. Breast Cancer Res. 2012;14(2):R56.
58. Long J, Cai Q, Sung H, Shi J, Zhang B, Choi JY, et al. Genome-wide association study in east Asians identifies novel susceptibility loci for breast cancer. PLoS Genet. 2012;8(2):e1002532.
59. Zheng W, Zhang B, Cai Q, Sung H, Michailidou K, Shi J, et al. Common genetic determinants of breast-cancer risk in east Asian women: a collaborative study of 23 637 breast cancer cases and 25 579 controls. Hum Mol Genet. 2013;22(12):2539–50.

Part VI
Next Generation Clinical Research

Chapter 26
Clinical Databases for Breast Cancer Research

Ki-Tae Hwang

Abstract

- Clinical database is a collection of clinical data related to patients, which can be used for analysis and research. Clinical data can be classified into several categories: patient-related, tumor-related, diagnostics-related, treatment-related, outcome-related, administration-related, and other clinical data. Clinical databases can be classified according to the data types of clinical databases, ranges of institutes, and accessibility to data.
- The numbers of papers and clinical trials are rapidly increasing. Recently, more than 9000 papers related to breast cancer have been published annually, and more than 7000 papers related to human breast cancer are published annually. The speed of increase is expected to be faster and faster in future. Now, almost 8000 clinical trials are registered world widely.
- Main research areas of breast cancer can be classified into followings; epidemiology, screening and prevention, diagnosis, treatment, and prognosis. Clinical databases that are available for breast cancer research are also introduced in this chapter.
- The analysis of big data is expected to be the mainstream of breast cancer research using clinical databases. As the technology of artificial intelligence (AI) is rapidly evolving, the technology of deep learning starts to be applied for breast cancer research. In near future, AI technology is predicted to penetrate deeply the field of breast cancer research.

Keywords Artificial intelligence · Big data · Breast cancer · Breast cancer research · Clinical data · Clinical database

---

K.-T. Hwang (✉)
Department of Surgery, Seoul Metropolitan Government Seoul National University Boramae Medical Center, Seoul, South Korea
e-mail: kiterius@snu.ac.kr

D.-Y. Noh et al. (eds.), *Translational Research in Breast Cancer*, Advances in Experimental Medicine and Biology 1187,
https://doi.org/10.1007/978-981-32-9620-6_26

26.1 Introduction

26.1.1 Definition of Clinical Database

'Data' is information that can be stored and used by a computer program. A 'database' is a collection of data that is stored in a computer and that can easily be used and added to. 'Clinical' means involving or relating to the direct medical treatment or testing of patients [1]. 'Clinical data' is a staple resource for most health and medical research. Clinical data is either collected during the course of ongoing patient care or as part of a formal clinical trial program [2]. 'Clinical database' can be defined as a collection of clinical data related to patients, which can be used for analysis and research. Sometimes, clinical database is used as the antonym of biological database that is collected from scientific experiments including genomics, proteomics, metabolomics, microarray gene expression, phylogenetics, and so on.

26.1.2 Classification of Clinical Data

Numerous clinical data can be generated during the course of health care services. Clinical data can be classified into one of the following categories (Table 26.1).

26.1.3 Classification of Clinical Databases

Clinical database can be classified according to the various viewpoints. Table 26.2 shows classification of clinical database according to the data types of clinical databases, ranges of institutes, and accessibility to data.

26.1.4 Research Databases and the HIPAA Privacy Rule

The website of Department of Health and Human Services (HHS) describes the following statements [3, 4].

> The Health Insurance Portability and Accountability Act (HIPAA) Privacy Rule establishes national standards to protect individuals' medical records and other personal health information and applies to health plans, health care clearinghouses, and those health care providers that conduct certain health care transactions electronically. The Rule requires appropriate safeguards to protect the privacy of personal health information, and sets limits and conditions on the uses and disclosures that may be made of such information without patient authorization. The Rule also gives patients rights over their health information, including rights to examine and obtain a copy of their health records, and to request corrections.

Table 26.1 Classification of clinical data

Title	Data type	Main clinical data	Institute	Access	Research area	Subject No	Reference
The influences of peritumoral lymphatic invasion and vascular invasion on the survival and recurrence according to the molecular subtypes of breast cancer	Electronic health records	Tumor-related clinical data outcome-related clinical data	Single institute	Limited	Prognostic factor	820	[13]
Prognostic influence of preoperative fibrinogen to albumin ratio on breast cancer	Electronic health records	Diagnostics-related clinical data outcome-related clinical data	Single institute	Limited	Prognostic factor	793	[14]
Prognostic influence of BCL2 expression in breast cancer	Electronic health records	Tumor-related clinical data outcome-related clinical data	Multiple institutes	Limited	Prognostic factor	7230	[15]
Prognostic influence of BCL2 on molecular subtypes of breast cancer	Electronic health records	Tumor-related clinical data outcome-related clinical data	Multiple institutes	Limited	Prognostic factor	9468	[16]
Education level is a strong prognosticator in the subgroup aged more than 50 years regardless of the molecular subtype of breast cancer: study based on the Nationwide Korean breast cancer registry database	Patient/disease registry	Patient-related clinical data outcome-related clinical data	Nationwide	Limited	Prognostic factor	64,129	[17]
Poor prognosis of lower inner quadrant in lymph node negative breast cancer patients who received no chemotherapy: a study based on Nationwide Korean breast cancer registry database	Patient/disease registry	Patient-related clinical data outcome-related clinical data	Nationwide	Limited	Prognostic factor	63,388	[18]
BCL2 regulation according to the molecular subtypes of breast cancer by analysis of the cancer genome atlas database	Other data types	Outcome-related clinical data biological data	Multiple institutes	Open	Prognostic factor	1096	[19]

Her2 human epidermal growth factor receptor 2

Table 26.2 Classification of clinical databases

Classification	Categories	Description
Data type[a]	Electronic health record	The purest type of electronic clinical data which is obtained at the point of care at a medical facility, hospital, clinic or practice
	Administrative data	Primarily hospital discharge data reported to a government agency, often associated with electronic health records
	Claims data	Data describing the billable interactions (insurance claims) between insured patients and the healthcare delivery system
	Patient/disease registry	Clinical information systems that collect clinical data for targeted disease entities
	Health surveys	Health surveys of the targeted chronic conditions, generally conducted to provide prevalence estimates
	Clinical trials data	Clinical data which is collected during the course of clinical trials
	Other data types	Other data types
Institute	Single institute	A database collected from a single institute
	Multiple institutes	A database collected from multiple domestic institutes
	Nation-wide	A database collected from nation-wide institutes
	International	A database collected from international multiple institutes
	Global	A database collected from global institutes
Access	Open	Open access to database
	Limited	Limited access to database

[a]According to classification by Health Sciences Library (University of Washington) [2]

Researchers in medical and health-related disciplines require access to many sources of health information, from archived medical records and epidemiological databases to disease registries, tissue repositories, hospital discharge records, and government compilations of vital and health records. As the Privacy Rule is implemented, researchers are asking how these rules might affect research that uses records within databases and repositories. In response to a congressional mandate in HIPAA of 1996, HHS issued regulations entitled, Standards for Privacy of Individually Identifiable Health Information. For most covered entities, compliance with these regulations, known as the Privacy Rule, was required as of April 14, 2003. The Privacy Rule was not intended to impede research using records within databases and repositories that include individuals' health information, but the Privacy Rule does place new conditions on the use and disclosure of protected health information (PHI) by covered entities for research. The creation of a research database or repository, and the use or disclosure of PHI from a database or repository for research, may each be considered a research activity under the Privacy Rule.

26.2 Review of Past Studies

26.2.1 Quantitative Volume of Published Papers in Breast Cancer Research

The number of papers that have been registered in PubMed is rapidly increasing annually [5]. The trend of increasing number of papers regarding breast cancer research is depicted in Fig. 26.1.

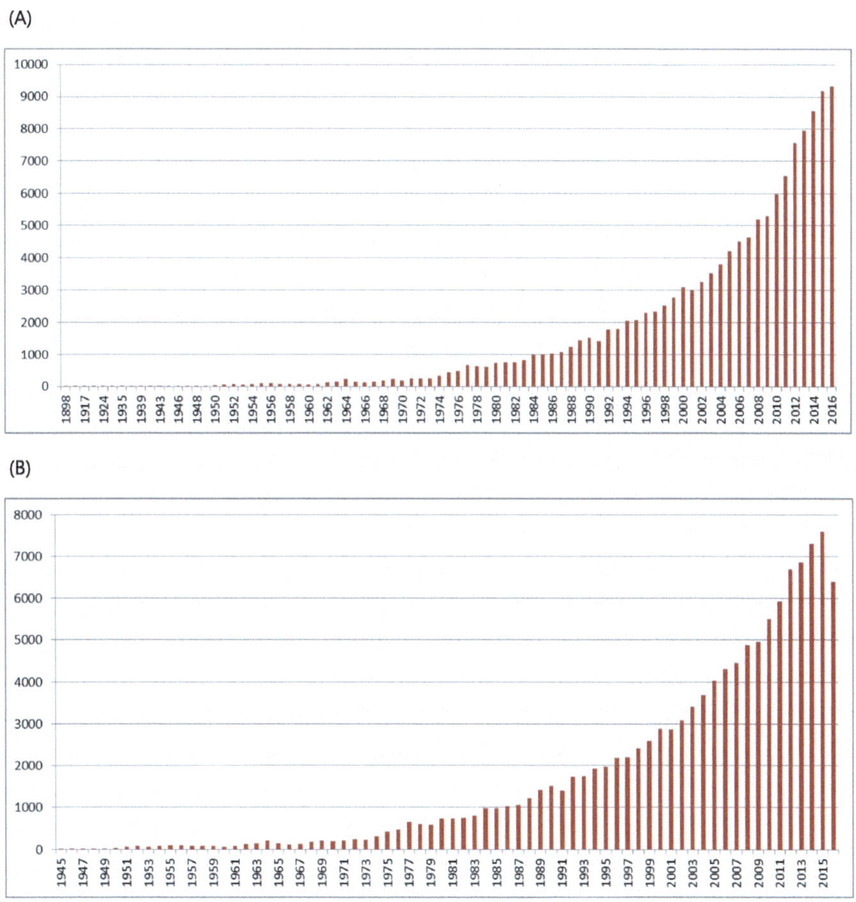

Fig. 26.1 The number of annual papers searched by PubMed (access date: Dec. 13th, 2017). (**a**) Search conditions: breast cancer[title] (number of total papers: 143,039), (**b**) search conditions: breast cancer[title] and humans (number of total papers: 123,709)

26.2.2 Quantitative Volume of Clinical Trials in Breast Cancer Research

The number of clinical trials that have been registered in clinicaltrials.gov is also rapidly increasing [6]. It is depicted in Fig. 26.2.

26.3 Current Evidence and Concepts

26.3.1 Breast Cancer Research Using Clinical Databases

Breast cancer research has been performed to elaborate new knowledges, and the main areas of breast cancer research are described in Table 26.3.

26.3.2 Clinical Databases for Breast Cancer Research

The main clinical databases available for breast cancer research are listed with description and reference websites in Table 26.4.

Especially, the Surveillance, Epidemiology, and End Results (SEER) database is open database and many studies using this database were published. SEER Data (1973–2014) were released on March 31th, 2017, and the number of all cases is 9,675,661 (8,662,369 patients for malignant cases and 9,429,379 patients for malignant and in situ cases) [7]. Case numbers of patients according to cancer types and data files are described in Table 26.5.

26.3.3 Examples of Breast Cancer Research Using Clinical Databases

Examples of breast cancer research using clinical databases are summarized in Table 26.6.

26.3.3.1 Clinical Database of a Single Institute

The influences of peritumoral lymphatic invasion and vascular invasion on the survival and recurrence according to the molecular subtypes of breast cancer [13]

- Data type: electronic health records.

(A)

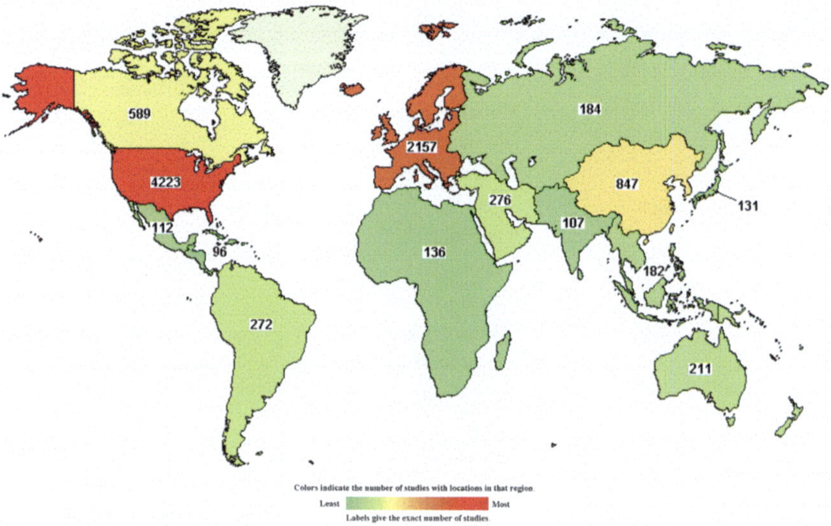

(B)

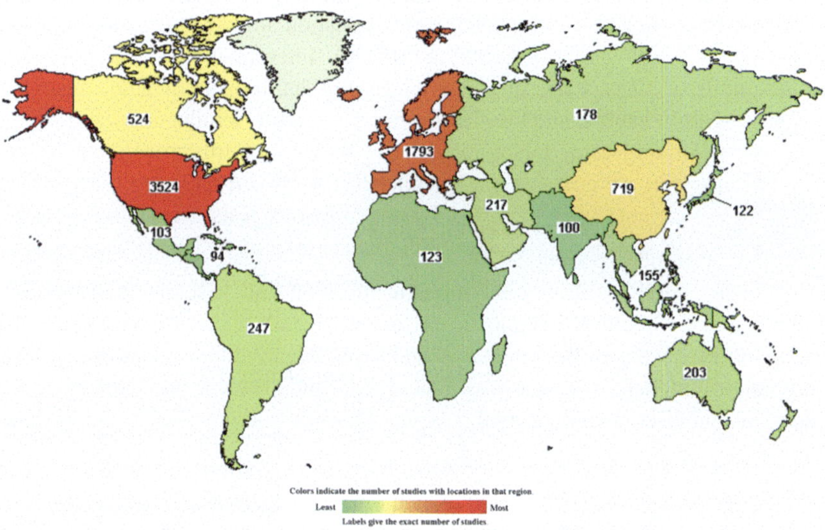

Fig. 26.2 The number of clinical trials by clinicaltrials.gov (access date: Dec. 22th, 2017). (**a**) All studies: 7891 (Interventional studies + Observational studies), (**b**) Interventional studies: 6411

- Main clinical data: tumor-related clinical data (peritumoral lymphatic invasion and vascular invasion) and outcome-related clinical data (overall survival and disease-free survival).
- Institute: a single institute (Seoul National University Boramae Medical Center).

Table 26.3 Main areas of breast cancer research using clinical databases

Category	Subcategory	Note
Epidemiology	Incidence	
	Prevalence	
	Mortality	
	Risk factor	
	Others	
Screeng and prevention	Screening	
	Prevention	
Diagnosis	Radiology	Current diagnositcs
	Pathology	New diagnostics
	Laboratory test	Companion diagnostics
	Tumor markers	Other diagnostics
	Other diagnosis	
Treatment	Current treatment	Surgery
	New treatment method	Chemotherapy
	Predictive factor	Anti-Her2 therapy
	Others	Radiation therapy
		Endorine therapy
		Other treatments
Prognosis	Prognostic factor	
	Prognostic modeling	
	Others	

Her2 human epidermal growth factor receptor 2

- Access: limited.
- Main areas of breast cancer research: prognostic factor.
- Number of enrolled patients: 820.
- Conclusion: Both peritumoral lymphatic invasion and vascular invasion were significant, unfavorable prognostic factors of overall survival and disease-free survival, especially in the luminal A and triple negative breast cancer subtypes. Although lymphatic invasion was a significant independent predictor of overall survival and disease-free survival, vascular invasion was not after the multivariate analyses.

Prognostic influence of preoperative fibrinogen to albumin ratio on breast cancer [14]

- Data type: electronic health records.
- Main clinical data: diagnostics-related clinical data (laboratory test: preoperative serum fibrinogen and albumin level) and outcome-related clinical data (overall survival).
- Institute: a single institute (Seoul National University Boramae Medical Center).
- Access: limited.
- Main areas of breast cancer research: prognostic factor.
- Number of enrolled patients: 793.

Table 26.4 Representative clinical databases for cancer research including breast cancer

Clinical databases	Description	Reference
SEER	The surveillance, epidemiology, and end results (SEER) program of the National Cancer Institute (NCI) is an authoritative source of information on cancer incidence and survival in the United States. SEER currently collects and publishes cancer incidence and survival data from population-based cancer registries covering approximately 28 percent of the US population	[7]
NCTN	On march 1, 2014, after several years of extensive consultation and coordination with many stakeholders, NCI transformed its longstanding cooperative group program into the new National Clinical Trials Network (NCTN). After approval of a signed data use agreement (DUA), researchers can download patient level clinical datasets and their associated data dictionaries	[8]
NCORP	The NCI Community oncology research program (NCORP) is a national NCI-supported network that brings cancer prevention clinical trials and cancer care delivery research (CCDR) to people in their communities. NCORP is comprised of 7 research bases and 46 community sites, 12 of which are designated as minority/underserved (MU) community sites. NCORP MU Community sites have a patient population comprised of at least 30% racial/ethnic minorities or rural residents	[9]
CCTG	The Canadian Cancer trials group (CCTG) is a cooperative oncology group which carries out clinical trials in cancer therapy, supportive care and prevention across Canada and internationally. It is one of the national programmes and networks of the Canadian Cancer Society Research Institute (CCSRI), and is supported by the Canadian Cancer society (CCS). After approval of a signed data use agreement (DUA), researchers can download patient level clinical datasets and their associated data dictionaries	[10]
DBCG	The Danish breast Cancer cooperative group (DBCG) was initiated by the Danish surgical society in 1976 and has since 1977 prepared guidelines for diagnostic and therapeutic procedures in primary invasive breast cancer later supplemented with guidelines for in situ carcinomas and hereditary breast cancer on a nationwide basis in Denmark	[11]
KBCR	Since 1996, the Korean Breast Cancer Society has collected nationwide data for breast cancer patients in the Republic of Korea by developing the Korean Breast Cancer Registry (KBCR) program and retrospective data collection was also allowed when a participating hospital had its own breast cancer database. The total number of patients registered in the Korean Breast Cancer Registry (KBCR) is 172,515 (access date: Dec. 18th, 2017). Data access is limited for patient data to members of KBCS	[12]

SEER surveillance, epidemiology, and end results, *NCTN* National Clinical Trials Network, *NCORP* NCI Community Oncology Research Program, *CCTG* Canadian Cancer Trials Group, *DBCG* Danish Breast Cancer Cooperative Group, *KBCR* Korean Breast Cancer Registry

Table 26.5 Case numbers of patients according to cancer types and data files in SEER database

Cancer types	Data files				
	YR1973_2014.SEER9[a]	YR1992_2014.SJ_LA_RG_AK[b]	YR2000_2014.CA_KY_LO_NJ_GA[c]	YR2005.LO_2ND_HALF[d]	Sum
Breast	798,624	200,250	547,920	1405	1,548,199
Colon and rectum	541,683	118,024	322,915	1185	983,807
Other digestive	378,680	104,566	262,073	800	746,119
Female genital	445,025	88,328	189,580	497	723,430
Lymphoma of all sites and leukemia	396,485	98,688	269,313	902	765,388
Male genital	654,149	168,219	456,115	1406	1,279,889
Respiratory	662,987	127,728	463,765	1766	1,256,246
Urinary	332,964	74,598	246,320	834	654,716
All other sites	826,710	206,909	682,472	1776	1,717,867
Sum	5,037,307	1,187,310	3,440,473	10,571	9,675,661

SEER surveillance, epidemiology, and end results

[a]YR1973_2014.SEER9: This directory contains the SEER November 2016 Research Data files from nine SEER registries for 1973–2014. The SEER 9 registries are Atlanta, Connecticut, Detroit, Hawaii, Iowa, New Mexico, San Francisco-Oakland, Seattle-Puget Sound, and Utah. Data are available for cases diagnosed from 1973 and later for these registries with the exception of Seattle-Puget Sound and Atlanta. The Seattle-Puget Sound and Atlanta registries joined the SEER program in 1974 and 1975, respectively

[b]YR1992_2014.SJ_LA_RG_AK: This directory contains the SEER November 2016 Research Data files from the San Jose-Monterey, Los Angeles, Rural Georgia, and Alaska Natives SEER registries for 1992–2014

[c]YR2000_2014.CA_KY_LO_NJ_GA: This directory contains the SEER November 2016 Research Data files from the Greater California, Kentucky, Louisiana, New Jersey, and Greater Georgia SEER registries for 2000–2014. For the year 2005, only January–June diagnoses are included for Louisiana. Hurricane Katrina had a large impact on Louisiana's population for the July–December 2005 time period. For most SEER reporting, Louisiana cases diagnosed in the latter half of 2005 are not analyzed

[d]YR2005.LO_2ND_HALF: This directory contains the July–December 2005 diagnoses for Louisiana from their November 2016 SEER submission. Hurricane Katrina had a large impact on Louisiana's population for this 6 month time period. For most SEER reporting, Louisiana cases diagnosed during this 6 month period are not analyzed. These data are considered a supplement to the SEER Research Data

Table 26.6 Examples of breast cancer research using clinical databases

Title	Data type	Main clinical data	Institute	Access	Research area	Subject No	Reference
The influences of peritumoral lymphatic invasion and vascular invasion on the survival and recurrence according to the molecular subtypes of breast cancer	Electronic health records	Tumor-related clinical data outcome-related clinical data	Single institute	Limited	Prognostic factor	820	[13]
Prognostic influence of preoperative fibrinogen to albumin ratio on breast cancer	Electronic health records	Diagnostics-related clinical data outcome-related clinical data	Single institute	Limited	Prognostic factor	793	[14]
Prognostic influence of BCL2 expression in breast cancer	Electronic health records	Tumor-related clinical data outcome-related clinical data	Multiple institutes	Limited	Prognostic factor	7230	[15]
Prognostic influence of BCL2 on molecular subtypes of breast Cancer	Electronic health records	Tumor-related clinical data outcome-related clinical data	Multiple institutes	Limited	Prognostic factor	9468	[16]
Education level is a strong prognosticator in the subgroup aged more than 50 years regardless of the molecular subtype of breast Cancer: Study based on the Nationwide Korean breast Cancer registry database	Patient/disease registry	Patient-related clinical data utcome-related clinical data	Nation-wide	Limited	Prognostic factor	64,129	[17]
Poor prognosis of lower inner quadrant in lymph node negative breast Cancer patients who received no chemotherapy: a study based on Nationwide Korean breast Cancer registry database	Patient/disease registry	Patient-related clinical data outcome-related clinical data	Nation-wide	Limited	Prognostic factor	63,388	[18]
BCL2 regulation according to the molecular subtypes of breast cancer by analysis of the cancer genome atlas database	Other data types	Outcome-related clinical data biological data	Multiple institutes	Open	Prognostic factor	1096	[19]

- Conclusion: Preoperative fibrinogen to albumin ratio was a strong independent prognostic factor in breast cancer. Its prognostic effect was more prominent in the stage II/III subgroup and in the luminal A-like subtype. Therefore, preoperative fibrinogen to albumin ratio can be utilized as a useful prognosticator for breast cancer patients. Further studies are needed to validate its applications in clinical settings.

26.3.3.2 Clinical Database of Multiple Institutes

Prognostic influence of BCL2 expression in breast cancer [15]

- Data type: electronic health records.
- Main clinical data: tumor-related clinical data (other immunohistochemical markers: BCL2) and outcome-related clinical data (overall survival and disease-free survival).
- Institute: multiple institutes (Seoul National University Boramae Medical Center and Seoul National University Hospital).
- Access: limited.
- Main areas of breast cancer research: prognostic factor.
- Number of enrolled patients: 7230.
- Conclusion: BCL2 had a strong influence on the established prognostic models, including the St. Gallen model, the Nottingham prognostic index model, and the TNM model. BCL2 was a powerful independent prognostic factor for breast cancer and had a strong influence on the current prognostic models. Favorable clinicopathologic features and a strong correlation with the hormonal receptor are suggested as the causes of superior survival in patients with BCL2 positive breast cancer.

Prognostic Influence of BCL2 on Molecular Subtypes of Breast Cancer [16]

- Data type: electronic health records.
- Main clinical data: tumor-related clinical data (other immunohistochemical markers: B-cell CLL/lymphoma 2 (BCL2)) and outcome-related clinical data (overall survival and breast cancer-specific survival).
- Institute: multiple institutes (Seoul National University Boramae Medical Center and Seoul National University Hospital).
- Access: limited.
- Main areas of breast cancer research: prognostic factor.
- Number of enrolled patients: 9468.
- Conclusion: The prognostic influence of BCL2 was different across molecular subtypes of breast cancer, and it was largely dependent on hormonal receptor (HR), human epidermal growth factor receptor 2 (HER2), Ki-67, and the stage of cancer. BCL2 had a strong favorable prognostic impact only in HR(+)/HER2(−) or luminal A and luminal B/HER2(−) subtypes, particularly in advanced stages. Further investigations are needed to verify the prognostic influence of BCL2 on

molecular subtypes of breast cancer and to develop clinical applications for prognostication using BCL2.

26.3.3.3 Clinical Database of Nation-Wide Clinical Database

Education Level is a Strong Prognosticator in the Subgroup Aged More Than 50 Years Regardless of the Molecular Subtype of Breast Cancer: Study Based on the Nationwide Korean Breast Cancer Registry Database [17]

- Data type: patient/disease registry (Korean Breast Cancer Registry database).
- Main clinical data: patient-related clinical data (education level) and outcome-related clinical data (overall survival).
- Institute: nation-wide.
- Access: limited.
- Main areas of breast cancer research: prognostic factor.
- Number of enrolled patients: 64,129.
- Conclusion: The education level is a strong independent prognostic factor for breast cancer in the subgroup aged >50 years regardless of the molecular subtype, but not in the subgroup aged ≤ 50 years. Favorable clinicopathologic features and active treatments can explain the main causality of the superior prognosis in the high education level group.

Poor Prognosis of Lower Inner Quadrant in Lymph Node Negative Breast Cancer Patients Who Received No Chemotherapy: a Study Based on Nationwide Korean Breast Cancer Registry Database [18]

- Data type: patient/disease registry (Korean Breast Cancer Registry database).
- Main clinical data: patient-related clinical data (tumor location) and outcome-related clinical data (overall survival).
- Institute: nation-wide.
- Access: limited.
- Main areas of breast cancer research: prognostic factor.
- Number of enrolled patients: 63,388.
- Conclusion: Lower inner quadrant showed a worse prognosis despite having more favorable clinicopathologic features than other tumor locations, and it was more prominent for lymph node-negative patients who received no chemotherapy. The hypothesis of possible hidden internal mammary node metastasis could be suggested to play a key role in lower inner quadrant lesions.

26.3.3.4 Clinical Database as a Part of Biological Database

BCL2 Regulation According to the Molecular Subtypes of Breast Cancer by Analysis of The Cancer Genome Atlas Database [19]

- Data type: other data types (clinical database as a part of biological database; The Cancer Genome Atlas database).
- Main clinical data: outcome-related clinical data (overall survival) and biological data (reverse phase protein array (RPPA), mRNA sequencing (mRNA-seq), mRNA microarray, methylation, copy number alteration (CNA) linear, CNA nonlinear, and mutation data).
- Institute: multiple institutes.
- Access: open.
- Main areas of breast cancer research: prognostic factor.
- Number of enrolled patients: 1096.
- Conclusion: The regulation of BCL2 was mainly associated with methylation across the molecular subtypes of breast cancer, and luminal A and luminal B subtypes showed upregulated expression of BCL2 protein, mRNA, and hypomethylation. Although CNA may have played a minor role, mutation status was not related to BCL2 regulation. Upregulation of BCL2 was associated with superior prognosis than downregulation of BCL2.

26.4 Future Research Direction

26.4.1 Big Data

Along with the development of science and technology, the volume of data with which the researcher can deal is also rapidly increasing. Advancement of electronic medical record systems enables us to generate, store, and process the huge amount of clinical data. The various projects of nation-wide registry, survey, and clinical trials are being initiated in many countries. Huge amount administrative data claims data are being accumulated. Standardization of clinical trials enables the researcher to combine many independent clinical trials into single entity, which could be analyzed as a whole. International or global clinical trials are being initiated in many places in the world. A large number of biological databases are generated, processed, and analyzed in research field, and clinical data are also merged in the analysis of biologic data. Wearable devices will constantly generate data of vital signs of breast cancer survivors or healthy people [20]. Social network services are producing huge amount of information, which may be useful to study life patterns of breast cancer survivors [21–24]. The analysis of big data is one of the major keywords in future breast cancer research using clinical databases.

The Observational Health Data Sciences and Informatics (or OHDSI, pronounced "Odyssey") tries to collect all possible health information of the world by adoption of a Common Data Model (CDM) known as the Observational Medical Outcomes Partnership (OMOP) CDM [25]. Recently, they reported that

> At last count, 52 databases, with a total of 682 million patient records, had been created using the CDM; this number may include duplicate records for databases with overlapping populations. This study used 11 of those databases with more than 250 million records [26].

26.4.2 *Artificial Intelligence*

Now that the technology of artificial intelligence (AI) is rapidly evolving, the technology of deep learning starts to be applied for breast cancer research. As deep learning algorithm is a kind of machine learning techniques based on pixel-by-pixel evaluation of the data from images, it can be easily applied in the fields of diagnostic radiology and diagnostic pathology [27]. Wang et al. evaluated the performance of deep learning-based models for the diagnostic accuracy of microcalcifications, and they reported that deep learning model achieved a discriminative accuracy of 87.3% if microcalcifications were characterized alone, compared to 85.8% with a support vector machine [28]. Recently, Ehteshami et al. assessed the performance of automated deep learning algorithms at detecting metastases in hematoxylin and eosin-stained tissue sections of lymph nodes of women with breast cancer and compare it with pathologists' diagnoses in a diagnostic setting. For the whole-slide image classification task, the best algorithm (AUC, 0.994; 95% CI, 0.983–0.999) performed significantly better than the pathologists with time constraint in a diagnostic simulation (mean AUC, 0.810; range, 0.738–0.884; $P < 0.001$), and that algorithm performance was comparable with an expert pathologist interpreting whole-slide images without time constraints [29]. These studies are regarded as just the beginnings of AI research in breast cancer. In near future, AI technology is predicted to penetrate deeply the field of breast cancer research.

26.5 Summary

- Clinical database is a collection of clinical data related to patients, which can be used for analysis and research. Clinical database can be classified according to the data types of clinical databases, ranges of institutes, and accessibility to data.
- The numbers of papers and clinical trials are rapidly increasing. The speed of increase is expected to be faster and faster in future.
- Main research areas of breast cancer are listed in this chapter, and clinical databases that are available for breast cancer research are also introduced in this chapter.
- "Big data" and "artificial intelligence" are two important key words for future direction of breast cancer research using clinical databases.

References

1. Collins English Dictionary: https://www.collinsdictionary.com/dictionary/english
2. University libraries, University of Washington: http://guides.lib.uw.edu/hsl/data/findclin
3. Research databases and the HIPAA Privacy Rule: https://privacyruleandresearch.nih.gov/research_repositories.asp

4. U.S. Department of Health & Human Services: https://www.hhs.gov/hipaa/for-professionals/privacy/index.html
5. PubMed: https://www.ncbi.nlm.nih.gov/pubmed
6. Clinicaltrials.gov: https://clinicaltrials.gov
7. SEER (Surveillance, Epidemiology, and End Results Program). https://seer.cancer.gov
8. NCTN (NCI's National Clinical Trials Network). https://www.cancer.gov/research/areas/clinical-trials/nctn
9. NCORP (NCI's Community Oncology Research Program) Data Archive: https://ncorp.cancer.gov
10. CCTG (Canadian Cancer Trials Group): https://www.ctg.queensu.ca
11. DBCG (Danish Breast Cancer Cooperative Group): http://www.dbcg.dk
12. KBCR (Korean Breast Cancer Society): http://www.kbcs.or.kr
13. Hwang KT, Kim YA, Kim J, Chu AJ, Chang JH, Oh SW, Hwang KR, Chai YJ. The influences of peritumoral lymphatic invasion and vascular invasion on the survival and recurrence according to the molecular subtypes of breast cancer. Breast Cancer Res Treat. 2017;163:71–82.
14. Hwang KT, Chung JK, Roh EY, Kim J, Oh S, Kim YA, Rhu J, Kim S. Prognostic influence of preoperative fibrinogen to albumin ratio for breast Cancer. J Breast Cancer. 2017;20:254–63.
15. Hwang KT, Woo JW, Shin HC, Kim HS, Ahn SK, Moon HG, Han W, Park IA, Noh DY. Prognostic influence of BCL2 expression in breast cancer. Int J Cancer. 2012;131: E1109–19.
16. Hwang KT, Han W, Kim J, Moon HG, Oh S, Song YS, Kim YA, Chang MS, Noh DY. Prognostic influence of BCL2 on molecular subtypes of breast Cancer. J Breast Cancer. 2017;20:54–64.
17. Hwang KT, Noh W, Cho SH, Yu J, Park MH, Jeong J, Lee HJ, Kim J, Oh S, Kim YA, Korean Breast Cancer Society. Education level is a strong prognosticator in the subgroup aged more than 50 years regardless of the molecular subtype of breast Cancer: a study based on the Nationwide Korean breast Cancer registry database. Cancer Res Treat. 2017;49:1114–26.
18. Hwang KT, Kim J, Kim EK, Jung SH, Sohn G, Kim SI, Jeong J, Lee HJ, Park JH, Oh S, Korean Breast Cancer Society. Poor prognosis of lower inner quadrant in lymph node-negative breast cancer patients who received no chemotherapy: a study based on nationwide korean breast cancer registry database. Clin Breast Cancer. 2017;17:e169–84.
19. Hwang KT, Kim K, Chang JH, Oh S, Kim YA, Lee JY, Jung SH, Choi IS. BCL2 regulation according to molecular subtype of breast Cancer by analysis of the Cancer genome atlas database. Cancer Res Treat. 2017;50(3):658–69. https://doi.org/10.4143/crt.2017.134.
20. Nguyen NH, Hadgraft NT, Moore MM, Rosenberg DE, Lynch C, Reeves MM, Lynch BM. A qualitative evaluation of breast cancer survivors' acceptance of and preferences for consumer wearable technology activity trackers. Support Care Cancer. 2017;25:3375–84.
21. Huesch M, Chetlen A, Segel J, Schetter S. Frequencies of private mentions and sharing of mammography and breast Cancer terms on Facebook: a pilot study. J Med Internet Res. 2017;19:e201.
22. Abramson K, Keefe B, Chou WY. Communicating about cancer through Facebook: a qualitative analysis of a breast cancer awareness page. J Health Commun. 2015;20:237–43.
23. Diddi P, Lundy LK. Organizational twitter use: content analysis of tweets during breast Cancer awareness month. J Health Commun. 2017;22:243–53.
24. Thackeray R, Burton SH, Giraud-Carrier C, Rollins S, Draper CR. Using twitter for breast cancer prevention: an analysis of breast cancer awareness month. BMC Cancer. 2013;13:508.
25. Hripcsak G, Duke JD, Shah NH, Reich CG, Huser V, Schuemie MJ, Suchard MA, Park RW, Wong IC, Rijnbeek PR, van der Lei J, Pratt N, Norén GN, Li YC, Stang PE, Madigan D, Ryan PB. Observational health data sciences and informatics (OHDSI): opportunities for observational researchers. Stud Health Technol Inform. 2015;216:574–8.
26. Hripcsak G, Ryan PB, Duke JD, Shah NH, Park RW, Huser V, Suchard MA, Schuemie MJ, DeFalco FJ, Perotte A, Banda JM, Reich CG, Schilling LM, Matheny ME, Meeker D, Pratt N,

Madigan D. Characterizing treatment pathways at scale using the OHDSI network. Proc Natl Acad Sci U S A. 2016;113:7329–36.

27. Golden JA. Deep learning algorithms for detection of lymph node metastases from breast Cancer: helping artificial intelligence be seen. JAMA. 2017;318:2184–6.
28. Wang J, Yang X, Cai H, Tan W, Jin C, Li L. Discrimination of breast cancer with microcalcifications on mammography by deep learning. Sci Rep. 2016;6:27327.
29. Ehteshami Bejnordi B, Veta M, van Johannes Diest P, van Ginneken B, Karssemeijer N, Litjens G, van der Laak JAWM, the CAMELYON16 consortium, Hermsen M, Manson QF, Balkenhol M, Geessink O, Stathonikos N, van Dijk MC, Bult P, Beca F, Beck AH, Wang D, Khosla A, Gargeya R, Irshad H, Zhong A, Dou Q, Li Q, Chen H, Lin HJ, Heng PA, Haß C, Bruni E, Wong Q, Halici U, Öner MÜ, Cetin-Atalay R, Berseth M, Khvatkov V, Vylegzhanin A, Kraus O, Shaban M, Rajpoot N, Awan R, Sirinukunwattana K, Qaiser T, Tsang YW, Tellez D, Annuscheit J, Hufnagl P, Valkonen M, Kartasalo K, Latonen L, Ruusuvuori P, Liimatainen K, Albarqouni S, Mungal B, George A, Demirci S, Navab N, Watanabe S, Seno S, Takenaka Y, Matsuda H, Ahmady Phoulady H, Kovalev V, Kalinovsky A, Liauchuk V, Bueno G, Fernandez-Carrobles MM, Serrano I, Deniz O, Racoceanu D, Venâncio R. Diagnostic assessment of deep learning algorithms for detection of lymph node metastases in women with breast Cancer. JAMA. 2017;318:2199–210.

Chapter 27
Care for Breast Cancer Survivors

Su Min Jeong and Sang Min Park

Abstract The number of cancer survivors is increasing globally. More than 15.5 million Americans in 2016 and 1.3 million Koreans in 2013 were living with cancer history. This growing population is expected to increase due to marked development of cancer treatment and early detection. Especially, breast cancer is the second most common cancer in Korean women with relatively favorable 5-year survival rate. Cancer survivors generally face various physical, psychological, and social problems including late-effect or long-term effect after cancer treatment and high risk for second primary cancer and comorbid chronic diseases such as cardiovascular disease and bone health. Breast cancer survivors also encounter wide range of health problems. To satisfy their complex needs, comprehensive supports are required. We categorized the strategy of comprehensive care for breast cancer survivors into (1) Surveillance for primary cancer, (2) Screening of second primary cancer, (3) Management of comorbid health condition, (4) Promoting healthy lifestyle behaviors, and (5) Preventive care. In the future, studies for providing best comprehensive care for breast cancer survivors are needed according to the individuals' demand.

Keywords Breast cancer survivors · Comprehensive care · Surveillance · Comorbidity · Lifestyle behaviors

27.1 Introduction

The term 'cancer survivor' refers to a person who has been diagnosed with cancer in any time of his or her life [1]. The number of cancer survivors is increasing globally. More than 15.5 million Americans in 2016 and 1.3 million Koreans in 2013 were living with cancer history [2, 3]. Cancer survivors are expected to grow because of

S. M. Jeong · S. M. Park (✉)
Seoul National University Hospital, Seoul, South Korea

D.-Y. Noh et al. (eds.), *Translational Research in Breast Cancer*, Advances in Experimental Medicine and Biology 1187,
https://doi.org/10.1007/978-981-32-9620-6_27

advanced aging population as well as marked advance of treatment and early detection. Especially, breast cancer is the second most common cancer in Korean women, next to thyroid cancer. According to the statistics of the National Cancer Registration, the age-standardized incidence rate of breast cancer is rapidly growing from 24.5 in 1999 to 55.9 per 100,000 people in 2015 among Korean women [4]. Meanwhile, 5-year relative survival rate and 10-year survival rate in breast cancer reached 92.3% and 86.6% in 2015, which is steadily improving. Therefore, the number of people with long-term breast cancer significantly increased.

Cancer survivors generally face various physical, psychological, and social problems including late-effect or long-term effect after cancer treatment, comorbid chronic diseases such as cardiovascular disease (CVD), high risk for second primary cancer (SPC), and anxiety and depression. The 2006 Institute of Medicine report suggested four essential components of survivorship care: [1] Prevention of new cancers, [2] Surveillance for cancer recurrence or secondary cancers, [3] Intervention for consequences of cancer or its treatment, and [4] Coordination between specialists and primary care [5]. In addition, American Cancer Society/American Society of Clinical Oncology Breast Cancer Survivorship Care Guideline provided recommendations aligned to these four components [6].

However, most cancer survivors receive limited care that does not extend beyond primary cancer-related surveillance for recurrence. Previous randomized clinical trials in United Kingdom and Canada have demonstrated the equivalent outcomes of early stage breast cancer survivors with follow-up of either an oncologist or a primary-care physician in terms of recurrence [7]. Furthermore, breast cancer survivors were more satisfied when they were followed by general practice than hospital clinics [8]. In this context, shared-care models for cancer survivorships were suggested (Fig. 27.1) [9]. Shared-care model means complementary role between primary care physician and oncologist according to the timing of cancer journey.

As a consequence, it is necessary to provide comprehensive care to satisfy demand of cancer survivors according to the cancer journey as the survival of cancer improves. However, it is still insufficient to adopt cancer survivorship care in primary care [10].

Based on literature review and our experience of practice in cancer survivorship clinic, we can categorize following five health care areas (Table 27.1): (1) Surveillance for primary cancer, (2) Screening of second primary cancer, (3) Management of comorbid health condition, (4) Promoting healthy lifestyle behaviors, and (5) Preventive care. In this chapter, we will discuss comprehensive care for breast cancer survivors.

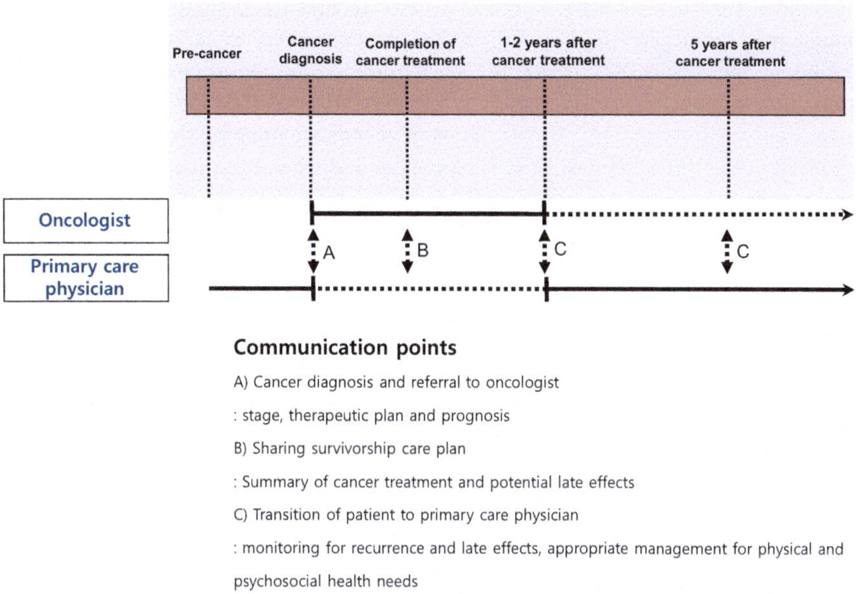

Fig. 27.1 Delivering survivorship care: shared care model caption: Solid line indicates primary responsibility and dashed line indicates secondary responsibility for cancer survivors between oncologist and primary care physician

Table 27.1 Strategy for providing comprehensive care to cancer survivors

Area	Contents
1. Surveillance for primary cancer	History taking, physical examination, and regular checkup including test
2. Screening of second primary cancer	Recommendation for general population at least
3. Management of comorbid health condition	
3.1 Physical	Cardiovascular disease, bone health, and late-effect of cancer treatment
3.2 Psychosocial	Psychologic distress (anxiety and depression), social support, and occupational problems
4. Promoting healthy lifestyle behaviors	Diet, alcohol, physical activity, and weight
5. Preventive care	Vaccination

27.2 Review of Past Studies

27.2.1 Surveillance for Primary Cancer

Surveillance for primary cancer can be individualized based on age, diagnosis, and treatment history through history taking, physical examination, and annual test.

Guidelines for surveillance for breast cancer recurrence commonly recommend annual mammography [6, 11]. While, breast sonography is more sensitive than mammography (91–97% vs 45–87%), most guidelines do not state the use of breast sonography because of insufficient evidence that improves the long-term survival of breast cancer survivors [12]. Breast magnetic resonance imaging (MRI) shows high sensitivity (95–100%). Breast MRI is recommended when life-time risk of developing secondary breast cancer (>20%) [6].

27.2.2 Screening of Second Primary Cancer

Cancer that occurs in cancer survivors after primary cancer treatment is called second primary cancer (SPC), which is different from recurrence or metastasis of original cancer [13]. The number of patients experiencing SPC is increasing as the cancer treatment is developing. In the United States, 8.1% of cancer survivors developed SPC [14], and in Korea, SPC risk of cancer survivors is known to be 2.3-fold higher than that of general population [15]. The risk of SPC is expected to be high due to genetic predisposition, behavioral risk factors, and long term side effects of chemotherapy, radiotherapy, and hormone therapy. Prediagnosis smoking history, obesity, and insulin resistance were associated with SPC [15]. A large cohort study for 239,615 Korean male cancer survivors suggested that magnitude of prediagnosis obesity was stronger in cancer survivors (adjusted hazard ratio [HR], 1.41; 95% confidence interval [CI], 1.15–1.74) than in the general population (adjusted HR, 1.12; 95% CI, 1.09–1.16).

High risks of SPC were reported as standardized incidence ratio (SIR) 1.2 ~ 1.4 [16–19]. In Korea, incidence of SPC in breast cancer survivors was 2.8% with high SIR (1.56; 95% CI, 1.26–1.91) in all sites in Korea [20]. Endometrial cancer (5.65; 95% CI 2.06–12.31), biliary tract cancer (3.96; 95% CI 1.19–8.60), and thyroid cancer (2.29; 95% CI 1.67–3.08) were associated with higher incidence in breast cancer survivors. Especially, tamoxifen treatment of breast cancer is associated with 2.4-fold increased endometrial cancer due to estrogenic effect on uterus [21]. In the case of BRCA 1 or BRCA 2 mutation, 10-year risk of ovarian cancer was 6.8–12.7% after breast cancer [22]. Radiotherapy in breast cancer is related to approximately two-fold high risk of lung cancer [23]. In addition, breast cancer survivors are recommended to adhere guidelines for SPC screening as recommendation in general population [6].

However, lack of physicians' advice for SPC screening and limited knowledge of cancer survivors could be barrier for screening of SPC [24]. Only 37% of cancer survivors had undergone appropriate SPC screening tests [25]. Thus, physicians as well as cancer survivors need proper education for SPC and SPC screening so that SPC screening can be provided with considering of individuals risk.

27.2.3 *Management of Comorbid Health Condition*

27.2.3.1 Risk for Cardiovascular Disease

The most common cause of noncancer death in long-term cancer survivors was disease of the circulatory system [26]. Breast cancer survivors are at increased risk of death from CVD after the treatment of breast cancer such as radiotherapy, chemotherapy, target therapy, and use of aromatase inhibitors (AI) [27]. A population-based study in United Kingdom confirmed that breast cancer survivors had an elevated incidence of heart failure (HR, 1.95; 95% CI, 1.27–3.01) and coronary artery disease (HR, 1.27; 95% CI, 1.11–1.44) [28]. Hypertension, diabetes, and dyslipidemia are representative risk factors for CVD and are known to be of high prevalence in breast cancer survivors [29]. However, management of diabetes in cancer survivors was not optimal compared to general population [30]. In particular, AI use was associated with increase in the odds of hypercholesterolemia (odds ratio [OR], 2.36; 95% CI, 2.15–2.60) [31] and increase risk of coronary artery disease (HR, 3.23; 95% CI, 1.26–8.25) [32] compared with tamoxifen use. Anthracycline and trastuzumab are known to have cardiotoxicity [33]. Therefore, lifestyle modification to lower cardiovascular risk should be encouraged in breast cancer survivors and examination such as blood lipid profile should be considered, if necessary.

27.2.3.2 Bone Health

Chemotherapy and endocrine treatment can induce the early menopause in premenopausal women and estrogen depletion in postmenopausal women, which accelerates the bone loss and increases the fracture risk [34]. About 80% of breast cancer survivors experience the bone loss [35]. Tamoxifen treatment had different effect according to the menopausal state, bone loss in premenopausal women, and against bone loss in postmenopausal women [36]. Guidelines also recommend the biennial dual-energy x-ray absorptiometry scan for women who are taking an aromatase inhibitor, premenopausal women who are taking tamoxifen and/or a gonadotropin-releasing hormone agonist, and women who have chemotherapy-induced premature menopause [6].

27.2.3.3 Psychosocial Effects

Psychologic distress refers to unpleasant emotional, psychological, social, or spiritual experience. Prevalence of high level of stress and depressive symptoms was 25% and 16% in cancer survivors, which are higher than general population [37]. Especially, depression occurrence was high those who had cancer diagnosis within past 5 years [38]. In addition, 29% of breast cancer survivors complained of fear of cancer recurrence [39]. Positive psychologic intervention can promote positive changes such as enhanced quality of life and well-being in breast cancer survivors [40]. Therefore, it is desirable to provide appropriate support to breast cancer survivors who need to help.

27.2.4 Promoting Healthy Lifestyle Behaviors

Lifestyle factors including diet, physical activity, and body weight have been closely associated with development of many cancers, prognosis of cancers, and health consequences for cancer survivors [41].

27.2.4.1 Diet

Dietary pattern and nutrient components could be linked to breast cancer survival. A High intake of prudent diet pattern (high in fruits, vegetables, whole grains, legumes, poultry, and fish) and low Western diet pattern was associated with low relative risks of death from causes other than breast cancer [42]. Furthermore, a study of post-menopausal breast cancer survivors in Germany suggested that 'healthy' dietary pattern was inversely associated with breast cancer recurrence [43].

A review study revealed that high dietary fat intake was inversely associated with breast cancer survival [44]. In addition, high intakes of saturated fat before cancer diagnosis were associated with worse prognosis of breast cancer [45]. Some of the studies found the vegetable intakes or nutrient (beta-carotene and vitamin C) supplied by fruit and vegetables may have protective effect [45–47] There were two representative diet intervention trials on whether dietary change toward low-fat [48] or increased vegetable and fruit intake [49] can influence the prognosis of breast cancer. Intervention through reducing fat intake with decreased body weight showed significantly better disease-free survival of breast cancer [48].

High protein intake was associated with better breast cancer survival regardless of amino acid types [46, 50, 51]. The association between soy intake and breast cancer risk is inconclusive, since soy foods have known to be both antiestrogenic and estrogen-like properties. A large population-based cohort study reported that [52]A meta-analysis reported that high soy intake was associated with modest reduction of breast cancer risk (OR, 0.86; 95% CI, 0.75–0.99) [53]. In addition, higher dietary isoflavone intake was associated with 21% decreased all-cause mortality in breast cancer survivors [54]. Effect of pomegranates on breast cancer was limited to animal studies or in vitro studies [55, 56]. There was potential to prevent breast cancer through reducing tumor proliferation [57].

In conclusion, healthy diet pattern with high intake of vegetables and fruits and limited intake of saturated fat is recommended to breast cancer survivors.

27.2.4.2 Alcohol

Alcohol consumption even light to moderate dose has been linked to increased risk of many cancers [58]. Moderate alcohol (5.0 ~ 9.9 g alcohol per day) was associated with increased breast cancer risk (relative risk [RR], 1.15; 95% CI, 1.06–1.24) [59]. A 10-g increase in alcohol intake significantly increased the relative risk of hormone receptor-positive breast cancer by 10% [60]. Acetaldehyde, a toxic metabolite of ethanol, can act as a carcinogen, and breast tissue may be more susceptible to it than other organs [58]. Alcohol also increases the secretion of estrogens and androgens in the body [59], which may increase the incidence of breast cancer. The life after cancer epidemiology (LACE) study in breast cancer survivors investigated that intake of ≥6 g alcohol a day increased the risk of breast cancer recurrence [61]. Therefore, it is desirable to limit alcohol consumption in breast cancer survivors.

27.2.4.3 Physical Activity

Physical activity after breast cancer diagnosis has benefit from breast cancer death as well as all-cause mortality [62–64]. The Nurses' Health study (NHS) demonstrated that breast cancer survivors who engaged in 9 or more metabolic equivalent task [MET] hours per week of physical activity, the equivalent of walking 3–5 h per week at an average pace had 50% lower risk of death from breast cancer death compared to breast cancer survivors who engaged in less than 3-MET-hours per week of physical activity [62]. A population-based Shanghai Cancer Registry suggested that exercise was inversely associated with 40% decreased risk of breast cancer recurrence [65]. In addition, a systemic review indicated that exercise may have positive effects on health-related quality of life including cancer-specific concerns, body image/self-esteem, emotional well-being, sexuality, sleep disturbance, social functioning, anxiety, fatigue, and pain [66]. Thus, regular physical activity at least 150 min per week in breast cancer survivors is recommended consistent with the guidelines for cancer survivors [67].

27.2.4.4 Weight

Obesity is a well-established risk factors for breast cancers and associated with high mortality or poor prognosis of breast cancer [68]. A meta-analysis found that weight gain (≥5% of body weight) compared to maintenance (< ±5% of body weight) was associated with increased all-cause mortality (HR, 1.12; 95% CI, 1.03–1.22) [69]. A retrospective study in Korea, mean weight gain was 0.32 kg and 21.3% of breast cancer survivors had gained more than 5% of body weight at diagnosis [70]. Obese patients with a body mass index (BMI) >30 kg/m^2 are more likely to have postoperative lymphedema (OR, 2.93; 95% CI, 1.03–8.31) compared with those with a

BMI of <25 kg/m [2] [71]. Furthermore, obesity in breast cancer survivors is associated with increased risks of contralateral breast (RR, 1.37), endometrial (RR, 1.96), and colorectal (RR, 1.89) SPC [72]. However, direct evidence of weight loss intervention on breast cancer prognosis is insufficient [73, 74]. Maintenance of healthy and proper weight should be achieved.

27.2.5 Preventive Care

27.2.5.1 Vaccination

Cancer survivors are considered to be vulnerable to infectious disease owing to reduce immunity after cancer treatment. The National Comprehensive Cancer Network (NCCN) recommended that following vaccines should be considered and encouraged for all cancer survivors: influenza vaccine; pneumococcal vaccine; tetanus, diphtheria, and pertussis; and human papilloma virus (in survivors aged ≤26 years) [75].

Influenza in cancer survivors is associated with high mortality [76]. Breast cancer survivors are much susceptible to influenza than general population free of cancer, and elder breast cancer survivors were relate to long stay of hospitalization [77]. In particular, influenza infection could be prevented through influenza vaccination. In Korea, 55% of cancer survivors were vaccinated for influenza [78], in spite of annual recommendation for annual influenza vaccination in cancer survivors [79]. Even though cancer survivors more than 65 years old showed high rate of vaccination, more than 76%, only 36% of cancer survivors aged less than 65 years old was vaccinated [80]. Among cancer survivors, those with chronic condition, elderly and rural dwellers were more likely to receive influenza vaccination [80].

Pneumococcal vaccines should be administrated to newly diagnosed cancer patients and elderly (≥ 65 years old) [79]. In the US, 48.3% of cancer survivors reported ever receiving a pneumococcal vaccination [81]. 13-valent pneumococcal conjugate vaccine (PCV13) and pneumococcal polysaccharide vaccine-23 (PPSV 23) should be combined with proper interval.

In terms of live attenuated vaccine, such as zoster vaccine, it could be considered for cancer survivors, unless they have received chemotherapy or radiation within the past 3 months or at least 4 weeks before initiation of cancer treatment [75].

27.3 Current Evidence and Concepts

27.3.1 Prognosis of Breast Cancer Survivors

Late recurrence rate of breast cancer is substantial, a prospective study reported that late recurrence accounts for 5.8% at ≥10 years of follow-up [82]. The well-established factors related to recurrence are known to be cancer stage (positive lymph node or tumor size), molecular type, and hormonal receptor status. Meanwhile, multigene expression profiling assays, such as Oncotype Dx, have been recently used to assess prognosis to stratify the groups that are beneficial from additional treatment or extended treatment in early breast cancer [83]. However, these assays have limitation to predict late recurrence. Meanwhile, circulating tumor cells (CTCs) detected in blood can be associated with late recurrence after 5 years of diagnosis as independent prognostic information according to the recent ECOG-ACRIN cancer research group [84]. A single positive CTC assay was associated with increased recurrence risk after 5 years of treatment (HR, 18.3; 95% CI 5.7–58.2). As precise medicine is developing, comprehensive cancer survivorship plans could be individualized according to the results.

On the other hand, individuals with SPC could have genetic susceptibility. Multiple complex genetic pathways such as DNA damage repair, oxidative stress, and cell cycle control likely contribute to the development of SPC. For example, *BRCA1* and *BRCA2* mutation carriers in breast cancer survivors have increased risk for second ovarian cancer or contralateral breast cancer [85, 86]. NCCN guidelines also recommend test for *BRCA1* and *BRCA2* mutation in breast cancer survivors who are diagnosed with ovarian cancer and diagnosed with breast cancer before 45 years old. Besides, the genes which increase the risk of SPC include PTEN, CHEK2, and p53 [87]. Practical approach to screen SPC can reflect individual genetic susceptibility as genetic alteration that may contribute to risk of SPC has been identified.

27.4 Future Research Direction

Survivorship care plan contains the summary of treatment course, recommendation for subsequent cancer surveillance, management of late effects, and strategies for health promotion [88]. Clinically, optimal cancer survivorship care models are uncertain and require further researches. Powered randomized controlled intervention for each element and cancer survivorship care model itself can be conducted.

27.5 Summary

27.5.1 The Bench

Individualized risk assessment, such as multigene profiling assays or circulating tumor cell detection, can be applied to cancer survivorship plan.

27.5.2 *Translation*

Precise strategy for cancer survivorship care should be provided encompassing comprehensive area such as surveillance for primary cancer, screening of second primary cancer, management of comorbid health condition, promoting healthy lifestyle behaviors, and preventive care.

27.5.3 *The Bedside*

To meet complex needs of breast cancer survivors, coordinated and collaborative care models are needed considering diverse practical settings.

References

1. Fairley TL, Pollack LA, Moore AR, Smith JL. Addressing cancer survivorship through public health: an update from the Centers for disease control and prevention. J Women Health. 2009;18(10):1525–31.
2. Miller KD, Siegel RL, Lin CC, et al. Cancer treatment and survivorship statistics, 2016. CA Cancer J Clin. 2016;66(4):271–89.
3. Seo HJ, Noh DY. Care pathway for Cancer survivorship in Korea: trend of breast Cancer pathway from 2003 to 2010. Healthcare Inform Res. 2017;23(2):119–25.
4. Korea National Cancer Center. Cancer Registry Korea; 2015 [cited 2018 Jan 5] Available from: http://www.ncc.re.kr/cancerStatsView.ncc?bbsnum=68&searchKey=total&searchValue=&pageNum=3 cJAf.
5. Institute of Medicine and National Research Council of the National Academies. FromCancer Patient to Cancer Survivor: Lost in Transition. Committee on Cancer Survivorship: Improving Care and Quality of Life. <IOM_2006_report.pdf>.
6. Runowicz CD, Leach CR, Henry NL, et al. American Cancer Society/American Society of Clinical Oncology breast Cancer survivorship care guideline. CA Cancer J Clin. 2016;66(1):43–73.
7. Grunfeld E, Levine MN, Julian JA, et al. Randomized trial of long-term follow-up for early-stage breast cancer: a comparison of family physician versus specialist care. J Clin Oncol. 2006;24(6):848–55.
8. Grunfeld E, Fitzpatrick R, Mant D, et al. Comparison of breast cancer patient satisfaction with follow-up in primary care versus specialist care: results from a randomized controlled trial. Br J Gen Pract. 1999;49(446):705–10.
9. Oeffinger KC, McCabe MS. Models for delivering survivorship care. J Clin Oncol. 2006;24(32):5117–24.
10. Rubinstein EB, Miller WL, Hudson SV, et al. Cancer survivorship Care in Advanced Primary Care Practices: a qualitative study of challenges and opportunities. JAMA Intern Med. 2017;177(12):1726–32.
11. Senkus E, Kyriakides S, Penault-Llorca F, et al. Primary breast cancer: ESMO Clinical Practice Guidelines for diagnosis, treatment and follow-up. Ann Oncol: Official J Eur Soc Med Oncol. 2013;24(Suppl 6):7–23.

12. Yoon JH, Kim MJ, Kim E-K, Moon HJ. Imaging surveillance of patients with breast Cancer after primary treatment: current recommendations. Korean J Radiol. 2015;16(2):219–28.
13. Coyte A, Morrison DS, McLoone P. Second primary cancer risk - the impact of applying different definitions of multiple primaries: results from a retrospective population-based cancer registry study. BMC Cancer. 2014;14(1):272.
14. Donin N, Filson C, Drakaki A, et al. Risk of second primary malignancies among cancer survivors in the United States, 1992 through 2008. Cancer. 2016;122(19):3075–86.
15. Park SM, Lim MK, Jung KW, et al. Prediagnosis smoking, obesity, insulin resistance, and second primary Cancer risk in male Cancer survivors: national health insurance corporation study. J Clin Oncol. 2007;25(30):4835–43.
16. Lee K-D, Chen S-C, Chan CH, et al. Increased risk for second primary malignancies in women with breast Cancer diagnosed at young age: a population-based study in Taiwan. Prevention. 2008;17:2647–55.
17. Tanaka H, Tsukuma H, Koyama H, Kinoshita Y, Kinoshita N, Oshima A. Second primary cancers following breast cancer in the Japanese female population. Jpn J Cancer Res: Gann. 2001;92(1):1–8.
18. Mellemkjaer L, Friis S, Olsen JH, et al. Risk of second cancer among women with breast cancer. Int J Cancer. 2006;118(9):2285–92.
19. Molina-Montes E, Requena M, Sanchez-Cantalejo E, et al. Risk of second cancers cancer after a first primary breast cancer: a systematic review and meta-analysis. Gynecol Oncol. 2015;136 (1):158–71.
20. Jung HK, Park S, Kim NW, et al. Development of second primary cancer in Korean breast cancer survivors. Ann Surg Treat Res. 2017;93(6):287–92.
21. Swerdlow AJ, Jones ME. Tamoxifen treatment for breast Cancer and risk of endometrial Cancer: a case–control study. JNCI: J Natl Cancer Inst. 2005;97(5):375–84.
22. Metcalfe KA, Lynch HT, Ghadirian P, et al. The risk of ovarian cancer after breast cancer in BRCA1 and BRCA2 carriers. Gynecol Oncol. 2005;96(1):222–6.
23. Zablotska LB, Neugut AI. Lung carcinoma after radiation therapy in women treated with lumpectomy or mastectomy for primary breast carcinoma. Cancer. 2003;97(6):1404–11.
24. Park SM, Lee J, Kim YA, et al. Factors related with colorectal and stomach cancer screening practice among disease-free lung cancer survivors in Korea. BMC Cancer. 2017;17(1):600.
25. Shin DW, Kim YW, Oh JH, et al. Knowledge, attitudes, risk perception, and cancer screening behaviors among cancer survivors. Cancer. 2011;117(16):3850–9.
26. Shin DW, Ahn E, Kim H, Park S, Kim YA, Yun YH. Non-cancer mortality among long-term survivors of adult cancer in Korea: national cancer registry study. Cancer Causes Control. 2010;21(6):919–29.
27. Hooning MJ, Aleman BM, van Rosmalen AJ, Kuenen MA, Klijn JG, van Leeuwen FE. Cause-specific mortality in long-term survivors of breast cancer: a 25-year follow-up study. Int J Radiat Oncol Biol Phys. 2006;64(4):1081–91.
28. Khan NF, Mant D, Carpenter L, Forman D, Rose PW. Long-term health outcomes in a British cohort of breast, colorectal and prostate cancer survivors: a database study. Br J Cancer. 2011;105(Suppl 1):S29–37.
29. Lenihan DJ, Cardinale DM. Late cardiac effects of Cancer treatment. J Clin Oncol. 2012;30 (30):3657–64.
30. Choi K-H, Park S, Lee K, Kim KH, Park J-S, Ho Han S. *Prevalence, Awareness, Control, and Treatment of Hypertension and Diabetes in Korean Cancer Survivors: A Cross-Sectional Analysis of the Fourth and Fifth Korea National Health and Nutrition Examination Surveys.* Vol 142013.
31. Amir E, Seruga B, Niraula S, Carlsson L, Ocaña A. Toxicity of adjuvant endocrine therapy in postmenopausal breast Cancer patients: a systematic review and meta-analysis. JNCI: J Natl Cancer Inst. 2011;103(17):1299–309.
32. Seruga B, Zadnik V, Kuhar CG, et al. Association of aromatase inhibitors with coronary heart disease in women with early breast cancer. Cancer Investig. 2014;32(4):99–104.

33. Curigliano G, Cardinale D, Suter T, et al. Cardiovascular toxicity induced by chemotherapy, targeted agents and radiotherapy: ESMO clinical practice guidelines. Ann Oncol: Official J Eur Soc Med Oncol. 2012;23(Suppl 7):155–66.
34. Guise TA. Bone loss and fracture risk associated with cancer therapy. Oncologist. 2006;11 (10):1121–31.
35. Chen Z, Maricic M, Pettinger M, et al. Osteoporosis and rate of bone loss among postmenopausal survivors of breast cancer. Cancer. 2005;104(7):1520–30.
36. Powles TJ, Hickish T, Kanis JA, Tidy A, Ashley S. Effect of tamoxifen on bone mineral density measured by dual-energy x-ray absorptiometry in healthy premenopausal and postmenopausal women. J Clin Oncol. 1996;14(1):78–84.
37. Choi K-H, Park SM. Psychological status and associated factors among Korean cancer survivors: a cross-sectional analysis of the fourth & amp; fifth Korea National Health and nutrition examination surveys. J Korean Med Sci. 2016;31(7):1105–13.
38. Kim KH, Cho YY, Shin DW, Lee JH, Ko YJ, Park SM. Comparison of physical and mental health status between cancer survivors and the general population: a Korean population-based survey (KNHANES II-IV). Support Care Cancer. 2013;21(12):3471–81.
39. Liu Y, Perez M, Schootman M, Aft RL, Gillanders WE, Jeffe DB. Correlates of fear of cancer recurrence in women with ductal carcinoma in situ and early invasive breast cancer. Breast Cancer Res Treat. 2011;130(1):165–73.
40. Casellas-Grau A, Font A, Vives J. Positive psychology interventions in breast cancer. a systematic review. Psycho Oncol. 23(1):9–19.
41. Ligibel J. Lifestyle factors in cancer survivorship. J Clin Oncol. 2012;30(30):3697–704.
42. Kroenke CH, Fung TT, Hu FB, Holmes MD. Dietary patterns and survival after breast Cancer diagnosis. J Clin Oncol. 2005;23(36):9295–303.
43. Vrieling A, Buck K, Seibold P, et al. Dietary patterns and survival in German postmenopausal breast cancer survivors. Br J Cancer. 2013;108(1):188–92.
44. Rock CL, Demark-Wahnefried W. Nutrition and survival after the diagnosis of breast Cancer: a review of the evidence. J Clin Oncol Off. 2002;20(15):3302–16.
45. Jain M, Miller AB, To T. Premorbid diet and the prognosis of women with breast cancer. J Natl Cancer Inst. 1994;86(18):1390–7.
46. Rohan TE, Hiller JE, McMichael AJ. Dietary factors and survival from breast cancer. Nutr Cancer. 1993;20(2):167–77.
47. Ingram D. Diet and subsequent survival in women with breast cancer. Br J Cancer. 1994;69 (3):592–5.
48. Chlebowski RT, Blackburn GL, Thomson CA, et al. Dietary fat reduction and breast cancer outcome: interim efficacy results from the Women's intervention nutrition study. J Natl Cancer Inst. 2006;98(24):1767–76.
49. Pierce JP, Natarajan L, Caan BJ, et al. Influence of a diet very high in vegetables, fruit, and fiber and low in fat on prognosis following treatment for breast cancer: the Women's healthy eating and living (WHEL) randomized trial. JAMA. 2007;298(3):289–98.
50. Goodwin PJ, Ennis M, Pritchard KI, Koo J, Trudeau ME, Hood N. Diet and breast Cancer: evidence that extremes in diet Are associated with poor survival. J Clin Oncol. 2003;21 (13):2500–7.
51. Holmes MD, Wang J, Hankinson SE, Tamimi RM, Chen WY. Protein intake and breast Cancer survival in the nurses' health study. J Clin Oncol. 2017;35(3):325–33.
52. Shu XO, Zheng Y, Cai H, et al. Soy food intake and breast cancer survival. JAMA. 2009;302 (22):2437–43.
53. Trock BJ, Hilakivi-Clarke L, Clarke R. Meta-analysis of soy intake and breast Cancer risk. JNCI: J Natl Cancer Inst. 2006;98(7):459–71.
54. Zhang FF, Haslam DE, Terry MB, et al. Dietary isoflavone intake and all-cause mortality in breast cancer survivors: the breast Cancer family registry. Cancer. 2017;123(11):2070–9.

55. Mehta R, Lansky EP. Breast cancer chemopreventive properties of pomegranate (Punica granatum) fruit extracts in a mouse mammary organ culture. Eur J Cancer Prev. 2004;13 (4):345–8.
56. Kim ND, Mehta R, Yu W, et al. Chemopreventive and adjuvant therapeutic potential of pomegranate (Punica granatum) for human breast cancer. Breast Cancer Res Treat. 2002;71 (3):203–17.
57. Vini R, Sreeja S. Punica granatum and its therapeutic implications on breast carcinogenesis: A review. BioFactors. 2015;41(2):78–89.
58. Cao Y, Willett WC, Rimm EB, Stampfer MJ, Giovannucci EL. Light to moderate intake of alcohol, drinking patterns, and risk of cancer: results from two prospective US cohort studies. BMJ. 2015;351:h4238.
59. Chen WY, Rosner B, Hankinson SE, Colditz GA, Willett WC. Moderate alcohol consumption during adult life, drinking patterns, and breast cancer risk. JAMA. 2011;306(17):1884–90.
60. Zhang SM, Lee IM, Manson JE, Cook NR, Willett WC, Buring JE. Alcohol consumption and breast cancer risk in the Women's health study. Am J Epidemiol. 2007;165(6):667–76.
61. Kwan ML, Kushi LH, Weltzien E, et al. Alcohol consumption and breast cancer recurrence and survival among women with early-stage breast cancer: the life after cancer epidemiology study. J Clin Oncol. 2010;28(29):4410–6.
62. Holmes MD, Chen WY, Feskanich D, Kroenke CH, Colditz GA. Physical activity and survival after breast cancer diagnosis. JAMA. 2005;293(20):2479–86.
63. Pierce JP, Stefanick ML, Flatt SW, et al. Greater survival after breast cancer in physically active women with high vegetable-fruit intake regardless of obesity. J Clin Oncol. 2007;25 (17):2345–51.
64. Holick CN, Newcomb PA, Trentham-Dietz A, et al. Physical activity and survival after diagnosis of invasive breast Cancer. Prevention. 2008;17(2):379–86.
65. Chen X, Lu W, Zheng W, et al. Exercise after diagnosis of breast cancer in association with survival. Cancer Prev Res. 2011;4(9):1409–18.
66. Mishra SI, Scherer RW, Geigle PM, et al. Exercise interventions on health-related quality of life for cancer survivors. Cochrane Database Syst Rev. 2012;8(8):Cd007566.
67. Rock CL, Doyle C, Demark-Wahnefried W, et al. Nutrition and physical activity guidelines for cancer survivors. CA Cancer J Clin. 2012;62(4):243–74.
68. Protani M, Coory M, Martin JH. Effect of obesity on survival of women with breast cancer: systematic review and meta-analysis. Breast Cancer Res Treat. 2010;123(3):627–35.
69. Playdon MC, Bracken MB, Sanft TB, Ligibel JA, Harrigan M, Irwin ML. Weight gain after breast cancer diagnosis and all-cause mortality: systematic review and meta-analysis. J Natl Cancer Inst. 2015;107(12):djv275.
70. Koo H-Y, Seo Y-G, Cho M-H, Kim M-J, Choi H-C. Weight change and associated factors in long-term breast Cancer survivors. PLoS One. 2016;11(7):e0159098.
71. Helyer LK, Varnic M, Le LW, Leong W, McCready D. Obesity is a risk factor for developing postoperative lymphedema in breast cancer patients. Breast J. 2010;16(1):48–54.
72. Druesne-Pecollo N, Touvier M, Barrandon E, et al. Excess body weight and second primary cancer risk after breast cancer: a systematic review and meta-analysis of prospective studies. Breast Cancer Res Treat. 2012;135(3):647–54.
73. Chlebowski RT, Aiello E, McTiernan A. Weight loss in breast Cancer patient management. J Clin Oncol. 2002;20(4):1128–43.
74. Playdon M, Thomas G, Sanft T, Harrigan M, Ligibel J, Irwin M. Weight loss intervention for breast Cancer survivors: a systematic review. Current Breast Cancer Rep. 2013;5(3):222–46.
75. Denlinger CS, Ligibel JA, Are M, et al. Survivorship: immunizations and prevention of infections, version 2.2014: clinical practice guidelines in oncology. J Natl Comprehensive Cancer Network: JNCCN. 2014;12(8):1098–111.
76. Cooksley CD, Avritscher EB, Bekele BN, Rolston KV, Geraci JM, Elting LS. Epidemiology and outcomes of serious influenza-related infections in the cancer population. Cancer. 2005;104 (3):618–28.

77. Heo J, Chun M, Oh YT, Noh OK, Kim L. Influenza among breast cancer survivors in south korea: a nationwide population-based study. In vivo. 2017;31(5):967–72.
78. Oh MG, Han MA, Yun NR, et al. A population-based, Nationwide cross-sectional study on influenza vaccination status among Cancer survivors in Korea. Int J Environ Res Public Health. 2015;12(8):10133–49.
79. Rubin LG, Levin MJ, Ljungman P, et al. IDSA clinical practice guideline for vaccination of the Immunocompromised host. Clin Infect Dis. 2014;58(3):e44–e100.
80. Choi KH, Park SM, Lee K, Lee JH, Park JS. Influenza vaccination and associated factors among Korean cancer survivors: a cross-sectional analysis of the fourth & fifth Korea National Health and nutrition examination surveys. J Korean Med Sci. 2014;29(8):1061–8.
81. Underwood JM, Townsend JS, Stewart SL, et al. Surveillance of demographic characteristics and health behaviors among adult cancer survivors--Behavioral Risk Factor Surveillance System, United States, 2009. MMWR Surveill Summ. 2012;61(1):1–23.
82. Nishimura R, Osako T, Nishiyama Y, et al. Evaluation of factors related to late recurrence--later than 10 years after the initial treatment--in primary breast cancer. Oncology. 2013;85 (2):100–10.
83. Chang MC, Souter LH, Kamel-Reid S, et al. Clinical utility of multigene profiling assays in early-stage breast cancer. Curr Oncol. 2017;24(5):e403–22.
84. Sparano JA ONA, Alpaugh K, Wolff AC, Northfelt DW, Dang C, Sledge, Jr. GW, Miller KD (2017) Circulating tumor cells (CTCs) five years after diagnosis are prognostic for late recurrence in operable stage II-III breast cancer. San Antonio Breast Cancer Symposium 2017
85. Schmidt MK, van den Broek AJ, Tollenaar RAEM, et al. Breast cancer survival of BRCA1/ BRCA2 mutation carriers in a hospital-based cohort of young women. JNCI: J Natl Cancer Inst. 2017;109(8):djw329.
86. Metcalfe K, Lynch HT, Ghadirian P, et al. Contralateral breast cancer in BRCA1 and BRCA2 mutation carriers. J Clin Oncol. 2004;22(12):2328–35.
87. Cybulski C, Nazarali S, Narod SA. Multiple primary cancers as a guide to heritability. Int J Cancer. 2014;135(8):1756–63.
88. Ganz PA, Hahn EE. Implementing a survivorship care plan for patients with breast cancer. J Clin Oncol. 2008;26(5):759–67.

Chapter 28
Considerations in Oncoplastic Surgery

Min Kyoon Kim and Jaihong Han

Abstract The development of oncoplastic surgery (OPS) is one of the greatest achievements for the treatment of breast cancer. OPS combines oncological resection with plastic surgery techniques in a single procedure to allow the excision of tumors without compromising cosmetic outcome. It allows better aesthetic–functional outcomes and consequently an improvement of the psychological aspects of patients with breast cancer.

OPS begins with preoperative design considering breast volume, tumor size, and location and distance from nipple of the tumor, with clinical breast examination and image studies. Various techniques of volume replacement and volume displacement methods described here can help the decision-making process so the best results concerning the aesthetic–functional aspects can be achieved.

The outcome measurement of the oncoplastic breast surgery consisted of local recurrence, cosmesis, and patients satisfaction. In OPS for breast cancer patients, aesthetic assessment could be performed by various methods. And questionnaires on quality of life can be applied as a scientific method to assess results. In this chapter, we introduced our results of assessment of both aesthetic and QOL outcomes in OPS patients.

Keywords Breast conserving surgery · Oncoplastic surgery · Mammoplasty · Cosmesis · Oncologic safety

M. K. Kim (✉)
Department of Surgery, Chung-Ang University College of Medicine, Seoul, South Korea

J. Han
National Cancer Center, Goyang-si, South Korea

D.-Y. Noh et al. (eds.), *Translational Research in Breast Cancer*, Advances in Experimental Medicine and Biology 1187,
https://doi.org/10.1007/978-981-32-9620-6_28

28.1 Introduction

Breast-conserving surgery followed by radiotherapy is standard treatment in breast cancer. The aim of surgeons doing breast-conserving surgery is to acquire acceptable cosmesis and secure adequate safety margins [1]. With the advance of radiotherapy and systemic therapies, the local recurrence rate is very low with less than 5%. Therefore, demand for good cosmetic result is increasing with quality of life of the breast cancer survivors are getting more and more important [2].

Oncoplastic surgery (OPS) is a well-established approach that combines conserving treatment for breast cancer and plastic surgery techniques. It allows wide excisions and prevents breast deformities by the immediate reconstruction of large resection defects, improving cosmetic outcomes even in case of large quadrantectomies. Compared with standard quadrantectomy or lumpectomy, OPS achieves more accurate tumor resection and free resection margins. Therefore, OPS might be useful to extend the indications for breast conservation [3].

There are various techniques for OPS regarding tumor location or breast shape. Also, there should be considerations for patients' perspective. Because of that, it is important not simply to preserve life but also to preserve a good quality of life for the patients. For those women who are deemed suitable candidates for whole or partial breast reconstruction, both the timing and the options for reconstructive surgery should be considered and discussed with the patient.

This chapter will deal with considerations and practical techniques for oncoplastic surgery in breast cancer, in order to achieve the best oncologic and aesthetic outcomes and to reduce errors. And we will introduce our analysis of aesthetic and quality of life evaluation after oncoplastic breast-conserving surgery.

28.2 Review of Past Studies

28.2.1 Definition of Oncoplastic Surgery

Oncoplastic surgery (OPS) is reconstruction of defect using various plastic surgical techniques after resection of the tumor with adequate margins [4]. It usually makes possible to acquire wider resection margins than standard BCS and to improve cosmetic result [5]. However, OPS is more complex and time-consuming than lumpectomy and quadrantectomy. Thus, the selection of patients from the oncologic, aesthetic, and psychological point of view is critical.

OPS includes

1. Excision of the cancer with adequate wide free margins.
2. Immediate remodeling of the defect to improve cosmetic result.
3. Contralateral breast symmetrization and reconstruction of the nipple-areola complex, when needed.
4. Immediate and late reconstruction after mastectomy.

28.2.2 Advantages and Oncological Safety of OPS (Table 28.1).

A number of studies have shown that OPS techniques are oncologically safe. But, there is no prospective randomized study comparing OPS vs conventional BCS for this issue. So it is hard to say that OPS is "better" than conventional BCS to decrease local recurrence after breast cancer surgery and adjuvant therapies.

Anyway OPS could achieve resection of larger breast volumes, wider tumor-free margins, lower re-excision rate, lower conversion rate to secondary mastectomy, and lower rate of secondary reconstruction [6].

On the other hand, the disadvantages of OPS are longer surgery time, more visible scars due to bigger incision, and requirement of experienced breast surgeon and/or plastic surgeon. There are some studies that OPS techniques such as aggressive glandular mobilization can increase fat necrosis of the breast especially in diabetes patients and heavy smokers [7, 8].

28.2.3 Indications of OPS

The general principles of doing OPS are same as those of conventional BCS. Tumor-free resection margin is mandatory, and the patients are able to get adequate radiation

Table 28.1 Studies reporting oncologic safety of oncoplastic surgery for breast cancer patients

Reference (Year)	No. patients	Mean age, y (range)	Median follow-up, mo (range)	Mean tumor size in mm (range)	Margin involvement
Clough et al. (2003)	101	53 (31–91)	46 (7–168)	32(10–70)	7%
Rietjans et al.(2007)	148	50 (31–71)	74 (10–108)	22 (3–100),	2.02%
Gulcelik et al.(2007)	101	52.2	Every 3 mo, first year	Stage I and II	6%
Giacalone et al.(2007)	31	51.3	Not reported	5–20 mm = 20 20–30 mm =8 30–40 mm = 1 >40 mm =2	21%
Fitoussi et al. (2010)	540	52(28–90)	49(6–262)	29.1(4 ~ 100)	18.9%
Bong et al. (2010)	167	55.6 (33–85)	Not reported	<2 cm = 74 (55.2%) >2 cm = 60 (44.8%)	22.2%
Chan et al. (2013)	162	52(20–96)	1–3	Not reported	Not reported

therapy. And the final result of the OPS should be cosmetically acceptable. However, with OPS technique, breast conservation can be done for larger size tumor. Unfavorable tumor locations that expected poor cosmetic result, such as lower part of breast and periareolar area, are good indication of OPS rather than conventional BCS. Especially, patients who have ptotic breast and who should consider reduction mammoplasty can be a best candidate for OPS than standard BCS.

28.2.4 Preoperative Consideration

There are various kind of oncoplastic procedures available, but basic principles are similar across the techniques. The more familiar with each technique and the more experiences the surgeon has, the more choices and indications will be possible. Tumor size, tumor location, and breast size of the patients should be considered [9]. Table 28.2 is showing the preferred procedures according to the location of tumor [10].

28.2.5 Technical Details of OPS Procedures in BCS

1. Volume Displacement Techniques: Rearrangement of local (dermo)glandular flaps into the defect (advancement, rotation, or transposition)
    1. Round block.
    2. Grisotti flap.
    3. Batwing incision.
    4. Tennis racket incision.
    5. Matrix rotation flap.
    6. S-shape oblique reduction mammoplasty.
    7. Sup pedicle mammoplasty, Inf. Pedicle mammoplasty.
    8. B-Plasty, J-mammoplasty V-mammoplasty. Etc.

Table 28.2 OPS procedures according to tumor location

Tumor location	Preferred procedure
Center	Grisotti flap, purse string suture
Periareolar	Round block, batwing technique
Upper	Inf. Pedicle mammoplasty, S-shape oblique reduction mammoplasty
Upper outer, outer	Latissimus dorsi flap or mini-flap, tennis racket incision
Upper inner	Matrix rotation, tennis racket incision
Lower	Sup pedicle mammoplasty
Lower inner	Omental flap

2. Volume replacement techniques: Use of distant autologous tissue flaps for tissue defect (LD flap, mini-LD flap, thoracodorsal artery perforator flap, Intercostal artery perforator flap, etc).
1. Latissimus dorsi mini-flap(Mini-LD flap).
2. Omental flap (laparoscopically harvested omental flap).

28.2.6 General Principles of OPS

OPS combines oncological resection with plastic surgery techniques in a single procedure to allow the excision of larger tumors without compromising cosmetic outcome. It begins with preoperative design considering breast volume, tumor size, and location and distance from nipple of the tumor, with clinical breast examination and image studies. OPS allows wide excision of the lesion with free margins, usually with larger length of incision. In this perspective, OPS is different from minimal invasive surgery. Sufficient mobilization of the gland is a key component of breast reshaping after wide excision in OPS.

General procedure of OPS are as follows:

1. Preoperative design.
2. Skin incision.
3. A full-thickness glandular excision with free margin.
4. Rearrangement of glandular flaps into the defect.
5. De-epithelialization and the NAC repositioning.
6. Skin closure.

28.2.7 Round block (Doughnut mastopexy)

The round block technique can be used in patients with any size of breast and tumors of any location only if not too far from NAC and not invading nipple [11]. It is relatively simple and easy technique with fair result.

Preoperatively, surgeon draws two circular skin markings surrounding the NAC. The inner circle is made on the areolar border. It would be better to make the circle smaller than real areolar line because the areola would become larger than original one after round block procedure. The external circle should be made at 1–2 cm distant from inner one. The distance between the two circles varies depending on the tumor size and location, the relationship of mass and nipple, and the degree of ptosis and size of breast. The distance would be wider in patients with higher grade ptosis and larger size breast. Sometimes they are not concentric to remove skin overlying tumor. After incisions are made along skin markings, de-epithelialization of skin between the two lines is done. During the de-epithelialization, surgeons must be careful not to injure vessels of dermis, because the blood supply of NAC is from the dermal vessels. Also, full-thickness incision of skin should not be larger than 50% of

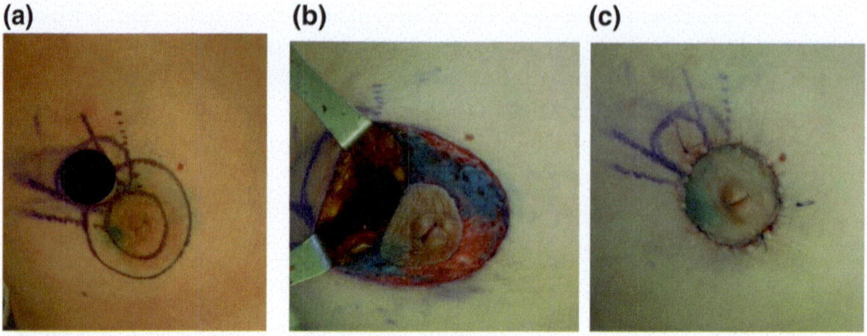

Fig. 28.1 Round block (**a**) Concentric circle incision around the NAC. (1–2 cm distance between two circles) (**b**) De-epithelization of the skin between two incisions. Resection with adequate margins. (**c**) The skin is closed with interrupt absorbable suture and finally closed with subcuticular suture

the NAC circumference. Tumor and surrounding parenchyma are removed securing adequate resection margins. Subareolar tissue can be removed without threatening the NAC blood supply, but wide subareolar tissue removal would result in poor cosmetic outcome. After undermining and mobilization of remaining breast tissues, the defect can be closed. The dermis of two skin incisions is closed with some interrupted sutures. Final skin closure is done using a subcuticular running suture with 4-0 or 5-0 monocryl (Fig. 28.1).

28.2.8 Grisotti Flap

The Grisotti flap technique can be used for tumors requiring nipple sacrifice in patients with moderate to large-sized breasts. The skin marking is done outlining the NAC. A circle for new NAC is drawn just below the original NAC. After drawing the inframammary fold, both sides of two circles (native and new NAC) are extended and connected to inframammary fold (IMF). Central lumpectomy including tumor and native NAC is done. Then, de-epithelize the flap excluding skin island preserved for reconstruction of new NAC. Full-thickness skin incision is done at the medial border of the skin flap. The defect is filled using rotation of the flap, and areolar is replaced with the skin island that is mobilized (Fig. 28.2).

28.2.9 Batwing Technique (Inverted V or Omega Plasty)

Batwing technique may be used for lesions in the upper breast around the nipple. This procedure uses a semicircular incision at the upper margin of the NAC. After measuring the height of the skin resection, another semicircular incision which is

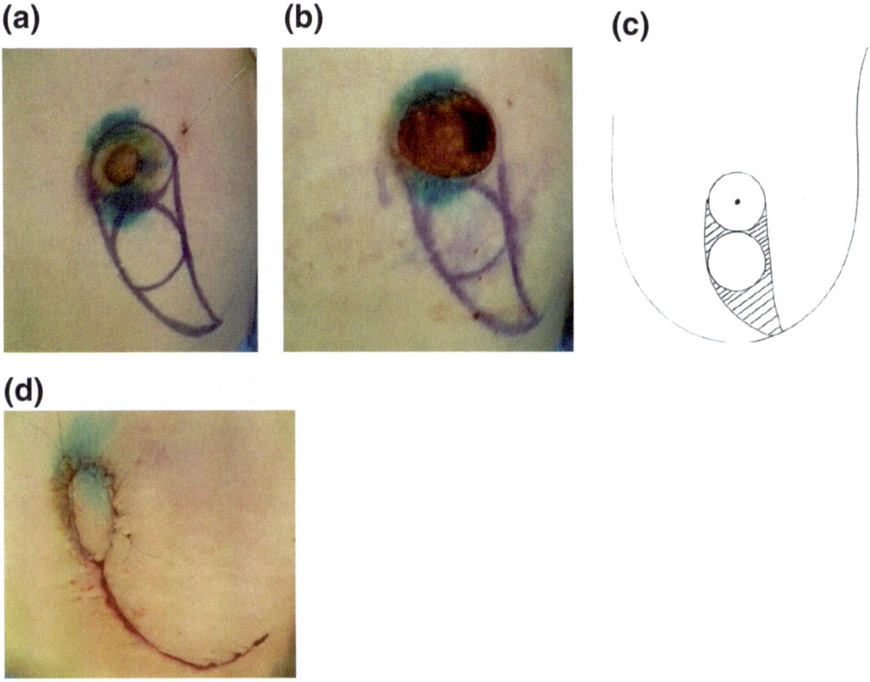

Fig. 28.2 Grisotti flap (**a**) Circumareolar skin incision and new NAC marking. (**b**) Excision of NAC and central quadrantectomy. (**c**) De-epithelization of the flap and a skin island preservation. (**d**) Glandular mobilization & Skin (new NAC circle) closure

parallel to the previous incision is made. Two triangular incisions are made at both sides of the two semicircular incisions. After resection of the tumor and overlying skin, the defect is filled by pulling up the inferior breast and the both side of angled incisions is sutured vertically side by side. It is very simple and easy technique. However, in small non-ptotic breast, it makes hyper-elevation of nipple (Fig. 28.3).

28.2.10 Tennis Racket Incision

Tennis racket incision is simple and very effective method for tumors in upper outer quadrant and lateral region of the breast, when the tumor size is rather large that simple lumpectomy would make serious defect. For segmentally distributed cancer (or DCIS) in a large breast, long resection (tumor size 5–10 cm, even larger than 10 cm) is possible. Sometimes, this method can be used for tumor in upper inner quadrant.

Concentric incisions are made around NAC just like the round block method described above. Then, long wedge-shaped resection including lesion and skin is done. De-epithelization between the two circular incisions is done. The defect is

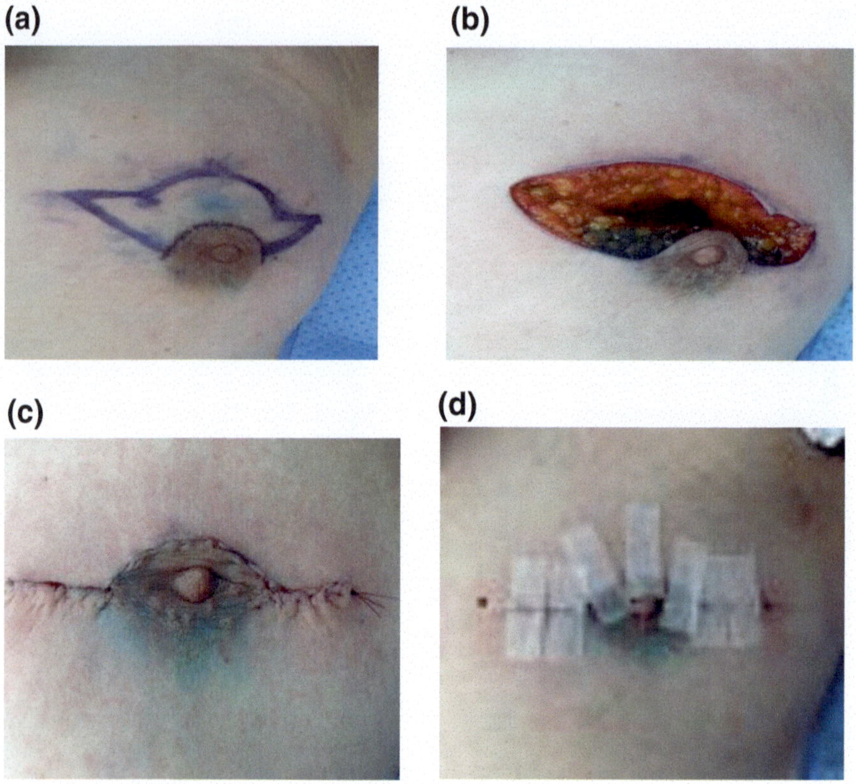

Fig. 28.3 Batwing mastopexy. (**a**) Skin marking with batwing form. (**b**) Resection of the tumor. (**c**) Reshaping by pulling up the inferior breast tissue. (**d**) Suture the incision vertically

closed with absorbable sutures by approximating the surrounding breast tissues after undermining and mobilization. Sometimes intramammarian flap technique should be used. Final skin closure is done using a subcuticular suture with 4-0 or 5-0 monocryl (Fig. 28.4).

28.2.11 Matrix Rotation Flap

This rotation flap technique uses lateral pedicle to fill the defect in UIQ. Two lines connecting between outer circumareolar incision and its arc indicate the range of resection. Burow's triangle incision near axilla should be made and used also for axillary lymph node surgery. After resection, de-epithelialization of periareolar skin is required, and then, the outer portion of breast tissue is extensively mobilized from deep fascia and rotated to fill in the defect. This method is useful for large tumor in

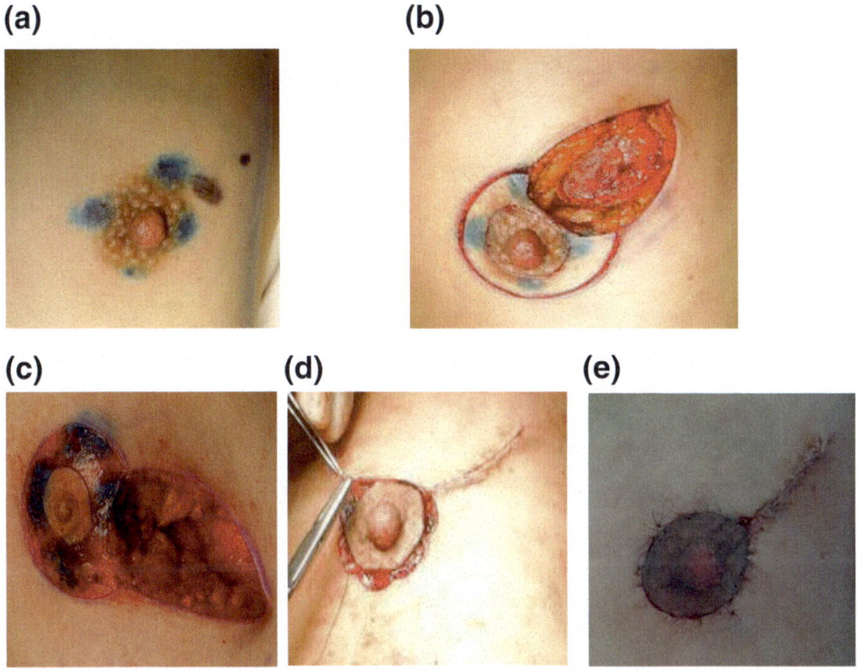

Fig. 28.4 Tennis racket incision. (**a**) Skin marking of racket shape. (**b**) Resection the tumor (**c**) glandular mobilization and de-epithelization. (**d**) NAC reposition was performed by interrupt suture with absorbable suture material (**e**) Finally skin closure with a subcuticular suture.

upper inner area of medium to large-sized breast. Large visible scar is a weakness of this technique. However, there are few choices for UIQ lesion (Fig. 28.5).

28.2.12 S-Shape Oblique Reduction Mammoplasty

S-shape oblique reduction mammoplasty allows removing tumor widely located in upper portion of breast. This technique can be applied for multifocal lesions horizontally located along the incision line. Moderate to large breast with ptosis is the best candidate for this technique. Two curved (S-shaped) lines are made from axilla toward medio-inferior portion of the breast. The distance between two incision lines is decided by the width of tumor resection and breast size. If the distance is too large, NAC can be elevated to too high position. Resection of the skin and tumor with adequate margins is done. Then, some area which is still covered with skin in lateral and medial side is de-epithelized. The upper and lower portion of excised tissue is dissected and mobilized to fill the defect. The wound is closed (Fig. 28.6).

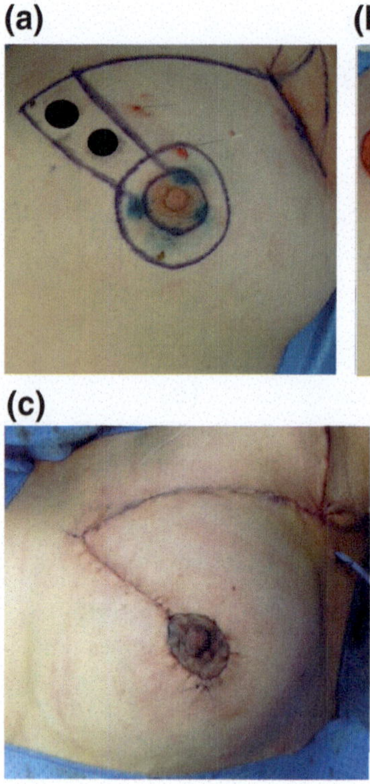

Fig. 28.5 Matrix rotation flap. (**a**) skin marking (**b**) resection and glandular tissue dissection (**c**) flap rotation and closure

28.2.13 Sup. Pedicle Mammoplasty (Inverted T Incision)

This technique is indicated for inferior area tumor (5–7 o'clock). It is best for large ptotic breast. However, because tumor in lower pole of breast usually makes worst breast contour and nipple dislocation, this technique can be applied to moderate-sized breast to prevent severe depression in lower pole. It needs several anatomical remarks the same as routine superior pedicel reduction mammoplasty. There should be a vertical line from midclavicular point to the nipple and extending to inframammary fold (IMF). A new nipple position should be marked with a new areolar line of about 4 cm diameter. Two vertical lines from areolar to new IMF make a mosque-like figure at the inferior end of breast. In a common Asian women with moderate-sized breast, the elevation of nipple is not needed, and in that case, two circumferential lines around nipple are enough. Skin is incised along the drawings, and skin of superior pedicle and around areola is de-epithelialized. The subdermal plexus should be preserved cranially while they can be incised medially and laterally. Resection of tumor is done with normal tissues within the lines.

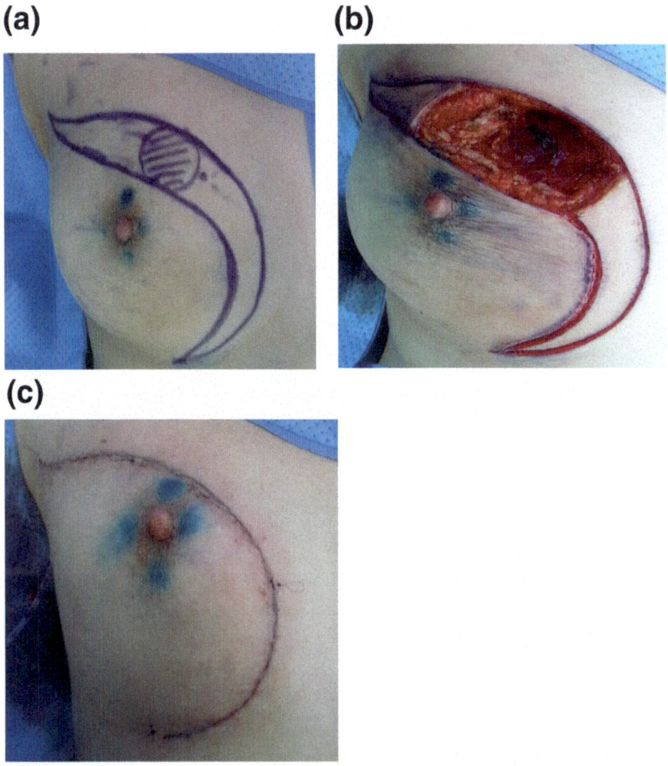

Fig. 28.6 S-shape oblique (**a**) skin marking (**b**) resection and dissection the flap (**c**) mobilization and filling the defect and closure

Glandular mobilization is usually required to make better shape. Skin is closed in two layers (Fig. 28.7).

28.2.14 Latissimus Dorsi Mini-Flap (Mini-LD Flap)

Originally, latissimus dorsi (LD) myocutaneous flaps are used to fill the wide defects incorporating overlying skin, but this conventional LD flap leaves a scar on the back and requires time and effort to change patient's position during operation. Mini-LD flap is a useful volume replacement method for tumors in upper or outer portion of breast irrespective of size of the breast. It is especially useful for diffuse in situ cancer and invasive cancer when the skin removal is not required. Skin drawing is made in upright position before operation. All operation procedure is done in lateral position of the patient. Skin incision is made along mid-axillary line from axilla to lower outer part of breast. Extensive dissection through breast parenchyme and pectoralis fascia is done. Then, superficial dissection through subcutaneous fat and breast

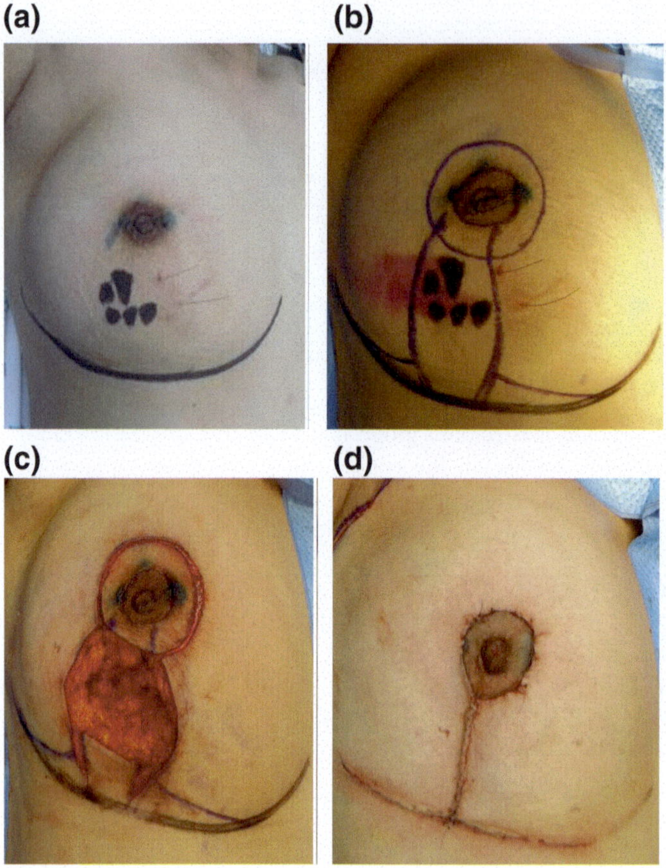

Fig. 28.7 Sup. pedicle mammoplasty (**a**) tumor location, (**b**) Skin marking. (**c**) Resection and glandular mobilization (pedicle elevation), (**d**) Transposition and closure

parenchyme is done to over the tumor site. It would be helpful to insert localization hook wire or inject charcoal at the inner and lower margin of the resection plane before operation. After removal of tumor and breast tissue, sentinel lymph node biopsy is done and identify thoracodorsal vascular bundle being careful not to injure it. Dissection of LD muscle can be easily done through the same incision. Preserving the pedicle, dissected LD muscle is repositioned to the breast resection defect and loosely sutured to breast parenchymal cavity wall. After meticulous hemostasis and drain insertion, skin closure is done (Fig. 28.8).

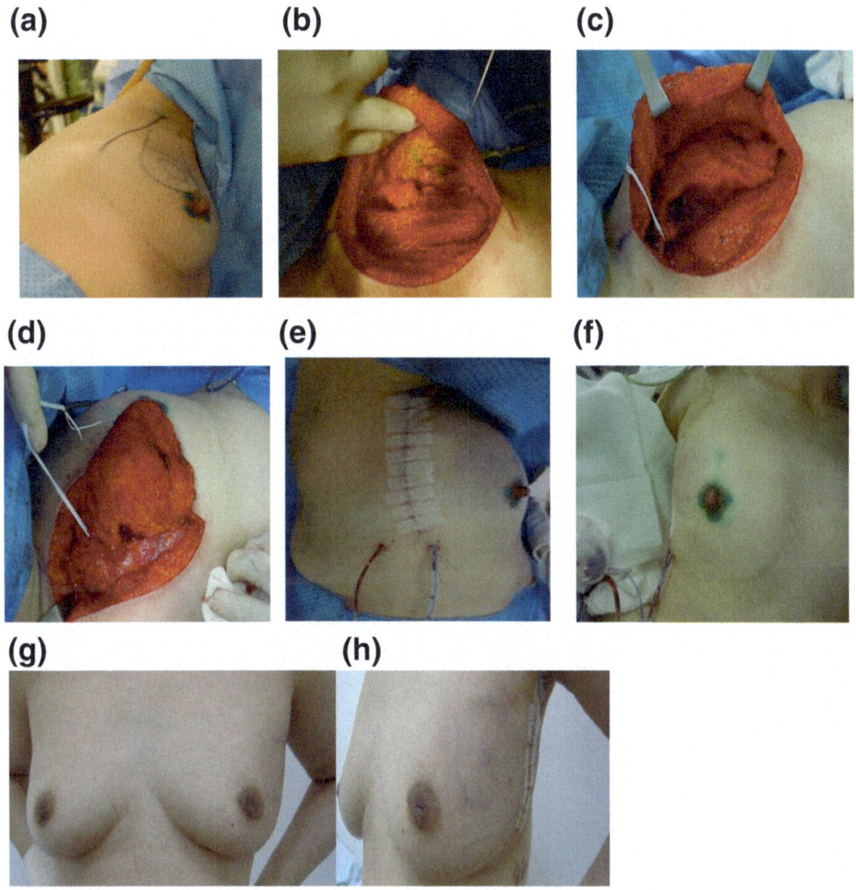

Fig. 28.8 Mini-LD flap. (**a**) Skin incision, (**b**)–(**c**) resection of breast tumor, (**d**) The mini-LD flap harvest, (**f**) fill the defect with the flap and closure, (**g**) postoperative status

28.2.15 Omental Flap (Laparoscopically Harvested Omental Flap)

Omental flap is a useful volume replacement technique for large tumor in inferior or medial region of the breast. It is especially good for diffuse in situ or invasive cancer not requiring removal of overlying skin. When breast size is not too large and expected omental volume is enough, total mastectomy and total replacement are also possible. The best skin incision is along inframammary fold, but radial incision on the tumor is also possible. After resection of the entire inferomedial quadrant of breast or wide local excision, dissection is done to the xiphoid and subcostal angle. Laparoscopy for harvesting greater omentum was then performed. Omental dissection is done using one umbilical camera port and three 5-mm ports. Harmonic

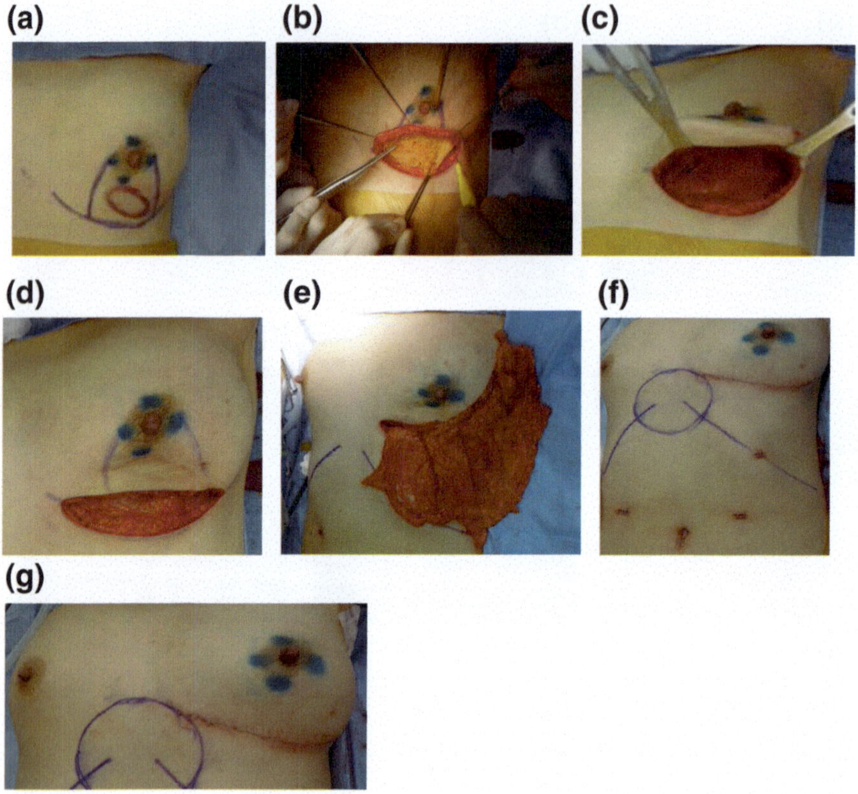

Fig. 28.9 Omental flap. (**a**) Inframammary skin incision (**b**)–(**d**) Resection of breast tumor (**e**) An omental flap harvest (**f**) Fill the defect with the flap. (**g**) Closure

Scalpel (Ethicon Endo-Surgery Inc., Cincinnati, OH) is useful as other laparoscopic surgery. It is important to preserve the roots of the gastroepiploic vessels as a pedicle. About two-finger width tunnel is made just lateral to xiphoid process connecting into the abdominal cavity. It is important to make enough size of tunnel not to strangulate the pedicle. Omental flap is carefully brought into breast cavity avoiding twist. Anchoring suture of the omental flap to cavity wall or muscle is not usually required. The wound of breast is closed in two layers, and laparoscopy wound is closed as routine manner. Be careful not to press pedicle with compression dressing or Surgi-Bra (Fig. 28.9).

28.3 Current Evidence and Concepts

There are many gaps concerning satisfaction and quality of life between patients undergoing breast cancer treatment and surgeons.

The essential and central element of the breast surgeon is the duty to obtain a good aesthetic outcome without compromising oncologic control. The outcome measurement of the OPS consisted of local recurrence, cosmesis, and patients satisfaction. We will discuss the three aspects of outcome measures after oncoplastic breast-conserving surgery here.

28.3.1 Local Recurrence Rate After OPS

Lorenz et al. reported local and distant recurrence rate after OPS recently [12]. Between 2000 and 2008, in the European Institute of Oncology (IEO) Breast Cancer Institutional Database, they identified 454 consecutive patients who underwent an oncoplastic approach for primary invasive breast tumors. They described the events in both groups, with a median follow-up of 7.2 years. The overall survival is similar within the two groups, being 91.4% and 91.3% at 10-year in the OPS group and in the control group respectively. The disease-free survival is slight lower in the OPS group (69% vs.73.1% at 10-year). The difference is not statistically significant.

The incidence of local events is slightly higher in the OPS group (3.2% vs. 1.8% at 5-year, 6.7% vs. 4.2% at 10-year); the incidence of regional events (3.1% vs. 2.8% at 10-year) and distant events (12.7% vs.11.6% at 10-year) is similar in the two groups. Lymphovascular infiltration and in situ component, both of which may have an influence on locoregional recurrence rates, were present respectively in 39.6% and in 66.7% of the relapsed patients.

They also reported that, in the OPS group, early complication occurred within 3 months from surgery at the side of quadrantectomy and in the healthy breast in 10.3% and 2.8%, respectively. They included infection (2.8% vs. 0.4%), wound dehiscence (3.5% vs. 0.6%), hematoma formation (2.4% vs. 1.3%), skin necrosis (1.3% vs. 0.4%), liponecrosis (2.6% vs. 1.1%), and others (3.7% vs. 0.8%). This difference seemed quite acceptable considering their larger tumor size compared to conventional BCS.

Another study compared local recurrence rate between OPS group and matched total mastectomy group in pT2-patients(larger than 2 cm tumors) [13]. The OS is similar within the two groups: 87.3% and 87.1% at 10 years in the OPS group and control group, respectively ($p = 0.74$, adjusted for multifocality and tumor size). The DFS also is similar in both groups: 60.9% and 56.3% at 10 years in the OPS group and control group, respectively. The incidence of local events is slightly higher in the OPS group (7.3% vs. 3% at 10 years), whereas the incidence of regional events is slightly higher in the mastectomy group (8% vs. 2.2% at 10 years). These differences are not statistically significant. The cumulative incidence of distant events is similar within the two groups (18.9% vs. 19.6% at 10 years in the OPS group and mastectomy group, respectively).

These results showed slightly higher local recurrence rate compared to earlier studies which reported that rate around 3% [7].

However, these results provided the best available evidence to suggest that OPS is a safe and reliable treatment for managing invasive pT1-2 breast cancers.

28.3.2 Cosmesis Measurement After OPS

Differences of contour, shape, position, or volume of the breast are the most important factors which define breast symmetry and influence cosmesis and patient satisfaction after breast surgery. There are three categories of cosmesis evaluation. First one is the patients' self-evaluation, which has several advantages like reflecting more psychosocial adaptation of patients to aesthetic result. But the reproducibility of self-evaluation is low. They are depended on patients' age and socioeconomic status. Observer's evaluation is the second one, which is like Harvard scale or Harris four-point scale. Patients' scar visibility, breast size, breast shape, nipple position, and skin color would be measured directly by one or several observers.

Conventional methods for aesthetic evaluation of breast-conserving surgery include assessment of patient's appearance directly, or through photographs, by one or more observers. Direct observation allows not only global appreciation but also other factors not visualized in captured images (skin atrophy, edema of breast and arm). However, Indirect evaluation through photographs has several advantages that the images can be saved permanently, visualized when necessary, and easily analyzed by different observers.

The third method is objective evaluation by specific tools. Objective methods attempt to measure differences between the right and the left breast according to linear distances like anthropomorphic measurements [14] or volume measurements using techniques like water displacement, [15] casting techniques, mammography or CT and MRI measurements. In addition, two software systems called breast analyzing tool (BAT) [16] and the Breast Cancer Conservative Treatment cosmetic result (BCCT.core) [17] were developed to objectively evaluate the aesthetic surgical outcome using patient's frontal two-dimensional (2-D) photographs. The BAT evaluates breast symmetry by comparing breast area, breast circumference, and nipple position between the breasts. The BCCT.core analyzes color differences and scar appearance in addition to calculate asymmetry.

A recent comparison of them on the same set of cases showed a similar performance on low-quality images and a superior performance of the BCCT.core software on higher quality images. This was attributed to the inclusion of color and scar features.

28.3.3 Patients Satisfaction and Quality of Life.

The impact of the disease and interventions on quality of life (QoL) in cancer patients has been increasingly recognized. Post-treatment QoL is particularly important for breast cancer patients, whose 5-year survival rates exceed 88% [18, 19]. Factors that impact patient QoL are multidimensional and difficult to define. For example, breast-specific concerns, such as altered sense of femininity, feelings of decreased attractiveness, and changes in body image and sexuality, as well as factors associated with many types of cancer, including pain, fear of recurrence, and fatigue, could affect general QoL [20, 21].

We attempted to clarify the relationships among aesthetic results and patient QoL in women who have undergone breast cancer surgery [22]. The impact of objectively measured breast cosmetic results and patient reported body image on QoL was analyzed a median 2.1 years after BCS or TMIR (total mastectomy with immediate reconstruction). We found that breast symmetry, measured objectively by BCCT. core software and panel judgment, did not correlate with patients' general QoL. In contrast, patient self-reported body image scale (BIS) was significantly associated with almost all general QoL outcomes.

In our study, the mean BIS among the 531 patients in the BCS and TMIR groups was 17.9 ± 5.4. Dichotomization relative to mean score showed that 365 patients (67.0%) could be classified as having good and 166 (34%) as having poor BIS. As expected, BIS was significantly better in the BCS and TMIR groups than in the total mastectomy (TM) group. Objectively measured cosmetic results, using both the BCCT.core and panel score, however, did not correlate significantly with BIS. However, BIS was significantly associated with almost all QoL factors of the QLQ-C30, QLQ-BR23, and HADS. This correlation was observed not only in the BCS and TMIR groups, but in the TM group, indicating that body image perception differs among individuals in all three groups.

Surgeons usually assume that patients want better cosmetic outcomes after surgery and that outcomes directly correlate with QoL. Thus, efforts are underway to develop oncoplastic and reconstructive surgical techniques. However, our results do not strongly indicate that superior surgical cosmetic outcomes translate into improved QoL. These findings support previous reports advocating TM over BCS on the basis of lower fear of the future and mood disturbances in patients who underwent mastectomy [23–25].

There is no consensus about whether postoperative QoL differs according to type of surgery (e.g., BCS vs. TM vs. TMIR). [26–28] Our study found that patient body image perception was better following BCS than following TMIR or TM. Also, patient QoL was better in the BCS or TMIR group than in the TM group, as shown by multiple QLQ factors.

28.4 Future Research Direction

The introduction of three-dimensional (3-D) surface imaging enabled quantitative linear distance measurements, surface and volumetric calculations of the breast region [29] and objective breast symmetry evaluations between the left and the right breast by virtually superimposing the mirrored breasts over each other.

The benefit of this 3-D evaluation protocol for breast surgeons can be easily expanded to other clinical applications: short and long lasting results after fat grafting to determine the resorption rate for reconstruction purposes over time, the temporal effect on skin envelope enlargement and volume increase after expander inflation for breast implant reconstruction, comparison between competitive surgical techniques in breast reduction (short scar vs. inverted T, central pedicled vs. superior–/medial or inferior pedicled) or breast augmentation (round vs. anatomical implants, choice of pocket, incision techniques) could be quantified. Actual clinical studies demonstrated the innovative character and clinical benefit of the technique, especially in plastic and reconstructive breast surgery. The 3-D application for objective breast symmetry evaluation is easily applicable, sufficiently fast, observer independent, and more precise than 2-D measurements [30].

Also, there are many research opportunities to be explored in oncoplastic surgery, such as how improve oncoplastic surgery training, how to decrease re-excision rates, how to decrease complication rates, how to decrease recurrence rates, how to optimize operating room time, how to optimize aesthetic outcomes, how to reduce costs of treatment, and analysis of the aesthetic and psychological benefits of the techniques.

It has become evident that surgeons working to aid the woman with breast cancer must become sensitive to the potential for a negative impact of the breast cancer experience on any one of many domains of quality of life and must discuss sufficiently with the patients about the results and appearance of breast cancer surgery.

28.4.1 The Bench

- Oncoplastic BCS requires combined skills, knowledge, and understanding of both oncological and plastic surgeries, which may be optimally delivered by a single oncoplastic surgeon.
- Proper surgery type should be selected by considering breast size, tumor location, and patient's opinion about contralateral breast surgery.

28.4.2 Translation

- Cosmetic result and satisfaction of oncoplastic BCS was very good, almost 80-90% patients were scored high with acceptable oncologic results.
- Oncoplastic BCS could be considered preferentially than SSM with reconstruction if it is possible.

28.4.3 The Bedside

- Beyond the original OPS techniques, new attempts like minimal invasive surgery or fat transplantation should be further developed.
- Further research regarding cosmesis and quality of life in breast cancer patients could help breast cancer patients' early recovery to their daily life.

References

1. Kaur N, Petit JY, Rietjens M, Maffini F, Luini A, Gatti G, et al. Comparative study of surgical margins in oncoplastic surgery and quadrantectomy in breast cancer. Ann Surg Oncol. 2005;12 (7):539–45.
2. Haloua MH, Krekel NM, Winters HA, Rietveld DH, Meijer S, Bloemers FW, et al. A systematic review of oncoplastic breast-conserving surgery: current weaknesses and future prospects. Ann Surg. 2013;257(4):609–20.
3. Bogusevicius A, Cepuliene D, Sepetauskiene E. The integrated evaluation of the results of oncoplastic surgery for locally advanced breast cancer. Breast J. 2014;20(1):53–60.
4. Berry MG, Fitoussi AD, Curnier A, Couturaud B, Salmon RJ. Oncoplastic breast surgery: a review and systematic approach. J Plast Reconstr Aesth Surg: JPRAS. 2010;63(8):1233–43.
5. Giacalone PL, Roger P, Dubon O, El Gareh N, Rihaoui S, Taourel P, et al. Comparative study of the accuracy of breast resection in oncoplastic surgery and quadrantectomy in breast cancer. Ann Surg Oncol. 2007;14(2):605–14.
6. Clough KB, Lewis JS, Couturaud B, Fitoussi A, Nos C, Falcou MC. Oncoplastic techniques allow extensive resections for breast-conserving therapy of breast carcinomas. Ann Surg. 2003;237(1):26–34.
7. Rietjens M, Urban CA, Rey PC, Mazzarol G, Maisonneuve P, Garusi C, et al. Long-term oncological results of breast conservative treatment with oncoplastic surgery. Breast. 2007;16 (4):387–95.
8. Fitoussi AD, Berry MG, Fama F, Falcou MC, Curnier A, Couturaud B, et al. Oncoplastic breast surgery for cancer: analysis of 540 consecutive cases [outcomes article]. Plast Reconstr Surg. 2010;125(2):454–62.
9. Gulcelik MA, Dogan L, Camlibel M, Karaman N, Kuru B, Alagol H, et al. Early complications of a reduction mammoplasty technique in the treatment of macromastia with or without breast cancer. Clin Breast Cancer. 2011;11(6):395–9.
10. Clough KB, Kaufman GJ, Nos C, Buccimazza I, Sarfati IM. Improving breast cancer surgery: a classification and quadrant per quadrant atlas for oncoplastic surgery. Ann Surg Oncol. 2010;17 (5):1375–91.
11. Yang JD, Bae SG, Chung HY, Cho BC, Park HY, Jung JH. The usefulness of oncoplastic volume displacement techniques in the superiorly located breast cancers for Korean patients with small to moderate-sized breasts. Ann Plast Surg. 2011;67(5):474–80.
12. De Lorenzi F, Hubner G, Rotmensz N, Bagnardi V, Loschi P, Maisonneuve P, et al. Oncological results of oncoplastic breast-conserving surgery: long term follow-up of a large series at a single institution: a matched-cohort analysis. Eur J Surg Oncol. 2016;42(1):71–7.
13. De Lorenzi F, Loschi P, Bagnardi V, Rotmensz N, Hubner G, Mazzarol G, et al. Oncoplastic breast-conserving surgery for tumors larger than 2 centimeters: is it Oncologically safe? A matched-cohort analysis. Ann Surg Oncol. 2016;23(6):1852–9.
14. Smith DJ Jr, Palin WE Jr, Katch VL, Bennett JE. Breast volume and anthropomorphic measurements: normal values. Plast Reconstr Surg. 1986;78(3):331–5.

15. Schultz RC, Dolezal RF, Nolan J. Further applications of Archimedes' principle in the correction of asymmetrical breasts. Ann Plast Surg. 1986;16(2):98–101.
16. Fitzal F, Krois W, Trischler H, Wutzel L, Riedl O, Kuhbelbock U, et al. The use of a breast symmetry index for objective evaluation of breast cosmesis. Breast. 2007;16(4):429–35.
17. Cardoso MJ, Cardoso J, Amaral N, Azevedo I, Barreau L, Bernardo M, et al. Turning subjective into objective: the BCCT.Core software for evaluation of cosmetic results in breast cancer conservative treatment. Breast. 2007;16(5):456–61.
18. Sprangers MA, Groenvold M, Arraras JI, Franklin J, te Velde A, Muller M, et al. The European Organization for research and treatment of cancer breast cancer-specific quality-of-life questionnaire module: first results from a three-country field study. J Clin Oncol Off J Am Soc Clin Oncol. 1996;14(10):2756–68.
19. Brady MJ, Cella DF, Mo F, Bonomi AE, Tulsky DS, Lloyd SR, et al. Reliability and validity of the functional assessment of Cancer therapy-breast quality-of-life instrument. J Clin Oncol Off J Am Soc Clin Oncol. 1997;15(3):974–86.
20. Waljee JF, Hu ES, Ubel PA, Smith DM, Newman LA, Alderman AK. Effect of esthetic outcome after breast-conserving surgery on psychosocial functioning and quality of life. J Clin Oncol Off J Am Soc Clin Oncol. 2008;26(20):3331–7.
21. Avis NE, Crawford S, Manuel J. Quality of life among younger women with breast cancer. J Clin Oncol Off J Am Soc Clin Oncol. 2005;23(15):3322–30.
22. Kim MK, Kim T, Moon HG, Jin US, Kim K, Kim J, et al. Effect of cosmetic outcome on quality of life after breast cancer surgery. Eur J Surg Oncol. 2015;41(3):426–32.
23. Nissen MJ, Swenson KK, Ritz LJ, Farrell JB, Sladek ML, Lally RM. Quality of life after breast carcinoma surgery: a comparison of three surgical procedures. Cancer. 2001;91(7):1238–46.
24. Nold RJ, Beamer RL, Helmer SD, McBoyle MF. Factors influencing a woman's choice to undergo breast-conserving surgery versus modified radical mastectomy. Am J Surg. 2000;180 (6):413–8.
25. Collins ED, Moore CP, Clay KF, Kearing SA, O'Connor AM, Llewellyn-Thomas HA, et al. Can women with early-stage breast cancer make an informed decision for mastectomy? J Clin Oncol Off J Am Soc Clin Oncol. 2009;27(4):519–25.
26. Markopoulos C, Tsaroucha AK, Kouskos E, Mantas D, Antonopoulou Z, Karvelis S. Impact of breast cancer surgery on the self-esteem and sexual life of female patients. J Int Med Res. 2009;37(1):182–8.
27. Avis NE, Crawford S, Manuel J. Psychosocial problems among younger women with breast cancer. Psychooncology. 2004;13(5):295–308.
28. Poulsen B, Graversen HP, Beckmann J, Blichert-Toft M. A comparative study of post-operative psychosocial function in women with primary operable breast cancer randomized to breast conservation therapy or mastectomy. Eur J Surg Oncol. 1997;23(4):327–34.
29. Nahabedian MY, Galdino G. Symmetrical breast reconstruction: is there a role for three-dimensional digital photography? Plast Reconstr Surg. 2003;112(6):1582–90.
30. Eder M, Waldenfels FV, Swobodnik A, Kloppel M, Pape AK, Schuster T, et al. Objective breast symmetry evaluation using 3-D surface imaging. Breast. 2012;21(2):152–8.

Chapter 29
Diet Before and After Breast Cancer

Jung Eun Lee

Abstract The incidence of breast cancer has dramatically increased recently in several Asian countries. This region has experienced rapid economic growth and demographic and environmental changes. Breast cancer rates vary substantially among countries, with a lower incidence in developing countries than that in Western countries. Given the upward trend of breast cancer incidence in Asian countries and the large variation in incidence around the world, dietary changes may contribute to breast cancer development. In particular, nutrients and foods from animal sources have drawn attention as potential causes of breast cancer given that obesity and energy balance appear to be important factors associated with breast cancer risk. However, prospective cohort and intervention studies do not support the hypothesis that diet in middle life influences breast cancer development. However, recent studies have provided better insight into the roles of dietary factors in specific types of breast cancers, such as estrogen receptor-negative (ER-) breast cancer. Some studies suggest that diet in early life may play a substantial role in breast cancer development, but data and evidence remain limited.

Although etiologic and epidemiologic studies have long studied modifiable risk factors for breast cancer incidence, much remains to be explored regarding the role of diet after a breast cancer diagnosis. Several epidemiologic studies have explored the factors that improve breast cancer survival rates, including diet, physical activity, and body mass index (BMI). While there is evidence of the effect of BMI on breast cancer mortality, the effects of changing dietary habits after a breast cancer diagnosis on survival or recurrence are less clear. A report of the World Cancer Research Fund stated that evidence was not sufficient to draw firm conclusions about the effect of diet and nutrition on breast cancer prognosis, but it did suggest a link between diet and breast cancer survival.

The global burden of breast cancer is increasing and breast cancer is a major and emerging health problem in both developed and developing countries. For example, the five-year survival rate for Korean breast cancer patients has improved from

J. E. Lee (✉)
Department of Food and Nutrition, Seoul National University, Seoul, South Korea
e-mail: jungelee@snu.ac.kr

D.-Y. Noh et al. (eds.), *Translational Research in Breast Cancer*, Advances in Experimental Medicine and Biology 1187,
https://doi.org/10.1007/978-981-32-9620-6_29

78.0% in 1993–1995 to 92.7% in 2012–2016. This improvement emphasizes the importance of supportive care, diet, and quality of life for breast cancer survivors. However, we have limited data of non-Western breast cancer survivors. There is a need to examine the role of diet in breast cancer survival in both Western and non-Western regions.

Keywords Diet · Breast cancer incidence · Breast cancer survival · Cohort study · Intervention study

29.1 Introduction

The incidence of breast cancer has dramatically increased in recent years in several Asian countries, where there has been rapid economic growth and demographic and environmental changes. In Korea, the incidence of breast cancer is the highest in women in 2016. The age-standardized incidence rate of breast cancer has steadily increased, reaching 54.9 per 100,000 in 2016 with an average annual increase of 7.8% from 1999 to 2016 [1]. However, the incidence rate in Korea remains still lower than that of Western countries. The age-standardized incidence rates of breast cancer (per 100,000) were 105.0 in Denmark, 95.0 in U.K., 92.9 in the US, and 86.0 in Australia in 2012 [2]. This large international variation in incidence, with incidence lower in developing countries than in Western countries, and the rapid upward trend in parts of Asia may suggest the important roles of dietary factors in breast cancer development.

The association between dietary factors and breast cancer risk has long been studied in epidemiologic research. Accumulating evidence suggests that maintaining healthy body weight and abstaining from alcohol can help to prevent breast cancer [3]. However, there is limited evidence regarding the association of diet in adulthood, including intake of fruit and vegetables, dairy products, and micronutrients. Future research should examine the role of soy products, vitamin D, diet during childhood and adolescence, and the interaction of diet with genetic and microbiological effects. In particular, dietary exposure in early life is of great interest.

Early detection, treatment improvement, and social support have contributed to improvement of breast cancer outcomes. The global comparison of population-based cancer survival (CONCORD)-2 study showed that five-year survival from breast cancer has increased steadily in most developed countries and the age-standardized 5-year survival from breast cancer was 80% or higher in 34 countries in women diagnosed between 2005–2009, including Korea [4]. Survival statistics based on the Korea Central Cancer Registry data linked to mortality data from Ministry of the Interior and Safety reported that five-year survival rate for Korean breast cancer patients has improved from 78.0% in 1993–1995 to 92.7% in 2012–2016 [1]. Global survival improvements emphasize the importance of supportive care, diet, and quality of life for breast cancer survivors. However, although evidence that maintaining a healthy weight and engaging in regular physical activity improved breast cancer prognosis, the association between diet after breast cancer diagnosis and survival or recurrence of breast cancer is less clear.

29.2 Diet before Breast Cancer and Breast Cancer Risk

29.2.1 Fat Intake

Ecologic studies suggested that dietary fat was associated with an increased risk of breast cancer, and several case-control studies supported this hypothesis [5]. However, total fat intake did not appear to prevent breast cancer in several prospective cohort studies [6], which are less prone to recall bias and selection bias than case-control studies. In a pooled analysis of seven prospective cohort studies, including 4980 cases from studies involving 337,819 women, RR (95% CI) for comparing the highest and the lowest quintiles was 1.05 (0.94–1.16) [6]. When different latencies between total fat intake and occurrence of breast cancer (0–4, 4–8, 8–12, 12–16, and 16–20 years) were taken into account, there was still no association between total fat intake and breast cancer in a cohort study [7]. The Women's Health Initiative Dietary Modification Trial found that reducing dietary fat did not reduce the risk of breast cancer in 48,835 postmenopausal women, randomly assigned to the dietary modification intervention group ($n = 19{,}541$) or the comparison group ($n = 29{,}294$) [8].

Regarding types of fat, the Pooling Project, an international consortium of prospective cohort studies, reported a weak positive association between saturated fat and breast cancer risk (RR = 1.09; 1.00–1.19 for 5% energy increment from saturated fat), but no such association for monounsaturated or polyunsaturated fat intake [9]. When investigators in the Nurses' Health Study analyzed diet only during premenopausal period, animal fat intake was associated with increasing risk of breast cancer (RR = 1.33 for the highest vs. the lowest quintiles), but vegetable fat intake was not [10].

In summary, considerable evidence supports that fat intake in middle life does not increase the risk of breast cancer, but fat from animal sources in early adulthood may be associated with breast cancer risk. The important effects of diet in early adulthood warrant further research.

29.2.2 Fruits and Vegetables

Prospective cohort studies indicate that total fruit and total vegetable intake in adulthood do not appear to prevent breast cancer [11, 12]. However, a recent cohort study found that this association might vary by type of breast cancer. A pooled analysis of 20 cohort studies including 993,466 women followed for 11 to 20 years found an inverse association between total fruit and vegetable intake and risk of ER−breast cancer, but there was no association with risk of breast cancer overall or estrogen receptor (ER) + tumors [13]; RRs (95% CIs) for the highest vs. the lowest quintiles of total vegetable intake were 0.82 (0.74–0.90) for ER− breast cancer and 1.04 (0.97–1.11) for ER+ breast cancer. In the European Prospective Investigation into Cancer and Nutrition (EPIC) cohort, including 10,197 incident invasive breast cancers with a median follow-up of 11.5 years, total vegetable intake had a stronger association with a lower risk of ER− progesterone receptor (PR)-breast cancer (RR = 0.74; 95% CI = 0.57–0.96 for the highest vs. the lowest quintiles) than ER +PR+ breast cancer [14].

29.2.3 Carbohydrate and Carbohydrate Quality

The hypothesis that cancer arises partly through insulin and the insulin-like growth factor axis has inspired research on the associations of carbohydrate and carbohydrate quality, as measured by glycemic index and glycemic load, with breast cancer risk. Although individual cohort studies have reported contradictory findings, a recent meta-analysis suggested a potential link of carbohydrate intake and glycemic load with ER-breast cancer [15]. As part of the World Cancer Research Fund/ American Institute for Cancer Research Continuous Update Project, Schlesinger S et al. conducted a systematic review and meta-analysis and found that glycemic load and carbohydrate intake were positively associated with breast cancer in postmenopausal women with ER− tumors; summary RRs (95% CIs) were 1.28 (1.08–1.52) for per 50 units/day of glycemic load and 1.13 (1.02–1.25) for per 50 g/day of carbohydrate intake [15].

29.2.4 Soy Product

Soy products have potential anti- and pro-estrogenic effects due to isoflavones, the major flavonoids of soy products. Isoflavones have been suggested to stimulate tumor growth [16, 17] because of their structural similarity to estrogen and high affinity for the estrogen receptor [18]. In vitro and in vivo studies suggested that isoflavones might exert anti-estrogenic effects on breast tissue by competing with the estrogen receptor, therefore blocking the action of endogenous estrogens, or other mechanisms including antioxidative potency [19] or inhibition of angiogenesis [20] or inhibition of tyrosine kinase [21]. Several cohort studies examined whether isoflavones were associated with breast cancer risk; however, the results were not consistent [22–24]. A recent report from the World Cancer Research Fund concluded that there is limited evidence to support the benefit or harm of soy products for breast cancer prevention [3].

29.2.5 Dietary Patterns

Dietary patterns have been attractive for both researchers and public because it deals with the effects of diet as a whole rather the effects of individual nutrients or foods. People often want to hear how to eat overall to improve their health, and dietary pattern analysis identifies overall diets that lower the risk of poor health outcomes [25]. The US Nurses' Health Study observed no significant association for either Prudent or Western dietary patterns in relation to overall breast cancer risk. However, when investigators categorized breast cancers into ER− and ER+ breast cancers, they found an inverse association between the Prudent dietary pattern and ER− breast cancer risk [26]. Likewise, a priori dietary quality indices (Alternate Healthy Eating Index, Recommended Food Score, and the alternate Mediterranean Diet Score) were inversely associated with ER− breast cancer risk; RRs for the highest vs. the lowest quintiles ranged from 0.69 to 0.79 for these indices with a statistically significant trend [27]. The PREDIMED study, a randomized, single-blind, controlled trial conducted in Spain, found that a Mediterranean diet lowered primary breast cancer risk [28]. The association between dietary patterns and breast cancer incidence remains to be explored in terms of the effect modification by other health-related behaviors, histological types, genetic and metabolic profiles.

29.2.6 Micronutrients

Dietary calcium has been suggested to prevent breast cancer as intake of dairy products showed an inverse association with breast cancer [29]. Also, dietary intake and circulating levels of vitamin D, which is often added to dairy products in the US, were associated with a lower risk of breast cancer in some observational studies [30–32], but not in others [33, 34]. The World Cancer Research Fund suggested that diets high in calcium may be inversely associated with the risk of premenopausal breast cancer, but there is limited evidence to draw conclusions about vitamin D [3]. In the Women's Health Initiative trial, calcium and vitamin D supplementation did not reduce breast cancer incidence among postmenopausal women [35].

Carotenoids, known for their antioxidant properties, are abundant in fruits and vegetables. Many observational studies have examined the role of carotenoids in cancer prevention. A pooled analysis of 18 prospective cohort studies found that inverse associations for α-carotene, β-carotene, and lutein/zeaxanthin intakes were limited to ER− breast cancer, whereas no associations were noted for ER+ breast cancer risk [36]. In a pooled analysis of prospective data, circulating levels of carotenoids were inversely associated with overall breast cancer risk and inverse associations were more apparent for ER− breast cancer than ER+ breast cancer for α-carotene and β-carotene [37]. Similarly, the European Prospective Investigation into Cancer and Nutrition cohort showed that higher concentrations of plasma β-carotene and α-carotene were associated with a lower risk of ER− breast cancer

[38]. Other antioxidant nutrients, including vitamins C and E and selenium, did not show consistent results in prospective cohort studies [3].

29.2.7 *Diet in Early Life*

In the 1980s, Willett [39] and DeWaard and Trichopoulos [40] proposed a relationship between breast cancer risk with an energy-rich diet during puberty and adolescence. Taller height, which reflects childhood nutrition, is an independent risk factor for breast cancer [41]. The potential plausible explanation is that early life around the time of mammary gland development may be a critical period in breast cancer development. A prospective cohort study in Denmark found that high stature at 14 years of age and peak growth at an early age were associated with the risk of breast cancer [42], suggesting that growth during adolescence is an important factor for breast cancer.

Limited prospective cohort studies have reported a potential link between diet in early life and breast cancer risk. Red meat intake in adolescence was significantly associated with a higher premenopausal breast cancer risk (RR = 1.43; 95%CI, 1.05–1.94 for the highest vs. the lowest quintiles), but not with postmenopausal breast cancer risk [43]. Total fruit intake [44] and dietary fiber intake [45] in adolescence lowered the risk of breast cancer. Whole-grain intake during adolescent and early adulthood was inversely associated with premenopausal breast cancer risk (RR = 0.74; 95% CI 0.56–0.99 for the highest vs. the lowest quintiles), but not with overall or postmenopausal breast cancer risk [46]. A comparison of the findings on dietary factors in adolescence and adulthood in relation to breast cancer incidence in the Nurses' Health Study I and II is presented in Table 29.1.

29.3 Diet after Breast Cancer and Breast Cancer Survival

Several prospective cohort and intervention studies have investigated the role of diet in breast cancer prognosis (Table 29.2). Although evidence regarding diet and breast cancer survival has been accumulating, the data are mainly from studies of Western populations. Few Asian studies have explored the association between diet and breast cancer survival.

29.3.1 *Dietary Patterns*

Recent prospective cohort studies reported that dietary patterns are an important component in addressing a healthy diet for breast cancer survivors (Table 29.3). Relatively consistent findings showed that healthy dietary patterns lowered the risk

Table 29.1 Comparison of the results; dietary factors during adolescence and during adulthood in relation to breast cancer incidence in the Nurses' Health Study I and II

Dietary factors	Study Characteristics	Dietary intake during mid-life or later adulthood	Dietary intake during adolescence
Meat	First author	Holmes MD [47]	Farvid MS [43]
	No. of participants	88,647 women	44,231 premenopausal women
	No. of breast cancer cases	4107 cases	1132 cases
	Follow-up period	1980–1998	1998–2011
	Results	• RR (95% CI) for the highest vs. the lowest quintile of red meat intake = 0.94 (0.84–1.05)	• RR (95% CI) for the highest vs. the lowest of red meat intake = 1.43 (1.05–1.94) for premenopausal breast cancer • RR (95%CI) for replacement of one serving/day of total red meat with one serving of combination of poultry, fish, legumes, and nuts = 0.85 (0.74–0.96) for overall breast cancer and 0.77 (0.64–0.92) for premenopausal breast cancer
Fruit and vegetable	First author	Smith-Warner SA [11]	Farvid MS [44]
	No. of participants	89,046 women in the NHS I (a) and 68,817 women in the NHS I (b)	44,223 premenopausal women
	No. of breast cancer cases	1023 cases in the NHS I (a) and 1638 cases in the NHS I (b)	1347 cases
	Follow-up period	1980–1986 in the NHS I (a) and 1986–1996 in the NHS I (b)	1998–2013
	Results	• RR (95% CI) for 100 g/day intake increment of total fruits = 0.98 (0.95–1.02) NHS I (a) and 0.98 (0.95–1.01) NHS I (b) • RR (95% CI) for 100 g/day intake increment of total vegetables = 1.01 (0.95–1.07) NHS I (a) and 1.01 (0.98–1.05) NHS I (b)	• RR (95% CI) for the highest vs. the lowest of total fruit intake = 0.75 (0.62–0.90). • RR (95% CI) for the highest vs. the lowest of total vegetable intake = 0.85 (0.71–1.01)
Dietary fiber	First author	Holmes MD [48]	Farvid MS [45]
	No. of participants	88,678 women	44,263 premenopausal women
	No. of breast cancer cases	4092 cases	1118 cases
	Follow-up period	1980–1998	1998–2011

(continued)

Table 29.1 (continued)

Dietary factors	Study Characteristics	Dietary intake during mid-life or later adulthood	Dietary intake during adolescence
	Results	• RR (95% CI) for the highest vs. the lowest quintile of total fiber intake = 0.98 (95% CI: 0.87, 1.11)	• RR (95% CI) for the highest vs. the lowest quintile of total fiber intake = 0.84 (0.70–1.01)

Investigators divided Nurses' Health Study (NHS) I into two studies; NHS I (a) and NHS I (b)

of non-breast cancer deaths in observational studies of breast cancer survivors. The US Nurses' Health Study (NHS), a large cohort study of female nurses from 11 US states, found that adherence to healthy dietary guidelines, the Dietary Approaches to Stop Hypertension (DASH) and the Alternative Healthy Eating Index (AHEI)-2010, after breast cancer diagnosis was associated with reduced risk of non-breast cancer mortality in women with breast cancer, but not with the risk of breast cancer death or recurrence [52]. Similarly, other cohort studies found a lower risk of death from non-breast cancer causes with healthy dietary pattern [58, 61, 62]. Inflammatory potential of diet after breast cancer diagnosis was associated with mortality from cardiovascular disease, but not with breast cancer-specific mortality or all-cause mortality among women diagnosed with invasive breast cancer in the Women's Health Initiative (WHI) [67]; compared to high inflammatory diet, low inflammatory diet (low vs. high quartile) had a 56% lower risk of cardiovascular disease mortality among breast cancer survivors.

29.3.2 Soy Products

A recent pooled analysis of three cohort studies (Life After Cancer Epidemiology, Shanghai Breast Cancer Survival Study, and Women's Healthy Eating and Living) suggested a potential benefit of consuming soy products for breast cancer survival; hazard ratio (HR)s (95% CIs) for comparing $\geq$10 mg/day of isoflavones vs. <4 mg/day were 0.87 (0.70–1.10) for all-cause mortality, 0.83 (0.64–1.07) for breast cancer-specific mortality, and 0.75 (0.61–0.92) for breast cancer recurrence [68]. In that study, the inverse association was slightly stronger among women with ER− breast cancer. When stratified by tamoxifen use, although the test for interaction was not statistically significant, an inverse association between isoflavone intake and breast cancer recurrence was stronger for tamoxifen users than non-users. The Breast Cancer Family Registry, containing 6235 women with breast cancer enrolled, found that post-diagnostic isoflavone intake reduced the risk of all-cause deaths [69]. Two Chinese cohort studies of breast cancer survivors in which investigators examined a larger contrast of soy product intake compared to Western studies observed an inverse association of isoflavone intake with breast

Table 29.2 Intervention and prospective cohort studies regarding post-diagnostic diet and breast cancer survival

Intervention study				
Study name	*Location*	*Design article or example article*	*Baseline number of breast cancer survivors*	*Intervention*
Women's Intervention Nutrition Study (WINS)	US	Chlebowski RT et al. [49]	2437	Reduction in fat intake
Women's Healthy Eating and Living (WHEL)	US	Pierce JP et al. [50]	3088	Increase in vegetable, fruit, and fiber intake and a decrease in dietary fat intake
Prospective cohort study				
Study name	*Location*	*Design article or example article*	*Baseline number of breast cancer survivors*	*Method and timing of dietary assessment*
DietCompLyf	UK	Swann R et al. [51]	3159	FFQ at baseline for pre and post-diagnosis FFQs at 1-year, 1.5-year, and every year up to 6-year post-diagnosis
Nurses' Health Study (NHS)	US	Izano MA et al. [52]	More than 2000 (increasing across time because new cases occur during follow-up)	FFQs at various time points before and after diagnosis
Health, Eating, Activity, and Lifestyle (HEAL)	US	Belle FN et al. [53]	1183	FFQ at 24 months after diagnosis
Shanghai Breast Cancer Survival Study (SBCSS)	China	Shu XO et al. [54]	5042	FFQs at 6-, 18-, 36-, and 60-month post-diagnosis
Women's Healthy Eating and Living (WHEL)	US	Caan BJ et al. [55]	3088	FFQ at baseline post-diagnosis
Life After Cancer Epidemiology Study (LACE)	US	Caan B et al. [56]	2321	FFQs at baseline post-diagnosis
Collaborative Women's Longevity Study (CWLS)	US	Beasley JM et al. [57]	5791	FFQ (42% of women completed within 5 years of diagnosis of breast cancer; range: 1–16 years)
Women's Health Initiative	US	George SM et al. [58]	More than 2000 (increasing across time because new cases occur during follow-up)	FFQs administered, on average, 1.5 years after diagnosis

(continued)

Table 29.2 (continued)

The Pathways Study	US	Kwan ML et al. [59]	1539	FFQs at baseline, 6 and 24 months after baseline
After Breast Cancer Pooling Project[a]	US and China	Nechuta SJ et al. [60]	More than 18,000 (increasing across time because new cases occur during follow-up)	FFQs after diagnosis
American Cancer Society's Cancer Prevention Study-II (CPS-II) Nutrition Cohort	US	McCullough ML et al. [61]	2152	FFQs after diagnosis

[a]After Breast Cancer Pooling Project is a collaborative work of SBCSS, LACE, WHEL, and NHS

cancers-specific mortality [70] or with breast cancer recurrence among postmenopausal patients [71]. A summary of the results is presented in Table 29.4.

29.3.3 Fruits and Vegetables and their Components

Total fruit and vegetable intake was not associated with breast cancer survival in observational [57, 61, 72] and intervention studies [73]. A recent meta-analysis of nine cohort studies and one randomized trial reported no associations between pre- or post-diagnostic intake of vegetables and fruits and overall survival among breast cancer survivors; HRs (95% CIs) of overall survival comparing the highest vs. the lowest categories were 1.01 (0.72–1.42) for vegetables and fruits combined, 0.96 (0.83–1.12) for vegetables alone, and 0.99 (0.89–1.11) for fruit alone [74]. In a randomized controlled trial of the Women's Healthy Eating and Living Study, an intervention that promoted a diet high in vegetables, fruits, and fiber and low in fat did not improve breast cancer prognosis [50]. Also, the After Breast Cancer Pooling Project did not support any association between cruciferous vegetable intake after diagnosis and breast cancer prognosis [75].

Although the evidence does not suggest benefit of overall fruit and vegetable intake for breast cancer prognosis, the results regarding components abundant in fruits and vegetables are mixed. The Women's Healthy Eating and Living (WHEL) study found that plasma levels of total carotenoids, measured from blood samples during the baseline visit, were inversely associated with breast cancer recurrence among women with a history of early-stage breast cancer [73]; HR (95% CI) was 0.57 (0.37–0.89) for the highest vs. the lowest quartiles of plasma total carotenoid levels. However, intakes of carotenoids were not associated with breast cancer prognosis in other observational studies [57, 72].

The association between dietary fiber intake and breast cancer survival was examined in several cohort studies of breast cancer survivors. These studies reported

Table 29.3 The association between dietary patterns and breast cancer survival

Authors, year	Study name	Location	Baseline number of women with breast cancer	Follow-up period	Results
Kwan ML et al. [62]	LACE	US	1901	Median follow-up of 3.17 years	Healthy dietary pattern was associated with improved overall survival and non-breast cancer survival
Kroenke CH et al. [63]	NHS	US	2619	Median follow-up of 9 years	A higher intake of the prudent pattern and a lower intake of the Western pattern were associated with lower risk of death from causes other than breast cancer
Izano MA et al. [52]	NHS	US	4103	Median follow-up of 112 months	Healthy dietary choices after breast cancer were associated with reduced risk of non-breast cancer mortality
Kim EH et al. [64]	NHS	US	2729	1978–1998 to 2004	A higher alternate Mediterranean Diet Score was associated with a lower risk of non-breast cancer death in women with low physical activity
George SM et al. [65]	HEAL	US	670	6 years	Women consuming better quality diets, as defined by higher Healthy Eating Index-2005 scores, had a reduced risk of death from any cause and a reduced risk of death from breast cancer
George SM et al. [58]	WHI	US	2317	Median follow-up of 9.6 years	Better quality diet had a lower risk of death from any cause and death from non-breast cancer causes
Vrieling A et al. [66][a]	N/A	Germany	2522	Median of 5.5 years	Increasing consumption of an unhealthy dietary pattern was associated with an increased risk of non-breast cancer mortality
McCullough ML et al. [61]	CPS-II nutrition	US	2152	Mean of 3.3 years	Diets consistent with guidelines for cancer prevention were associated with non-breast cancer mortality

Study abbreviations: *LACE* Life After Cancer Epidemiology Study, *HEAL* Health, Eating, Activity, and Lifestyle, *NHS* Nurses' Health Study; and *CPS-II Nutrition* American Cancer Society's Cancer Prevention Study-II Nutrition Cohort

[a]A follow-up of cases from a case-control study

no statistically significant association with overall survival [53, 57] or with breast cancer-specific survival [76], and a statistically significant inverse association with overall survival [72, 77] or with recurrence among women with late stage breast cancer [78].

29.3.4 Fats

The possible link between total fat intake and breast cancer survival has long been the focus of attention. However, the evidence remains inconclusive [79]. For types of fat, several cohort studies examining the associations between intakes of saturated fat, unsaturated fat, and trans-fat and breast cancer-specific and overall mortality among breast cancer survivors had inconsistent findings. The Collaborative Women's Longevity Study reported an increased risk of overall mortality with increasing intakes of saturated fat and trans-fat, but no association for mono- or polyunsaturated fat intake [57]. Other studies have reported no statistically significant associations [72, 76] or increased risk of all-cause mortality for increasing saturated fat intake [77, 80], A U-shaped association has been reported for the polyunsaturated to saturated ratio [81]. Marine fatty acids from food were associated with a reduced risk of recurrences and deaths in the in the Women's Healthy Eating and Living (WHEL) Study. Women with higher intakes of EPA and DHA from food had a 28% lower risk of breast cancer recurrence (HR comparing top vs. bottom tertiles = 0.72 (95% CI = 0.57–0.90)) and 41% lower risk of all-cause mortality (HR comparing top vs. bottom tertiles = 0.59 (95% CI = 0.43–0.82) [82]. Further research is warranted on omega-3 fatty acids.

29.3.5 Vitamin D

Vitamin D has been hypothesized to decrease cancer risk from ecologic [83] and observational studies [84] because of its anti-carcinogenic properties, including inhibition of angiogenesis and proliferation and promotion of differentiation and apoptosis. Goodwin PJ et al. reported that breast cancer survivors with low prognostic levels of 25-hydroxyvitamin D ($<$50 nmol/L), a good indicator of vitamin D status, had 1.71 times higher risk of distant recurrence and 1.60 times higher risk of death compared to those with sufficient levels ($\geq$72 nmol/L) [85]. A meta-analysis involving five studies of 4413 women with breast cancer reported that pooled hazard ratios (95% confidence intervals) comparing the highest with lowest categories were 0.62 (0.49–0.78) for all-cause mortality and 0.58 (0.38–0.84) for breast cancer-specific mortality [86].

Table 29.4 Prospective cohort studies regarding the association between isoflavones or soy products and breast cancer survival

Authors, year	Study name	Location	Ethnicity	Baseline number of women with breast cancer	Follow-up period	No. of endpoints	Results (HR and 95% CI)
Shu XO et al. [54]	Shanghai Breast Cancer Survival Study (SBCSS)	China	Asian	5042	2002–2009 (median follow-up of 3.9 years)	444 deaths 534 recurrence or breast cancer-related death	Soy food intake All-cause deaths: 0.71 (95% CI, 0.54–0.92) for ≥15.31 g/day vs. ≤5.31 g/day Recurrence/breast cancer-specific deaths: 0.68 (95% CI, 0.54–0.87) for ≥15.31 g/day vs. ≤5.31 g/day Isoflavones All-cause deaths: 0.79 (95% CI, 0.61–1.03) for ≥62.68 mg/day vs. ≤20.00 mg/day Recurrence/breast cancer-specific deaths: 0.77 (95% CI, 0.60–0.98) for ≥62.68 mg/day vs. ≤20.00 mg/day
Nechuta SJ et al. [68]	After Breast Cancer Pooling Project	US and China	White, Black, Asian, Hispanic, and other	9514	Mean follow-up of 7.4 years	1171 total deaths 881 breast cancer-specific deaths 1348 recurrences	Isoflavones All-cause deaths: 0.87 (95% CI, 0.70–1.10) for ≥10 mg/day vs. <4 mg/day Breast cancer-specific deaths: 0.83 (95% CI, 0.64–1.07) for ≥10 mg/day vs. <4 mg/day Recurrence: 0.75 (95% CI, 0.61–0.92) for ≥10 mg/day vs. <4 mg/day

(continued)

Table 29.4 (continued)

Authors, year	Study name	Location	Ethnicity	Baseline number of women with breast cancer	Follow-up period	No. of endpoints	Results (HR and 95% CI)
Zhang YF et al. [70]	N/A	China	Asian	616	2004–2006 to 2011	79 breast cancer-specific deaths	Isoflavones Breast cancer-specific deaths: 0.62 (95% CI, 0.42–0.90) for >28.83 mg/day vs. <7.56 mg/day Soy protein Breast cancer-specific deaths: 0.71 (95% CI, 0.52–0.98) for >13.03 mg/day vs. <2.12 mg/day
Kang X et al. [71]	N/A	China	Asian	524	2002–2003 to 2008	154 overall deaths 185 recurrence	Isoflavones Among premenopausal patients ($n = 248$) All-cause mortality: 1.05 (95% CI, 0.78–1.71) for >42.3 mg/day vs. <15.2 mg/day Recurrence: 0.88 (95% CI, 0.61–1.23) for >42.3 mg/day vs. <15.2 mg/day Among postmenopausal patients ($n = 276$) All-cause mortality: 0.88 (95% CI, 0.56–1.24) for >42.3 mg/day vs. <15.2 mg/day Recurrence: 0.67 (95% CI, 0.54–0.85) for >42.3 mg/day vs. < 15.2 mg/day

Zhang FF et al. [69]	The Breast Cancer Family Registry	US	White 58.5% Hispanics 16.6% Blacks 12% Asians 11.1% other 1.8%	6235	Median of 9.4 years	1224 deaths	Pre-diagnostic total isoflavones ($n = 4769$) All-cause mortality: 0.84 (0.66–1.06) for $\geq$1.494 mg/day vs. $<$0.342 mg/day Post-diagnostic total isoflavones ($n = 1466$) All-cause mortality: 0.65 (0.41–1.00) for $\geq$1.494 mg/day vs. $<$0.342 mg/day

After Breast Cancer Pooling Project included data from 2 US cohorts (WHEL and LACE) and 1 Chinese cohort (SBCSS)
N/A not applicable

29.3.6 *Dietary Supplement*

Cancer survivors tended to use dietary supplements more than general populations, and the prevalence of dietary supplement use was relatively higher in breast cancer survivors than survivors of cancer in other sites [87, 88]. The American Cancer Society guidelines suggests that taking a dietary supplement should be considered only when there is a nutrient deficiency and cancer survivors need to obtain nutrients mainly from dietary sources [89]. Evidence for dietary supplements improving prognosis after a cancer diagnosis is lacking. For example, the After Breast Cancer Pooling Project suggested a better prognosis with vitamins C and E, but an attenuated association of vitamins C and E with recurrence after mutual adjustment [90].

29.4 Research in Asia

Breast cancer in Asian individuals has a different profile than breast cancer in Western individuals. For example, the incidence of newly diagnosed breast cancer was the highest among women aged 40–49 years and the median age at diagnosis was 50 years in Korea, which is younger than Western women [91]. Given that Asian women have different patterns of breast cancer compared to Western women and breast cancer incidence is predicted to continue to increase in Asian regions, it is important to identify a healthy diet after diagnosis that is customized to Asian women.

However, evidence on the effect of diet on breast cancer survival in Asia is limited. The Shanghai Breast Cancer Survival Study [54] and a few Chinese [70, 71] and Japanese hospital-based study [92] have examined the relationship between dietary factors and breast cancer prognosis among breast cancer survivors. Soy products and isoflavones are of particular interest in Asian studies because these foods are widely consumed in Asia. This research has contributed to the understanding of the roles of soy products and isoflavones in breast cancer prognosis [54, 70, 71]. A few cross-sectional studies or small scale intervention studies reported on diet and quality of life among breast cancer survivors in Korea [93–95]. However, these studies warrant further prospective cohort and large-scale intervention studies to provide evidence on how Korean diet and dietary behaviors affect breast cancer survival.

29.5 Future Research Direction

Breast cancer is a major and emerging health problem in both developed and developing countries. The high incidence and prevalence of breast cancer and improved cancer treatment require a better understanding of breast cancer risk factors and lifestyle management for breast cancer survivors. Given that a few, limited cohort studies suggest that diet in early life may play a critical role in breast cancer development, further long-term follow-up studies are needed. The effects of pre- and post-diagnostic diet on quality of life, recurrence, and mortality among breast cancer survivors need to be characterized. In particular, little is known about dietary guidelines for Asian breast cancer survivors, who have different diagnostic, genetic, and anthropometric profiles from Western women. Survival strategies for breast cancer survivors may differ by genetic profiles and treatment type, but data on interaction factors are sparse. In conclusion, identifying the role of diet in breast cancer prevention and prognosis and its interaction with clinical and genetic factors remain important as the global burden of breast cancer is increasing.

29.6 Summary

The global burden of breast cancer is increasing and it is a major and emerging health problem in both developed and developing countries. Therefore, identifying the role of diet in breast cancer prevention and prognosis and its interaction with clinical and genetic factors are of great importance.

References

1. Jung KW, Won YJ, Kong HJ, Lee ES. Cancer statistics in Korea: incidence, mortality, survival, and prevalence in 2016. Cancer Res Treat. 2019;51(2):417–30.
2. Ferlay J, Soerjomataram I, Ervik M, Dikshit R, Eser S, Mathers C, et al. GLOBOCAN 2012 v1.1, cancer incidence and mortality worldwide: IARC CancerBase no. 11 [internet]. International Agency for Research on Cancer: Lyon; 2013. http://globocan.iarc.fr
3. World Cancer Research Fund/American Institute for Cancer Research. Continuous update project report: diet, nutrition, physical activity and breast cancer. 2017. wcrf.org/breast-cancer-2017. All CUP reports are available at wcrf.org/cupreports.
4. Allemani C, Weir HK, Carreira H, Harewood R, Spika D, Wang XS, et al. Global surveillance of cancer survival 1995-2009: analysis of individual data for 25,676,887 patients from 279 population-based registries in 67 countries (CONCORD-2). Lancet (Lond). 2015;385 (9972):977–1010.
5. Boyd NF, Stone J, Vogt KN, Connelly BS, Martin LJ, Minkin S. Dietary fat and breast cancer risk revisited: a meta-analysis of the published literature. Br J Cancer. 2003;89(9):1672–85.
6. Hunter DJ, Spiegelman D, Adami HO, Beeson L, van den Brandt PA, Folsom AR, et al. Cohort studies of fat intake and the risk of breast cancer--a pooled analysis. N Engl J Med. 1996;334 (6):356–61.
7. Kim EH, Willett WC, Colditz GA, Hankinson SE, Stampfer MJ, Hunter DJ, et al. Dietary fat and risk of postmenopausal breast cancer in a 20-year follow-up. Am J Epidemiol. 2006;164 (10):990–7.
8. Prentice RL, Caan B, Chlebowski RT, Patterson R, Kuller LH, Ockene JK, et al. Low-fat dietary pattern and risk of invasive breast cancer: the Women's Health Initiative Randomized Controlled Dietary Modification Trial. JAMA. 2006;295(6):629–42.

9. Smith-Warner SA, Spiegelman D, Adami HO, Beeson WL, van den Brandt PA, Folsom AR, et al. Types of dietary fat and breast cancer: a pooled analysis of cohort studies. Int J Cancer. 2001;92(5):767–74.
10. Cho E, Spiegelman D, Hunter DJ, Chen WY, Stampfer MJ, Colditz GA, et al. Premenopausal fat intake and risk of breast cancer. J Natl Cancer Inst. 2003;95(14):1079–85.
11. Smith-Warner SA, Spiegelman D, Yaun SS, Adami HO, Beeson WL, van den Brandt PA, et al. Intake of fruits and vegetables and risk of breast cancer: a pooled analysis of cohort studies. JAMA. 2001;285(6):769–76.
12. van Gils CH, Peeters PH, Bueno-de-Mesquita HB, Boshuizen HC, Lahmann PH, Clavel-Chapelon F, et al. Consumption of vegetables and fruits and risk of breast cancer. JAMA. 2005;293(2):183–93.
13. Jung S, Spiegelman D, Baglietto L, Bernstein L, Boggs DA, van den Brandt PA, et al. Fruit and vegetable intake and risk of breast cancer by hormone receptor status. J Natl Cancer Inst. 2013;105(3):219–36.
14. Emaus MJ, Peeters PH, Bakker MF, Overvad K, Tjonneland A, Olsen A, et al. Vegetable and fruit consumption and the risk of hormone receptor-defined breast cancer in the EPIC cohort. Am J Clin Nutr. 2016;103(1):168–77.
15. Schlesinger S, Chan DSM, Vingeliene S, Vieira AR, Abar L, Polemiti E, et al. Carbohydrates, glycemic index, glycemic load, and breast cancer risk: a systematic review and dose-response meta-analysis of prospective studies. Nutr Rev. 2017;75(6):420–41.
16. Allred CD, Allred KF, Ju YH, Goeppinger TS, Doerge DR, Helferich WG. Soy processing influences growth of estrogen-dependent breast cancer tumors. Carcinogenesis. 2004;25 (9):1649–57.
17. Hsieh CY, Santell RC, Haslam SZ, Helferich WG. Estrogenic effects of genistein on the growth of estrogen receptor-positive human breast cancer (MCF-7) cells in vitro and in vivo. Cancer Res. 1998;58(17):3833–8.
18. Martin PM, Horwitz KB, Ryan DS, McGuire WL. Phytoestrogen interaction with estrogen receptors in human breast cancer cells. Endocrinology. 1978;103(5):1860–7.
19. Jha HC, von Recklinghausen G, Zilliken F. Inhibition of in vitro microsomal lipid peroxidation by isoflavonoids. Biochem Pharmacol. 1985;34(9):1367–9.
20. Su SJ, Yeh TM, Chuang WJ, Ho CL, Chang KL, Cheng HL, et al. The novel targets for anti-angiogenesis of genistein on human cancer cells. Biochem Pharmacol. 2005;69(2):307–18.
21. Spinozzi F, Pagliacci MC, Migliorati G, Moraca R, Grignani F, Riccardi C, et al. The natural tyrosine kinase inhibitor genistein produces cell cycle arrest and apoptosis in Jurkat T-leukemia cells. Leuk Res. 1994;18(6):431–9.
22. Horn-Ross PL, Hoggatt KJ, West DW, Krone MR, Stewart SL, Anton H, et al. Recent diet and breast cancer risk: the California Teachers Study (USA). Cancer Causes Control. 2002;13 (5):407–15.
23. Yamamoto S, Sobue T, Kobayashi M, Sasaki S, Tsugane S. Soy, isoflavones, and breast cancer risk in Japan. J Natl Cancer Inst. 2003;95(12):906–13.
24. Grace PB, Taylor JI, Low YL, Luben RN, Mulligan AA, Botting NP, et al. Phytoestrogen concentrations in serum and spot urine as biomarkers for dietary phytoestrogen intake and their relation to breast cancer risk in European prospective investigation of cancer and nutrition-Norfolk. Cancer Epidemiol Biomark Prev. 2004;13(5):698–708.
25. Hu FB. Dietary pattern analysis: a new direction in nutritional epidemiology. Curr Opin Lipidol. 2002;13(1):3–9.
26. Fung TT, Hu FB, Holmes MD, Rosner BA, Hunter DJ, Colditz GA, et al. Dietary patterns and the risk of postmenopausal breast cancer. Int J Cancer. 2005;116(1):116–21.
27. Fung TT, Hu FB, McCullough ML, Newby PK, Willett WC, Holmes MD. Diet quality is associated with the risk of estrogen receptor-negative breast cancer in postmenopausal women. J Nutr. 2006;136(2):466–72.

28. Toledo E, Salas-Salvado J, Donat-Vargas C, Buil-Cosiales P, Estruch R, Ros E, et al. Mediterranean diet and invasive breast cancer risk among women at high cardiovascular risk in the PREDIMED trial: a randomized clinical trial. JAMA Intern Med. 2015;175(11):1752–60.
29. Dong JY, Zhang L, He K, Qin LQ. Dairy consumption and risk of breast cancer: a meta-analysis of prospective cohort studies. Breast Cancer Res Treat. 2011;127(1):23–31.
30. Bertone-Johnson ER, Chen WY, Holick MF, Hollis BW, Colditz GA, Willett WC, et al. Plasma 25-hydroxyvitamin D and 1,25-dihydroxyvitamin D and risk of breast cancer. Cancer Epidemiol Biomark Prev. 2005;14(8):1991–7.
31. Engel P, Fagherazzi G, Boutten A, Dupre T, Mesrine S, Boutron-Ruault MC, et al. Serum 25 (OH) vitamin D and risk of breast cancer: a nested case-control study from the French E3N cohort. Cancer Epidemiol Biomark Prev. 2010;19(9):2341–50.
32. Shin MH, Holmes MD, Hankinson SE, Wu K, Colditz GA, Willett WC. Intake of dairy products, calcium, and vitamin d and risk of breast cancer. J Natl Cancer Inst. 2002;94 (17):1301–11.
33. Freedman DM, Chang SC, Falk RT, Purdue MP, Huang WY, McCarty CA, et al. Serum levels of vitamin D metabolites and breast cancer risk in the prostate, lung, colorectal, and ovarian cancer screening trial. Cancer Epidemiol Biomark Prev. 2008;17(4):889–94.
34. McCullough ML, Stevens VL, Patel R, Jacobs EJ, Bain EB, Horst RL, et al. Serum 25-hydroxyvitamin D concentrations and postmenopausal breast cancer risk: a nested case control study in the Cancer Prevention Study-II Nutrition Cohort. Breast Cancer Res. 2009;11 (4):R64.
35. Chlebowski RT, Johnson KC, Kooperberg C, Pettinger M, Wactawski-Wende J, Rohan T, et al. Calcium plus vitamin D supplementation and the risk of breast cancer. J Natl Cancer Inst. 2008;100(22):1581–91.
36. Zhang X, Spiegelman D, Baglietto L, Bernstein L, Boggs DA, van den Brandt PA, et al. Carotenoid intakes and risk of breast cancer defined by estrogen receptor and progesterone receptor status: a pooled analysis of 18 prospective cohort studies. Am J Clin Nutr. 2012;95 (3):713–25.
37. Eliassen AH, Hendrickson SJ, Brinton LA, Buring JE, Campos H, Dai Q, et al. Circulating carotenoids and risk of breast cancer: pooled analysis of eight prospective studies. J Natl Cancer Inst. 2012;104(24):1905–16.
38. Bakker MF, Peeters PH, Klaasen VM, Bueno-de-Mesquita HB, Jansen EH, Ros MM, et al. Plasma carotenoids, vitamin C, tocopherols, and retinol and the risk of breast cancer in the European Prospective Investigation into Cancer and Nutrition cohort. Am J Clin Nutr. 2016;103 (2):454–64.
39. Willett WC. Implications of total energy intake for epidemiologic studies of breast and large-bowel cancer. Am J Clin Nutr. 1987;45(1 Suppl):354–60.
40. de Waard F, Trichopoulos D. A unifying concept of the aetiology of breast cancer. Int J Cancer. 1988;41(5):666–9.
41. van den Brandt PA, Spiegelman D, Yaun SS, Adami HO, Beeson L, Folsom AR, et al. Pooled analysis of prospective cohort studies on height, weight, and breast cancer risk. Am J Epidemiol. 2000;152(6):514–27.
42. Ahlgren M, Melbye M, Wohlfahrt J, Sorensen TI. Growth patterns and the risk of breast cancer in women. N Engl J Med. 2004;351(16):1619–26.
43. Farvid MS, Cho E, Chen WY, Eliassen AH, Willett WC. Adolescent meat intake and breast cancer risk. Int J Cancer. 2015;136(8):1909–20.
44. Farvid MS, Chen WY, Michels KB, Cho E, Willett WC, Eliassen AH. Fruit and vegetable consumption in adolescence and early adulthood and risk of breast cancer: population based cohort study. BMJ (Clin Res). 2016;353:i2343.
45. Farvid MS, Eliassen AH, Cho E, Liao X, Chen WY, Willett WC. Dietary fiber intake in young adults and breast cancer risk. Pediatrics. 2016;137(3):e20151226.
46. Farvid MS, Cho E, Eliassen AH, Chen WY, Willett WC. Lifetime grain consumption and breast cancer risk. Breast Cancer Res Treat. 2016;159(2):335–45.

47. Holmes MD, Colditz GA, Hunter DJ, Hankinson SE, Rosner B, Speizer FE, et al. Meat, fish and egg intake and risk of breast cancer. Int J Cancer. 2003;104(2):221–7.
48. Holmes MD, Liu S, Hankinson SE, Colditz GA, Hunter DJ, Willett WC. Dietary carbohydrates, fiber, and breast cancer risk. Am J Epidemiol. 2004;159(8):732–9.
49. Chlebowski RT, Blackburn GL, Thomson CA, Nixon DW, Shapiro A, Hoy MK, et al. Dietary fat reduction and breast cancer outcome: interim efficacy results from the women's intervention nutrition study. J Natl Cancer Inst. 2006;98(24):1767–76.
50. Pierce JP, Natarajan L, Caan BJ, Parker BA, Greenberg ER, Flatt SW, et al. Influence of a diet very high in vegetables, fruit, and fiber and low in fat on prognosis following treatment for breast cancer: the Women's Healthy Eating and Living (WHEL) randomized trial. JAMA. 2007;298(3):289–98.
51. Swann R, Perkins KA, Velentzis LS, Ciria C, Dutton SJ, Mulligan AA, et al. The DietCompLyf study: a prospective cohort study of breast cancer survival and phytoestrogen consumption. Maturitas. 2013;75(3):232–40.
52. Izano MA, Fung TT, Chiuve SS, Hu FB, Holmes MD. Are diet quality scores after breast cancer diagnosis associated with improved breast cancer survival? Nutr Cancer. 2013;65(6):820–6.
53. Belle FN, Kampman E, McTiernan A, Bernstein L, Baumgartner K, Baumgartner R, et al. Dietary fiber, carbohydrates, glycemic index, and glycemic load in relation to breast cancer prognosis in the HEAL cohort. Cancer Epidemiol Biomark Prev. 2011;20(5):890–9.
54. Shu XO, Zheng Y, Cai H, Gu K, Chen Z, Zheng W, et al. Soy food intake and breast cancer survival. JAMA. 2009;302(22):2437–43.
55. Caan BJ, Natarajan L, Parker B, Gold EB, Thomson C, Newman V, et al. Soy food consumption and breast cancer prognosis. Cancer Epidemiol Biomark Prev. 2011;20(5):854–8.
56. Caan B, Sternfeld B, Gunderson E, Coates A, Quesenberry C, Slattery ML. Life After Cancer Epidemiology (LACE) Study: a cohort of early stage breast cancer survivors (United States). Cancer Causes Control. 2005;16(5):545–56.
57. Beasley JM, Newcomb PA, Trentham-Dietz A, Hampton JM, Bersch AJ, Passarelli MN, et al. Post-diagnosis dietary factors and survival after invasive breast cancer. Breast Cancer Res Treat. 2011;128(1):229–36.
58. George SM, Ballard-Barbash R, Shikany JM, Caan BJ, Freudenheim JL, Kroenke CH, et al. Better postdiagnosis diet quality is associated with reduced risk of death among postmenopausal women with invasive breast cancer in the women's health initiative. Cancer Epidemiol Biomark Prev. 2014;23(4):575–83.
59. Kwan ML, Ambrosone CB, Lee MM, Barlow J, Krathwohl SE, Ergas IJ, et al. The pathways study: a prospective study of breast cancer survivorship within Kaiser Permanente Northern California. Cancer Causes Control. 2008;19(10):1065–76.
60. Nechuta SJ, Caan BJ, Chen WY, Flatt SW, Lu W, Patterson RE, et al. The after breast cancer pooling project: rationale, methodology, and breast cancer survivor characteristics. Cancer Causes Control. 2011;22(9):1319–31.
61. McCullough ML, Gapstur SM, Shah R, Campbell PT, Wang Y, Doyle C, et al. Pre- and postdiagnostic diet in relation to mortality among breast cancer survivors in the CPS-II Nutrition Cohort. Cancer Causes Control. 2016;27(11):1303–14.
62. Kwan ML, Weltzien E, Kushi LH, Castillo A, Slattery ML, Caan BJ. Dietary patterns and breast cancer recurrence and survival among women with early-stage breast cancer. J Clin Oncol. 2009;27(6):919–26.
63. Kroenke CH, Fung TT, Hu FB, Holmes MD. Dietary patterns and survival after breast cancer diagnosis. J Clin Oncol. 2005;23(36):9295–303.
64. Kim EH, Willett WC, Fung T, Rosner B, Holmes MD. Diet quality indices and postmenopausal breast cancer survival. Nutr Cancer. 2011;63(3):381–8.
65. George SM, Irwin ML, Smith AW, Neuhouser ML, Reedy J, McTiernan A, et al. Postdiagnosis diet quality, the combination of diet quality and recreational physical activity, and prognosis after early-stage breast cancer. Cancer Causes Control. 2011;22(4):589–98.

66. Vrieling A, Buck K, Seibold P, Heinz J, Obi N, Flesch-Janys D, et al. Dietary patterns and survival in German postmenopausal breast cancer survivors. Br J Cancer. 2013;108(1):188–92.
67. Zheng J, Tabung FK, Zhang J, Liese AD, Shivappa N, Ockene JK, et al. Association between post-cancer diagnosis dietary inflammatory potential and mortality among invasive breast cancer survivors in the women's health initiative. Cancer Epidemiol Biomark Prev. 2018;27 (4):454–63.
68. Nechuta SJ, Caan BJ, Chen WY, Lu W, Chen Z, Kwan ML, et al. Soy food intake after diagnosis of breast cancer and survival: an in-depth analysis of combined evidence from cohort studies of US and Chinese women. Am J Clin Nutr. 2012;96(1):123–32.
69. Zhang FF, Haslam DE, Terry MB, Knight JA, Andrulis IL, Daly MB, et al. Dietary isoflavone intake and all-cause mortality in breast cancer survivors: The Breast Cancer Family Registry. Cancer. 2017;123(11):2070–9.
70. Zhang YF, Kang HB, Li BL, Zhang RM. Positive effects of soy isoflavone food on survival of breast cancer patients in China. Asian Pac J Cancer Prev. 2012;13(2):479–82.
71. Kang X, Zhang Q, Wang S, Huang X, Jin S. Effect of soy isoflavones on breast cancer recurrence and death for patients receiving adjuvant endocrine therapy. Can Med Assoc J. 2010;182(17):1857–62.
72. Holmes MD, Stampfer MJ, Colditz GA, Rosner B, Hunter DJ, Willett WC. Dietary factors and the survival of women with breast carcinoma. Cancer. 1999;86(5):826–35.
73. Rock CL, Flatt SW, Natarajan L, Thomson CA, Bardwell WA, Newman VA, et al. Plasma carotenoids and recurrence-free survival in women with a history of breast cancer. J Clin Oncol. 2005;23(27):6631–8.
74. Peng C, Luo WP, Zhang CX. Fruit and vegetable intake and breast cancer prognosis: a meta-analysis of prospective cohort studies. Br J Nutr. 2017;117(5):737–49.
75. Nechuta S, Caan BJ, Chen WY, Kwan ML, Lu W, Cai H, et al. Postdiagnosis cruciferous vegetable consumption and breast cancer outcomes: a report from the After Breast Cancer Pooling Project. Cancer Epidemiol Biomark Prev. 2013;22(8):1451–6.
76. Rohan TE, Hiller JE, McMichael AJ. Dietary factors and survival from breast cancer. Nutr Cancer. 1993;20(2):167–77.
77. McEligot AJ, Largent J, Ziogas A, Peel D, Anton-Culver H. Dietary fat, fiber, vegetable, and micronutrients are associated with overall survival in postmenopausal women diagnosed with breast cancer. Nutr Cancer. 2006;55(2):132–40.
78. Saxe GA, Rock CL, Wicha MS, Schottenfeld D. Diet and risk for breast cancer recurrence and survival. Breast Cancer Res Treat. 1999;53(3):241–53.
79. World Cancer Research Fund/American Institute for Cancer Research. Continuous update project expert report 2018. Diet, nutrition, physical activity and breast cancer survivors. dietandcancerreport.org.
80. Zhang S, Folsom AR, Sellers TA, Kushi LH, Potter JD. Better breast cancer survival for postmenopausal women who are less overweight and eat less fat. The Iowa Women's Health Study. Cancer. 1995;76(2):275–83.
81. Goodwin PJ, Ennis M, Pritchard KI, Koo J, Trudeau ME, Hood N. Diet and breast cancer: evidence that extremes in diet are associated with poor survival. J Clin Oncol. 2003;21 (13):2500–7.
82. Patterson RE, Flatt SW, Newman VA, Natarajan L, Rock CL, Thomson CA, et al. Marine fatty acid intake is associated with breast cancer prognosis. J Nutr. 2011;141(2):201–6.
83. Garland CF, Garland FC. Do sunlight and vitamin D reduce the likelihood of colon cancer? Int J Epidemiol. 1980;9(3):227–31.
84. Giovannucci E. The epidemiology of vitamin D and cancer incidence and mortality: a review (United States). Cancer Causes Control. 2005;16(2):83–95.
85. Goodwin PJ, Ennis M, Pritchard KI, Koo J, Hood N. Prognostic effects of 25-hydroxyvitamin D levels in early breast cancer. J Clin Oncol. 2009;27(23):3757–63.

86. Maalmi H, Ordonez-Mena JM, Schottker B, Brenner H. Serum 25-hydroxyvitamin D levels and survival in colorectal and breast cancer patients: systematic review and meta-analysis of prospective cohort studies. Eur J Cancer (Oxf). 2014;50(8):1510–21.
87. Velicer CM, Ulrich CM. Vitamin and mineral supplement use among US adults after cancer diagnosis: a systematic review. J Clin Oncol. 2008;26(4):665–73.
88. Song S, Youn J, Lee YJ, Kang M, Hyun T, Song Y, et al. Dietary supplement use among cancer survivors and the general population: a nation-wide cross-sectional study. BMC Cancer. 2017;17(1):891.
89. Rock CL, Doyle C, Demark-Wahnefried W, Meyerhardt J, Courneya KS, Schwartz AL, et al. Nutrition and physical activity guidelines for cancer survivors. CA Cancer J Clin. 2012;62 (4):243–74.
90. Poole EM, Shu X, Caan BJ, Flatt SW, Holmes MD, Lu W, et al. Postdiagnosis supplement use and breast cancer prognosis in the After Breast Cancer Pooling Project. Breast Cancer Res Treat. 2013;139(2):529–37.
91. Park EH, Min SY, Kim Z, Yoon CS, Jung KW, Nam SJ, et al. Basic facts of breast cancer in Korea in 2014: the 10-year overall survival progress. J Breast Cancer. 2017;20(1):1–11.
92. Kyogoku S, Hirohata T, Nomura Y, Shigematsu T, Takeshita S, Hirohata I. Diet and prognosis of breast cancer. Nutr Cancer. 1992;17(3):271–7.
93. Song S, Hwang E, Moon HG, Noh DY, Lee JE. Adherence to guidelines for cancer survivors and health-related quality of life among Korean breast cancer survivors. Nutrients. 2015;7 (12):10307–19.
94. Lee MK, Yun YH, Park HA, Lee ES, Jung KH, Noh DY. A web-based self-management exercise and diet intervention for breast cancer survivors: pilot randomized controlled trial. Int J Nurs Stud. 2014;51(12):1557–67.
95. Kim N-H, Song S, Jung S-Y, Lee E, Kim Z, Moon H-G, et al. Dietary pattern and health-related quality of life among breast cancer survivors. BMC Womens Health. 2018;18(1):65.

Chapter 30
Current Trends in and Indications for Endoscopy-Assisted Breast Surgery for Breast Cancer

Hyukjai Shin

Abstract Endoscopic oncoplastic breast surgery represents a minimal invasive approach with the aim of both safe excision of cancer and preserving the breast shape. It has less noticeable scar, excellent cosmetic outcomes, high patient satisfaction rate. Recently, relative long-term follow-up results have been reported to be very safe (Soybir and Fukuma, J Breast Health 11:52–58, 2015; Fan et al., Chin Med J 122:2945–2950, 2009; Jiang, Zhonghua Wai Ke Za Zhi 45:439–441, 2007).

Operative techniques for both endoscopic breast-conserving surgery and endoscopic nipple/areola/skin-sparing mastectomy have been described in detail. Two different working planes in which one of them is subcutaneous and the other one is sub-mammary planes are being used during the surgery. Surgical technique needs some instruments such as endoscopic retractor, light guided specific mammary retractor, wound protector, and energy device such as bipolar scissor, Harmonic Scalpel, LigaSure, Thunderbeat. Endoscopic breast retractors provide magnified visualization and extensive posterior dissection facility. Tunneling method and the hydro-dissection simplify the technique in the subcutaneous field (Soybir and Fukuma, J Breast Health 11:52–58, 2015; Fan et al., Chin Med J 122:2945–2950, 2009). Oncoplastic reconstruction techniques are also applied after the tumor resection by endoscopic method. The complication rate of endoscopic breast surgery is similar with the rate of open breast surgery. Quite successful local recurrence, distant metastasis, and overall survival rates have been declared. However, it looks reasonable to wait for the results with longer follow-up before having a judgement about oncologic efficiency and safety of the endoscopic breast cancer surgery (Tamaki et al., Nihon Geka Gakkai Zasshi 103(11):835–838, 2002; Leff et al., Breast Cancer Res Treat 125(3):607–625, 2011; Fukuma, Nihon Geka Gakkai Zasshi 116 (5):316–319, 2015).

Recently some surgeons reported about robotic nipple sparing mastectomy and immediate breast reconstruction with Gel implant procedure. Nevertheless, experience with application of a robotic surgery platform in the management of breast

H. Shin (✉)
Hyanyang University College of Medicine, Ansan, Gyeonggi-do, South Korea

D.-Y. Noh et al. (eds.), *Translational Research in Breast Cancer*, Advances in Experimental Medicine and Biology 1187,
https://doi.org/10.1007/978-981-32-9620-6_30

cancer is limited. From the preliminary experiences, R-NSM and IBR with Gel implant is a safe procedure, with good cosmetic results, and could be a promising new technique for breast cancer patients indicated for mastectomy (Lai et al., Ann Surg Oncol 26(1):42–52, 2019).

Keywords Breast cancer · Endoscopic-assisted breast surgery · Oncoplastic surgery · Nipple sparing mastectomy · Robotic nipple sparing mastectomy · Immediate breast reconstruction

30.1 Introduction

Historically, modified radical mastectomy was the preferred method for treating operable.

Sentinel lymph node biopsy is now performed in most patients thereby sparing the need for axillary lymph node dissection in clinical node negative patients. Another important advancement in the field of breast surgery has been the development of oncoplastic breast surgery, a breast-conserving technique that combines wide tumor excision with immediate partial breast reconstruction using either volume displacement or volume replacement techniques [1–3].

Sentinel lymph node biopsy is now performed in most patients thereby sparing the need for axillary lymph node dissection in clinical node negative patients. Another important advancement in the field of breast surgery has been the development of oncoplastic breast surgery, a breast-conserving technique that combines wide tumor excision with immediate partial breast reconstruction using either volume displacement or volume replacement techniques.

Nonetheless, mastectomy is still indicated for some patients, especially for women with large tumors or multi-centric lesions. Fortunately, recent advances in the field now allow for nipple sparing mastectomy with immediate breast reconstruction to be performed, which results in much better cosmetic outcome and quality of life than conventional mastectomy. Endoscopic surgery, a technique that optimizes cosmetic outcome because it is performed through small wounds hidden in inconspicuous areas, is widely used in the gastrointestinal, urologic, and thoracic surgical fields. Endoscopy-assisted breast surgery, which is performed through minimal axillary and/or peri-areolar incisions, was initially developed to facilitate breast augmentation, but is now increasingly used to excise benign breast tumors, resect malignant breast tumors, and to assist in SLNB. EABS has been shown to be an effective breast-conserving technique for early breast cancer. In addition, endoscopic approaches can be used to perform skin-sparing mastectomy and NSM followed by IBR with implants or autologous flaps. EABS is used as an alternative to conventional surgery in select patients with early stage breast cancer in a few Western countries and in some Asian countries, such as Japan, China, and Korea. However, the use of EABS in the management of breast cancer has yet to become a mainstream treatment modality mainly because there is an absence of randomized level I clinical evidence showing that EABS achieves oncologic outcomes equivalent to open surgery [2, 4–7].

30.2 Endoscopy-Assisted Breast Surgery

30.2.1 Indication and Patient Selection

Breast-Conserving Surgery is performed for T1–T2 tumors. The skin, pectoral muscle, and chest wall invasions are contraindications. It cannot be performed in cases of multifocal tumors [8]. The exclusion criteria include tumor close to skin, thoracic deformity, hemorrhagic diathesis, elderly age, poor health condition, and patient's reluctance towards this method. The other limitations of breast-conserving surgery are applicable for this, as well. Some studies cited clinically positive axilla as a contraindication. There are also studies limiting the technique to cases that would have less than 20% of volume loss. If the potential loss of volume in the breast is estimated at 20–40%, volume replacement techniques may be more appropriate in place of volume displacement method.

EAO-BCS is rather targeted at Cup A and Cup B breasts. Also, the location of tumor is important, too. For tumors located in the inner or lower part of the breast, the spaces to emerge following excision have to be filled in via volume displacements [9] through peri-areolar and axillary incision. Oil necrosis may be frequent especially when reconstruction is performed with wide-ranging mobilization and volume displacement in old patients with low breast density [2, 3].

Mastectomy Skin-sparing mastectomy and nipple–/areola-sparing mastectomy can be performed with the assistance of endoscopy. Both techniques can be employed in breast cancer, ductal carcinoma in situ, risk-reducing mastectomy, large Phyllodes tumor, and benign breast diseases that would require mastectomy. When mastectomy is required, EA-NSM is preferred with priority. The patient selection criteria are the same as in open surgery [10, 11].

For endoscope-assisted subcutaneous mastectomy, the skin, pectoral muscle, and chest wall invasions are contraindications. Tumor that is close to skin, inflammatory cancer, thoracic deformity hemorrhagic diathesis, elderly age, poor health condition, and the patient's reluctance towards the method are accepted as exclusion criteria. Large <Cup C or above> breast and breasts that are too flabby are not eligible for EASM. As for EA-NSM, the other exclusion criteria reported in the literature are as follows: tumor larger than 3 cm, tumor that is more than 2 cm near the tumor, bleeding nipple, tumor near the area under the nipple, Paget's disease, and large central tumor. Furthermore, clinically positive axilla, local recurrence and tumor with negative estrogen and progesterone receptors with a high potential for distant metastasis are accepted as exclusion criteria in many clinics. No consensuses are present for patients that would receive preoperative or post-operative radiotherapy. The results indicate that this technique can be performed in such patients [7, 11, 12].

30.2.2 Marking

30.2.2.1 Breast-Conserving Surgery

The projections of tumors or lesions on the skin are marked before surgery under ultrasound guidance (Fig. 30.1). The excision margins are determined at 1–2 cm away from the tumor margins. At the beginning of surgery, all-round color stain injections are performed at the excision margins (Fig. 30.2). Since the blue stain is generally used for marking sentinel lymph nodes, the marking should be done using a stain that is not mixed with the blue stain in EAO-BCS. The stains used according to the literature include Gentian Violet, Diagnogreen, Indigo Carmine, and

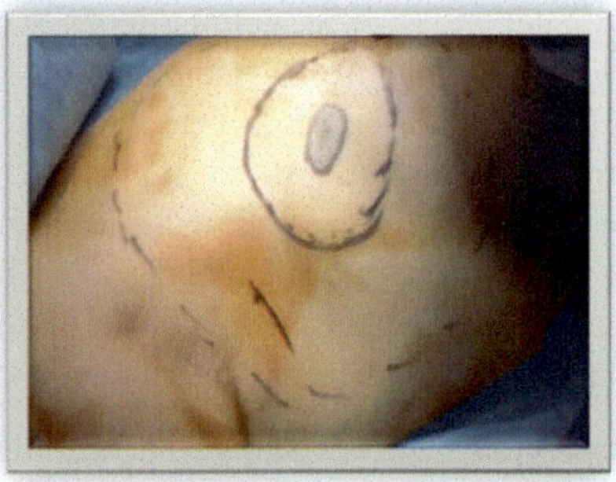

Fig. 30.1 Marking and drawing on the breast. The tumor margins (innermost), excision margins (middle ring), margins of dissection and mobilization to be performed in the anterior and posterior sites (outermost) and the lymph node incision in the axilla are shown

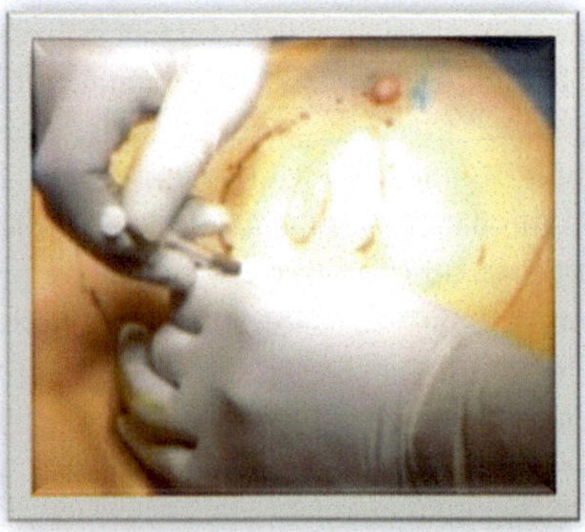

Fig. 30.2 Subcutaneous stain injections at several points on the excision margins are seen reconstruction

Pyoctanin. Furthermore, these stains are used by being mixed with gel <1% Lidocaine Gel or Xylocaine Gel> at a ratio of 1/1 in order to prevent the injected stain from being absorbed and spreading [13].

30.2.2.2 Mastectomy

The projections of tumors or lesions on the skin are marked by drawings prior to surgery. The all-round margins of breast tissue are also included in marking. Furthermore, the marking of internal thoracic and artery branches on the breast in the parasternal area would be beneficial for the preservation of blood flow during dissection [6].

30.2.3 Incision

Axillary and peri-areolar incisions are the most frequently used incisions in both mastectomy and breast-conserving surgery. The incision used in axilla is a generally an incision that is 2 cm, which is made for sentinel lymph node, and it is used for dissection performed in the posterior part of the breast. To create a skin flap, a peri-areolar incision is used. In addition to this incision, an additional skin excision in the shape of half moon is used to enlarge the incision, thereby facilitating the removal of excised tissue through here. The site for peri-areolar incision is determined on the basis of the location of tumor in the breast. The incision is kept at a size that is approximately 2/5 of the perimeter of areola. Since work is done through a small incision with EAO-BCS, the skin around the incision during the procedure may be injured. To prevent this, a wound protector (Alexis; Hakko Co; Johnson & Johnson) is used (Fig. 30.3) [14].

Although there are recommendations in the literature for mastectomy such as long (5–10 cm), single axillary incision and lateral breast incision, these are not currently used at an extensive rate. A comparative series demonstrated that 5.5 cm axillary incision had superiority over open skin-conserving mastectomy. Peri-areolar incision is performed laterally on the breast. This ensures facilitation in the placement of implant or expander and in the creation of a pocket.

Another technique used in EASM is the endoscopic technique where trocars are also used. With this technique, the working area is created via insufflation over a single-port entry on a single axillary incision of 4–6 cm, and then an anterior site dissection is performed followed by a posterior site dissection. In this series of 10 cases, the average operation time was reported as 250 min, rate of partial nipple necrosis corrected with medical treatment as 30%, hematoma as 10%, and infection as 10%.

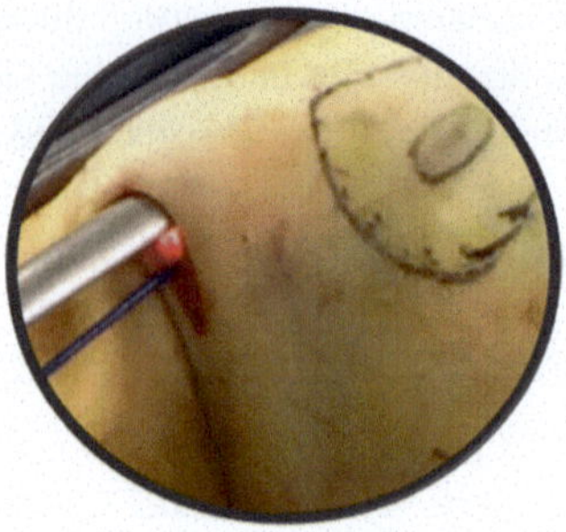

Fig. 30.3 The dissection performed using special lighted breast retractor in deep sites while the skin flap is prepared in the posterior site is observed. Wound protective material is also used for areola dissection

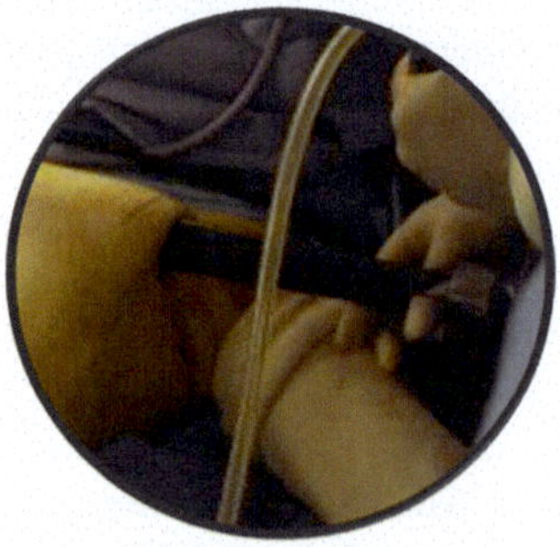

Fig. 30.4 Endoscope (retractor) is inserted through the axillary incision and the posterior site is dissected with electro-cautery as seen. Here, endoscope is also used as a retractor

30.2.4 Posterior Dissection

Dissection in the retromammary space is performed between the posterior face of the breast and the pectoral muscle (Fig. 30.4). Retractors with optical systems (Vein Harvest, Ultra Retractor, Vein Retractor) are also used for blunt dissection while bipolar scissors or electro-cautery is used for coagulation (Figs. 30.5 and 30.6). Techniques for creating the work area using pre-peritoneal dissection balloon or insufflation were used in the past as part of posterior dissection; however, they are not preferred today [6, 14, 15].

In cases of Breast-Conserving Surgery, mobilization is performed in such a way as to cover an area further beyond the tumor margins in order to facilitate especially volume displacements. In cases that will undergo mastectomy, the dissection site is consistent with the anatomic margins of the breast [2].

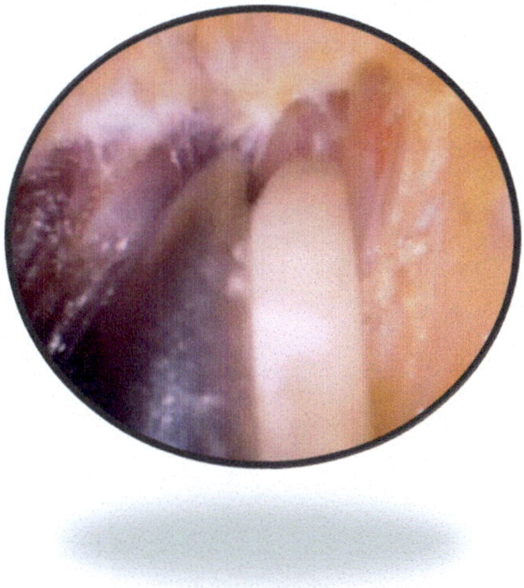

Fig. 30.5 Dissection in the posterior site is seen in the monitor. Sharp dissection is performed with a pair of bipolar scissors in the plane between the breast tissue and pectoral muscle under imaging guidance and the breast tissue is mobilized

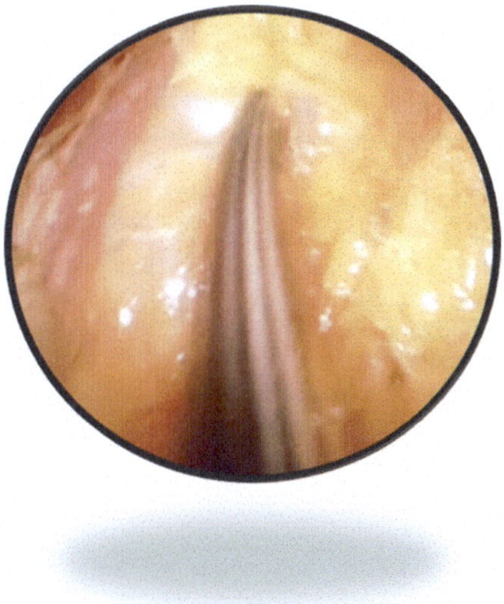

Fig. 30.6 Dissection using a pair of bipolar scissors under endoscopic guidance in the posterior site is seen in the monitor. The breast tissue is mobilized in the space between the breast tissue and pectoral muscle and at the edge of the pectoral muscle in the outer lateral side

30.2.5 Anterior Dissection (Creation of a Skin Flap)

This dissection is performed between the breast and skin and peri-areolar incision is used (Fig. 30.7). Before the dissection, injections of physiological saline solution with Epinephrine at a ratio of 1/1,000,000 (approximately 150 cc) are administered in this plane (Fig. 30.8). This technique is termed the "Tumescent Technique" or "Hydro-dissection" and it not only facilitates dissection, but also ensures that they are performed with less bleeding. Following the hydro-dissection, the dissection is completed by using an optical system and bipolar scissors between the subcutaneous

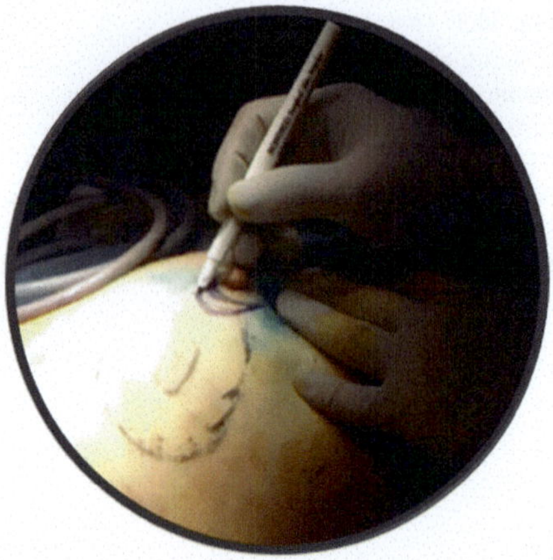

Fig. 30.7 The periareolar incision line is drawn before anterior site dissection is started. The incision entrance will have been slightly enlarged with a skin incision in a half moon shape

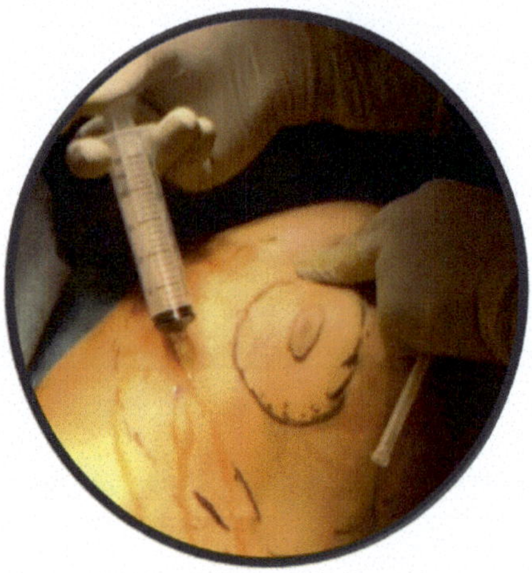

Fig. 30.8 Before starting dissection in the anterior site, injections of physiological saline solution with epinephrine at a ratio of 1/1.000.000 are performed in the previously marked mobilization area. This procedure would ensure a dissection that is not only easy, but also causes relatively less bleeding

plane and the breast tissue (Fig. 30.9). Attention should be shown during dissection to make sure that the flap is not too thin. Very thin flaps increase the potential for ischemia and necrosis in the skin. For dissection, "harmonic scalpel" or electrocautery may also be used (Fig. 30.10). The flap is gently retracted using a special lighted breast retractor (Mamma Retractor-Four Medics, Tokyo; Cold Light

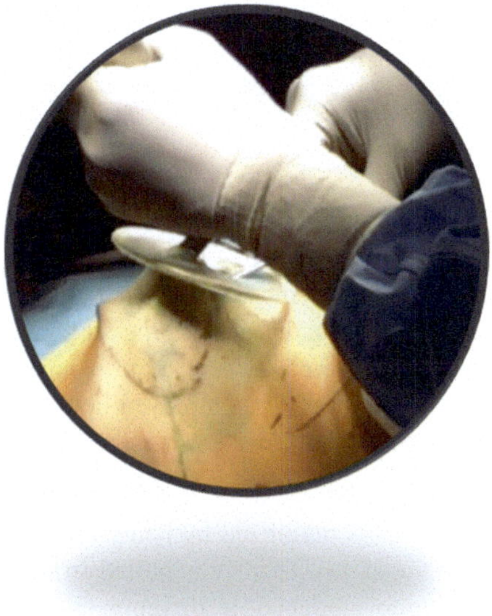

Fig. 30.9 Working through the periareolar incision, the skin traction is ensured, advancement in the subcutaneous plane is made and the breast tissue is separated from the skin

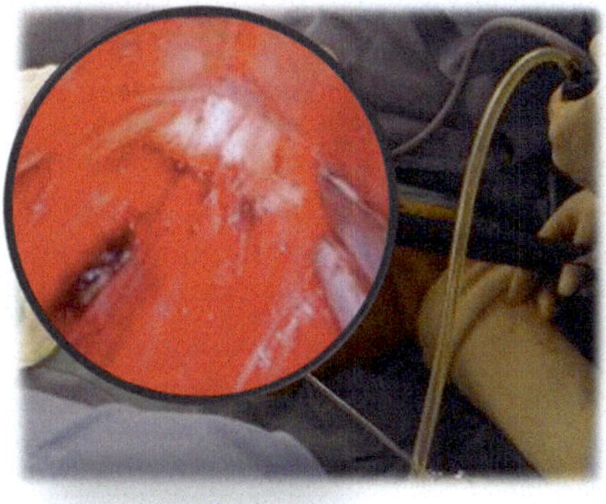

Fig. 30.10 After the completion of the mobilization of skin flap in the anterior site, the tumor tissue has been excised in line with the margins and hemostasis control is achieved in the tumor bed as accompanied by endoscopy. At the same time, breast tissue with enough mobilization for the volume displacement procedure is prepared

Retractor-Komagowa, Spain; Oral Retractor- TISE) in order to facilitate the dissection.

Subcutaneous dissection is made easier by the tunnel method. With this technique, a multiple tunnel is opened using scissors on the subcutaneous plane in a radial way towards the periphery from the nipple. Then, the septa between tunnels are cut. One of the different methods employed as part of the tunnel method is the creation of tunnels using bladeless trocars "Optiview, Bladeless Trocar, Endopath, Visiport Plus" [1, 2, 8, 13, 14, 16].

One of the techniques for subcutaneous dissection, which is recommended in the literature, yet has not been widely adopted in practice, is the use of traction sutures placed on the skin to facilitate dissection or the use of needles stuck on the skin in order to delineate the excision margins.

30.2.6 Specimen Excision and Reconstruction

Breast-Conserving Surgery The tissue that has been excised is removed through the peri-areolar incision. Some surgeons use "Endo-catch" in order to remove the specimen. The cavity is marked using clips. All the oncoplastic techniques used in reconstruction can be employed here, as well. The most commonly used techniques include the volume displacement, volume replacement, and filling techniques [1, 2, 13].

Volume Displacement This is the most commonly used technique. The breast tissue that is mobilized by being removed over the pectoral muscle posteriorly and from the skin anteriorly is pulled from both sides towards the cavity in the middle under the guidance of imaging and stitched together using sutures. If plication develops on the skin following volume displacement, skin mobilization is performed on a wider area.

Volume Replacement If the excised tissue is 30% of the total breast or more or the cavity that emerged cannot be closed with volume displacement, the latissimus dorsi flap or lateral thoracic adipose tissue flap mobilized with endoscopic technique can be brought to the cavity by working through the axillary incision [9, 17, 18].

Mastectomy For reconstruction after EASM, the methods that are employed in the open technique are used. Reconstruction with implant is performed with priority. A technique with dual or single procedure is preferred depending on the case or the surgeon. During the EASM procedure, mastectomy is completed and then work is done through the peri-areolar incision. An endoscopic retractor is used to start dissection of the pectoralis major muscle from its lateral margin with the aid of imaging, the area under the muscle is entered with sharp dissection and a pocket for implant is created using an expander. An implant or expander is inserted in the pocket through the axillary incision [1, 10, 11].

30.2.7 Operation Time

In general, longer times are reported for the endoscopic surgeries of the breast. The operation times are closely related with the reconstruction technique that is used. The endoscopic procedures performed at the beginning bring about an additional 30–40 min on average to the conventional surgical times. However, this time is associated with the learning curve. Operation times equal to those of open surgery when the learning process was completed have been reported.

30.2.8 Cost

The increased cost is associated with the materials that are used. Single-use instruments increase the cost. Re-usable instruments reduce the average cost. A study reported that the essential setup cost of the system to be able to start endoscopic breast surgery in addition to open surgery was $10,000. In another study where a rough cost analysis was performed, the cost of endoscopic lumpectomy was reported as $1150 and open lumpectomy as $500 [19, 20].

30.2.9 Cosmetic Results

Generally speaking, reasonable aesthetic results are reported with EAO-BCS. Two studies reported better results as compared to open surgery. A significant difference is achieved especially in terms of scars. For a comprehensive and objective assessment, a 4-point-scoring aesthetic evaluation should be made, and the quality of life should also be questioned. The assessment methods appropriate for this include the "Breast Cancer-Specific Quality of Life Questionnaire" (EORTC-QLQ-BR23) or "Patient Satisfaction Rate" (FACT-B) by EORTC (European Organization for Research and Treatment).

In the "5-item" system, which is commonly used in cosmetic assessment (ABNSW), the important assessment parameters include asymmetry, breast shape, nipple shape, skin condition, and wound scar. The scoring is done using a 4-points scoring system (excellent = 3, good = 2, moderate = 1, poor = 0). A score of 11 points in total or above is considered as good or excellent breast aesthetics.

The Japanese Breast Cancer Society, on the other hand, uses an 8-item classification. The themes used include the breast size, breast shape, breast scar, breast hardness, nipple and areola size, nipple and areola shape, nipple and areola color, nipple and areola position, and inframammary groove condition. Every theme is scored according to a 3-point system (good: 2 points, moderate: 1 point, poor: 0 points). In total, a score of 11–12 points is considered an excellent cosmetic result, 8–10 points good, 5–7 points moderate, and 0–4 points a poor cosmetic result. The results of endoscopic-assisted breast surgeries are generally reported as minimal scar and excellent cosmetic results. Kitamura reported an excellent result of 85% with the endoscopic technique and of 60% with the open technique in a study comparing this technique with open surgery. As for the questionnaire studies related to patient satisfaction, it is seen that the majority of patients receiving EOSM are pleased with the result [20, 21].

30.2.10 Complications

The complications reported with endoscopic breast surgery are generally the same in type and equal in rate with open surgery. Fan reported in his comparative series that the complication rates were equal for endoscopic and open technique and that they varied according to the surgical technique and type of reconstruction performed. The most frequently encountered complication is the development of seroma. Superficial or deep skin burns and ecchymoses due to the inadequate protection of skin are also often encountered. The wound site infection rates range between 1% and 9% and they are not higher than in open breast surgery. The infection rates are higher for mastectomy and implant procedures. The requirement to remove the prosthesis due to infection develops in approximately 10% cases where implants were used. When the insufflation technique is used to create a surgical working area, subcutaneous emphysema is often seen in the breast and surrounding tissues. Furthermore, asymmetry, deformity, and skin plication may develop in the breast and nipples depending on the reconstruction technique and procedure. There are no studies comparing endoscopic breast surgery with open surgery in relation to post-operative pain and the use of analgesics [14].

Nipple Necrosis It is one of the serious complications developing with EA-NSM. The rates reported in the literature are in the range of 0–20%. Full or partial necrosis may develop. The ratio of complete necrosis is below 10%. The reason why different rates are seen in the literature is that the tissue left in the tissue with EA-NSM is variable. No standard tissue thicknesses exist on which consensus has been achieved. Leaving a tissue with a thickness of 5 mm on an area with a width of 2 cm has been recommended. Another factor influencing the rate of complications is the use of cautery in dissection. For the dissection of the area below the nipple, the use of scissors rather than cautery is recommended [11].

An important factor in nipple necroses that develop following EA-NSM is the incision performed. Radial or lateral incisions should be preferred rather than medial incisions. For transareolar incisions, nipple necrosis develops at the highest frequency with a rate of 80%. Partial or full necrosis develops at a rate of 17% in periareolar incisions and a rate of 4–8% in radial or inframammary incisions.

One of the factors effective in the development of nipple necrosis following EA-NSM is the "coring" technique which is performed in certain centers. The tissue under the nipple is completely excised by being cored with oncological concerns and only the nipple skin is left behind. The rates of necrosis in cases where the nipple is cored amounts to 40% and nearly 24% of them are complete necrosis.

The most important factors influencing nipple necrosis are the ones that pertain to the patient. Patients who have diabetes, vascular disease, and smoke have higher rates of nipple necrosis. Nipple necrosis secondary to perfusion disturbance in large (Cup C and above) and overly flappy breasts also have higher rates. Most of the nipple necrosis, especially partial ones, improve with medical treatment and do not require excision.

30.2.11 Loss of Sensation in the Nipple/Areola

The loss of sensation in the skin, nipple, and areola following endoscopic breast-conversing surgery is rare. It is reported to generally improve in a period of 6 months to 1 year in patients receiving mastectomy [14].

30.2.12 Loss of Blood

In the initial periods when endoscopic technique entered into use, Kitamura reported that the endoscopic mastectomy group had more bleeding in his study where he reported the early results. In the consequent years, three different studies were performed in relation to intraoperative bleeding and post-operative drainage with the EASM technique and no differences were found between endoscopic and open methods. A study where reconstruction was made using the filling method following EAO-BCS found that bleeding was lower than with the open method.

30.2.13 Oncological Results

Breast-Conserving Surgery Rates that are equal to those of open surgery are reported with respect to local recurrence, distant metastasis, and overall survival while certain studies report better oncological results. However, the average follow-up durations are between 12 and 40 months and this is a rather short period to make a clear decision about oncological results [7].

Local Recurrence There are six studies assessing local recurrence following EAO-BCS. The studies where local recurrence is cited in the range of 0–4% have average follow-up durations of 12–38 months. Nakajima specified tumor size as a risk factor for local recurrence in EAO-BCS with local recurrence rates of 3.7% for T1 tumors and 5.1% for T2 tumors in his series. To date, local recurrence on peri-areolar or axillary incision in any of the EAO-BCS cases has not been reported [22].

Distant Metastasis Three studies related to the development of distant metastasis in patients who received EAO-BCS have been reported. In the study with an average follow-up period of 40 months, it was reported that the distant metastasis rate was associated with the tumor diameter. In a study with 244 cases, no differences were found in terms of distant metastasis among patients undergoing EAO-BCS and open surgery. Another study citing a metastasis rate of 10%, distant metastasis was attributed to the high axillary involvement ratio (41%) and high tumor load was blamed [22].

Overall Survival Five studies related to overall survival in patients undergoing EAO-BCS have been reported. The follow-up periods of the studies are short, but the results look excellent. A study citing data sorted by the tumor diameter reported an overall survival rate of 97.3% for T1 tumors and 95.7% for T1 tumors. Another study demonstrated that there were no differences in terms of survival among State I and Stage II patients who underwent EAO-BCS [22].

Mastectomy As in the open nipple-conserving mastectomy technique, discussions on the oncological risk of breast tissue left behind the nipple with EAO-BCS are also ongoing [9]. The collection and examination of biopsy from the tissue under the nipple during EAO-BCS constitutes a method that is rather widely implemented. However, suspicion of tumor or marginal positivity at the nipple are identified at rates amounting to 9% in the paraffin wax cross-sections in post-operative period in spite of this procedure, which may require these cases to undergo nipple excision in the aftermath. There are also studies recommending radiotherapy during or after surgery for the breast tissue remaining behind the nipple.

Local Recurrence Eight of the published papers cited the local recurrence rates. No recurrences were reported in studies with an average follow-up period of 2 years on average and in non-prospective studies. It is obvious that studies with longer follow-up periods are required in the light of studies indicating that recurrence is increased especially after the third year. A non-randomized study compared EASM and open, skin-conserving mastectomy cases in terms of local recurrence and it was reported that none of the cases had recurrence. Another study compared EASM and open breast-conserving surgery and no was demonstrated with the rate being 1.9% for open breast-conserving surgery and 8% for EASM [14].

Distant Metastasis Three studies in the literature cited distant metastasis rates and a rate in the range of 4.5–10% with the longest follow-up period being 38 months was reported. No differences in terms of distant metastasis were identified among EASM and open skin-conserving mastectomy patients in 2 studies with 143 patients in total [14].

Overall Survival One of the studies where EASM was performed and overall survival was reported, no significant differences were identified between EASM and open skin-conserving mastectomy. In other studies, a survival rate of 100% was reported for EASM with an average follow-up period of 12 months to 4 years [19].

30.2.14 Advantages

The most important advantages of endoscopically assisted breast surgery are “less scar,” “better cosmetic,” and “more patient satisfaction” [8].

30.2.15 Disadvantages

Longer Operation Time The reason behind is that work is done on a more limited surgical site. Furthermore, an influencing factor is that it is a new technique and requires training. The learning period also influences the learning period. The "Tumescent Technique" reduced the operation time.

Additional Cost EASM technique requires a new group of instruments and materials. The single-use instruments used in other laparoscopic surgeries have not yet been approved for endoscopic breast surgery. This deficiency creates a cost- and legislation-related problem in the implementation of this technique. For the solution, simple and re-usable instruments should be developed for the field of endoscopic breast surgery. In five studies reported in the literature, re-usable endoscopic retractors were used [4, 6, 15, 22, 23].

30.3 Robotic Nipple Sparing Mastectomy

Robotic surgery, which incorporates a three-dimensional imaging system, as well as flexibility of the robotic arm and instruments, has been increasingly used in different fields of surgeries. Robotic nipple sparing mastectomy (R-NSM), which introduces the da Vinci surgical platform through a small axillary wound to perform NSM with or without IBR, was reported to have the potential to overcome the technique difficulty of E-NSM, showed promising cosmetic outcome. In Hung-Wen Lai's study, they report on the preliminary experience and clinical outcome of the R-NSM and IBR with Gel implant procedure in breast cancer patients [24].

In their results, a total of 22 patients who received 23 R-NSM and IBR with Gel implant procedures were analyzed. The mean operation time for R-NSM was 118.8 $\pm$ 50.6 min, and 74.5 $\pm$ 26.6 min for Gel implant reconstruction. Docking time quickly dropped from 20 to 6–8 min, and the time needed to complete R-NSM was usually completed within 100 min after accumulation of case experience. Mean blood loss was 37 $\pm$ 38.2 mL, and the positive surgical margin rate was 0%. Three (13%) patients had transit nipple ischemia change, and no total nipple-areolar complex necrosis cases were observed. No local recurrence or mortality was found during a mean 6.9 $\pm$ 3.5 months of follow-up. All 22 patients were satisfied with the post-operative aesthetic outcome.

From their preliminary experience, R-NSM and IBR with Gel implant is a safe procedure, with good cosmetic results, and could be a promising new technique for

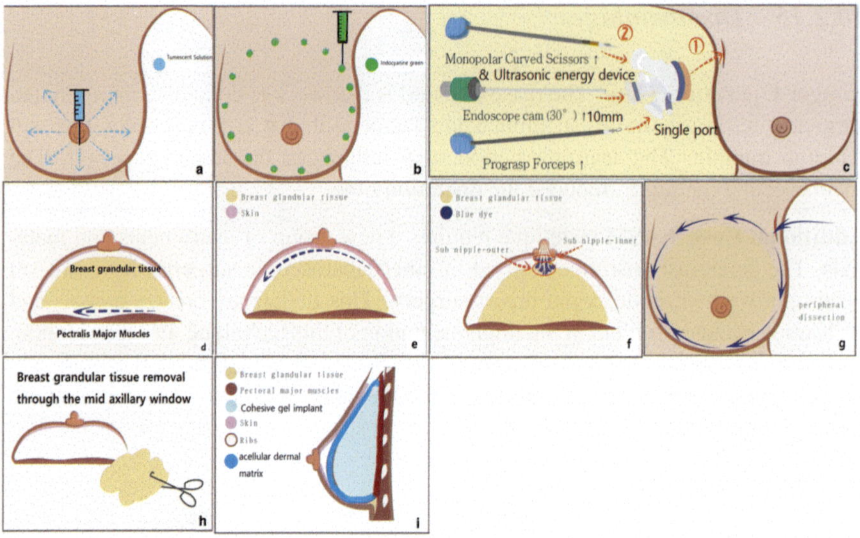

Fig. 30.11 Cartoon pictures to depict robotic nipple-sparing mastectomy and immediate breast reconstruction with Gel implant. (**a**) Hydrodissection with subcutaneous injection of saline solution (containing adrenaline and lidocaine) was performed in the whole breast to minimize bleeding. A physiological saline solution containing lidocaine 0.05% and epinephrine 1:1,000,000 was used in the current study. (**b**) Injection of jelly containing methylene blue as a guide to mark the boundary of resection. (**c**) Insertion of a single port, and robotic surgical platform with the da Vinci Si system (video camera, monopolar scissor, and ProGrasp forceps). (**d**) Subcutaneous skin flap dissection was performed by dissection between the skin flaps and breast glandular tissue. The septa between the skin flap and parenchyma were dissected using monopolar scissors. (**e**) Intraoperative sub-nipple biopsy was performed by taking two separate specimens (inner and outer part) under the nipple-areolar complex, which were sent for frozen section pathologic analysis. (**f**) Peripheral dissection was performed using ProGrasp forceps and monopolar scissors for dissection of breast tissue, and detached from the peripheral skin flap and chest wall. (**g**) Posterior subglandular dissection was performed using ProGrasp forceps and monopolar scissors for dissection of the plane between the pectoral muscle fascia and deep (inferior) part of the breast parenchyma. The penetrating vessels were coagulated and cut with monopolar scissors to ensure a clear visual field and to maintain hemostasis. (**h**) After completion of all the dissections, the entire breast specimen was removed through the axillary wound. (**i**) Breast reconstruction was performed with dissection of the subpectoral muscular pocket, which was formed by the pectoralis major, serratus anterior, and fascia of the external oblique muscle, using ProGrasp forceps and monopolar scissors. The Gel implant was inserted from the axillary wound and placed in the muscular pocket

breast cancer patients indicated for mastectomy. Women with small- to medium-sized breasts, node negative, and tumor located in the upper outer quadrant, with adequate skin to tumor distance (3 mm), are good candidates for R-NSM (Fig. 30.11).

The two main limitations of R-NSM were the longer operation time and the higher cost of robotic surgery. We observed that 10–12 cases were needed to decrease the robotic mastectomy time and, after that, R-NSM could usually be completed within 100 min, which was close to the conventional NSM operation time. There is inevitable increase in cost when performing R-NSM compared with conventional mastectomy. According to their estimation, it would cost US $10,000–12,000 to perform an R-NSM and IBR with Gel implant procedure. The cost of using the da Vinci surgical platform varied according to different institutions; however, in his institution, approximately US $6000 per use was required. Nonetheless, the cost effectiveness of robotic surgery in the management of breast disease remains to be analyzed [24].

30.4 Conclusion

Endoscopy is commonly used in the gastrointestinal, thyroid and endocrine surgery, urologic, and thoracic surgical fields but has yet to become a mainstream technique in the field of breast surgery. This is mainly because of the limited working space, the superficial nature of breast lesions, the low morbidity rate, and low levels of pain associated with breast surgery. The longer operation time than conventional surgery and the fact that breast tumors can commonly be accessed through small incisions were also the reasons why EABS is not widely performed.

Although those are valid reasons for not performing EABS for early stage breast cancer, which can be easily managed with partial breast excision followed by radiotherapy, in patients for whom mastectomy is indicated, EABS is an ideal surgery for cosmetic reasons because the wounds required for endoscopic surgery are much smaller than those needed for conventional surgery and can be hidden in inconspicuous locations.

The benefits of EABS with regard to incision size were more apparent in EATM than EPM.

BCS for patients with early stage breast cancer typically does not result in large scars. This might explain why EABS was more frequently performed in the setting of total mastectomy than partial mastectomy over the past 6 years in Taiwan (Fig. 30.13). However, compared with some oncoplastic breast surgery techniques (e.g., racket incision, batwing incision, and the round block technique), EAPM combined with volume displacement repair results in a smaller scar and better cosmetic outcome (Fig. 30.12) [5, 7, 14, 16].

EATM can be performed through a minimal incision without removing the skin envelope and NAC when there is no evidence of cancer cell invasion. This makes immediate, one-stage breast reconstruction feasible in most circumstances.

In Taiwan's EATM program, E-NSM was feasible in 74% of patients. Breast reconstruction after mastectomy is becoming more common worldwide. We found a similar increase in the use of EATM combined with IBR in their study (Fig. 30.13)

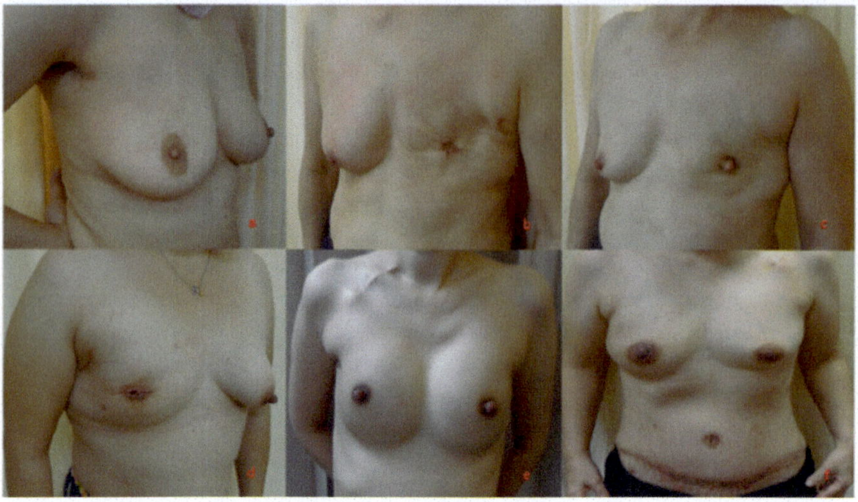

Fig. 30.12 Operative photos taken for representative techniques for robotic nipple-sparing mastectomy and immediate breast reconstruction with Gel implant. (**a**) An approximately 2.5–4 cm oblique axillary incision was made for lymph node surgery and insertion of a port. The axillary skin incision length depended on the size of the breast to be removed and the size of the Gel implant to be inserted. From our experience, when a breast specimen weighs 300 g (approximate breast cup size B), a 3.5 cm wound was usually sufficient; a breast specimen weighing 400 or 500 g (approximate breast cup size C or D) would require a 4 or 5 cm wound to retrieve the specimen. (**b**) After creation of the working space, the single port (Glove Port) was inserted over the operating axilla, and carbon dioxide (CO_2) inflation with air pressure was kept at 8 mmHg to create space for mastectomy. (**c**) The robotic side cart (da Vinci) is positioned posterior to the patient, with the two robotic arms and the endoscope extending over the patient in proximity to the ports. In this position, the arms are aligned with the plane of the breast, nearly parallel to the floor, and the ports are docked to the robotic arms. To prevent conflict during dissection, the elbows of robotic arms were opened as much as possible. (**d**) Anterior skin flap dissection was performed by dissection between the skin flaps and breast glandular tissue using the monopolar scissors. Intraoperative sub-nipple biopsy was performed by taking two separate specimens (inner and outer parts) under the nipple-areolar complex, which were then sent for frozen section pathologic analysis. (**e**) After mastectomy, the specimen was removed from the axillary wound, and the submuscular pocket, which was formed by the pectoralis major, serratus anterior, and fascia of the external oblique muscle, was then dissected for prosthesis breast reconstruction. The ProGrasp forceps were used to lift the pectoralis major muscles, and monopolar scissors were used for dissection of the submuscular space. By using the single port with one-way gas inflation and gas deflation in the opposite direction, a circulation air flow zone is created, which efficiently drains the smoke created when using monopolar scissors during dissection. (**f**) Immediately post-mastectomy before reconstruction, the wound was small and was hidden in the inconspicuous axilla region. (**g**) Immediate post-breast reconstruction outcome result, front view. The cohesive Gel implant (or tissue expander when indicated) used for breast reconstruction was inserted from the axillary wound and left in the subpectoral muscular pocket. Two drains were usually left (one beneath the skin flap and the other over the submuscular pocket).The drains were removed during the outpatient clinic follow-up, within 2 weeks postoperation

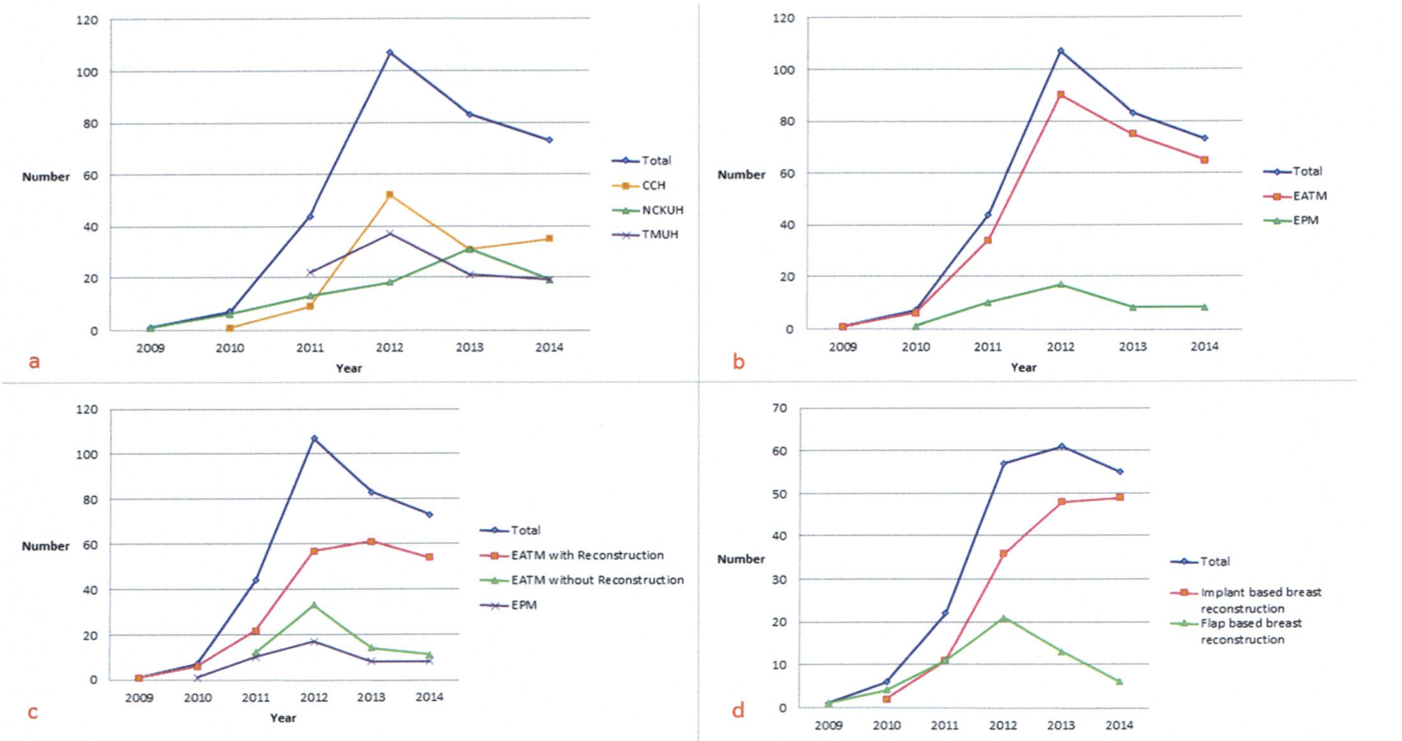

Fig. 30.13 Pre- and postoperative photos for patients receiving R-NSM and IBR with Gel implant. (**a**) Preoperative front view of a 49-year-old female with left breast ductal carcinoma in situ prepared for operation. The patient underwent left SLNB, and R-NSM and IBR with Gel implant. (**b**) Postoperative front view of the patient showing bilateral breast symmetry. The left breast nipple was well perfused, without sign of ischemia, and the wound was well hidden over the axilla. (**c**) Postoperative lateral view showing that the wound was small and well hidden in the inconspicuous axilla region. (**d**) Front view of a 59-year-old female with

[7]. Breast reconstruction following EATM normally involves the use of a tissue expander or implants (cohesive Gel or saline). E-NSM or E-SSM combined with IBR involving autologous pedicle TRAM flap is uncommon. In Taiwan's previous study, they found that EATM with autologous TRAM flap is a safe procedure and that it results in acceptable cosmetic outcome in women with early stage breast cancer.

During the six-year study period, we found a marked increase in the number of E-NSM procedures combined with reconstruction with Gel implants (Fig. 30.13). For women with small- to medium-sized breasts, BCS followed by radiotherapy, in some conditions, may not render a satisfying cosmetic result. E-NSM with IBR (Fig. 30.12) might provide an alternative option for patients because it does not involve radiotherapy and sometimes can result in better cosmetic outcome. This might explain why the number of EPM procedures decreased and the number of E-NSM procedures combined with Gel implant or TRAM flap for reconstruction increased during the study period (Fig. 30.13) [7].

Surgical margin, locoregional recurrence, distant metastasis, and overall survival are the major concerns regarding the oncologic safety of EABS in the management of breast cancer. Previous studies have demonstrated that EABS, either for BCS (E-PM) or total mastectomy.

(EATM), with or without preservation of the NAC, combined with delayed or immediate breast reconstruction, is associated with good cosmetic results and is oncological safe.

Nonetheless, larger patient numbers and longer follow-up are needed to establish the oncologic safety of the EABCS and E-NSM. Those from previous studies should help promote this under-used surgical technique in the field of breast cancer (Tables 30.1 and 30.2) [5–7, 10–15, 22, 24, 35].

Fig. 30.13 (continued) cancer of the left breast. R-NSM and SLNB were performed. Frozen biopsy revealed metastatic carcinoma, and axillary lymph node dissection was performed. Left R-NSM and IBR with Gel implant was performed. (**e**) Front view of the patient 3 months' postoperation, revealing bilateral breast symmetry. The nipple was well perfused, without sign of ischemia, and the wound was well hidden over the axilla. (**f**) Left lateral view, taken 11 months postoperation and after completion of a course of radiotherapy, showing that the wound was small and well hidden in the inconspicuous axillary region. (**g**) Relation of operation time and case experience accumulation in R-NSM and IBR with Gel implant. The 'time for docking' was defined as the time from the start of the insertion of a single port to completion of the set-up of a da Vinci surgical platform. The 'time for R-NSM' was defined as the time from set-up of a robotic surgical platform and starting skin flap dissection with monopolar scissors to the completion of robotic mastectomy and removal of the mastectomy specimen. The 'time for breast reconstruction' was defined as the time from removal of the mastectomy specimen to completion of the Gel implant insertion. The 'overall operation time' was defined as the time from the start of the skin incision to the end of the wound closure. The 'specimen weight' was the weight of the removed mastectomy specimen. R-NSM robotic nipple-sparing mastectomy, IBR immediate breast reconstruction, SLNB sentinel lymph node biopsy

Table 30.1 Oncologic safety of EABCS as reported in the literature

Author	Year	Journal	Number	OP method	margin positive	Follow-up (m)	Local recurrence	Distant metastasis	Death
Lee [25]	2006	World J Surg	20	E-PM	10% (2/20)	Cosmetic f/u 3 m			
Yamashita [23]	2006	J Nippon med Sch	82	E-PM	0%	25	0%	0%	
Yamashita [26]	2008	Am J Surg	20	E-PM	0%	12	0%	0%	
Nakajima [27]	2009	Ann Surg	551	E-PM	20.5% (113/551)	35	4.2% (23/551)	4.5% (25/551)	1.3% (7/551)
Park [3]	2011	J breast cancer	40	E-PM	5%	12	0%		
			681	BCS	10.6% (85/681)	12	0.3% (2/681)		
Ozaki [28]	2013	J Laparoendosc Adv Surg tech	73	E-PM	1.4% (1/73)	18.1 (12–30)	0%		
Takahashi [29]	2014	Surg today	100	E-PM	4%	23 (9–40)	0%	0%	0%

m months, *TM* total mastectomy, *f/u* follow-up, *E-PM* endoscopic-assisted partial mastectomy

Table 30.2 Oncologic safety of E-NSM as reported in the literature

Author	Year	Journal	Number	OP method	Reconstruction	margin positive	Nipple ischemia	Follow-up (m)	Local recurrence	Prothesis loss	Death
Nakajima [30]	2002	Biomed Pharmacother	17	E-NSM	LDMF	0 (0%)		14			
Ho [31]	2002	Surg endoscope	9	E-NSM	Prothesis, average 235 mL	0 (0%)					
Ito [32]	2008	ANZ J Surg	33	E-NSM	Prothesis, 30/33 (90.9%) average 235 mL	8 (24.3%) and excised NAC	3(9.1%) necrosis	51.2 (16–86)	0	9.1% (3/33) infection with prosthesis removed	
Fan [1]	2009	Chinese med J	43	E-NSM	Implant	0 (0%)	11.6% (5/43)	16.9 ± 11.2 (6–48)	0		0
Sakamoto [33]	2009	Ann Surg Oncol	87/89	E-NSM	No mention 0	0%, nipple involved 2 (2.2%)	18% (16/89)	52 (16–80)	0		
Tukenmez [34]	2014	J Laparoendosc Adv Surg tech	10/11	E-NSM	Prothesis, implant 4, Expander 6	0%, subnipple biopsy 1 (9.1%) positive	0%	3			

m months, *E-NSM* endoscopic-assisted nipple sparing mastectomy, *LDMF* latissimus dorsi myocutaneous flap

References

1. Fan LJ, Jiang J, Yang XH, Zhang Y, Li XG, Chen XC, et al. A prospective study comparing endoscopic subcutaneous mastectomy plus immediate reconstruction with implants and breast conserving surgery for breast cancer. Chin Med J (Engl). 2009;122(24):2945–50.
2. Hong YI, Shin H. Endoscopy-assisted breast conserving surgery for breast cancer: a preliminary clinical experience. J Breast Cancer. 2010;13(2):138–46.
3. Park HS, Lee JS, Lee JS, Park S, Kim S-I, Park B-W. The feasibility of endoscopy-assisted breast conservation surgery for patients with early breast cancer. J Breast Cancer. 2011;14 (1):52–7.
4. Jiang J. The assessment of safety of endoscopic surgery in the treatment of breast cancer. Zhonghua Wai Ke Za Zhi. 2007;45(7):439–41.
5. Fukuma E. Present situation and future of endoscopic breast surgery for breast disease. Nihon Geka Gakkai Zasshi. 2015;116(5):316–9.
6. Fukuma E. Endoscopic breast surgery for breast cancer. Nihon Geka Gakkai Zasshi. 2006;107 (2):64–8.
7. Lai HW, Chen ST, Chen DR, Chen SL, Chang TW, Kuo SJ, et al. Current trends in and indications for endoscopy-assisted breast surgery for breast cancer: results from a six-year study conducted by the Taiwan endoscopic breast surgery cooperative group. PLoS One. 2016;11(3): e0150310.
8. Ozaki S, Ohara M. Endoscopy-assisted breast-conserving surgery for breast cancer patients. Gland Surg. 2014;3(2):94–108.
9. Sanuki J, Fukuma E, Wadamori K, Higa K, Sakamoto N, Tsunoda Y. Volume replacement with polyglycolic acid mesh for correcting breast deformity after endoscopic conservative surgery. Clin Breast Cancer. 2005;6(2):175.
10. Friedlander LD, Sundin J, Bakshandeh N. Endoscopy mastectomy and breast reconstruction: endoscopic breast surgery. Aesthetic Plast Surg. 1995;19(1):27–9.
11. Du J, Liang Q, Qi X, Ming J, Liu J, Zhong L, et al. Endoscopic nipple sparing mastectomy with immediate implant-based reconstruction versus breast conserving surgery: a long-term study. Sci Rep. 2017;7:45636.
12. Satake T, Narui K, Muto M, Ishikawa T, Maegawa J. Endoscopic nipple-sparing mastectomy with immediate multi-stage fat grafting for Total breast reconstruction: a new combination for minimal scar breast cancer surgery. Plast Reconstr Surg. 2018;142:816–8.
13. Fukuma E, Sakamoto N. Endoscopic breast conserving surgery for breast cancer. Nihon Geka Gakkai Zasshi. 2009;110(1):34–6.
14. Soybir G, Fukuma E. Endoscopy assisted oncoplastic breast surgery (EAOBS). J Breast Health. 2015;11(2):52–8.
15. Tamaki Y, Miyoshi Y, Noguchi S. Application of endoscopic surgery for breast cancer treatment. Nihon Geka Gakkai Zasshi. 2002;103(11):835–8.
16. Singh S, Agarwal AA, Singh KR, Sonkar AA, Khuswaha JK, Singh A, Takahashi H, et al. Usefulness of endoscopic breast-conserving surgery for breast cancer. Surg Today. 2015;45 (8):1071–2.
17. Pomel C, Missana MC, Lasser P. Endoscopic harvesting of the latissimus dorsi flap in breast reconstructive surgery. Feasibility study and review of the literature. Ann Chir. 2002;127 (5):337–42.
18. Bognar G, Novak A, Ledniczky G, Istvan G. Breast reconstruction surgery with endoscopic assisted latissimus dorsi muscle flap. Magy Seb. 2017;70(2):147–50.
19. Leff DR, Vashisht R, Yongue G, Keshtgar M, Yang GZ, Darzi A. Endoscopic breast surgery: where are we now and what might the future hold for video-assisted breast surgery? Breast Cancer Res Treat. 2011;125(3):607–25.
20. Kitamura K, Ishida M, Inoue H, Kinoshita J, Hashizume M, Sugimachi K. Early results of an endoscope-assisted subcutaneous mastectomy and reconstruction for breast cancer. Surgery. 2002;131(1 Suppl):S324–9.

21. Jinno H, Inokuchi M, Ito T, Kitamura K, Kutomi G, Sakai T, et al. The Japanese Breast Cancer Society clinical practice guideline for surgical treatment of breast cancer. Breast Cancer. 2015;23(3):367–77.
22. Sawai K, Nakajima H, Mizuta N, Sakaguchi K, Hachimine Y. Progress in endoscopic surgery for breast cancer. Gan To Kagaku Ryoho. 2005;32(9):1240–3.
23. Yamashita K, Shimizu K. Endoscopic video-assisted breast surgery: procedures and short-term results. J Nippon Med Sch. 2006;73(4):193–202.
24. Lai HW, Chen ST, Lin SL, Chen CJ, Lin YL, Pai SH, et al. Robotic nipple-sparing mastectomy and immediate breast reconstruction with gel implant: technique, preliminary results and patient-reported cosmetic outcome. Ann Surg Oncol. 2019;26(1):42–52.
25. Lee E-K, Kook S-H, Park Y-L, Bae W-G. Endoscopy-assisted breast-conserving surgery for early breast cancer. World J Surg. 2006;30(6):957–64.
26. Yamashita K, Shimizu K. Transaxillary retromammary route approach of video-assisted breast surgery enables the inner-side breast cancer to be resected for breast conserving surgery. Am J Surg. 2008;196(4):578–81.
27. Nakajima H, Fujiwara I, Mizuta N, Sakaguchi K, Hachimine Y. Video-assisted skin-sparing breast-conserving surgery for breast cancer and immediate reconstruction with autologous tissue. Ann Surg. 2009;249(1):91–6.
28. Ozaki S, Ohara M, Shigematsu H, Sasada T, Emi A, Masumoto N, et al. Technical feasibility and cosmetic advantage of hybrid endoscopy-assisted breast-conserving surgery for breast cancer patients. J Laparoendosc Adv Surg Tech A. 2013;23(2):91–9.
29. Takahashi H, Fujii T, Nakagawa S, Inoue Y, Akashi M, Toh U, et al. Usefulness of endoscopic breast-conserving surgery for breast cancer. Surg Today. 2014;44(11):2037–44.
30. Nakajima H, Sakaguchi K, Mizuta N, Hachimine T, Ohe S, Sawai K. Video-assisted total glandectomy and immediate reconstruction for breast cancer. Biomed Pharmacother. 2002;56:205–8.
31. Ho WS, Ying SY, Chan AC. Endoscopic-assisted subcutaneous mastectomy and axillary dissection with immediate mammary prosthesis reconstruction for early breast cancer. Surg Endosc. 2002;16(2):302–6.
32. Ito K, Kanai T, Gomi K, Watanabe T, Ito T, Komatsu A, et al. Endoscopic-assisted skin-sparing mastectomy combined with sentinel node biopsy. ANZ J Surg. 2008;78(10):894–8.
33. Sakamoto N, Fukuma E, Higa K, Ozaki S, Sakamoto M, Abe S, et al. Early results of an endoscopic nipple-sparing mastectomy for breast cancer. Ann Surg Oncol. 2009;16(12):3406–13.
34. Tukenmez M, Ozden BC, Agcaoglu O, Kecer M, Ozmen V, Muslumanoglu M, et al. Videoendoscopic single-port nipple-sparing mastectomy and immediate reconstruction. J Laparoendosc Adv Surg Tech A. 2014;24(2):77–82.
35. Tajima T. Endoscopic surgery for breast diseases: the present state of art and outlook for the future. Nihon Geka Gakkai Zasshi. 2002;103(10):713–6.

Chapter 31
Minimal Invasive and Individualizing Management of the Axillary Nodes

Jun Won Min and Jihyoung Cho

Abstract The status of the axillary lymph nodes is one of the most important prognostic factors for patients with breast cancer. For over 100 years, axillary lymph node dissection was the standard approach to obtain and manage axillar lymph node, but now, sentinel lymph node biopsy has become a standard approach with less morbidity and equal accuracy in clinical node-negative patients. In addition, numerous studies are on the way to omit axillary lymph node dissection in specific patient subgroups. The recent trials like the ACOSOG Z0011 showed the evidence that omitting an ALND in patients with low burden nodal disease is safe in patients receiving whole-breast radiation. To reduce the use of ALND is the goal to consider when selecting an axillary management strategy.

Keywords Breast cancer · Axillary lymph node · Axillary lymph node dissection · Sentinel lymph node biopsy · Neoadjuvant chemotherapy

31.1 Introduction

In patients with breast cancer, the surgical management divides as breast and axillar part. The surgical management of breast cancer has undergone continuous and profound changes over the half decades. The recent trends have shifted from morbid radical resections to conservative multimodal approaches. The goals of axillary surgery are staging to decide the use and type of systemic therapy, and the locoregional control. Axillary lymph node dissection (ALND) was the standard approach of breast cancer throughout the last century, but has been largely replaced over the past decade by sentinel lymph node (SLN) biopsy [1, 2]. SLN biopsy for

J. W. Min (✉)
Department of Surgery, Dankook University College of Medicine, Cheonan-si, South Korea

J. Cho
Department of Surgery, Keimyung University school of Medicine, Daegu, South Korea

D.-Y. Noh et al. (eds.), *Translational Research in Breast Cancer*, Advances in Experimental Medicine and Biology 1187,
https://doi.org/10.1007/978-981-32-9620-6_31

breast cancer was first reported by Krag et al. in 1993 and Giuliano et al. in 1994 [3, 4]. Since SLN biopsy was developed, management of the axilla has been evolving rapidly in recent years. Numerous studies have demonstrated that aggressive surgical management of the axilla can be omitted for some breast cancer patients with not only negative SLNB results but also positive SLNB results.

31.2 Sentinel Lymph Node Biopsy

The sentinel lymph node is defined by the first lymph node which receives lymphatic drain from the anatomic site of the primary tumor [5]. The concept of SLN biopsy is based on that the tumor status of the SLN reflects the tumor status of the nodal basin. SLN biopsy was first introduced in the penile cancer and malignant melanoma [6]. The feasibility of identifying SLN and the capability of SLN biopsy to accurately predict the status of the entire axillary basin was demonstrated in 1994 [4]. SLN biopsy is performed using a blue dye or radioisotope, and the most commonly used agents are isosulfan blue dye and filtered technetium sulfur colloid. Numerous studies have shown that the combination of blue dye and radioisotope increases the SLN identification rate. However, in only one prospective randomized trial comparing the method, the number of cases done by an individual surgeon was a most significant predictor of SLN identification regardless of the method [7].

31.3 Clinically Negative Axilla (cN0)

In AJCC cancer staging, clinical categorization of cancer is based on findings of history, physical examination, and any imaging studies that are done [8]. Routine preoperative axillary ultrasonography for staging of clinical lymph node is controversial. Meta-analyses suggest that among patients who prove to have positive nodes, clinically occult axillary nodal metastases can be detected in about half on preoperative ultrasound evaluation [9, 10]. However, other studies suggest that abnormal node appearance on ultrasonography did not meet criteria for ALND in 70% of cases [11], and a needle biopsy specimen found to be positive tumor triggers an unnecessary ALND in 33% to 59% of cases [12]. Therefore, most guidelines do not recommend routine preoperative ultrasound evaluation, and clinical trials examining alternatives to ALND have defined eligibility based on physical examination alone.

In the clinically node-negative patient with invasive breast cancer, SLN biopsy should routinely be performed for axillary staging. Multiple randomized controlled trials have compared the overall and disease-free survival with the rate of identification rate of SLN and false negative rate (FNR) between SLN biopsy along with SLN biopsy plus ALND in patients with pathologically negative axilla. In most of these trials, the rate of identification of SLN was $\geq 95\%$, and the FNR ranging from 6.7% to 9.8% [2, 13–15]. The survival statistics from these trials showed the equivalent overall and disease-free survival rate to ALND, but associated with much less morbidity [2, 13, 15–18]. These studies led to SLN biopsy replacing ALND as the standard procedure in staging the axilla in clinically negative axilla patients.

31.3.1 *Neoadjuvant Chemotherapy in cN0*

The use of neoadjuvant chemotherapy (NAC) is increasing for patient with operable breast cancer to allow less invasive surgery in the breast and axilla [19]. In early studies about SLN biopsy after NAC, the accuracy of SLN biopsy was low, identification rates ranging from 63% to 100%, as well as FNR ranging from 0% to 33% [20, 21]. However, recently, various methods such as the use of dual tracer have been developed and the accuracy has increased. Also, many studies examining the accuracy of SLNB after NAC in patients with cN0 reported similar identification rates and FNRs to those seen in the upfront surgery setting [22, 23]. A single institution retrospective study of patients with cN0 and cN1 from Seoul National University Hospital (SNUH) include 281 patients who underwent SLN biopsy following NAC. The identification rate of SLNB after NAC was 93.6% and the false negative rate was 10.4% [24].

The timing of SLN biopsy when the patients have the plan of NAC has been debated extensively, with each approach having its advantages and disadvantages. The strongest advantage of SLN biopsy before NAC is to provide accurate axillary staging, which can be helpful to determine the loco-regional treatment, mainly radiotherapy (RT). There is a population-based study, which compared SLN biopsy in patients with cN0 axilla before NAC ($n = 980$) and after ($n = 203$) [25]. They reported that a higher proportion of patients had a negative SLN biopsy when assessed after NAC compared to before (67% vs. 54%, $p = 0.001$) and had lesser chance of undergoing ALND (33% vs. 45%, $p = 0.006$). These results indicate that SLN biopsy after NAC in patients with cN0 axilla is a feasible treatment option, and additional axillary treatment is not necessary in those with negative SLN [25].

31.3.2 *Positive Sentinel Lymph Node*

In the clinically negative axilla patients, SLN biopsy is considered the gold standard surgery for axillar management. If the SLN biopsy is positive for metastasis, then axillary lymph node dissection is warranted, and if it is negative, no additional axillary surgery is needed. However, many clinicians founded that the additional metastatic lymph node was often not founded when ALND was subsequently performed [26]. So, they designed the prospective randomized studies to investigate whether ALND can also be omitted for some breast cancer patients with positive SLN biopsy results. There were five randomized clinical trials with T1 or T2 clinically node negative breast cancers and one or two metastases in SLN that compared with [1] ALND or no further axillary treatment (ACOSOG Z0011,

Table 31.1 Studies of axillary lymph node dissection versus other treatment (observation or Ax RT) in cT1-2 N0 with one or two sentinel lymph node metastases

	ACOSOG Z0011 [28]	IBCSG 23-01 [29]	AATRM [30]	AMAROS [31]	OTOASOR [32]
No. of patients	856	933	233	1425	474
Randomization	Observation vs ALND	Observation vs ALND	Observation vs ALND	Ax RT vs ALND	Ax RT vs ALND
Breast conservation	100%	91%	88%	83%	84%
Size of SLN mets (%)	50% macromets	100% micromets	100% micromets	60% macromets	68% macromets
Follow-up	9.25 years	5 years	5.1 years	6.1 years	8 years
Additional positive nodes	27.3%	13%	13%	32.8%	38.5%
Axillary recurrence	ALND 0.5% observation 1.5%	ALND 0.2% observation 1%	ALND 1.0% observation 1.7%	ALND 0.4% Ax RT 1.2%	ALND 2% Ax RT 1.7%

IBCSG 23-01, AATRM) [27–30] or [2] ALND or axillary radiotherapy (AMAROS, OTOASOR) [31, 32] (Table 31.1).

ACOSOG Z0011, OTOASOR, and AMAROS trials recruited patients with limited macro-metastasis to the axilla. ACOSOG Z0011 study that was a phase 3 trial in which T1 or T2 patients undergoing breast-conserving surgery with one or two positive sentinel nodes were randomized either to completion ALND ($n = 445$) or observation ($n = 446$). ACOSOG Z0011 reported no additional benefit in regional control of the axilla for completion of ALND in this specific group of patients with low recurrence risk (1.5% vs. 0.5%, $p > 0.05$) [28]. The study was criticized because of lack of homogeneity in the whole breast radiotherapy tangents, early accrual closure, and too many ER-positive patients. However, it remains a very well-designed trial and the trial led to practice changing. AMAROS trial enrolled a patient population similar with ACOSOG Z0011. The difference with ACOSOG Z0011 was that mastectomy patients were included in AMAROS trial. They compared treating SLN biopsy-positive patients with ALND versus radiation treatment to the axilla. Five-year axillary recurrence was 0·43% ALND versus 1.19% after axillary radiotherapy. This trial also reported no additional benefit of ALND compared to RT in DFS (86.9% in the ALND group vs. 82.7% in the RT group, $p = 0.18$) [31]. The OTOASOR (Optimal Treatment Of the Axilla - Surgery Or Radiotherapy) trial compared ALND to regional nodal irradiation in patients with SLN metastasis in stage I or II breast cancer. Mean follow-up was 97 months. Axillary recurrence was 2.0% in ALND group vs. 1.7% in RTx group. Overall survival at 8 years was 77.9% vs. 84.8%, and DFS was 72.1% in ALND group and 77.4% after RTx group [32]. In conclusion, these trials have provided data that SLN biopsy alone in patients undergoing breast-conserving surgery found to have minimal disease burden in the axilla (micrometastases, one or two positive lymph nodes) is not inferior to a complete ALND. So, we can omit ALND in patients with low-burden axillary disease undergoing breast-conserving therapy with adjuvant whole-breast radiation.

However, an ALND should still be performed in patients who have three or more positive sentinel lymph nodes, or have fixed matted nodes, and in patients who are undergoing a mastectomy with any positive axillary lymph nodes. The POSNOC trial is now recruiting patients with limited axillary disease and will provide more reliable evidence on the comparison of axillary clearance vs. no further surgery to axilla [33]. The trial contained the patients who undergo either breast conservation or mastectomy. The trial can resolve the question whether ACOSOG Z0011 outcomes are reproducible to patients undergoing mastectomy.

31.4 Clinically Positive Axilla

Patients with palpable and suspicious appearing lymph nodes on imaging at the time of diagnosis should undergo needle biopsy or aspiration biopsy to confirm the presence of cancer. Patients with lymph node proven as metastasis by core biopsy or FNA are considered as clinically node-positive patients. In the presence of palpable nodal metastases, the only option to avoid ALND is the use of neoadjuvant chemotherapy (NAC). Although NAC does not improve survival compared with adjuvant therapy, one of the significant benefits of NAC is to preserve the breast and avoid the ALND after down-staging of the tumor [34]. The use of NAC has rapidly increased in operable breast cancer, and the rate of nodal response to NAC has reached up to 50–75% by the improvement of chemotherapy and targeted therapy [24, 35]. The increasing use of NAC has raised the question about the accuracy for patients who were clinically positive before NAC but became clinically negative. There are three clinical trials that investigated the validity of SLNB after NAC for those patients (Table 31.2). The ACOSOG-Z1071 trial enrolled 756 patients to investigate the validity of SLN biopsy after NAC and the primary endpoint was to determine the false negative rate of SLN biopsy with resection of at least two SLNs [36]. The predetermined threshold for the trial was a FNR of <10%, and they failed

Table 31.2 Prospective studies of sentinel node biopsy after neoadjuvant chemotherapy in cN+ axilla

	ACOSOG Z1071 [36]	SENTINA [37]	SN FNAC [38]
No. of patients	649	592 (cN+)[a]	153
Mapping	Dual tracer (79%)	Technetium required	Technetium required
Pre-OP biopsy	Yes	Not required (25%)	Yes
Nodal Pcr	41%	52% ypN0	35%
Identification rate (%)	92.7%	80.1%	87.6%
False negative rate (%)	12.6%	14.2%	9.6%
1 SLN	31.5%	24.3%	18.2%
2 SLN	21.1%	18.5%	4.9%
≥3 SLN	9.1%	7.3%	

[a]1737 patients enrolled in four-arm multicenter trial. 592 ARM C were cN+ to cN

to meet the threshold by the overall FNR was 12.6%. However, in further subgroup analysis, a significant reduction in the FNR was seen with the use of dual tracer mapping (11% vs 20%) and with the removal of at least three SLNs (9%). The SENTINA trial was the second prospective multicenter trial investigating SLNB after NAC in patients, who were clinically positive in Germany and Austria between 2009 and 2012 [37]. The trial had four study arms, and one of them (arm C) had 592 clinically node-positive patients that converted to a clinically and ultrasound node-negative axillar after NAC. They found an IR of 80.1% and an FNR of 14.2%. They showed a lower FNR with the use of dual agents (8.6% vs 16.0%) and when more SLN were removed (24.3% with one node, 18.5% with two nodes, and 4.9% with at least three nodes). The last prospective multicenter trial was the SN-FNAC study in Canada [38]. The difference from the two previous studies was that they included patients with isolated tumor cells (ITCs) on immunohistochemistry in the SLN as node positive. In this study, an IR of 87.6% and an overall FNR of 8.4% was reported. They also showed that removing more SLNs was associated with a lower FNR (18.2% with one SLN vs 4.9 with at least two SLNs). The use of dual tracers decreased the FNR. These three studies demonstrated that SLNB can be safely performed in patients who converted from node positive to clinically negative after NAC with usage of dual tracer and removal of at least two SLNs. Additional methods have been investigated to improve the FNR after NAC like [1] pre-NAC clipping and removing the clip-bearing node [39] and [2] marking the axillary nodes with radioactive seeds (MARI procedure) [40].

The last remaining question when performing only SLN biopsy after NAC was the long-term outcome, especially local recurrence, in patients who convert from clinically node positive to negative (SLN). All prospective studies required a back-up ALND to calculate the FNR, the information on nodal recurrence was not available from these studies. There is a multicenter retrospective study that we can address the issue [41]. They reviewed the records of 1247 patients who had breast cancer with clinically axillary lymph node-positive status and negative conversion after NAC. They compared the axillary node recurrence and distant recurrence-free survival with patients who underwent axillary operations with SLN biopsy-guided decision (Group A, 428 patients) and who underwent complete ALND without sentinel lymph node biopsy (Group B, 819 patients). The recurrence-free survivals were not significantly different between Groups A and B (4-year axillary recurrence-free survival: 97.8 vs. 99.0%; $p = 0.148$).

At present, SLN biopsy after NAC for clinical node-positive patients is being considered across dedicated breast units and is implemented in the last edition of the NCCN guidelines (Level 2b) [42].

31.5 Conclusion

The trend of management of axillar in breast cancer is moving toward less aggressive surgery in the axilla and individualizing the surgical approach to the axilla. The optimal approach to achieve this goal will depend on the type of breast surgery, nodal status, tumor biology (hormone receptor and ERBB2/HER2 status), and response to therapy.

References

1. Mansel RE, Fallowfield L, Kissin M, Goyal A, Newcombe RG, Dixon JM, et al. Randomized multicenter trial of sentinel node biopsy versus standard axillary treatment in operable breast cancer: the ALMANAC trial. J Natl Cancer Inst. 2006;98:599–609.
2. Veronesi U, Paganelli G, Viale G, Luini A, Zurrida S, Galimberti V, et al. A randomized comparison of sentinel-node biopsy with routine axillary dissection in breast cancer. N Engl J Med. 2003;349:546–53.
3. Krag DN, Weaver DL, Alex JC, Fairbank JT. Surgical resection and radiolocalization of the sentinel lymph node in breast cancer using a gamma probe. Surg Oncol. 1993;2:335–40.
4. Giuliano AE, Kirgan DM, Guenther JM, Morton DL. Lymphatic mapping and sentinel lymphadenectomy for breast cancer. Ann Surg. 1994;220:391–401.
5. Wong JH, Cagle LA, Morton DL. Lymphatic drainage of skin to a sentinel lymph node in a feline model. Ann Surg. 1991;214:637–41.
6. D'Angelo-Donovan DD, Dickson-Witmer D, Petrelli NJ. Sentinel lymph node biopsy in breast cancer: a history and current clinical recommendations. Surg Oncol. 2012;21:196–200.
7. Morrow M, Rademaker AW, Bethke KP, Talamonti MS, Dawes LG, Clauson J, et al. Learning sentinel node biopsy: results of a prospective randomized trial of two techniques. Surgery. 1999;126:714–20; discussion 720–2.
8. American Joint Committee on Cancer (AJCC). AJCC cancer staging manual. 8th ed. New York: Springer; 2017.
9. Houssami N, Diepstraten SC, Cody HS 3rd, Turner RM, Sever AR. Clinical utility of ultrasound- needle biopsy for preoperative staging of the axilla in invasive breast cancer. Anticancer Res. 2014;34:1087–97.
10. Diepstraten SC, Sever AR, Buckens CF, Veldhuis WB, van Dalen T, van den Bosch MA, et al. Value of preoperative ultrasound-guided axillary lymph node biopsy for preventing completion axillary lymph node dissection in breast cancer: a systematic review and meta-analysis. Ann Surg Oncol. 2014;21:51–9.
11. Pilewskie M, Jochelson M, Gooch JC, Patil S, Stempel M, Morrow M. Is preoperative axillary imaging beneficial in identifying clinically node-negative patients requiring axillary lymph node dissection? J Am Coll Surg. 2016;222:138–45.
12. Pilewskie M, Mautner SK, Stempel M, Eaton A, Morrow M. Does a positive axillary lymph node needle biopsy result predict the need for an axillary lymph node dissection in clinically node-negative breast cancer patients in the ACOSOG Z0011 era? Ann Surg Oncol. 2016;23:1123–8.
13. Mansel RE, Fallowfeld L, Kissin M, Goyal A, Newcombe RG, Dixon JM, et al. Randomized multicenter trial of sentinel node biopsy versus standard axillary treatment in operable breast cancer: the ALMANAC trial. J Natl Cancer Inst. 2006;98:599–609.
14. Krag DN, Anderson SJ, Julian TB, Brown AM, Harlow SP, Ashikaga T, et al. Technical outcomes of sentinel-lymph-node resection and conventional axillary-lymph-node dissection in

patients with clinically node-negative breast cancer: results from the NSABP B-32 randomised phase III trial. Lancet Oncol. 2007;8:881–8.
15. Canavese G, Catturich A, Vecchio C, Tomei D, Gipponi M, Villa G, et al. Sentinel node biopsy compared with complete axillary dissection for staging early breast cancer with clinically negative lymph nodes: results of randomized trial. Ann Oncol. 2009;20:1001–7.
16. Ashikaga T, Krag DN, Land SR, Julian TB, Anderson SJ, Brown AM, et al. Morbidity results from the NSABP B-32 trial comparing sentinel lymph node dissection versus axillary dissection. J Surg Oncol. 2010;102:111–8.
17. Veronesi U, Viale G, Paganelli G, Zurrida S, Luini A, Galimberti V, et al. Sentinel lymph node biopsy in breast cancer: ten-year results of a randomized controlled study. Ann Surg. 2010;251:595–600.34.
18. Krag DN, Anderson SJ, Julian TB, Brown AM, Harlow SP, Costantino JP, et al. Sentinel-lymph-node resection compared with conventional axillary-lymph-node dissection in clinically node-negative patients with breast cancer: overall survival findings from the NSABP B-32 randomised phase 3 trial. Lancet Oncol. 2010;11:927–33.
19. Bear HD, Anderson S, Brown A, Smith R, Mamounas EP, Fisher B, et al. The effect on tumor response of adding sequential preoperative docetaxel to preoperative doxorubicin and cyclophosphamide: preliminary results from National Surgical Adjuvant Breast and Bowel Project Protocol B-27. J Clin Oncol. 2003;21:4165–74.
20. Xing Y, Foy M, Cox DD, Kuerer HM, Hunt KK, Cormier JN. Meta-analysis of sentinel lymph node biopsy after preoperative chemotherapy in patients with breast cancer. Br J Surg. 2006;93:539–46.
21. van Deurzen CH, Vriens BE, Tjan-Heijnen VC, van der Wall E, Albregts M, van Hilligersberg R, et al. Accuracy of sentinel node biopsy after neoadjuvant chemotherapy in breast cancer patients: a systematic review. Eur J Cancer. 2009;45:3124–30.
22. Mamounas EP, Brown A, Anderson S, Smith R, Julian T, Miller B, et al. Sentinel node biopsy after neoadjuvant chemotherapy in breast cancer: results from National Surgical Adjuvant Breast and Bowel Project Protocol B-27. J Clin Oncol. 2005;23:2694–702.
23. Classe JM, Bordes V, Campion L, Mignotte H, Dravet F, Leveque J, et al. Sentinel lymph node biopsy after neoadjuvant chemotherapy for advanced breast cancer: results of Ganglion Sentinelle et Chimiotherapie Neoadjuvante, a French prospective multicentric study. J Clin Oncol. 2009;27:726–32.
24. Han A, Moon HG, Kim J, Ahn SK, Park IA, Han W, et al. Reliability of sentinel lymph node biopsy after neoadjuvant chemotherapy in breast cancer patients. J Breast Cancer. 2013;16:378–85.
25. de Munck L, Sonke GS, van Dalen T, van Diest PJ, van den Bongard HJ, Peeters PH, Rutgers EJ, et al. Population based study on sentinel node biopsy before or after neoadjuvant chemotherapy in clinically node negative breast cancer patients: identification rate and influence on axillary treatment. Eur J Cancer. 2015;51:915–21.
26. Chagpar AB. Clinical significance of minimal sentinel node involvement and management options. Surg Oncol Clin N Am. 2010;19:493–505.
27. Giuliano AE, Hunt KK, Ballman KV, Beitsch PD, Whitworth PW, Blumencranz PW, et al. Axillary dissection vs no axillary dissection in women with invasive breast cancer and sentinel node metastasis: a randomized clinical trial. JAMA. 2011;305:569–75.
28. Giuliano AE, Ballman K, McCall L, Beitsch P, Whitworth PW, Blumencranz P, et al. Locoregional recurrence after sentinel lymph node dissection with or without axillary dissection in patients with sentinel lymph node metastases: long-term follow-up from the American College of Surgeons Oncology Group (Alliance) ACOSOG Z0011 randomized trial. Ann Surg. 2016;264:413–20.
29. Galimberti V, Cole BF, Zurrida S, Viale G, Luini A, Veronesi P, et al. Axillary dissection versus no axillary dissection in patients with sentinel-node micrometastases (IBCSG 23-01): a phase 3 randomised con-trolled trial. Lancet Oncol. 2013;14:297–305.

30. Solá M, Alberro JA, Fraile M, Santesteban P, Ramos M, Fabregas R, et al. Complete axillary lymph node dissection versus clinical follow-up in breast cancer patients with sentinel node micrometastasis: final results from the multicenter clinical trial AATRM 048/13/2000. Ann Surg Oncol. 2013;20:120–7.
31. Donker M, van Tienhoven G, Straver ME, Meijnen P, van de Velde CJH, Mansel RE, et al. Radiotherapy or surgery of the axilla after a positive sentinel node in breast cancer (EORTC 10981-22023 AMAROS): a randomised, multicentre, open-label, phase 3 non- inferiority trial. Lancet Oncol. 2014;15:1303–10.
32. Sávolt Á, Péley G, Polgár C, Udvarhelyi N, Rubovszky G, Kovács E, et al. Eight-year follow up result of the OTOASOR trial: the Optimal Treatment of the Axilla - surgery or Radiotherapy after positive sentinel lymph node biopsy in early-stage breast cancer: a randomized, single centre, phase III, non-inferiority trial. Eur J Surg Oncol J Eur Soc Surg Oncol Br Assoc Surg Oncol. 2017;43:672–9.
33. Goyal A, Dodwell D. POSNOC: a randomised trial looking at axillary treatment in women with one or two sentinel nodes with macrometa- stases. Clin Oncol R Coll Radiol G B. 2015;27:692–5.
34. Rastogi P, Anderson SJ, Bear HD, Geyer CE, Kahlenberg MS, Robidoux A, et al. Preoperative chemotherapy: updates of National Surgical Adjuvant Breast and Bowel Project Protocols B-18 and B-27. J Clin Oncol. 2008;26:778–85.
35. Mamtani A, Barrio AV, King TA, Van Zee KJ, Plitas G, Pilewskie M, et al. How often does Neoadjuvant chemotherapy avoid axillary dissection in patients with histologically confirmed nodal metastases? Results of a prospective study. Ann Surg Oncol. 2016;23:3467–74.
36. Boughey JC, Suman VJ, Mittendorf EA, Ahrendt GM, Wilke LG, Taback B, et al. Sentinel lymph node surgery after neoadjuvant chemotherapy in patients with node-positive breast cancer: the ACOSOG Z1071 (Alliance) clinical trial. JAMA. 2013;310:1455–61.
37. Kuehn T, Bauerfeind I, Fehm T, Fleige B, Hausschild M, Helms G, et al. Sentinel-lymph-node biopsy in patients with breast cancer before and after neoadjuvant chemotherapy (SENTINA): a prospective, multicentre cohort study. Lancet Oncol. 2013;14:609–18.
38. Boileau JF, Poirier B, Basik M, Holloway CM, Gaboury L, Sideris L, et al. Sentinel node biopsy after neoadjuvant chemotherapy in biopsy-proven node-positive breast cancer: the SN FNAC study. J Clin Oncol. 2015;33:258–64.
39. Caudle AS, Yang WT, Krishnamurthy S, Mittendorf EA, Black DM, Gilcrease MZ, et al. Improved axillary evaluation following neoadjuvant therapy for patients with node-positive breast cancer using selective evaluation of clipped nodes: implementation of targeted axillary dissection. J Clin Oncol. 2016;34:1072–8.
40. Donker M, Straver ME, Wesseling J, Loo CE, Schot M, Drukker CA, et al. Marking axillary lymph nodes with radioactive iodine seeds for axillary staging after neoadjuvant systemic treatment in breast cancer patients: the MARI procedure. Ann Surg. 2015;261:378–82.
41. Kang YJ, Han W, Park S, You JY, Yi HW, Park S, et al. Outcome following sentinel lymph node biopsy-guided decisions in breast cancer patients with conversion from positive to negative axillary lymph nodes after neoadjuvant chemotherapy. Breast Cancer Res Treat. 2017;166:473–80.
42. Gradishar WJ, Anderson BO, Balassanian R, Blair SL, Burstein HJ, Cyr A, et al. NCCN guidelines insights: breast cancer, version 1.2017. J Natl Compr Cancer Netw. 2017;15:433–51.

Chapter 32
Malignant Phyllodes of Breast

Cha Kyong Yom

Abstract Phyllodes tumors of breast (PTB) have been known to an uncommon and particular disease to handle owing to diagnostic ambiguity and unpredictable clinical outcome. Malignant phyllodes tumors (MPT) are diagnosed when there are marked stromal hypercellularity, atypia, increased mitoses of $\geq$10/10 HPFs, permeative tumor borders, and stromal overgrowth. The presence of a malignant heterologous element (MHE) places the tumor into the malignant category regardless of other histological features. Excision with negative margins should be achieved for recurrent and malignant phyllodes tumor. An ideal margin width remains to be determined, and may need to be considered in relation to factors such as tumor size and cosmesis. Without the convincing evidence of survival benefit, adjuvant RT has revealed more favorable local control rate compared with observation group. Stromal expression of Twist and Foxc2, epithelial–mesenchymal transition marker, was associated with high tumor grade and poor prognosis. Tumor-associated macrophage drives myoblast differentiation and malignant progression of PTB through a CCL18-driven signaling cascade amenable to antibody disruption. Recent targeted sequencing on PTBs provided insights into the molecular pathogenesis and genetic characterization with potential clinical implications.

Keywords Malignant phyllodes tumors (of breast) · (Factors associated with) distant metastasis · Risk stratification

32.1 Introduction

The term *"phyllodes"* originates from the latin root *"Phyllodium"* meaning leaf-like depicting its appearance on microscopy. Its days would fade away like a leaf, unfortunately, the reality to be faced tells a different story. Phyllodes tumor of breast

C. K. Yom (✉)
Yom Breast Clinic, Seoul, South Korea

D.-Y. Noh et al. (eds.), *Translational Research in Breast Cancer*, Advances in Experimental Medicine and Biology 1187,
https://doi.org/10.1007/978-981-32-9620-6_32

(PTB) constitutes an uncommon but complex group of mammary fibroepithelial lesions and is a biphasic breast tumor composed of cellular spindle stroma with epithelial elements. Accurate and reproducible grading of these tumors has long been challenging, owing to the need to assess multiple stratified histological parameters, which may be weighted differently by individual pathologists. Characteristics of malignant phyllodes tumor of breast (MPT) different from benign and borderline diseases can cause metastasis to other organs and there is no convincing adjuvant treatment modality. One-fourth of PTBs are classified as malignant. However, the clinical behavior of PTBs can be difficult to predict, as some MPT may never exhibit metastatic behavior, while those that do metastasis have an extremely poor clinical outlook. Therefore, well catch and organization of property and propensity of MPT will make it possible to obtain treatment direction and policy. From a diagnostic and management perspective, it is important to accurately recognize MPT, which should be surgically eradicated and effectively treated at diagnosis, as these tumors have a well-established but relatively infrequent risk of metastasis and death.

32.2 Review of Past Studies

32.2.1 Clinicopathological Features

The World Health Organization in 2012 revisited the division of subtypes of PTB. A MPT shows marked stromal cellularity and atypia, has permeative margins, and has mitotic activity of at least 10/10 HPFs. Stromal overgrowth is usually easily identified (Table 32.1) [1]. The perceived clinical relevance of grading PTBs is to predict clinical behavior. Clinical presentations are often preceded by a rapid increase in size but the growth rate has not been firmly associated with malignancy [2]. Although the

Table 32.1 Histologic features of phyllodes tumors (adopted from WHO classification book 2012)

	Benign	Borderline	Malignant
Tumor border	Well-defined	Well-defined, may be focally permeative	Permeative
Stromal cellularity	Cellular, usually mild, may be non-uniform or diffuse	Cellular, usually moderate, may be non-uniform or diffuse	Marked
Stromal atypia	Mild or none	Mild or moderate	Marked
Mitotic activity	Usually few (<5 per 10 HPF)	Usually frequent (5–9 per 10 HPF)	Usually abundant (>10 per HPF)
Stromal overgrowth	Absent	Absent or very focal	Often present
Malignant heterologous elements	Absent	Absent	May be present

Table 32.2 Metastatic rates in phyllodes tumors according to grade [3]

	Tumour grade, % (no.)		
Authors (case number), publication year	Benign	Borderline	Malignant
Chaney et al. (n = 101), 2000	1.7 (1/59)	0 (0/12)	26.7 (8/30)
Chen et al. (n = 172), 2005	0 (0/131)	0 (0/12)	10.3 (3/29)
Sotheran et al. (n = 50), 2005	0 (0/29)	0 (0/12)	11.1 (1/9)
Abdalla et al. (n = 79), 2006	3.2 (1/31)	11.1 (3/27)	28.6 (6/21)
Tan et al. (n = 37), 2006	0 (0/22)	0 (0/9)	50 (3/6)
Cheng et al. (n = 182), 2006	0 (0/138)	7.7 (1/13)	9.7 (3/31)
Belkacémi et al. (n = 443), 2008	0 (0/284)	2.5 (2/80)	16.5 (13/79)
Lenhard et al. (n = 33), 2008	0 (0/13)	0 (0/9)	27.3 (3/11)
Guillot et al. (n = 165), 2010	0 (0/114)	0 (0/37)	14.3 (2/14)
Tan et al. (n = 605), 2012	0 (0/440)	0 (0/111)	13 (7/54)
Jang et at. (n = 164), 2012	0 (0/82)	0 (0/42)	10 (4/40)
Sawalhi et al. (n = 42), 2013	0 (0/16)	0 (0/9)	35.3 (6/17)
Wang et al. (n = 227), 2014	0 (0/125)	1.8 (1/55)	10.6 (5/47)
Bumpers et al. (n = 50), 2015	0 (0/40)	0 (0/3)	28.5 (2/7)
Total	0.13 (2/1524)	1.62 (7/431)	16.71 (66/395)

guidelines may appear straightforward, their application can be fraught with equivocacy. Furthermore, how the subdivisions for each microscopic parameter interact to constitute the final grade is subjective. It is also not uncommon for PTB to show intratumoral heterogeneity, and harbor features that typify benign lesions in some areas, and characteristics of borderline and malignant lesions in other foci. (For instance, a PTB with marked stromal atypia and brisk mitotic activity, but without permeative margins or stromal overgrowth, may be considered by some pathologists to be borderline, whereas others may regard the tumor as malignant, owing to different weighting of the relevance of each feature, with prioritization of stromal atypia.) A practical approach is to grade a phyllodes tumor as malignant when it shows all of the histological changes of malignancy, and as borderline when not all malignant characteristics are present [3]. Unexpectedly, grade progression during local recurrence of PTB can occur. There have been several suggestions regarding why this happens, including a lack of representative sampling of the initial tumor, tumor heterogeneity with the presence of stromal subclones, and loss of stromal–epithelial interdependency. Recurrence rates for MPT alone are reported as 23–30% in the literature [4]. The mean time to recurrence of MPT is reported as 20.3 ± 19.0 months [5]. PTBs show commonly hematogenous spread not lymphogenic. The majority of the tumors metastasize to the lungs, followed by the skeleton, heart, and then liver. It has been reported to involve almost all other organs. Most patients with metastatic diseases dye within 3 years of initiation of treatment regardless of the regimen [6]. How often do PTB metastasize, and do benign tumors ever do so? Table 32.2 shows metastatic rates according to phyllodes tumor grades that have been described by various authors. It may be reasonably inferred that metastatic disease is a vanishingly rare occurrence in benign PTB, with the qualification that all tumors should be adequately sampled to account for intratumoral heterogeneity. Conversely, metastatic behavior is an established risk for MPT, albeit still uncommon, and pathological diagnosis should focus on accurately identifying this group of tumors [3].

32.2.2 Surgery

The recommended NCCN guideline treatment of MPT is complete surgical excision with 1 cm margins without sentinel lymph node biopsy. Mastectomy at the index surgery is only recommended in the cases if the inability to adequately obtain 1 cm margins or if changes in the cosmetics of the breast would be unacceptable to the patient [7]. The backbone of PTB management has generally consisted of surgical excision with wide margins of at least 10 mm. As convincing evidence for an appropriate margin width in surgically excised PTB remains elusive, it may be pragmatic to consider tumor on ink, or <1 mm as positive margin. Literature review from 2009 to 2016 of 12 studies with overall 1702 patients shows that there is no difference in recurrence rates between a 1 and a 10 mm margin. One millimeter is an acceptable margin for benign PTBs. The recurrence rate increases if there is focal margin involvement [8]. Taira et al. reported that a positive surgical stump was the only independent predictor of local recurrence (LR) in multivariate analysis (RR 0.086; 95% CI 0.01–0.743, $p = 0.012$). Stromal overgrowth was a predictive factor for LR in cases with a positive surgical margin ($p = 0.014$) [9].

To ensure a surgical margin of ≥ 1 cm for the effective treatment of all PTBs, a second resection has been recommended, but is it indispensible to obtain negative margins in all cases? PTB is still a problematic entity to identify those patients who need reoperation to obtain negative margins to avoid LR. Our recent study about reappraisal of conventional risk stratification for LR and optimal treatment based on clinical outcomes gave a proposal to draw paradigm shift in the treatment of PTB. We set out to determine the most appropriate surgical approach to PTB, especially with regard to aspects involving the question of eliminating the need for reoperation. Yom et al. retrospectively analyzed data on all 285 cases resected between June 1989 and December 2008 at the Department of Surgery of Seoul National University Hospital and affiliated hospital. Surgical treatment was categorized as the vacuum-assisted biopsy system (VABS), wide local excision, or mastectomy. The surgical margin was defined as positive if the tumor was present at or close to (<0.1 mm) the inked tissue edge on histological evaluation. The results show that mitoses ($p < 0.001$) and tumor size ($p = 0.021$) were independent prognostic factors for LR in multivariate analysis (Table 32.3). Neither margin status ($p = 0.758$) nor type of surgery ($p = 0.922$) had any significance for LR. In the risk stratification for LR, PTB ≤ 5 cm in size with ≥ 10 mitoses/10 HPF had the highest LR rate (55.6%) compared with all other subgroups ($p < 0.001$) (Table 32.4). Our results also show that margins <0.1 mm were not associated with greater LR ($p = 0.773$ for LR-free survival compared with the ≥ 0.1 mm group). That is, a clear surgical margin of

Table 32.3 Local recurrence-free survival of phyllodes tumor of breast by Cox-regression

Subgroup of patients	No recurrence		Recurrence		Univariate		Multivariate	
	n	%	*n*	%	HR	*p* value	HR	*p* value
Mitoses						0.012		<0.001
1–9/10 HPF	225	93.8	15	6.2				
>10/10 HPF	20	80.0	5	20.0	3.647		10.282	
Size (cm)						0.160		0.021
≤5	212	87.9	19	12.1	4.237		12.500	
>5	51	98.1	1	1.9				
Operation						0.957		0.922
WLE	229	93.1	17	6.9				
VABS	23	92.0	2	8.0	1.247	0.768	1.230	0.865
Mastectomy	13	92.9	1	7.1	1.055	0.959	0.658	0.709
Margin						0.886		0.758
Clear	202	93.1	15	6.9				
Close/involvement	42	93.3	3	6.7	0.983	0.979	1.223	

Yom et al. [10]
HR hazard ratio, *HPF* high-power fields, *WLE* wide local excision, *VABS* vacuum-assisted biopsy system

Table 32.4 Local recurrence rate according to subgrouping by tumor size and mitoses ($p < 0.001$) [10]

	Mitosis			
Tumor size (cm)	0–9/10 HPF		≥10/10 HPF	
≤5	Group 1		Group 2	
	$N = 204$	LRR = 6.9%	$N = 9$	LRR = 55.6%
		(14/204)		(5/9)
>5	Group 3		Group 4	
	$N = 36$	LRR = 2.8%	JV = 15	LRR = 0.0%
		(1/36)		(0/15)

0.1 mm is not inferior to a margin of 1 cm. Therefore, it is recommended a wide excision and clear margin of 1 cm be ascertained in only small PTB with frequent mitoses, if necessary by means of a second surgery, which could be considered in order to avoid the risk of LR in this distinct and limited group [10].

Because of the infrequency of nodal disease in PTBs, most investigators do not recommend routine axillary dissection [3]. Clinical lymphadenopathy has been said to be present in 20% of patients, but true metastatic locally advanced disease in the axilla is very rare although distant metastatic disease has been reported in up to 20% of MPT [11].

32.2.3 Radiation Therapy (RT)

Patients with MPT are routinely treated with surgery alone. Complete surgical excision has high rates of local control and disease-free survival [11, 12]. However, surgical resection alone yields long-term local control for the large majority of MPT patients. Richard et al. reported that five-year actuarial local control rates for patients with MPT treated by surgery alone were 91.2% in mastectomy and 79.4% in lumpectomy. This study demonstrated that local control was related to tumor size and type of surgery (Table 32.5). For mastectomy patients, local control rates exceed 85% for all patients except those with tumors >10 cm. For lumpectomy patients, local control rates exceeded 85% only for those with tumors <2 cm [13]. Analyses of LR for other malignancies such as breast cancer suggest that a 15% risk of LR would seem an appropriate level of concern to consider adjuvant RT. Based on these data, adjuvant RT should be evaluated for MPT patients if they underwent lumpectomy for tumors at least 2 cm in size or mastectomy for tumors at least 10 cm in size. The most persuasive role of RT is the adjuvant treatment for patients with positive or close resection margin. One study demonstrated that the 5-year disease-free survival rates were not different between BCS plus RT (tumor-free margin <1 cm) and BCS only (tumor-free margin 1 cm) groups [14]. In a recent meta-analysis of updated SEER 18 data (1983–2013), a total of 1974 patients with MPT were reviewed. Of these, 825 (42%) and 1149 (58%) patients underwent mastectomy and BCS, respectively. In each group, 130 (16%) and 122 (11%) patients with adverse risk factors including high grade and large tumor size received postoperative RT. Age (>50 years old), black ethnicity, tumor size (>5 cm), tumor invasion depth, and LN positivity were significantly correlated with cancer specific death in the mastectomy group while age and grade were significant in the BCS group. Neither postoperative RT impact on cancer-specific survival (CSS) in multivariate analysis, nor RT group was inferior to non-RT group on CSS even though RT group contained more adverse clinicopathologic features than the counterpart regardless the type of surgery [15]. Without the convincing evidence of survival benefit, however, the administration of postoperative RT for MPT has increased, and postoperative RT has revealed more favorable local control rate compared with the observation group [16, 17]. If adjuvant RT is recommended, it would be reasonable to use RT guidelines for soft tissue sarcomas. This might typically involve treatment of the breast or chest wall to approximately 50 Gy in 5–5.5 weeks followed by a local boost to the tumor bed (or mastectomy scar) for an additional 10–15 Gy in 1–2 weeks [13].

Table 32.5 Five-year actuarial local control rates for patients with malignant phyllodes tumors of the breast treated by surgery alone based on tumor size and type of surgery [13]

Tumor size	Lumpectomy	Mastectomy
0–2 cm	91% ($n = 23$)	100% ($n = 16$)
2–5 cm	85% ($n = 84$)	95% ($n = 59$)
5–10 cm	59% ($n = 24$)	88% ($n = 51$)
10–20 cm	None	85% ($n = 32$)
All cases	79.4% ($n = 169$)	91.2% ($n = 207$)

32.2.4 *Systemic Therapy*

ER and PR positivity have been described in 58% and 75% of PTB, respectively, but no defined benefit has been derived from hormone therapy [3]. Hormone receptors have confirmed their presence in epithelial tissue of all types of PTB. Unfortunately, the ER-β is the predominant receptor present rather than ER-α that is the most common ER present in typical invasive ductal carcinoma of the breast. At this point, hormone therapy has no role in the treatment of MPT and should be omitted [18–20]. Chemotherapy for MPT is controversial and there are no randomized clinical trials assessing the role of adjuvant chemotherapy with the poor prognosis of metastatic disease. In a large MPT, preoperative chemoembolization permits avoidance of skin graft after surgery [21].

32.3 Current Evidence and Concepts

Tumor size has been shown to be associated with distant metastasis in several studies that tumor size of >10 cm correlated with the development of distant metastases [22]. Koh et al. reported that a combination of large tumor size (≥90 mm) and the presence of malignant heterologous elements (MHE) had a statistically significant association with the development of distant metastasis. MHE were defined as malignant mesenchymal components such as liposarcoma, rhabdomyosarcoma, osteosarcoma, and chondrosarcoma. On multivariate analysis, large tumors harboring MHE are independently associated with poorer metastasis-free survival (HR 2.434, 95% CI 1.041–12.517, $p = 0.049$). The most common MHE was also liposarcoma being documented in this series [23]. Heterologous sarcomatous differentiation is a rare occurrence in PTB; its presence, however, immediately qualifies a PTB as malignant, even in the absence of other malignant histologic features [24]. The presence of a MHE such as liposarcoma, chondrosarcoma, or osteosarcoma relegates the tumor into the malignant category regardless of whether other histological parameters (stromal hypercellularity, atypia, mitotic rate, overgrowth, and nature of tumor borders) show changes characteristic of MPT.

The stroma is the most important aspect of the pathologic characteristics as it predicts the behavior pattern and metastatic potential of PTB. That is, the potentially recurring and metastatic behavior of PTB is attributed to the characteristics of stromall cells, mainly fibroblasts. Activated fibroblasts express the α-smooth muscle actin (α-SMA) as a hallmark and is so-called as myofibroblasts. Myofibroblasts were the major malignant component of PTB. The increased myofibroblast population drives the tumorigenicity of PTB. In addition, α-SMA can serve as an independent prognostic factor for PTB with better predictive values than histologic classification. The fibroblasts–myofibroblasts transition in PTB is driven by the elevated miR-21, whereas the mechanism of miR-21 upregulation and how it drives tumorigenicity of PTB remain unknown [25].

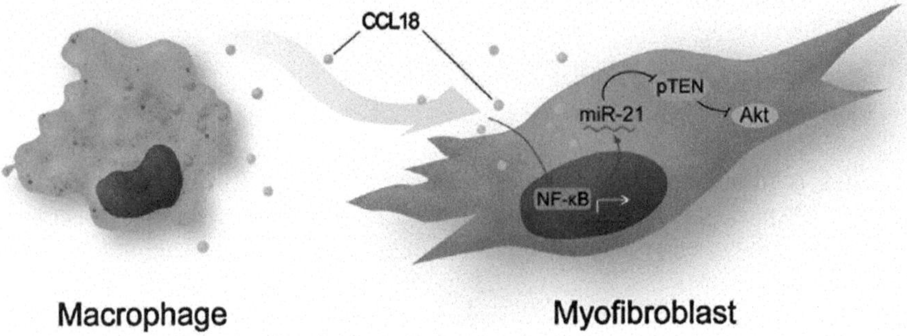

Fig. 32.1 The working model of how macrophages release CCL18 to promote phyllodes tumor tumorigenesis via NF-kB/miR-21/PTEN axis [30]

Epithelial–mesenchymal transition (EMT), an important process during embryonic development, is reportedly exploited during tumor progression. Aberrant expression of EMT-related molecules has been shown in many malignancies. Lim et al. reported that Twist and Foxc2 stromal nuclear expression was associated with tumor grade ($p = 0.038$ and 0.012). Foxc2 stromal nuclear expression was positively correlated with tumor relapse and metastasis ($p = 0.037$). Furthermore, stromal nuclear immunoreactivity of Twist and Foxc2 was interrelated ($p < 0.001$). Tumors expressing Foxc2 and those co-expressing both Twist and Foxc2 revealed a shorter time to recurrence ($p < 0.001$ and 0.001) and death ($p = 0.044$ and 0.015). Twist and Foxc2 stromal expression in PTB was significantly correlated with tumor grade and worse histological features. In addition, expression of Foxc2 and co-expression of Twist and Foxc2 in the stroma of PTs contributed to poorer prognosis [26]. Other recent study supported these results that expression of E-cadherin, Snail, Slug, and Twist were higher in epithelial cells from borderline and malignant tumors than those in benign tumors, where the expression of N-cadherin was apposite [27].

It is well established that tumor-associated macrophages (TAM) are one of the most abundant cell type in tumor microenvironment, which are involved in tumor metastasis and progression and a strong correlation between the increased TAMs density and poor prognosis in several types of cancer including breast cancer [28, 29]. Nie et al. report that TAMs induce myofibroblast differentiation and promote the proliferation and invasion of the phyllodes tumor cells and CCL18 is responsible for TAM-induced myofibroblast differentiation, proliferation, and invasion. CCL18 upregulates miR-21 expression, thus inducing myofibroblast differentiation via activating NF-kB, that is, promotes AKT activation in myofibroblasts through NF-kB/miR-21/PTEN axis. M2 macrophage-secreted CCL18 accelerates tumor growth, induces myofibroblast differentiation, and promotes metastasis of PTB xenografts. TAMs are essential for driving myofibroblast differentiation (fibro-myofibroblasts transition) in the malignant progression of PTB via the CCL18/NF-κB/miR-21/PTEN/AKT axis and targeting CCL18 is a promising strategy for treating PTB (Fig. 32.1). In this study, in vivo findings show that blocking CCL18 with neutralizing antibody effectively shrinks phyllodes tumors in mouse xenograft models, which suggests that antagonizing the CCL18 signaling may emerge as a promising strategy to treat phyllodes tumors. Together, these data suggest that the intercellular communication between TAMs and myofibroblasts via CCL18/NF-kB/miR-21/PTEN/AKT axis plays a central role in the tumorigenesis of PTB. Monitoring CCL18 level and targeting this pathway raise the possibility of precision diagnosis and treatment for breast phyllodes tumors [30].

Tan et al. reported genomic landscapes of breast fibroepithelial tumors by performing whole-exome sequencing of 22 matched tumor and normal fairs of PTBs and identified 333 nonsynonymous splice-site somatic mutations in 310 genes. These results show highly recurrent mediator complex subunit 12 (*MED12)* somatic mutation in exon 2 (73%) with most mutations occurring in codon 44 and *RARA* (32%) mutations in both fibroadenomas and PTB, emphasizing the importance of these mutations in fibroepithelial tumorigenesis. PTB exhibited mutations in *FLNA*, *SETD2,* and *KMT2D* that were rarely present in fibroadenomas, suggesting a role in driving phyllodes tumor development. In comparison to benign, borderline and malignant PTBs exhibited additional mutations coupled with putative CNAs in *NF1*, *RB1*, *TP53*, *PIK3CA*, *ERBB4,* and *EGFR*, which are known cancer driver genes that have transforming ability. These show canonical activating mutations in *PIK3CA* and high-level amplifications of *EGFR* exclusively in higher-grade phyllodes tumors, identifying a potential therapeutic opportunity for EGFR- and PI3K-targeted treatments. *RARA* mutations exhibited clustering in the portion of the gene encoding the ligand-binding domain, functionally suppressed RARA-mediated transcriptional activation and enhanced RARA interactions with transcriptional co-repressors. They investigated whether fibroadenomas might progress to malignant phyllodes tumors in a linear fashion. They sequenced paired concurrent fibroadenoma-like and phyllodes tumor regions isolated from the same patients ($n = 3$) also analyzed paired longitudinally acquired tumor samples from two more patients with initial fibroadenomas and subsequent phyllodes tumor recurrences. Even in the same patient, higher-grade phyllodes tumors harbored more mutations in cancer-associated genes than the paired fibroadenoma-like regions in concurrent samples. Taken collectively, these observations suggest that the development of these tumors may not always follow a strict linear progression from fibroadenomas to phyllodes tumors, but these tumors may also arise de novo [31].

In a recent study, a total of 17 PTBs including 13 MPTs were collected between 2001 and 2012 on targeted deep sequencing of PTB showing that the most frequently detected genetic alteration occurred in the *TERT* promoter region (70.6%), followed by *MED12* (64.7%), as in previous genetic studies. MPTs without genetic alterations in *MED12* and *TERT* promoter regions had variant genetic alterations. *EGFR* amplification and *TP53* and *DNMT3A* mutations were repeatedly observed, and they suggest that these mutations were possibly initiate tumorigenesis in the absence of *TERT* and *MED12* alterations. Genetic alterations of *RARA* and *ZNF703* were repeatedly found in PTB with local recurrence, and genetic alterations of *SETD2, BRCA2*, and *TSC1* were detected in PTB with distant metastasis. Especially, one case of MPT harboring *PTEN* and *RB1* copy number deletion showed rapid

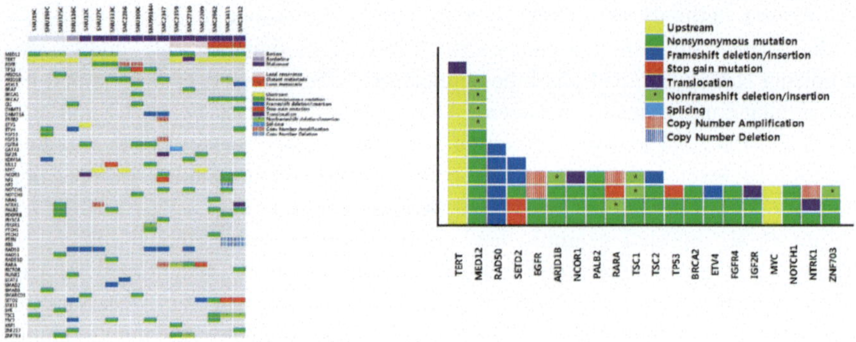

Fig. 32.2 Frequency of genetic alterations identified in phyllodes tumors ($N = 17$) [32]

disease progression despite exertive treatment including repeated metastatectomy, palliative chemotherapy, and RT. Target agents for these genetic alterations already exist. PARP inhibitor targeting *BRCA2* and mTOR/AKT inhibitor for *TSC1* would be potential target agents for the treatment of metastatic MPTs (Fig. 32.2) [32].

32.4 Future Research Direction

Interpretive subjectivity, overlapping histological diagnostic criteria, suboptimal correlation between histological classification and clinical behavior and the lack of robust molecular predictors of outcome make further investigation of the pathogenesis of these fascinating tumors a matter of active research. Further work in investigating predictive factors of distant metastasis will help in identifying the group of patients who are at higher risk of developing metastasis. That is, evaluation of EMT marker, tumor-associated macrophage, and α-SMA can serve the prognostic and predictive information of MPT. The intercellular communication between TAMs and myofibroblasts via CCL18/NF-kB/miR-21/PTEN/AKT axis plays a central role in the tumorigenesis of PTB. Therefore, monitoring CCL18 level and targeting this pathway raise the possibility of precision diagnosis and treatment for PTB. Canonical activating mutations in PIK3CA and high-level amplifications of EGFR exclusively in higher-grade PTB, identifying a potential therapeutic opportunity for EGFR- and PI3K-targeted treatments. Notable genetic alterations associating local recurrence and metastasis exhibiting malignant potential were detected. Therefore, large-scale comprehensive genetic studies and functional validation will provide a fundamental understanding of the genetic characteristics of PTB and clues to effective therapeutic strategies for this rare and potentially lethal disease.

32.5 Summary (the Bench—Translation—The Bedside)

Clinical relevance of expression of EMT-related molecules, evaluation of TAM with CCL18 and targeting this pathway, and to identify and validate the specific genes associated with tumor progression including metastasis and recurrence may be worthy of further investigation in PTB. These comprehensive approaches with clinical features can illuminate current murky condition and raise the possibility of precision diagnosis and treatment of PTB, especially for risky patients facing high-grade tumors.

References

1. Tavassoli FA, Devilee P. Pathology and genetics of tumours of the breast and female genital organs. In: World Health Organization classification of tumours. Lyon: International Agency for Research on Cancer (IARC) Press; 2003. p. 99–101.
2. Parker SJ, Harries SA. Phyllodes tumours. Postgrad Med J. 2001;77(909):428–35.
3. Tan BY, Acs G, Apple SK, Badve S, Bleiweiss IJ, Brogi E, et al. Phyllodes tumours of the breast: a consensus review. Histopathology. 2016;68:5–21. https://doi.org/10.1111/his.12876.
4. Tan PH, Thike AA, Tan WJ, Thu MM, Busmanis I, Li H, et al. Predicting clinical behaviour of breast phyllodes tumours: a nomogram based on histological criteria and surgical margins. J Clin Pathol. 2012;65:69–76.
5. Adesoye T, Neuman HB, Wilke LG, Schumacher JR, Steiman J, Greenberg CC. Current trends in the management of phyllodes tumors of the breast. Ann Surg Oncol. 2016;23(10):3199–205.
6. Tavassoli FA, Eusebi V. Chapter 14: biphasic tumor. In: AFIP atlas of tumor pathology series 4. Tumors of the mammary gland. Washington DC: America Registry of Pathology Press-Armed Forces of Institute of Pathology; 2009. p. 323–34.
7. National Comprehensive Cancer Network. NCCN guidelines version 2.2016. Breast cancer. https://www.nccn.org/professionals/physician_gls/pdf/breast_blocks.pdf. Accessed 21 Nov 2016.
8. Shaaban M, Barthelmes L. Benign phyllodes tumours of the breast: (over) treatment of margins - a literature review. Eur J Surg Oncol. 2017;43:1186–90.
9. Taira N, Takabatake D, Aogi K, Ohsumi S, Takashima S, Nishimura R, et al. Phyllodes tumor of the breast: stromal overgrowth and histological classification are useful prognosis-predictive factors for local recurrence in patients with a positive surgical margin. Jpn J Clin Oncol. 2007;37(10):730–6.
10. Yom CK, Han WS, Kim SW, Park SY, Park IA, Noh DY. Reappraisal of conventional risk stratification for local recurrence based on clinical outcomes in 285 resected phyllodes tumors of the breast. Ann Surg Oncol. 2015 Sep;22(9):2912–8.
11. Macdonald OK, Lee CM, Tward JD, Chapple CD, Gaffney DK. Malignant phyllodes tumor of the female breast: association of primary therapy with cause-specific survival from the surveillance, epidemiology, and end results (SEER) program. Cancer. 2006;107:2127–33.
12. Chaney AW, Pollack A, McNeese MD, et al. Primary treatment of cystosarcoma phyllodes of the breast. Cancer. 2000;89:1502–11.
13. Pezner RD, Schultheiss TE, Benjamin Paz I. Malignant phyllodes tumor of the breast: local control rates with surgery alone. Int J Radiat Oncol Biol Phys. 2008;71(3):710–3.
14. Mitus J, Reinfuss M, Mitus JW, Jakubowicz J, Blecharz P, Wysocki WM, et al. Malignant phyllodes tumor of the breast: treatment and prognosis. Breast J. 2014;20:639–44.

15. Kim YJ, Kim KB. Radiation therapy for malignant phyllodes tumor of the breast: an analysis of SEER data. Breast. 2017;32:26–32.
16. Barth RJ Jr, Wells WA, Mitchell SE, Cole BF. A prospective, multi-institutional study of adjuvant radiotherapy after resection of malignant phyllodes tumors. Ann Surg Oncol. 2009;16:2288–94.
17. Gnerlich JL, Williams RT, Yao K, Jaskowiak N, Kulkarni SA. Utilization of radiotherapy for malignant phyllodes tumors: analysis of the National Cancer Data Base, 1998-2009. Ann Surg Oncol. 2014;21:1222–30.
18. Tse GM, Lee CS, Kung FY, Scolyer RA, Law BK, Lau TS, et al. Hormonal receptors expression in epithelial cells of mammary phyllodes tumors correlates with pathologic grade of the tumor: a multicenter study of 143 cases. Am J Clin Pathol. 2002;118(4):522–6.
19. Sapino A, Bosco M, Cassoni P, Castellano I, Arisio R, Cserni G, et al. Estrogen receptor-beta is expressed in stromal cells of fibroadenoma and phyllodes tumors of the breast. Mod Pathol. 2006;19(4):599–606.
20. Kim YH, Kim GE, Lee JS, Lee JH, Nam JH, Choi C, et al. Hormone receptors expression in phyllodes tumors of the breast. Anal Quant Cytol Histol. 2012;34(1):41–8.
21. Hashimoto K, Mimura H, Arai Y, Doi M, Kojima Y, Tsugawa K, et al. Successful preoperative chemoembolization in the treatment of a giant malignant phyllodes tumor. Cardiovasc Intervent Radiol. 2016;39(7):1070–5.
22. Kapiris I, Nasiri N, A'Hern R, Healy V, Gui GP. Outcome and predictive factors of local recurrence and distant metastases following primary surgical treatment of high-grade malignant phyllodes tumours of the breast. Eur J Surg Oncol. 2001;27(8):723–30.
23. Koh VCY, Thike AA, Nasir NDM, Yip GWC, Bay BH, Tan PH. Size and heterologous elements predict metastases in malignant phyllodes tumours of the breast. Virchows Arch. 2018;472(4):615–21.
24. Hallin M, Thway K. Phyllodes tumor with heterologous liposarcomatous differentiation. Int J Surg Pathol. 2017;25(5):435–7.
25. Gong C, Nie Y, Qu S, Liao JY, Cui X, Yao H, et al. miR-21 induces myofibroblast differentiation and promotes the malignant progression of breast phyllodes tumors. Cancer Res. 2014;74:4341–52.
26. Lim JST, Koh VCY, Tan JSY, Tan WJ, Thike AA, Tan PH. Prognostic significance of epithelial–mesenchymal transition proteins twist and Foxc2 in phyllodes tumours of the breast. Breast Cancer Res Treat. 2015;150:19–29.
27. Feng X, Zhao L, Shen H, Liu X, Yang Y, Lv S, et al. Expression of EMT markers and mode of surgery are prognostic in phyllodes tumors of the breast. Oncotarget. 2017;8(20):33365–74.
28. Condeelis J, Pollard JW. Macrophages: obligate partners for tumor cell migration, invasion, and metastasis. Cell. 2006;124:263–6.
29. Pollard JW. Tumour-educated macrophages promote tumour progression and metastasis. Nat Rev Cancer. 2004;4:71–8.
30. Nie Y, Chen J, Huang D, Yao Y, Chen J, Ding L, et al. Tumor-associated macrophages promote malignant progression of breast phyllodes tumors by inducing myofibroblast differentiation. Cancer Res. 2017;77:3605–18.
31. Tan J, Ong CK, Lim WK, Ng CCY, Thike AA, Ng LM, et al. Genomic landscapes of breast fibroepithelial tumors. Nat Genet. 2015;47(11):1341–5.
32. Kim JY, Yu JH, Nam SJ, Kim SW, Lee SK, Park WY, et al. Genetic and clinical characteristics of phyllodes tumor of the breast. Transl Oncol. 2018;11(1):18–23.

Chapter 33
Next-Generation Clinical Trials and Research with Successful Collaborations

Masakazu Toi and Ravi Velaga

Abstract While clinical trials have evolved and improved over time, fundamental changes are needed to reflect the outcomes of great relevance to the institutions where they are performed, by integrating scientific rationale and society's movement to increase efficiency, accountability, and transparency by fast integrating the next-generation advances offered by omics technology and artificial intelligence. Several global clinical and exploratory collaborative studies that achieved successful outcomes in terms of patients' survival, drug toxicity, efficacy, safety, biomarkers, and consensus reached to improve good clinical practices are addressed in this article. Going forward, through collaborations, cooperation, and intellectual curiosity many more advances can be made in clinical trial approaches that can bring transparency, accountability, best outcomes, and develop friendship with trust among all the involved.

Keywords Breast cancer · Next generation · Clinical trial paradigm · Toxicity · EBCTCG · NSABP · BIG · APHINITY CREATE-X · BEATRICE · BOLERO-3 · FALCON · ADTree · Biomarker · Watson · Deep Mind · Hanover · KBCCC · Collaboration

33.1 Introduction

Next-generation clinical trial paradigms and systems that are more transparent and enterprising for novel translational research could be the way going forward to improve and achieve the best breast cancer management. Recent advances in

M. Toi (✉)
Graduate School of Medicine, Kyoto University, Kyoto, Japan
e-mail: toi@kuhp.kyoto-u.ac.jp

R. Velaga
Japan Breast Cancer Research Group, Kyoto University, Kyoto, Japan

D.-Y. Noh et al. (eds.), *Translational Research in Breast Cancer*, Advances in Experimental Medicine and Biology 1187,
https://doi.org/10.1007/978-981-32-9620-6_33

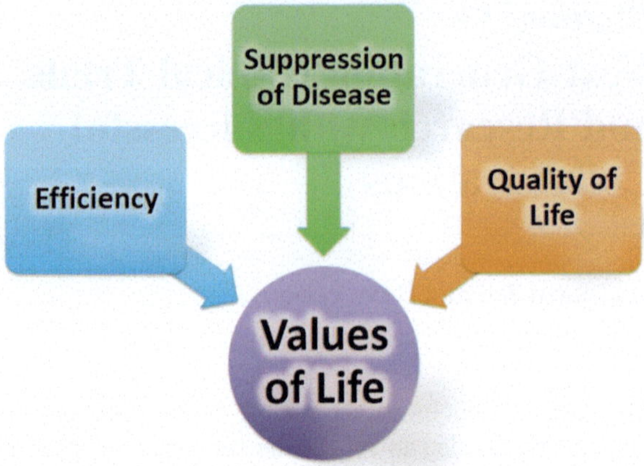

Fig. 33.1 Basis for clinical trial collaborations

diagnosis and treatment along with using qualified and standardized systemic and local treatments have influenced and dramatically changed the common practice of breast cancer, which enabled us to detect cancers in the very early stages and to achieve more than 80% overall survival (OS) rates by 10 years. With the paradigm shift in clinical trial approaches, gradual but progressive trend could be achieved further in a decade or two with more favorable survival outcomes. Though clinical trials have evolved and improved over the time, in order to further establish good clinical practices and develop novel diagnostics and therapeutics, not only for increasing drug efficacy and quality of life but also for decreasing treatment burden and toxicity, future paradigms should be reengineered so as to increase the values in life across the trial participants (Fig. 33.1). In this regard, collaborations, particularly international collaborations, are indispensable to make the approach more accountable, comprehensive, efficient, and transparent.

33.2 Collaboration Experiences

33.2.1 Global Clinical Trials with Improved Clinical Outcomes

Over the past two decades, we have participated in global clinical trial consortiums such as the Early Breast Cancer Trialists' Collaborative Group (EBCTCG), the National Surgical Adjuvant Breast and Bowel Project (NSABP), and the Breast International Group (BIG). A series of meta-analyses and its overview of prospective randomized clinical trials data particularly from adjuvant study results encouraged us to construct qualified platforms for good clinical practice and persuaded the standardized treatments for each individual patient, which in fact have improved survival outcomes enormously across the globe. Adjuvant study involving 88 clinical trials data from 62,923 estrogen receptor-positive women participants was published in 2017 by the EBCTCG group concluded that after 5 years of adjuvant endocrine therapy, breast-cancer recurrences continued to occur steadily throughout the study period from 5 to 20 years [1]. Improved outcomes were found in another global clinical investigation, APHINITY trial in which pertuzumab significantly improved the rates of invasive-disease-free survival among patients with HER2-positive, operable breast cancer when it was added to trastuzumab and chemotherapy [2]. Since the benefit of adjuvant chemotherapy in patients with residual invasive carcinoma who had poor prognosis after receiving neoadjuvant chemotherapy for human epidermal growth factor receptor 2 (HER2)-negative breast cancer remained questionable, CREATE-X trail was carried out [3]. CREATE-X trail concluded that disease-free and overall survivals among the patients can be prolonged after the standard neoadjuvant chemotherapy containing anthracycline, taxane, or both by safe and effective addition of adjuvant capecitabine therapy. BEATRICE phase 3 trial involving 2591 triple negative breast cancer patients across 360 sites in 37 countries was carried out and consensus was reached that, bevacizumab cannot be recommended as adjuvant treatment in unselected patients with triple-negative breast cancer [4]. In BOLERO-3 trail, scientific rationale that, disease progression in patients with HER2-positive breast cancer receiving trastuzumab might be associated with activation of the PI3K/Akt/mTOR intracellular signaling pathway formed the basis in performing a phase 3 trial among women with trastuzumab-resistant, human epidermal growth factor receptor 2 (HER2)-positive advanced breast cancer patients [5]. From the BOLERO-3 trail, the authors interpreted that the addition of everolimus to trastuzumab plus vinorelbine significantly prolongs progression-free survival in patients with trastuzumab-resistant and taxane-pretreated, HER2-positive, advanced breast cancer patients. Breast cancer patients from Asian countries have also participated in other ground-breaking global clinical trials like HERA trial [6] and FALCON study [7] which have been successfully carried out. Significant improvements in disease-free and progression-free survivals have been shown in a 11-year follow-up of trastuzumab after adjuvant chemotherapy in HER2-positive early breast cancer (HERA trial) and in a randomized, double-blind, phase 3 trial involving fulvestrant 500 mg versus anastrozole 1 mg for hormone receptor-positive advanced breast cancer (FALCON). Many such advanced clinical trials addressed drug efficacy and improved survival rates using CDK4/6 inhibitors like palbociclib, ribociclib, and abemaciclib in advanced or metastatic breast cancer patients that resulted in improvements of patient care.

33.2.2 *Studies to Elucidate Drug Toxicity Profiling, Efficacy, and Safety*

Since drug approval rates have increased in the past two decades, it remains paramount to assess the adverse effects, toxicity, and efficacy of the drugs used during the clinical trials. Still, information is lacking about racial differences in

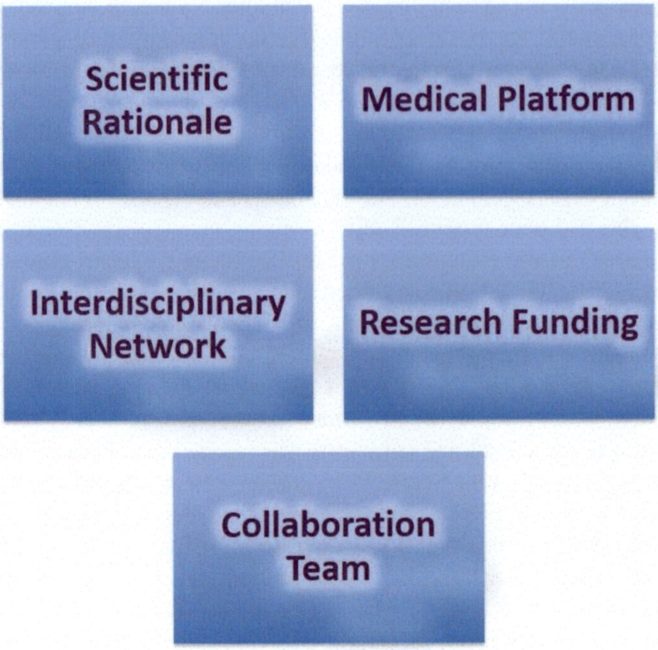

Fig. 33.2 Current collaboration scheme

treatment-related toxicities. Racial disparities in breast cancer outcomes stems from the differences in baseline tumor characteristics and biology, stage, age, ethnic background, and socioeconomic factors. To that effect, a recent study has emphasized that there is a need to validate safety of chemotherapeutic regimens in patients of different ethnicities by enhancing the participation of minorities in clinical trials [8]. Having achieved remarkable outcomes by being part of global clinical consortiums, the experience has motivated us to expand our collaborative activities further and beyond. Current and ingenious work flows (Fig. 33.2) have been followed and developed through these activities and a few new approaches have been implemented in clinical and translational research settings.

Several exploratory studies have been carried out by the Organisation for Oncology and Translational Research (OOTR) and Celecoxib Antiaromatase Neoadjuvant (CAAN) studies to evaluate and understand the drug safety and efficacy. In 2013, OOTR carried out a prospective study in which the efficacy and safety of the concurrent use of celecoxib (CXB) with 5-fluorouracil, epirubicin, and cyclophosphamide (FEC), followed by docetaxel (T) in the neoadjuvant setting was investigated [9]. The study concluded that the neoadjuvant use of FEC-T with concurrent CXB is active and safe for treatment of operable invasive breast cancer. Another OOTR study in 2017 tested the efficacy of neoadjuvant palbociclib therapy and evaluated its impact on cell cycle arrest and changes in EndoPredict (EP) scores before and after treatment [10]. The study concluded that, effective clinical response was demonstrated by neoadjuvant letrozole in combination with palbociclib. Also, the authors proposed that between the preoperative endocrine prognostic index (PEPI) and EndoPredict (EPclin), EPclin might serve as a better parameter to estimate prognosis after neoadjuvant therapy.

Owing to the significant role of Her2/neu in neoadjuvant endocrine therapy, an earlier CAAN study during 2004 determined whether the level of Her2/neu expression in advanced breast cancer changes after antiaromatase neoadjuvant treatment, as well as identified the relationship between Her2/neu expression and response to this kind of therapy [11]. In line with the previous findings, the study also suggested that Her2/neu expression and its change during the treatment might be predictive markers for this kind of therapy. Though, anti-aromatase therapy is considered as an important treatment approach for breast cancer in postmenopausal women, it leaves a long-standing effect on the bone mineral density (BMD) and osteoporosis. Combined efficacy of anti-aromatase therapy (exemestane) and COX-2 inhibitors neoadjuvantly in postmenopausal women with breast cancer was investigated and published as a proof of principle study [12], in which the groups showed significant difference among themselves ($p = 0.007$) for BMD at femur. Potential role of Cyclooxygenase-2 (COX-2) inhibitors in association with Ki-67 and p53 in breast cancer patients [13] was proposed and demonstrated.

33.2.3 Clinical Trials with Opportunity to Develop New Surgical Tools and Algorithms

Multiple new diagnostics and drugs have been developed successfully which contributed to increase diagnostic accuracy and prognostic outcomes significantly. It not only helps in patients having primary diseases but also in those having advanced diseases. Furthermore, studies on therapeutic and diagnostic algorithms or on the therapy guidelines have also been executed as part of collaborative activities that can also help to make practical platforms smarter and to promote standardization of the treatments. New algorithm for predicting positive resection margins in breast-conserving surgery [14] was one such proposed outcome resulted from collaboration. The study has shown that nomogram is useful to reduce frozen section biopsies (FSBs) without increasing reoperation rate for surgeons who perform routine FSBs and it can give useful information to most surgeons about the possibility of tumor-positive resection margins. A new data-mining model to predict axillary lymph node (AxLN) metastasis in primary breast cancer was successfully developed by using a decision tree-based prediction method—the alternating decision tree (ADTree) [15]. The authors demonstrated near-perfect accuracy levels in predicting nodal metastatsis in patients with breast cancer and commonly recorded clinical variables. A successful application of these tools and algorithms can permit the study of large samples of breast cancer patients as well as save time of the oncologists in the decision-making process before starting the treatment and cost to the patients.

33.3 Indispensable Role of Biomarkers in Breast Cancer Management

Precision medicine in oncology relies on rapid associations between unique patient-specific variations and targeted therapeutic efficacy. With the advances in technology, huge amount of literature characterizing cancer-associated molecular aberrations and therapeutic relevance has been published in the past decade. Genomic era has offered clinicians and researchers the ability to explore and utilize the clinical potential of the patients' molecular data and identify genetic markers that may have an impact on the clinical outcome and treatment choices. With the big clinical and molecular data banks generated and made available across the globe, accessing relevant information in a clinically acceptable time frame has turned out to be a daunting task, hampering the link between data available, clinicians, and patients to make an informed decision. Hence, clinical trials have formed to be an important therapeutic avenue for oncology patients to assess the strengths and weaknesses of the trials. To assist and improve the breast cancer management, biomarkers currently play an indispensable role in guiding and deciding the type of systemic therapy to be administered. Markers like, ER, PR, Her2, Ki67, and multigene signatures like Oncotype DX, MammaPrint, EndoPredict, Breast Cancer Index (BCI), and Prosigna (PAM50) which are developed using omics technology are being extensively used to predict the outcome and help adjunct therapy decision-making in breast cancer patients. Most of these markers are made by the normal cells as well as by cancer cells. Through a multicenter randomized trial of preoperative docetaxel with or without capecitabine after 4 cycles of 5-fluorouracil–epirubicin–cyclophosphamide (FEC) in early-stage breast cancer, we also identified Ki67 as a predictive biomarker for response to neoadjuvant chemotherapy [16]. Exploratory analyses during the same trial suggested that assessment of pretreatment Ki67LI may be a useful tool in the identification of responders to preoperative docetaxel/capecitabine in early-stage breast cancer. Though multigene signature biomarkers are proposed, there is still a large gap between initial biomarker discovery studies and their clinical translation due to the challenges in the process of cancer biomarker development. Also, regulatory issues and future perspectives in the era of big data analysis and precision medicine should be taken into consideration to before consensus is reached among the experts.

33.4 International Consortium and Kyoto Breast Cancer Consensus Conference (KBCCC)

To highlight and agree the contradictory or current best clinical practices, and for clinicians to interpret the guidelines, a consensus meeting was carried out among the international clinical experts and Kyoto Breast Cancer Consensus Conference [17]. During the meeting, the reviewed data showed that preoperative systemic therapy increases the likelihood of patients receiving localized surgery and individualized treatment regimens. Also, a consensus was reached to recognize nomograms that are used for predicting nodal status and drug sensitivity as a tool to support decision-making in the selection of surgical treatment. Likewise, in 2014, breast cancer international experts and KBCCC met again in two sessions [18, 19]. First, to discuss and reach an agreement on the loco-regional management of breast cancer is increasingly complex with application of primary systemic therapies, oncoplastic techniques, and genetic testing for breast cancer susceptibility. During the second session meeting, consensus were discussed and recommendations were made for radiation treatment, primary systemic therapies, and management of genetic predisposition.

33.5 Clinical Trial Paradigm

With collaborations among global clinicians, pharmaceutical companies, cooperation from the participating patients, intellectual curiosity among the clinicians and researchers involved made all the above studies and achievements possible (Fig. 33.3).

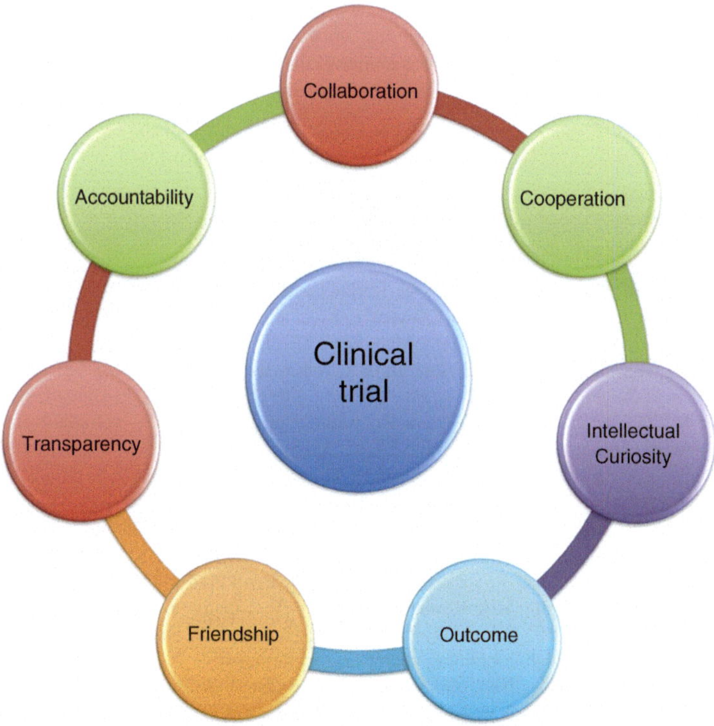

Fig. 33.3 Clinical trial paradigm

Along with trying to improve the quality and efficiency of clinical trials, the probability of success (POS) of a clinical trial in a time span is also critical for clinical researchers and investors to evaluate while making scientific and economic decisions. Accuracy and transparency among all the participants had been the corner stones while assessing the risk and value of drug development, leading to gain opportunities for both investors and patients. On one hand, with the next-generation optimism among all the clinical trial participants, an active and trustworthy relationships among the participants could help improve clinical trial outcomes. On the other hand, artificial intelligence (AI) is maturing into multiple disciplines that could result in a constellation of methods which can enable and improve our perception, learning, reasoning, and natural language understanding. Nonprofit organizations like the Partnership on AI, formed in 2017, by representatives from industry, academia, and civil society can discuss, frame, and recommend the best practices for developing and fielding AI technologies in all walks of life, including clinical trials. In the same breath, companies like IBM (Watson for Oncology), Google (Deep Mind–Deep Variant), and Microsoft (Hanover) have already developed oncology-related AI tools which are being widely used by oncologists across the globe to carry out modern-day clinical trials. AI when developed, guided, and used with care, collaboration, intellectual curiosity, and cooperation can be a powerful tool that can bring the clinical trial paradigm shift.

Acknowledgements We like to thank all the study participants, clinicians, researchers, and members from different pharmaceutical companies globally because of which progress has been achieved.

References

1. Pan H, Gray R, Braybrooke J, Davies C, Taylor C, McGale P, Peto R, Pritchard KI, Bergh J, Dowsett M, Hayes DF. EBCTCG. 20-year risks of breast-Cancer recurrence after stopping endocrine therapy at 5 years. N Engl J Med. 2017;377(19):1836–46.
2. von Minckwitz G, Procter M, de Azambuja E, Zardavas D, Benyunes M, Viale G, Suter T, Arahmani A, Rouchet N, Clark E, Knott A, Lang I, Levy C, Yardley DA, Bines J, Gelber RD, Piccart M, Baselga J. APHINITY steering committee and investigators. Adjuvant pertuzumab and trastuzumab in early HER2-positive breast Cancer. N Engl J Med. 2017;377(2):122–31.
3. Masuda N, Lee SJ, Ohtani S, Im YH, Lee ES, Yokota I, Kuroi K, Im SA, Park BW, Kim SB, Yanagita Y, Ohno S, Takao S, Aogi K, Iwata H, Jeong J, Kim A, Park KH, Sasano H, Ohashi Y, Toi M. Adjuvant capecitabine for breast cancer after preoperative chemotherapy. N Engl J Med. 2017;376(22):2147–59.
4. Cameron D, Brown J, Dent R, Jackisch C, Mackey J, Pivot X, Steger GG, Suter TM, Toi M, Parmar M, Laeufle R, Im YH, Romieu G, Harvey V, Lipatov O, Pienkowski T, Cottu P, Chan A, Im SA, Hall PS, Bubuteishvili-Pacaud L, Henschel V, Deurloo RJ, Pallaud C, Bell R. Adjuvant bevacizumab-containing therapy in triple-negative breast cancer (BEATRICE): primary results of a randomised, phase 3 trial. Lancet Oncol. 2013;14(10):933–42.
5. André F, O'Regan R, Ozguroglu M, Toi M, Xu B, Jerusalem G, Masuda N, Wilks S, Arena F, Isaacs C, Yap YS, Papai Z, Lang I, Armstrong A, Lerzo G, White M, Shen K, Litton J, Chen D, Zhang Y, Ali S, Taran T, Gianni L. Everolimus for women with trastuzumab-resistant, HER2-

positive, advanced breast cancer (BOLERO-3): a randomised, double-blind, placebo-controlled phase 3 trial. Lancet Oncol. 2014;15(6):580–91.
6. Cameron D, Piccart-Gebhart MJ, Gelber RD, Procter M, Goldhirsch A, de Azambuja E, Castro G Jr, Untch M, Smith I, Gianni L, Baselga J, Al-Sakaff N, Lauer S, McFadden E, Leyland-Jones B, Bell R, Dowsett M, Jackisch C. Herceptin adjuvant (HERA) trial study team. 11 years' follow-up of trastuzumab after adjuvant chemotherapy in HER2-positive early breast cancer: final analysis of the HERceptin adjuvant (HERA) trial. Lancet. 2017;389(10075):1195–205.
7. Robertson JFR, Bondarenko IM, Trishkina E, Dvorkin M, Panasci L, Manikhas A, Shparyk Y, Cardona-Huerta S, Cheung KL, Philco-Salas MJ, Ruiz-Borrego M, Shao Z, Noguchi S, Rowbottom J, Stuart M, Grinsted LM, Fazal M, Ellis MJ. Fulvestrant 500 mg versus anastrozole 1 mg for hormone receptor-positive advanced breast cancer (FALCON): an international, randomised, double-blind, phase 3 trial. Lancet. 2016;388(10063):2997–3005.
8. Han HS, Reis IM, Zhao W, Kuroi K, Toi M, Suzuki E, Syme R, Chow L, Yip AY, Glück S. Racial differences in acute toxicities of neoadjuvant or adjuvant chemotherapy in patients with early-stage breast cancer. Eur J Cancer. 2011;47(17):2537–45.
9. Chow LW, Tung SY, Ng TY, Im SA, Lee MH, Yip AY, Toi M, Glück S. Concurrent celecoxib with 5-fluorouracil/epirubicin/cyclophosphamide followed by docetaxel for stages II - III invasive breast cancer: the OOTR-N001 study. Expert Opin Investig Drugs. 2013;22 (3):299–307.
10. Chow LWC, Morita S, Chow CYC, Ng WK, Toi M. Neoadjuvant palbociclib on ER+ breast cancer (N007): clinical response and EndoPredict's value. Endocr Relat Cancer. 2018;25 (2):123–30.
11. Zhu L, Chow LW, Loo WT, Guan XY, Toi M. Her2/neu expression predicts the response to antiaromatase neoadjuvant therapy in primary breast cancer: subgroup analysis from celecoxib antiaromatase neoadjuvant trial. Clin Cancer Res. 2004;10(14):4639–44.
12. Chow LW, Yip AY, Chu WP, Loo WT, Toi M. Bone metabolism and quality-of-life of postmenopausal women with invasive breast cancer receiving neoadjuvant hormonal therapy: sub-analyses from celecoxib anti-aromatase neoadjuvant (CAAN) trial. J Steroid Biochem Mol Biol. 2011;125(1–2):112–9.
13. Chow LW, Loo WT, Wai CC, Lui EL, Zhu L, Toi M. Study of COX-2, Ki67, and p53 expression to predict effectiveness of 5-flurouracil, epirubicin and cyclophosphamide with celecoxib treatment in breast cancer patients. Biomed Pharmacother. 2005;59(Suppl 2): S298–301.
14. Lee ES, Han W, Shin HC, Takada M, Ryu HS, Cho N, Kim MK, Kim J, Yoo TK, Moon HG, Toi M, Moon WK, Park IA, Noh DY. Clinical benefit of nomogram for predicting positive resection margins in breast conserving surgery. Eur J Surg Oncol. 2016;42(8):1169–75.
15. Takada M, Sugimoto M, Naito Y, Moon HG, Han W, Noh DY, Kondo M, Kuroi K, Sasano H, Inamoto T, Tomita M, Toi M. Prediction of axillary lymph node metastasis in primary breast cancer patients using a decision tree-based model. BMC Med Inform Decis Mak. 2012;13 (12):54.
16. Ohno S, Chow LW, Sato N, Masuda N, Sasano H, Takahashi F, Bando H, Iwata H, Morimoto T, Kamigaki S, Nakayama T, Nakamura S, Kuroi K, Aogi K, Kashiwaba M, Yamashita H, Hisamatsu K, Ito Y, Yamamoto Y, Ueno T, Fakhrejahani E, Yoshida N, Toi M. Randomized trial of preoperative docetaxel with or without capecitabine after 4 cycles of 5-fluorouracil– epirubicin–cyclophosphamide (FEC) in early-stage breast cancer: exploratory analyses identify Ki67 as a predictive biomarker for response to neoadjuvant chemotherapy. Breast Cancer Res Treat. 2013;142(1):69–80.
17. Toi M, Benson JR, Winer EP, Forbes JF, von Minckwitz G, Golshan M, Robertson JF, Sasano H, Cole BF, Chow LW, Pegram MD, Han W, Huang CS, Ikeda T, Kanao S, Lee ES, Noguchi S, Ohno S, Partridge AH, Rouzier R, Tozaki M, Sugie T, Yamauchi A, Inamoto T. Preoperative systemic therapy in locoregional management of early breast cancer: highlights from the Kyoto Breast Cancer Consensus Conference. Breast Cancer Res Treat. 2012;136 (3):919–26.

18. Toi M, Winer EP, Benson JR, Inamoto T, Forbes JF, Von Minckwitz G, Robertson JF, Grobmyer SR, Jatoi I, Sasano H, Kunkler I. Personalization of loco-regional care for primary breast cancer patients (part 1). Future Oncol. 2015;11(9):1297–300.
19. Toi M, Winer EP, Benson JR, Inamoto T, Forbes JF, von Minckwitz G, Robertson JF, Grobmyer SR, Jatoi I, Sasano H, Kunkler I, Ho AY, Yamauchi C, Chow LW, Huang CS, Han W, Noguchi S, Pegram MD, Yamauchi H, Lee ES, Larionov AA, Bevilacqua JL, Yoshimura M, Sugie T, Yamauchi A, Krop IE, Noh DY, Klimberg VS. 2014 Kyoto breast cancer consensus conference. Personalization of loco-regional care for primary breast cancer patients (part 2). Future Oncol. 2015;11(9):1301–5.

Part VII
Epilogue

Chapter 34
Transformation of the Patient and Society: A Patient Survivors' Group and Breast Cancer Awareness Campaign

Dong-Young Noh

Abstract Most biomedical research has the same goal: to make human lives better and healthier. However, sometimes doctors forget their own mission while treating disease. Physicians should remember the old adage to treat the patient, not the disease. The doctor–patient relationship used to be a one-way affair, going from the doctor to the patient. Compared with doctors, society expects relatively little in terms of roles and duties from patients as well as the rest of the population. Thus, society could be a foundational place in which doctors, patients, and research can communicate with one another, or society itself could transform each of these components. The best way for physicians to provide better care is to listen to the needs of patients and society more broadly. We must reflect on whether this kind of transformation is happening in our current society.

Keywords Breast cancer · Survivor · Awareness · Good doctor · Pink Ribbon Campaign

34.1 The Venus Association

In 2000, I established a breast cancer survivors' group, the Korea Venus Association. This was not only a matter of patient need, but also a response to an increased number of breast cancer cases in Korea, which were associated with the growth of the economy at that time. I saw a need for better individual communication between patients and doctors as well as among patients themselves so that they could better help one another. The purpose of the survivors' group is to help patients understand

---

D.-Y. Noh (✉)
Department of Surgery, College of Medicine, Seoul National University, Seoul, South Korea

Gangnam CHA Medical Center, Seoul, South Korea
e-mail: dynoh@snu.ac.kr; dynoh@chamc.co.kr

D.-Y. Noh et al. (eds.), *Translational Research in Breast Cancer*, Advances in Experimental Medicine and Biology 1187,
https://doi.org/10.1007/978-981-32-9620-6_34

breast cancer better, to support one another, and to have a social impact through volunteering, such as in awareness campaigns and fundraising for poorer patients.

A couple of years later, in order to promote the website (koreavenus.com), I opened my own Questions and Answers corner [1]. I have continued to work on this every day, so that by the end of 2020 we had almost 50,000 Q&As. Questions come from all over the world—the USA, Europe, Japan—from Asian women who speak Korean, but of course, most are from Korea. The Q&A content is very valuable, not only because of the answers it provides, but also because it offers vital insights about patients' needs and experiences to doctors and society at large.

Several research articles were published based on the Q&As. The first was "Needs of Women with Breast Cancer as Communicated to Physicians on the Internet" by Juhee Cho et al., published in *Supportive Care in Cancer* in 2011 [2]. The researchers found that the information requested by site users covered a broad range of topics, from treatment (38.4%) and physical condition (31.7%), to lifestyle/self-care (24%). Requests for emotional support were often embedded in requests for information, with over 63% of women expressing concern and worry in their posts. Cho et al. concluded that online Q&A boards can be a valuable tool in assisting breast cancer patients to manage their physical and psychosocial needs, and also to communicate these needs to physicians. In other words, this kind of online interactive forum is a good means of bringing about transformation.

The informational needs of Korean women with breast cancer were strongly stressed by Myungsun Yi et al. in an earlier article published in *Asian Nursing Research* in 2007 [3]. There, they demonstrated that, to plan and execute educational interventions effectively, healthcare professionals must understand the domains of information that these women perceive to be important.

One picture in particular shows to me the kind of close patient–doctor relationship that can be achieved. The Venus Association used to hold an annual camp at a famous resort or beach, to which I was always invited. I remember posing for a photo with the patients group by the children's swimming pool at one of the resorts. I was the only man invited to take a group photo all in swimming suits there. Whenever I look back on this moment, I wonder if such relationships exist between patients and doctors in any other country. For me, the photo is a symbol of the closeness of my relationships with my patients, as well as the open-mindedness I have sought to maintain to their complaints, their welfare, and even their sorrows.

I think as time goes by, this kind of relationship has become more difficult to foster, especially in the very personalized and individualized society of the so-called Fourth Industrial Revolution. Now more than ever, however, physicians need to keep in mind the importance of the humanity of patients who suffer from disease or disability, and cultivate sympathy, basic affection, and consideration toward them.

The Venus Association has been involved in philanthropic activities such as fundraising through bazaars, Pink Ribbon activities to teach breast self-examination, and supplying free wigs for patients undergoing chemotherapy. They also organize a lot of activities, from their own choir group and yoga school, to mountain-climbing, group tutoring, and even laughing therapy. In this way, the Venus Association is a good example of a survivors' group, not only in the activities they organize but also in how they demonstrate ways of overcoming a devastating disease and making a new life.

I hope this model can spread all over the nation and be a positive influence on society to support the human rights of women with breast cancer. I say this because of the significant negative impact that diagnosis and treatment can have on patients within their family or workplace. In 2009, Eunmi Ahn et al. reported that the employment of their study subjects decreased from 47.6% to 33.2% after a breast cancer diagnosis [4]. Fatigue and exhaustion were frequent difficulties encountered by women during occupational work and housework. In addition, women who lived with a spouse were more likely to quit working after treatment than those without spouses. In other words, sociocultural factors as well as certain clinical characteristics influence Korean women's decisions to return to work or not after surviving breast cancer.

Some of the most memorable activities since 2000 have been a salsa dance performance with patients after 3 months of lessons to celebrate 10th anniversary, and also climbing high mountains with them, including Paektu in China (2774 m), Mount Tateyama in Japan (3000 m), and the Himalayas (5000 m). We shared and made many memories together—some very funny, some very dangerous and fraught with difficulties. Whenever I joined the group, I was like a team doctor and a good friend or brother.

We studied whether these kinds of activities influence the lifestyle or quality of life of breast cancer survivors, and found that those who are hopeful and have a clear purpose in life are more likely to be happy than those who do not [5]. We also concluded that setting proper life goals might be beneficial to help breast cancer survivors who experience persistent quality of life issues.

34.1.1 The Korea Breast Cancer Foundation and the Pink Ribbon Campaign

Officially, my greatest contribution to the patients and society more generally was my work to establish the Korea Breast Cancer Foundation (KBCF). After more than 2 years of engagement with business and government, and thanks to the motivation and support of Kyung-Bae Suh, CEO of Amorepacific, KBCF was finally launched in 2000. Its mission, like that of Susan G. Komen in the USA, is to improve women's health by fighting breast cancer.

KBCF, the first nonprofit organization of its kind, was established under the direction of a businessman, Mr. Suh, who had a love and hope for women with breast cancer, and a doctor who had both a calling and an affection for his patients. Prominent people in the fields of medicine, law, journalism, and politics joined the mission to eradicate breast cancer, and health seminars were held nationwide to spread information about breast cancer and raise public awareness. KBCF also provides funding for academic research and support for education and training to eliminate breast cancer.

In Seoul, Korea, in 2000, I also founded the Pink Ribbon Campaign, a breast cancer awareness campaign aimed at raising public awareness of breast cancer and the importance of early detection. KBCF initiatives include the annual Pink Ribbon Marathon (now Pink Run) in five major regions, as well as The Global Landmark Illuminations Initiative with Estée Lauder Korea, in which first Namsan Tower, and then later most landmark bridges and buildings (like the 123-floor Lotte World Tower) in major cities were symbolically lit in bright pink lights.

The results of these awareness campaigns and the promotion of early detection have been outstanding: the detection rate of early-stage breast cancer is high, and, as a result, Korea now has the world's highest rate of breast cancer survival. A 2015 national report cited the five-year survival rate of the whole treated group as over 90%. Moreover, the annual incidence of new cases between 2000 and 2015 increased from around 4000 to over 20,000 [6].

34.1.2 What Makes for a Good Doctor–Patient Relationship?

To summarize, then, in terms of transforming the doctor–patient relationship, how should the ideal relationship be characterized? First, there should be admiration from patients and affection from doctors. Second, doctors must do their best and ensure that patients benefit from their efforts. Third, in terms of cancer patients, the doctor must have a patient's life-long care in mind, even if there is no regular contact through the Outpatient Department. In other words, care should be provided through appropriate education, events, or social activities. Fourth, patients should respect and trust their physician and the hospital with which they are registered. Fifth, in order to encourage better doctor–patient relationships, individuals on both sides, and the societies in which they are involved, should engage in active communication with each other, sharing their opinions along with any difficulties or misunderstandings.

In my essay "Good Doctor and Good Patient," I ask, "What is a good doctor?" My answer is that, in general, a good doctor is one who is equipped with superior knowledge and skills, listens carefully to patients, and treats patients kindly. If I had to say which is the most important of these qualities, I would say that it varies according to individual circumstances. Occasionally, I wonder: do I qualify as a good doctor? It often bothers me to think that the answer could be "No."

Some say that what a person needs in life is a skillful doctor, lawyer, and a friend who will come whenever they are called. This indicates that health and disease are among our biggest concerns, affecting us throughout our lifetime. In fact, a doctor should study all his life to keep up-to-date with new information and technology, and professors like me cannot maintain their jobs if they neglect to conduct research and work on self-improvement continuously.

That said, I believe that a good doctor is also made by a good patient. Westerners tend to believe firmly that doctors are next to God. Of course, they are treated that way because their behavior encourages patients' and society's confidence and esteem. What, then, is a good patient? In short, a good patient is a person who firmly believes in and faithfully follows the doctor's words, and cultivates their own affection for the doctor.

From the standpoint of the doctor, the patient does not have to be "good," since the doctor has to see the patient no matter what. However, a good patient can in fact produce a good doctor. For instance, some patients go against their doctor's advice by simultaneously seeking alternative (or even conflicting) treatments; some refuse to listen to doctors' explanations; and some ask prying questions about the doctor's weaknesses. There have been many cases from which I would have shied away had I not been serving as a doctor. Once or twice a year, I get fractious and lose my temper in front of a patient, which I regret afterward. As might be expected, the most important qualities I desire in my patients are confidence and faith. Of course, in order to gain the esteem and confidence of my patients, I should first become a good doctor.

The most wonderful thing happens when a good doctor and a good patient meet. What I am describing is a kind of *joie de vivre*, in which they share warm and generous exchanges with each other that transcend disease. I have kept letters from previous patients that I treasure, which I think I will collect in a book when I retire. Among these letters, one in particular made me resolve to become a good doctor. I would like to share it here:

> I had a hunch that you were a good doctor.
>
> While facing pain and anxiety, and looking at this flower that is about to blossom into hardship and suffering, it is said that the one who knows pain is the noblest. Do you know what disease it is? Breast cancer... This one phrase was clearly the herald of a big event that could either kill me or save me. However, I was aware of who, although tearing parts of me off, would also heal me by stitching the tear. All of a sudden, I was looking at the hidden workings of the Lord, who also disciplined himself to this great extent.
>
> I yield the decisions regarding all treatments to my favorite professor, who was appointed by the Lord. It would be wonderful if the healer and the patient could forge an alliance to destroy these cunning enemies. I think we would make the "perfect duo," and work in total harmony.
>
> After passing through a long tunnel of pain, there may be an untreatable disease but no such "untreatable" patient. I feel confident that my hunch will prove right and I will give thanks to the Lord of hosts that my doctor is the nicest and the greatest in the world.

Acknowledgments English language corrections were kindly made by Mr. Sangwoo Kim (Imperial College, London).

References

1. Koreavenus website. http://www.koreavenus.com/.
2. Cho J, Smith KC, Roter D, Guallar E, Noh DY, Ford DE. Needs of women with breast cancer as communicated to physicians on the internet. Support Care Cancer. 2011;19(1):113–21.

3. Yi M, Cho J, Noh DY, Song MR, Lee JL, Juon HS. Informational needs of Korean women with breast cancer: cross-cultural adaptation of the Toronto informational needs questionnaire of breast cancer. Asian Nurs Res. 2007;1(3):176–86.
4. Ahn E, Cho J, Shin DW, Park BW, Ahn SH, Noh DY, et al. Impact of breast cancer diagnosis and treatment on work-related life and factors affecting them. Breast Cancer Res Treat. 2009;116(3):609–16.
5. Kang D, Kim IR, Choi EK, Yoon JH, Lee SK, Lee JE, et al. Who are happy survivors? Physical, psychosocial, and spiritual factors associated with happiness of breast cancer survivors during the transition from cancer patient to survivor. Psycho-Oncology. 2017;26(11):1922–8.
6. National Cancer Center Statistics. https://ncc.re.kr.

The manufacturer's authorised representative in the EU is Springer Nature Customer Service Centre GmbH, Europaplatz 3, 69115 Heidelberg, Germany. If you have any concerns regarding our products, please contact ProductSafety@springernature.com

Printed and bound by CPI Group (UK) Ltd, Croydon, CR0 4YY
30/09/2026
02225240-0015